Nutrition, Immunology, and Microbiology

Nutrition, Immunology, and Microbiology

The Critical Window of Development

J.E. Butler, Kirsten Bennett,

Larry Williams, and Ekhard Ziegler

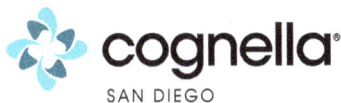

cognella®

SAN DIEGO

Bassim Hamadeh, CEO and Publisher
Amanda Martin, Executive Publisher
Amy Smith, Associate Editorial Manager
Rachel Kahn, Production Editor
Jess Estrella, Senior Graphic Designer
Kylie Bartolome, Licensing Specialist
Natalie Piccotti, Director of Marketing
Kassie Graves, Senior Vice President, Editorial
Alia Bales, Director, Project Editorial and Production

cognella® | ACADEMIC PUBLISHING
3970 Sorrento Valley Blvd., Ste. 500, San Diego, CA 92121

Brief Contents

Preface   xv

    Chapter 1   Biology and the Critical Window of Development   1

    Chapter 2   The Prepartum Maternal-Fetal Connections   23

    Chapter 3   The Role of Breast-Feeding in Infant Health   51

    Chapter 4   Infant Formulas as Breast Milk Alternatives   83

    Chapter 5   "A Little Help From Our Little Friends": Establishment of the Microbiome and Constituency in Health and Disease   99

    Chapter 6   Internal Protection: Immune Systems, Vaccination, and Antimicrobials   139

    Chapter 7   The Bumpy Road of Progress: The Certainty of Uncertainty   193

    Chapter 8   Mythology, Misconceptions, and Controversies in Healthcare   213

Appendix A-1: Molecular Genetics, Biotechnology, and Bioengineering   241

Appendix A-2: Mammalian Diversity and Animal Models   299

Appendix A-3: Further Information and Acronyms   345

Appendix A-4: The COVID-19 Teaching Model   353

Abbreviations and Glossary   373

Index   379

Detailed Contents

Preface   xv

CHAPTER 1   Biology and the Critical Window of Development   1

Parental Care, Species Survival, and Wellness   1
Establishment, Diversification, and Interdependence of Life   3
  Evolution, Diversification of Life, and Human Colonization   3
  Establishment of Life on Earth   3
  The Pyramid of Life and Life's Interdependence   5
  Human Colonization   8
  The Role of Subcellular Life Forms in Life's Interdependence   9
  Ancestors, Descendants, and the Biomass Pyramid   10
Emerging Diseases and the Critical Window   10
  The History of Emerging Diseases   10
  Emerging Disease and Human Behavior   12
Protection, Nutrition, Genetics: A Triad for Survival and Wellness   13
  Introduction   13
  Protection and Fecundity   13
  Internal Protection from Antibiotics and Bacteriophages   14
  Internal Protection Provided by the Immune System   15
Nutrition   16
  Introduction   16
  Nutrition of Human Offspring   16
  Nutrient Transfer and the Role of the Microbiome   17
Genetics and Health in the Critical Window   18
  Basic Principles   18

Gene Expression and Epigenetics   *18*

Rapid Genetic Changes in Pathogens Challenge Internal
Immune Protections and Compromise Human Health   *19*

Correction of Genetic Defect Through Bioengineering   *19*

The Place of Basic Science in Medicine   **20**

The "Go/No Go" Decision   *20*

The Role of Animal Models and Comparative Biology   *20*

Controversies, Misconceptions, and the Critical Window   *21*

Suggested Reading (SR)   **21**

References   **22**

CHAPTER 2   **The Prepartum Maternal-Fetal Connections**   **23**

Conception and Establishment
of the Maternal-Fetal Connection   **23**

Nutrient Supply, Fetal Growth, and Postnatal Outcomes   **25**

The Mechanisms of Transfer Across the Placenta   **27**

The Placenta: An Avenue From Mother to Fetus   *27*

Transfer of Passive Antibodies   *28*

Transfer of Regulatory Factors   *31*

Cellular Trafficking   *33*

Transfer of Pathogens and Congenital Infections   *33*

Placental Changes Associated With Infectious Disease   *36*

Transfer of Drugs and Other Substances   *37*

Allograft Incompatibility and Other Consequences
of Pregnancy   **42**

The Miracle of Fetal Survival   *42*

Complications That Threaten Hemi-Allograft Survival   *43*

Non-Infectious Diseases in the Fetus, Newborn, and Child   **44**

Genetic-Based Congenital Disease   *44*

Changes in the GI Tract at Birth   **46**

Changes in the Immune System at Birth   **47**

Summary   **47**

Suggested Readings (SR)   **48**

References   **48**

CHAPTER 3   **The Role of Breast-Feeding in Infant Health**   **51**

Breast-Feeding and Alternatives   **51**

The Role of Breast Milk for Newborns   *51*

The Importance of Breast-Feeding   *52*

Societal and Economic Issues and Breast-Feeding   *52*

Breast-Feeding and Later Health   *53*

When Breast-Feeding Is Not an Option   *54*

Physiology and Function of the Mammary Gland   55
  The Basic Structure of Milk   55
  Anatomy and Physiology of the Mammary Gland   56
  Changes in Mammary Gland Function During Lactation   60
  Energy From Milk Drives Infant Growth   62
  The Relationship Between Maternal Diet and Milk   63
The Role of Individual Milk Components   63
  The Complexity of Milk   63
  Caseins   64
  Lactoferrin   64
  α-Lactalbumin and β-Lactoglobulin   65
  Lysozyme and Defensins   65
  Antibodies and Immunoregulatory Factors   66
  Milk Fat and Milk Fat Globules (MFG)   66
  HMOs (Human Milk Oligosaccharides)   67
  Maternal Cells in Colostrum and Milk   68
  Bacteria in Milk   68
Passive Immunity and the Mammary Gland   69
  Transfer of Maternal Antibody   69
  Passive Antibody and Childhood Vaccinations   71
  Passive Transfer of Regulatory Factors   72
Transfer of Harmful Agents in Milk   75
  Pathogens in Milk   75
  Drugs and Environmental Contaminants in Milk   75
Breast Milk Supplementation   77
  Supplementation During Breast-Feeding   77
  Preterm Birth Presents a Special Situation   77
Summary   78
Suggested Readings (SR)   78
References   79

CHAPTER 4   Infant Formulas as Breast Milk Alternatives   83

The History of Surrogate Milks and Infant Formulas   83
Milks and Formulas in Special Medical Situations   86
  Premature Infants (Preterms)   86
  Formulas for Infants With Metabolic Diseases   87
  Formulas for Gastrointestinal Illnesses   87
  Formulas for Allergy to Milk   88
Consequences of Using Infant Formulas   89
  Short-Term Versus Long-Term Issues   89
  Why Might Immune-Related Maladies Be Associated
  With Formula Feeding?   89

Infant Formula Changes Over Time   91
  Composition and Regulation   91
  Recently Proposed Additions to Infant Formula   95
Conclusions   97
Suggested Readings (SR)   97
References   97

CHAPTER 5   "A Little Help From Our Little Friends": Establishment of the Microbiome and Constituency in Health and Disease   99

The Microbiome: Posterchild of Life's Interdependence   99
  Short Course in Bacteriology   103
  Role of the Bacteriophage   105
  Role of Mucosal Fungi   106
  The GI Tract Microbiome: The Good, the Bad and the Ugly   106
  Ethnic and Cultural Influences on Diet and Microbiome Diversity   107
  The "Ugly" Challenge the GI Tract Epithelial Barrier   109
  The Microbiome of the Reproductive Tract   111
  Establishment of the GI Tract Microbiome   112
  Origin of the Early Settlers   113
  The Maternal Diet and Other Influences on the Microbiome During Pregnancy   119
  Childhood Allergy and the Microbiome   120
  Disease and the Microbiome   122
  Pre-, Pro-, and Synbiotics and the Newborn   128
  Probiotic Mediation in Selected Adult Maladies   129
  Postnatal Feeding and the Microbiome   130
  Antibiotic Therapy and the Developing Neonatal Microbiome   131
Suggested Readings (SRs)   132
References   133
Chapter Reviewers   136

CHAPTER 6   Internal Protection: Immune Systems, Vaccination, and Antimicrobials   139

Section I: Basic Concepts Governing Immune Systems   139
  Immunology: "The Science of Self-/Non-Self-Discrimination"   140
  First Responders: The Innate Immune System   146
  Critical Messengers: Cytokines and Chemokines   149
  Antimicrobial Peptides (AMPs)   150

Why Adaptive Immunity Is Needed   150
Lymphocyte Interactions, MHC, and Making
"Better Antibodies"   154
Immunologic Memory   157
The Microbial Empire Strikes Back   157
Mucosal Immunity: Anatomical Distribution and Function   160
Passive Immunity   162
Section II: Immunological Tolerance and
Immunological Injury   163
The TSA and "Checkpoint Charlie": **Horror Autotoxicus** and
Immunological Tolerance   163
Oral Tolerance and Immune Homeostasis in the GI Tract   165
Immunologic Injury: Molecular Mimicry, Allergy, and
Autoimmunity   165
The Rise of Allergies   168
The Role of Viruses in Autoimmunity   171
Section III. Vaccines and Antimicrobials   172
The History of Vaccination   172
Vaccine Development, Diversity, and Administration   175
The Role of Adjuvants   178
The Story of Polio Vaccines: A Useful Model   179
Maternal Vaccination   180
Herd Immunity and the Anti-Vaccination Movement   182
"Hard Nuts to Crack"   183
Modern Vaccine Technology   183
Section IV. Protection Through Use of Antimicrobials   184
The Antibiotic Revolution: The Miracle Cure?   184
MDR Pathogens: Origin, STAT, and Bi-Directional Transfer   186
Antiviral Drugs   186
Suggested Readings (SR)   188
References   188
Chapter Reviewers   192

CHAPTER 7   The Bumpy Road of Progress: The Certainty
of Uncertainty   193

Evaluating Evidence: What Everyone Should Know   193
Hype and Uncertainty   194
The Hierarchy of Evidence: Weak Versus Strong   195
Randomized Controlled Trials (RCTs)   198
Observational Studies   199
Case Reports and Case Series   199
Lesser Evidence Levels   200

Vaccine Trials: Examples of Strong Studies   200
Making Health Decisions With Imperfect Knowledge   204
  Infant Formula Choices   *205*
  Vaccine Decisions   *207*
  Antibiotic Usage   *208*
  Nutritional Decision-Making   *209*
Summary   210
Suggested Readings (SR)   210
References   211

CHAPTER 8   Mythology, Misconceptions, and Controversies
in Healthcare   213

Best and Future Medical Practices in the Critical Window   213
Names Can Lead to Misconceptions   214
Misconceptions About the Actions and Uses of Antibiotics   215
STAT: Concerns, Misconceptions, and Adjustments   216
Prebiotics and Misconceptions About Probiotics   218
Vaccination Hesitancy, Herd Immunity, and Global Mobility   219
Misunderstandings About Vaccination Protocols   223
Hypotheses Masquerading as Facts   225
Programmed Gullibility   228
National Priorities   229
If It's Good Enough for Grandparents,
It's Good Enough for Grandchildren   229
Nature Versus Nurture   231
Food Allergy, Intolerance, and Food Aversion—A
"Can of Worms"?   232
  Allergy or Something Else?   *232*
  Food Intolerance   *233*
  Preventive Strategies   *234*
  Food Allergies in Other Mammals   *235*
  Synopsis and Conclusions   *235*
Human Health and Dietary Supplementation
in Food Animals   236
Misconceptions About Food Labeling   236
Summary   237
Suggested Readings (SR)   238
References   238
Acknowledgments   240

Appendix A-1: Molecular Genetics, Biotechnology, and Bioengineering   241

Appendix A-2: Mammalian Diversity and Animal Models   299

Appendix A-3: Further Information and Acronyms   345

Appendix A-4: The COVID-19 Teaching Model   353

Abbreviations and Glossary   373

Index   379

Preface

Healthcare training programs that require coursework in microbiology and immunology typically focus on diseases and maladies affecting the adult population, yet many of these illnesses can be traced to events in the **Critical Window of Development**, the period from conception to puberty. The relationship of early life events to later health is seldom presented and integrated in basic science textbooks used in healthcare training programs. Nutrition, a cornerstone of health in the Critical Window, is rarely included. This all-in-one book fills that gap by describing events in the **Critical Window** that impact neonatal and adult health. Among these are the interdependence of life on planet Earth, and the importance of understanding the linkage of medical practice and basic biology. We integrate nutrition, genetics, immunology, the microbiome, and lessons from comparative medicine. The textbook can therefore also serve pre-vet and veterinary students.

The book was written during the COVID-19 pandemic, when the public was deluged with information and misinformation via the Internet, social media, TV advertisements, news networks, and even the government. Erroneous information endangers the health and well-being of infants, children, and adults. Therefore, Chapter 8 is devoted to discussions of misinformation about topics like the: (1) anti-vaccine movement, (2) use of antibiotics and antivirals, (3) use of probiotics for healthy adults, (4) misuse of the term *allergy*, and (5) danger of accepting hypotheses masquerading as medical facts. Chapter 7 focuses on the nature and uncertainty of scientific progress, reviews the scientific method and the meaning of "fact" in medical science. This chapter explains the origin of evidence-based science guidelines provided by medical associations such as the American Academy of Pediatrics (AAP) and the World Health Organization (WHO).

The book is designed to achieve three educational objectives. The **first** begins with a focus on basic biology, on which all healthcare depends. This includes explaining the pyramid of life forms and, most importantly, the interdependence of life forms in health and disease. This objective also provides an opportunity to introduce the major life forms involved in human health that are regularly encountered. The **second** objective is teaching basic concepts that all health care students should master that include: (1) fetal development, (2) nutrition, infant health, and growth, (3) the impact of passive antibodies, pharmaceuticals, environmental contaminants, and pathogens transferred in utero or through breastfeeding, (4) the role of the microbiome in health, and (6) internal protection provided by immune systems. The **final** objective is to integrate the basic concepts with medical practice.

We avoid drowning beginning healthcare students with molecular and cellular details, which can interfere with mastery of the basic concepts. We do this by: (1) providing **enabling objectives** for the first eight chapters and (2) using a series of **appendices**. Appendix A-1 reviews basic genetics, mitosis, meiosis, horizontal gene transfer, and the molecular genetics of adaptive immunity, as well as modern biotechnology, bioengineering, and animal models. Appendix A-2 is devoted to animal models which requires describing mammalian diversity. Appendix A-3 list acronyms and other helpful details (see later) while Appendix A-4 uses COVID-19 as a teaching model for a viral infection, bringing students into direct contact with the most recent primary literature. Including these appendices should also make the book useful for graduate education in medicine, developmental biology, and veterinary science.

Names and acronyms can be a great hurdle for students in the life sciences and medicine. The story goes that when the first moon rock was brought to Earth, it was given to chemists to determine its composition, to physicists to determine how these chemicals formed rock, and to biologists to give it a name. Biologists and medical scientists specialize in assigning names, dating to the nomenclature established for all life forms by Linnaeus (which even puts federal bureaucracies to shame). While nomenclature is necessary, time spent deciphering the names can interfere with learning concepts. In this book we try to reduce nomenclature to a minimum, define abbreviations when first used, and provide both a glossary and, in Appendix A-3, a list of acronyms used throughout the book. This is an effort to soften the impact of the inevitable blizzard of terms and acronyms. We encourage students to avail themselves to PubMed and to online webinars and to consult free online resources like Wikipedia for definitions, but with caution, since not all sites are authoritative. They may also wish to access services provided by the Centers for Disease Control (CDC), Food and Drug Administration (FDA), and specialty medical societies, for the most current and accurate information. Since this is a textbook not a review article, we provide students with suggested readings and a few other citations included in the references. Information less frequently cited in the many articles on the topics we discuss may go without citations. We expect current students with unlimited Internet access, including PubMed in the libraries of the schools where they study, to investigate such comments if it is a great interest to them.

By exploring the information presented in this book our goal is that application of key concepts in everyday clinical care will positively impact healthcare practice and the way information related to the **Critical Window** is shared with clients, students and colleagues. Enjoy the journey of discovery!

CHAPTER 1

Biology and the Critical Window of Development

LEARNING OBJECTIVES

1. Learn how major life forms differ and define "Biological Big Bangs."

2. Provide examples of life's interdependence that are essential to human health.

3. Learn about the mechanisms used by life forms to provide species survival.

4. Discuss emerging diseases that impact events in the Critical Window and beyond.

5. Distinguish between Mendelian genetics and factors that alter Mendelian principles.

6. Learn about the procedures/practices that are critical in reducing infant and childhood mortality.

Parental Care, Species Survival, and Wellness

The health and survival of the offspring of all mammals, all warm-blooded vertebrates, and many other higher organisms depends on parental care; the survival of all life forms depends on their ability to replace themselves. In short, offspring survival depends on **nutrition**, **protection**, and **genetics**. Let's consider the backyard robin. Parents must produce a fertile egg, incubate and protect the egg for it to hatch, spend long hours collecting food for their nearly helpless fledglings, continue to find food for their offspring even after the young birds take flight, and protect and educate them on food selection. For the robin and other species to survive, the offspring must also have inherited the necessary genes to live long enough to mate and start the life cycle again. Hence, the most vulnerable period in the life of robins, humans, and all multicellular organisms is from conception to sexual maturity, which falls into the period that we call the **Critical Window of Development** (Figure 1.1). It is during this period that the highest rate of mortality and morbidity occurs. Two hundred years ago only one-third of infants lived beyond their third birthday; however, medical advances such as the use of vaccines, antibiotics, and better hygiene practices, have significantly reduced mortality, although childhood mortality rates of more than 20% are still common in underdeveloped countries. Every year worldwide, 13 million children still go without a single dose of vaccine and 9 million newborns, children, and recent mothers die from treatable illness. In developed countries, modern medical practices have allowed **survival** to reach 90%, so the primary emphasis in these countries has shifted from survival to the **wellness** of the survivors during the Critical Window. Ironically, in developed countries like the United States, wellness has worsened for certain diseases, as evidenced by dramatic increases in asthma (Burr; American Lung Association), inflammatory bowel disorders (Kaplan), obesity (Fryar), diabetes (CDC), and

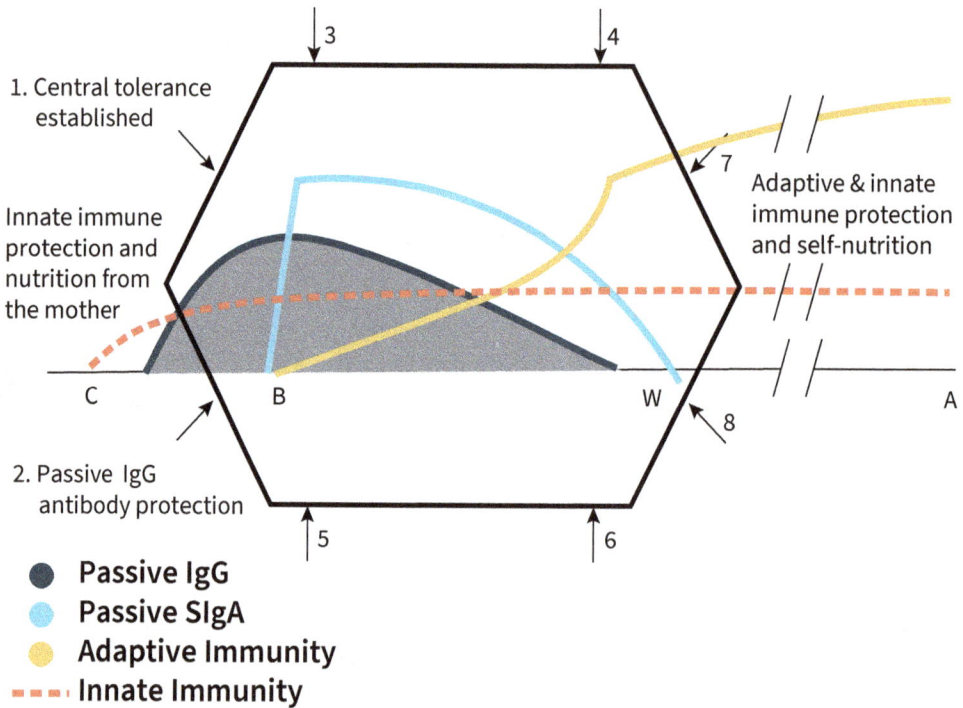

Figure 1.1   The Critical Window of Development. Numbered arrows highlight major events that occur within the Critical Window (black hexagon), each of which will be discussed throughout the book: 1=Central tolerance established; 2=Passive *in utero* IgG antibody protection; 3=Passive SIgA and colostral regulatory factors; 4=Waning of passive immunity; 5=Colonization of newborn, which stimulates development of adaptive immunity; 6=Peripheral tolerance becomes established; 7= Passive immunity replaced by adaptive immunity; 8=Rapid expansion of adaptive immunity. The capital letters on the horizontal axis are: C=conception, B=birth, W=weaning, and A=adulthood.

antibiotic resistance (Davies). Some of these increases raise questions about the impact of lifestyle in highly developed countries, including its association with diet and changes in the microbiome of the gastrointestinal (GI) tract. The often-cited parallel increases in autism spectrum disorder (ASD) may be largely due to a broadened definition of the disorder and an increase in reporting. Infectious diseases have been compounded by globalization and the increase in worldwide travel of humans and the products they produce.

We believe that medical practice also depends on understanding the nature and role of the various life forms on planet Earth, their interdependence, and their interactions. The next section reviews these topics. We believe it is necessary for aspiring professionals to understand how human colonization of planet Earth has influenced the interactions that affect human development and how these interactions have contributed to wellness or diseases.

Establishment, Diversification, and Interdependence of Life
Evolution, Diversification of Life, and Human Colonization

Human health depends on interactions among members of Earth's biomass; human life survives in an ecosystem, not a privileged vacuum. We begin by describing what is known about the sequential appearance of life on planet Earth. We emphasize that the two pro-karyotic groups, the Archaea and Eubacteria, comprise 85% of Earth's biomass and this greatly impacts the well-being of eukaryotes (like us humans), which comprise the remaining 15% of life on planet Earth. The interactions among life forms underlie the health of all life forms. Understanding their order of appearance helps to explain their metabolic and reproductive interdependence.

Establishment of Life on Earth

Life, defined by its contemporary molecular features, is believed to have inhabited planet Earth for slightly less than 4 billion years (Figure 1.2). Evidence suggests that life on Earth did not arrive or develop all at once. Even religious writing supports a gradual development, although we take a scientific approach and use a paleontological timescale. Measuring time by reference to a 12-hour clock, life appeared on Earth at circa 00:20 a.m., or 3.8 billion years ago. It is believed that the earliest life forms were members of the **Archaea**, or ancient bacteria. Systematists group Earth's life forms into three major categories: ancient bacteria (Archaea), true bacteria (**Eubacteria**), and the **eukaryotes**. The latter two groups are sometimes simply referred to as bacteria and eucarya (Pace, SR). All three major groups share a common biochemical and molecular genetic basis: surprisingly, humans and bacteria share approximately 90% of their genes. Eukaryotes include all life forms in which the genetic information and its regulation are contained in a cell organelle, called the **nucleus**, that contains a code for life based on deoxynucleic acid or DNA. Neither Archaea nor Eubacteria have such an organelle; the DNA in bacteria exists in a circular chromosome tethered to the cell wall. The early Archaea thrived on an oxygen-free planet (anaerobic) by obtaining their energy from the breakdown of hydrogen sulfide, CO_2, and other lifeless chemicals, typically products of volcanism. The environment of these organisms may be familiar to anyone who has visited an active volcano or a volcanic gas vent such as those in Yellowstone National Park. Archaea dominate the deep marine subsurface and are found in sediment deposited in these regions millions of years ago (Lipp). Descendants of the ancestral Archaea are present in the microbiome in oxygen-deprived regions of the GI tract (Chapter 5). Such bacteria are referred to as autotrophs, literally meaning an organism that does not depend on any other organism for their existence. Scientists believe this was the way of life on planet Earth 3.8 billion years ago, setting it apart from the current complexity and inter-dependence of life forms. About 3.6 billion years ago, Eubacteria (simply called bacteria by many) appeared and could utilize the metabolic products of the autotrophic Archaea as a source of food, although they still lived on a planet that lacked oxygen. The first evidence that oxygen was accumulating on the planet came 400 million years later, when it is believed certain Eubacteria acquired the ability to use solar energy (photoautotrophs) to break down carbon compounds, resulting in the release and slow accumulation of oxygen and resulting in what some call the first "Biological Big Bang" (BBB; Figure 1.2). Increasing exposure to oxygen probably caused a large die-off of terrestrial anaerobes for which oxygen was toxic. The next billion years of Earth's history witnessed a gradual increase in oxygen production and the dawn of a new era with the emergence of some Eubacteria (oxytrophs or obligate aerobic bacteria) that could now survive in, and even depended on, the presence of oxygen. The appearance of oxygen in the last 3 billion years is believed to be a major factor in the diversification of life on Earth and is associated with greater interdependence between life forms. Oxygen speeds up chemical reactions, which translates into more rapid growth and allowed for more rapid diversification of life forms in the last 1.5 billion years compared to the first 2 billion years (Figure 1.2). Oxygen availability, often called *oxygen pressure* or *tension*, also explains why certain pathogens of the GI tract gain an early "foothold" and why the constituency of the microbiome changes with age and differs among regions of the GI tract (Chapter 5).

It is estimated that life existed on planet Earth for 2 billion years before eukaryotes made an appearance (Figure 1.2) at a time when DNA and associated enzymes and other compounds necessary for genetic control became compartmentalized in a special organelle (*eu* = true, *karyo* = kernel or **nucleus**). This was the dawn and defining feature of eukaryotes and is often called the second BBB. This was also associated with the move to **multicellularity**. Multicellularity provided the opportunity for individual cells within colonies to diversify and for each type to perform a specific function. Colony formation is not unique to eukary-otes and occurs when Eubacteria grow into biofilms. These colonies can now behave as one organism, as exemplified by slime molds. The simple marine sponge exhibits many features associated with multicellularity. When two different species of sponges are dispersed into individual cells in the same dish, they reform according to their original species, suggesting sponge colonies possess a **self-recognition system**. In higher vertebrates, this morphed into differences among individuals of the same species, as demonstrated in tissue transplantation (Chapter 6), a barrier that needs to be overcome to allow fetal survival (Chapter 2).

Eucaryotes and Vertebrates Arrived Late in the Development of Life on Earth

Time expressed in billions of years (Ga) and converted to a 12-hour day

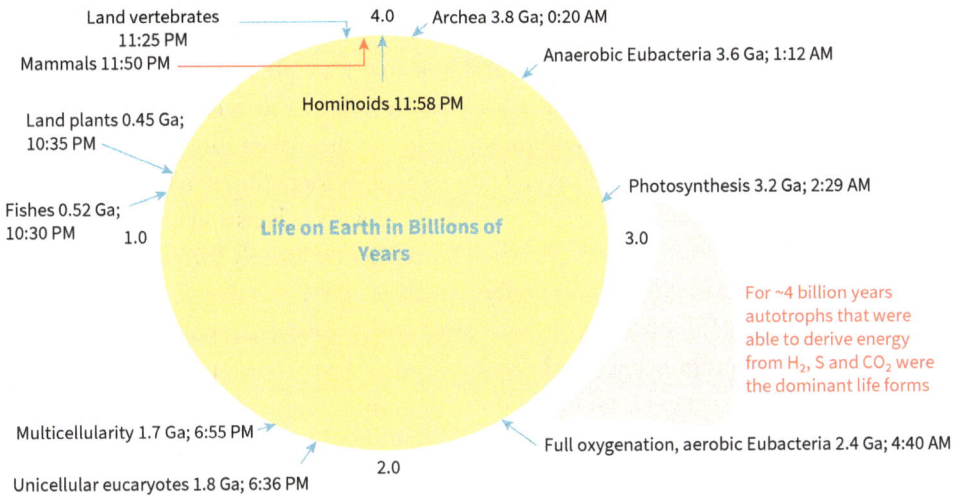

Land vertebrates
11:25 PM — 4.0 — Archea 3.8 Ga; 0:20 AM

Mammals 11:50 PM — Anaerobic Eubacteria 3.6 Ga; 1:12 AM

Hominoids 11:58 PM

Land plants 0.45 Ga;
10:35 PM

Photosynthesis 3.2 Ga; 2:29 AM

Fishes 0.52 Ga;
10:30 PM — 1.0 — **Life on Earth in Billions of Years** — 3.0

For ~4 billion years autotrophs that were able to derive energy from H_2, S and CO_2 were the dominant life forms

Multicellularity 1.7 Ga; 6:55 PM

Full oxygenation, aerobic Eubacteria 2.4 Ga; 4:40 AM

Unicellular eucaryotes 1.8 Ga; 6:36 PM — 2.0

Figure 1.2 Appearance of life on Earth. The appearance of life on planet Earth is illustrated, indicating when it is estimated that certain life forms first appeared. Time is expressed in billions of years and converted to a 12-hour clock.

The third BBB in the evolution of life on Earth was the appearance of sexual reproduction. Its appearance 1.8 billion years ago permitted a major increase in genetic diversity within a species. Prior to sexual reproduction, prokaryotes (Archaea and Eubacteria) reproduced by simple cell division that produced offspring identical to themselves. Apart from spontaneous mutation or **horizontal gene transfer (HGT)**, simple cell division limited genetic diversification in prokaryotes. If unfavorable conditions developed, it could be "sink or swim" for the identical daughter cells/offspring. Genetic details of sexual reproduction, spontaneous mutation, and HGT are provided in Appendix A-1.

The Pyramid of Life and Life's Interdependence

The result of life's colonization of planet Earth was a complex ecosystem and, after the appearance of the Eubacteria 3.6 billion years ago, interdependence became the way of life. Eubacteria marked the beginning of interdependence since they depend on organic products from autotrophs (ie, Archaea). This required that some Eubacteria acquire enzymes that degrade the proteins, carbohydrates, and other bio-organic compounds produced by the Archaea. The appearance of the Eubacteria also allowed for "reverse dependence." Namely, as autotroph populations increased, the products they produced, which could not be utilized, accumulated and retarded growth. Thus, they developed a dependence on the Eubacteria for "waste product" cleanup. One bacterium's waste become another bacterium's food. This simple scenario illustrates how primitive interdependence of life on Earth may have begun to build a fledgling biomass ecosystem.

Biologists have created names for the different types of life's interdependencies. **Mutualism** is perhaps the most ubiquitous form of commensalism, in which both life forms benefit. Schoolchildren are taught the story of lichens, a relationship in which a fungus (a multicellular eukaryote) provides support and moisture for a photosynthetic "blue-green algae" (actually, a eubacterium) in return for nutrients. When such mutualism is obligatory for both members, the term **symbiosis** is used. Because plants are immobile, many wildflowers depend on bees, butterflies, and hummingbirds for pollination for sexual reproduction, while "paying" for their service with food. As with lichens and blue-green algae, these symbiotic bonds are very tight. Monarch butterflies exclusively thrive on milkweeds during their long migration, which not only provide food for their larvae but a home for them to develop their full life cycle. Lilies evolved to rely on certain pollinators, notably hummingbirds and hummingbird moths equipped with the necessary proboscis (or bill) to reach the pollen. Plants have nectar for food and fragrant perfumes that are attractants for pollinators. In the tropics, certain trees and bromeliads are designed to allow only properly equipped hummingbirds or bats to carry out pollination. In fact, some only bloom at night, restricting pollination to certain bat species (Fleming). The lack of mobility of plants has led to many other clever adaptations needed for their reproduction. Certain flies and beetles are attracted to the stench of decaying vertebrates, which provide a home and nutrition for their offspring. As a result, some plants release a rotting-flesh odor so that these insects will gather their pollen. Symbiotic relationships can be more complicated since in some cases the stench is not made by the plant but by a bacterium living symbiotically with the plant or the decaying vertebrate.

One of the most complex and important symbiotic relationships involves the up to 10^{12} bacteria of more than 1,000 species that live on the surface of the epithelial cells (enterocytes) of the GI tract of human and other mammals; these are called the *microbiota* or *microbiome*. This translates into 10 bacteria for each human body cell. In insects such as termites and cockroaches, and in ruminant mammals, GI tract microbiota is essential for nutrition and survival. Larval termites that fail to obtain this microbiome from adult termites starve to death. Mice and piglets deprived of their microbiota thrive poorly and fail to develop protection against pathogens. So important is the symbiosis between the GI tract microbiome and the host that Chapter 5 is devoted to this topic.

Another example of life's interdependence is the microscopic ecosystem that makes up what we call the *soil*. Soil is a mixture of life forms and minerals broken down by physical forces from rocks produced during Earth's thermic origin and during periodic volcanism. No better example exists than the soil that forms the forest floor. In addition to minerals, the soil contains filamentous fungi linked to the roots of trees and plants with which they exchange food, water, and information, many Eubacteria, Archaea, and single-cell and multicellular eukaryotes that can only be seen with a scanning electron microscope. The latter include amoeba of all types (some that colonize into slime molds), and other protozoans, mites, rotifers, hairlike worms, and tardigrades. As in the GI tract microbiome, symbiosis is the norm. Plant photosynthesis converts solar energy into carbon-rich molecules that are released from plants' roots for use and further conversion by the microflora and microfauna described. In return, plant roots absorb micronutrients produced by the soil microflora and microfauna that are essential for proper growth and survival. It is well-documented that clear-cut forestry and industrial agricultural practices (the use of pesticides, herbicides, and excessive amounts of chemical fertilizer) kill members of the vital soil ecosystem and can destroy it.

While interdependences are necessary for the survival of almost all life forms, some may have negative consequences such as discomfort and disease. Parasitism (see next) is one example, and it often requires the interaction of several different life forms. In Chapter 5 we describe how certain viruses and some protozoans depend on insect vectors such as female mosquitoes, which in turn depend on certain volatiles from mammal skin and its microbiome to attract them to a host mammal that can provide the necessary environment needed for their reproduction and survival (Zhao & del Marmol).

Commensal interdependence that is not equal is called **parasitism**, in which one member is harmed at the expense of the other. Parasitism is a form of infectious disease and will be mentioned in the section on emerging diseases. It is a complex example of interdependence, since many parasites engage the services of three different life forms in completing their life cycle, one often serving as an unharmed vector (Table 1.1). In the case of malaria (caused by a protozoan), certain species of mosquitos are needed. In Rocky Mountain spotted fever a bacterium must be carried by certain tick species, much the same as Lyme disease in humans and their pets is caused by the bacteria *Borrelia burgdorferi*, which uses the deer tick as a vector. Certain worm parasites require an intermediary host not merely as a vector but also to provide a special environment where part of their development occurs. Many pathogens that can cause fatal infections in humans and other mammals are transmitted by insects, like female mosquitoes and vampire bats, that crave a blood meal. Infected mammals like raccoons, skunks, and foxes are prone to bite, allowing them to transmit rabies.

TABLE 1.1   Parasitism and Infectious Diseases Illustrate Life's Interdependence

Disease	Parasite or Microbe	Vector	Related Diseases
African sleeping sickness	Trypanosome (protozoan)	Tsetse fly (insect)	Chagas disease
Rocky Mt. spotted fever	*Rickettsia* (bacteria)	Various ticks (arachnid)	Lyme disease
West Nile fever	West Nile virus (flavivirus)	Mosquito (insect) Horse (mammal)	Rubella, yellow fever Dengue fever
Hemorrhagic fever	Hantavirus (bunyavirus)	Deer mouse (mammal)	La Crosse encephalitis
Ebola hemorrhagic fever	Ebola virus (filovirus)	Fruit bat (mammal)	Marburg fever
"Norwegian" tapeworm	Fish tapeworm (cestode)	Pike (teleost fish) Cyclops (crustacean)	Pork tapeworm Echinococcus

(Continued)

TABLE 1.1   Parasitism and Infectious Diseases Illustrate Life's Interdependence *(Continued)*

Disease	Parasite or Microbe	Vector	Related Diseases
Malaria	Plasmodium (protozoan)	Mosquito (insect)	Leishmaniasis Toxoplasmosis
African blood fluke	Schistosome (trematode)	Snail (mollusk)	"Swimmer's itch"
Sheep liver fluke	Fasciola (trematode)	Snail (mollusk)	Chinese liver fluke
Equine morbid disease	Hendra virus (paramyxovirus)	Fruit bat (mammal) Horse (mammal)	Canine distemper Measles, mumps
Bubonic plague	Yersinia pestis (Eubacteria)	House rat (mammal) Flea (insect)	Sylvatic plague
River blindness	Onchocerca (nematode)	Blackfly (insect)	Elephantiasis Trichinosis
Rabies	Rabies virus (rhabdovirus)	Canines (mammal)	Vesicular stomatitis

Human Colonization

Paleontological evidence suggests that anatomically modern humans have been on planet Earth for at least 300,000 years. In the last 100,000 years they dispersed out of Africa to inhabit the Artic, deserts, rainforests, and mountain environments. However, in the last 10,000 years, most human societies transitioned from hunting and gathering to agriculture, which resulted in dietary changes. Most lived in small rural communities in close contact with domesticated animals and relied on a variety of food sources: fruits, vegetables, and nuts, milk products, and, less often, meat. In many cultures glucose was a rare ingredient in food, mostly derived from honey. During this period humans worked manually and covered long distances on foot.

Especially in the last century, humans adapted to yet another environment. This involved a shift to professional occupations that required less physical activity. Change was driven by science, industry, and medicine and altered many aspects of life. The concentration in cities favored the spread of infectious agents and airborne pollutants that contribute to pulmonary disease. Urban centers also lacked large domestic animals, contributing to an overly strict hygienic condition that may have contributed to the increase in allergic diseases in urban industrialized cultures. The impact of this change is discussed in Chapter 6 as part of the **hygiene hypothesis**.

The shift to occupations that featured a sedentary office environment and the replacement of walking with mechanical transportation reduced muscular activity. Muscular activity increases myokine-mediated vascularization throughout the body so the body can more efficiently utilize oxygen (Ahn). This change was accompanied by a greater dependence on processed food containing more sugar and multiple additives (Winkler). Excess sugars are converted to fat and the hunger feeling then re-emerges, leading to further caloric intake. This may explain why more than 50% of the human population in industrialized countries is obese or overweight.

Particularly relevant to the Critical Window was the associated shift away from breast-feeding. This, along with other dietary changes, influenced the constituency of the microbiome of the developing neonate and later the adult. The impacts of these changes are a focus of Chapter 5.

The Role of Subcellular Life Forms in Life's Interdependence

The description of the three major life forms, their evolutionary debut, and their contribution to the biomass pyramid fails to mention the subcellular life forms that are also part of Earth's biomass and are present in diseases encountered within the Critical Window and beyond. These include viruses, plasmids, viroids, mitochondria, chloroplasts, and exosomes. None can live on their own but survive as intracellular **symbionts** or **parasites**. Viruses, plasmids, and mitochondria are able to reproduce inside the cells of their hosts, while other subcellular life forms replicate during cell division. Viruses are parasites of eukaryotic cells and are responsible for some of the major childhood diseases described later in this book. There are estimated to be 10^{31} viral particles in the world. Those that parasitize bacteria are called **bacteriophages**, and more than 142,000 bacteriophages are present in the genomes of the bacteria that comprise the GI tract microbiome (Chapter 5). As previously stated, true bacteria and Archaea are the dominant cellular life forms on Earth and account for 85% of the world's biomass (Figure 1.3). However, bacteriophages outnumber them by an order of magnitude (Krupovic, SR). These subcellular life forms contain nucleic acids, sometimes

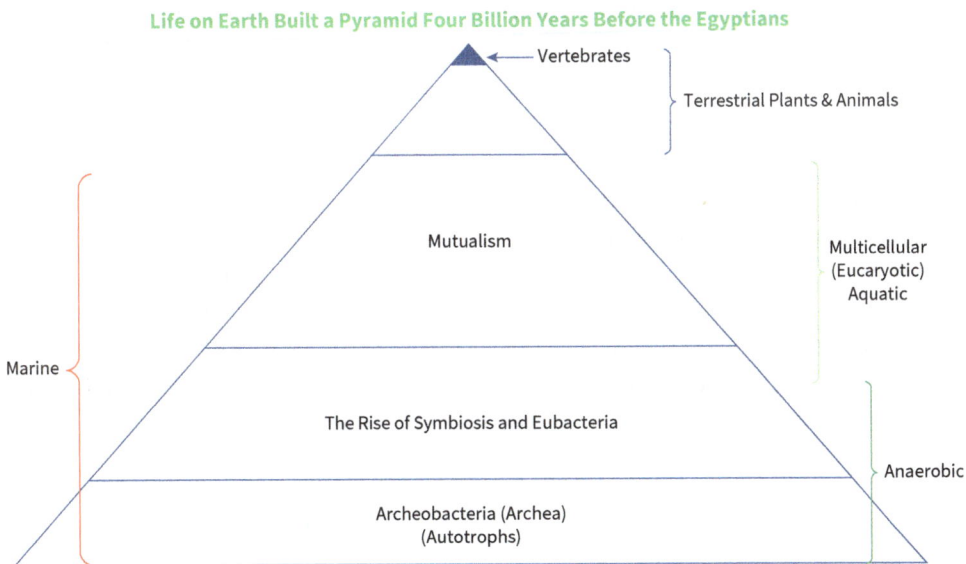

Life on Earth Built a Pyramid Four Billion Years Before the Egyptians

- Vertebrates
- Terrestrial Plants & Animals
- Mutualism
- Multicellular (Eucaryotic) Aquatic
- Marine
- The Rise of Symbiosis and Eubacteria
- Anaerobic
- Archeobacteria (Archea) (Autotrophs)

Figure 1.3   Life's pyramid on planet Earth. Life forms on planet Earth form a pyramid, the width of which represents the size of the population and shows that vertebrates like humans form the apex of the triangle but are very low in number in comparison to prokaryotes, invertebrates, and other simple multicellular life forms. Within the triangle, various ecological events are indicated, and the constituency at each stage is indicated.

RNA but predominately double-stranded DNA that instruct the host cell machinery to work for them, most of all using the host cell to produce their offspring (ie, more virus). **Plasmids** are associated with unicellular prokaryotes. These small, circular, self-replicating segments of nucleic acids are transferred horizontally among bacteria (HGT). Since subcellular life forms depend on cells, they must have appeared after the development of true cells. Theories abound, although we know that potential viral genomes become incorporated into the genome of higher organisms where they exist as **proviruses**. The nucleic acids of some plasmids use special enzymes (**integrases**) to become incorporated into the genome of the bacteria in which they thrive. Perhaps this process also explains the origins of proviruses in the eukaryote genome, since the human immunodeficiency virus (HIV) does exactly that. In any case, viruses belong to the collection of forms only visible by electron microscopy that are collectively referred to as *microbes*. Studies on them are called virology.

Ancestors, Descendants, and the Biomass Pyramid

No organism can be both ancestor and descendant, meaning that a contemporary life form that resembles an ancestor is at most a descendent and may be a new species resulting from the accumulation of many spontaneous genetic changes. Thus, the current biomass pyramid (Figure 1.3) contains only modern representatives of ancestors. Genome change in prokaryotes is rapid and extensive changes can result in new species. Such drastic changes in higher vertebrates that have huge genomes requires thousands of years before they are expressed as a substantially altered **phenotype** (Chapter 6). The term **phenotype** is "genetic speak" to describe overt physical structure or behavior of a life form. **Genotype** refers to changes in the genome that may or may not result in a new **phenotype**.

The biomass pyramid suggests that the proportional contribution of the different life forms is inversely proportional to their complexity. The autotrophic Archaea form the base of the pyramid and, together with the Eubacteria, comprise 85% of the entire biomass, of which 60% are marine (Lipp). Figures 1.2 and 1.3 together make clear that without the production of oxygen through photosynthesis, no aerobic eukaryotic life forms could survive on planet Earth. Since the autotrophs form the base of the pyramid and dominate the ocean floor, changes in their populations due to climate change and pollution linked to human activity could affect the entire pyramid. Factors that alter the base of the pyramid can be transmitted through the food chain to the apex of the pyramid (Figure 1.3).

Emerging Diseases and the Critical Window
The History of Emerging Diseases

The COVID-19 pandemic caused by the SARS-CoV-2 virus attracted the attention of the public to virology and immunology in a manner that may not otherwise have occurred. COVID-19 was a "wake-up call" to the public, especially for millennials and those who have not witnessed a previous **pandemic** or **epidemic** (Morens, SR). Pandemics may be a new experience even for the older public, but not to medical science. Emerging diseases and pandemics have threatened humans for 12,000 years, back to when hunter-gathers settled into villages and domesticated wild animals. Some believe that such domestication was the beginning of the manipulation of nature that brought humans and animals into close proximity, providing an opportunity for the spread of **zoonotic diseases**. Zoonotic diseases are those which can "jump" from one species to another; they account for 75% of all emerging pathogens. Proximity between humans and animals facilitated the spread of bubonic plague from rats to humans and influenza from birds and swine to humans. Civilization and the establishment of villages concentrated humans and their feces and caused them to be dependent on the same water supply. Common water sources have allowed the human-adapted *Aedes aegyptus* mosquito to develop an ecological niche in close proximity with humans and thus facilitate the spread of malaria, yellow fever, dengue, chikungunya, and Zika. The improper disposal of human waste has repeatedly led to cholera epidemics and to the spread of parasitic diseases. Some have warned that the greatest threat of a nuclear war is not radiation, but the rampant disease that might follow if sewer systems fail and water systems are contaminated. This prediction was based on the view that bacterial pathogens were the major threat, but the current threat comes from emerging viruses.

A hundred years ago, the 1918 influenza pandemic ("Spanish flu") killed 50 million people. Since 1981, human immunodeficiency virus (HIV) has killed 35 million, and recently SARS-CoV-2 has infected more than 50 million, causing more than 1 million deaths in the United States. This far exceeds all the American military casualties of WWII. Estimates suggest that greater than 6 million people worldwide will eventually die from COVID-19. In 1918 viruses were hardly understood, including the cause of the Spanish flu, an influenza virus. At that time, antibiotics were unknown and not available to treat secondary bacterial infections associated with this flu. The nearly tenfold lower number of deaths from COVID-19 reflects the advances made in medicine since 1918 (Goldstein). Viruses are very species-specific because their entry into a eukaryotic cell depends on recognition of species-specific cell receptors, such as ACE2 in the case of SARS-CoV-2 and CD4 in the case of HIV (Appendix A-4).

Evidence shows that the majority of viruses have developed a means to coexist in humans and quite often have their origin in some animal; waterfowl in the case of the 1918 Spanish flu, the civet cat for SARS-CoV-1, the camel for MERS, and possibly Asian fruit bats for SARS-CoV-2. In addition to influenza, HIV, and SARS-CoV-2, other viruses of zoonotic origin include varicella-zoster (VZV), herpes simplex, cytomegalovirus (CMV), and Epstein-Barr virus (though this is not a complete list).

Viruses are the most dangerous infectious microbes for developing offspring, since fetal mammals can encounter viruses through *in utero* transfer from the mother (*in utero* transfer of bacteria is possible but less common), making the mother the disease-causing vector. Examples include HIV, Zika, CMV, and VZV in humans (Chapter 2); parvoviruses, porcine reproductive and respiratory syndrome virus (PRRSV), and hog cholera in swine; equine arteriviruses in horses; bovine viral diarrhea viruses in cattle; and Border disease in sheep. While mostly deleterious, some benign viruses may be beneficial since a microbial encounter in fetal and newborn mammals is a trigger that initiates development of their **adaptive immune system** and allows them to combat these and many other pathogens (Chapter 6). In addition to viruses transmitted *in utero*, a number infect the infant shortly after birth (Chapter 3). Among these are *Varicella* (chicken pox), which can be life-threatening, particularly when **passive maternal immunity** is lacking (see later). Respiratory syncytial virus (RSV), a rather benign infection for adults, can cause severe generalized infection in infants, including neurological damage. While HIV is more often transmitted *in utero*, HIV-infected mothers may also transmit this virus to their offspring through breast milk (Chapter 3).

A bacterium, *Yersinia pestis*, was responsible for the bubonic plague, but current epidemics and pandemics are of viral origin. Human societies have learned that antibiotics can be used to control bacterial but not viral infections. The only permanent antidote for infectious viruses is the host's immune system (see "Internal Protection Provided by the Immune System" later). The ability of all microbes to adapt and cause disease in new hosts lies in the plasticity of their genomes, which is described in Chapter 6 and favors viruses, especially RNA viruses like influenza and SARS-CoV-2 (Appendix A-4).

Emerging Disease and Human Behavior

Globalization has allowed humans to travel the world and assemble in large groups, thereby spreading infectious diseases. Furthermore, populations migrate for survival and are driven by changes in food supply, climate, and water availability, slavery, politics, and war. Humans immigrated to the Americas from Europe, the Middle East, and Africa. These travelers brought along contagious diseases not common in their new environment. The story of Mayans and other Indigenous natives in the Americas who died from smallpox, syphilis, and other diseases introduced by European conquerors and settlers is well known. Current concentrations of immigrants from Africa, refugees in Europe, and those waiting to cross the Texas-Mexican border hoping to emigrate served as breeding grounds for diseases and their rapid spread. While immigrants bring along their pathogens, they also encounter new ones for which they lack an internal immune defense. Whether or not climate change is caused by humans, its effect on migration and the spread of disease is the same.

COVID-19 was not a total surprise since coronaviruses are ubiquitous in all mammals. They are responsible for the "common cold" and other less virulent diseases but also several recent epidemics. When any virus "jumps" to another species that lacks immune protection, it replicates rapidly and may become highly contagious (Morens, SR). The increased rate of genome replications, made possible by the move to a new species that lacks immunity to the pathogen (and therefore has no established co-existence with it), offers a greater chance for spontaneous mutation, since spontaneous mutation occurs during reproduction when of DNA and RNA duplicate (Figure A1.2; Chapter 6). The prevailing opinion has been that "species jumping" was the origin of the COVID-19 pandemic, which allowed SARS-CoV-2 to mutate into many virulent variants (Appendix A-4). Mutant variants of SARS-CoV-2 are naturally selected if they favor greater transmission, but greater transmission is not necessarily linked to greater virulence. Usually, a rapid rate of mutation indicates an unstable genome, so highly virulent forms are courting their own destruction, since "good parasites don't kill their hosts." Perhaps SARS-CoV-2 will eventually mutate into a variant that may be highly contagious, but with such low virulence that it will resemble coronaviruses responsible for the common cold. In Appendix A-4, we use SARS-CoV-2 as a teaching model for virology, immunology, and epidemiology that could be helpful in each field's views on infectious disease and its treatment.

Surprisingly and given the experience gained from earlier SARS outbreaks (ie, SARS-CoV-1 and MERS-CoV), America and European countries seemed poorly prepared for the impact of the "jump" of SARS-CoV-2 to humans. Countries in Southeast Asia that had experienced SARS-CoV-1 were somewhat more prepared. Fortunately, the scientific resources were in place, since a SARS-CoV-1 vaccine was produced in 2005, a world record for the time that was repeated for SARS-CoV-2 in Operation Warp Speed (Appendix A-4). Sadly, not all world leaders were transparent about the danger of a SARS-CoV-2 pandemic. However, they were not pioneers in their ignorance, nor were they representatives of a particular political party, since Woodrow Wilson (a Democrat) did the same during the 1918 influenza pandemic. Nevertheless, politics, religion, and failures in education too often tend to override science, with dangerous consequences to human health. The reluctance of Americans to take precautions to curb the spread of SARS-CoV-2 was similar to their attitude in 1918. The much-quoted statement of Churchill: "Those who fail to learn from history are prone to repeat it" is still appropriate more than 100 years later. Those contemplating a career in healthcare need to understand the history of emerging diseases and their actions, depend on evidence-based information, and employ best practices in disease management (Chapter 8).

Protection, Nutrition, Genetics: A Triad for Survival and Wellness

Introduction

Figure 1.1 summarized eight events that occur within humans' Critical Window of Development and are necessary for our survival. The timing and mechanisms of the Critical Window vary among mammals (Appendix A-2). Invertebrates and lower vertebrates have also evolved ways to assure the survival of their offspring. In any case, the same triad of factors needed for offspring survival and wellness is a feature of all life forms.

Protection and Fecundity

Increases in protection parallel increases in complexity of life forms, and protection becomes favored over fecundity. Plants and less complex animals depend on safety in numbers by producing millions of offspring that, with few exceptions, forgo the protection factor, leaving survival to chance. Consider the success rate of the millions of winged maple seeds that spiral down in parks and backyards; the thousands of maple seedlings that arise in your lawn, garden, and roof gutters; and the seemingly overwhelming number of mosquito larvae that appear in standing water. Yet several months later, only a handful of maple seedlings have taken root in a place where they can survive long enough to reproduce, and adult mosquitoes may one day become an endangered species in the United States due to eradication measures. However inefficient, this system still enables adults to replace themselves and maintain a stable population. In these examples, protection plays a minor role. As complexity in the animal kingdom increased, systems evolved in which offsprings' survival was dependent on protection. Protection is so effective in elephants and some whales and sharks that their populations remain stable even when parents produce just one offspring every 2 to 5 years. Birds and reptiles physically protect their developing offspring by encasing them in a shell, and mammals do it by sheltering them in the womb of the mother. Many snakes provide additional protection since the developing eggs are carried inside the body of the female until they hatch. Humans and higher vertebrates also utilize a variety of behaviors to provide physical protection for offspring after birth. The common killdeer encourages potential predators to join it in a merry chase to draw them away from the nest or the young killdeer; loons use a similar tactic. Other bird species and mammals have developed similar but less conspicuous guarding behavior. However, these mere physical or behavioral methods cannot protect against the threat posed by bacterial, fungal, and viral pathogens.

Protection is more than external protection and more than "skin deep"; it also includes **internal protection**. Internal protection against pathogens depends on having a healthy bacterial microbiome in the GI tract that can block colonization by bacterial pathogens; this is often called **colonization resistance** (Chapter 5). Internal protection against pathogens also depends heavily on the **innate immune system**, which can discriminate "dangers" from "benign" microbes and can respond appropriately (Chapter 6). The innate immune system is common to almost all life forms. In higher vertebrates, its activation stimulates development of another form of internal protection, the **adaptive immune system**, which, like sexual maturity, is delayed in development (Figure 1.1). To compensate for this delay, **passive adaptive immune protection** is provided *in utero* to human infants (Chapter 2) and then after birth via suckling in all mammals (see next and Chapter 3).

Internal Protection from Antibiotics and Bacteriophages

Many bacteria and fungi produce "antimicrobial" substances call **antibiotics**, not to be confused with **antibodies**, the latter being a tool of the **adaptive immune system**. Antibiotics interfere with the metabolism of bacteria, causing their death. The discovery and identification of **antibiotics** that could kill pathogenic bacteria was regarded as the "miracle cure" of the 1940s (Chapter 6). However, these antibiotics only interdict the metabolism of bacteria, which is sometimes misunderstood. This has resulted in their prescription for all sorts of infectious diseases, too often for viral infections, for which they have no direct effect. Overuse of antibiotics has resulted in multidrug-resistant (MDR) bacteria. MDR bacteria are regarded by the WHO as a major threat to human health worldwide (Blaser, SR; Chapters 6 and 8). Currently protection against viral diseases depends on vaccines and, in special cases, antiviral drugs. We described bacteriophages as viruses that infect bacteria instead of eukaryotic cells. Many cause lysis of the bacteria and a hundred years ago they were even being considered as a way to control bacterial infection, a precursor of vaccines. However, phage therapy declined in the 1930s as antibiotics and vaccines took center stage. However, in light of MDR bacteria, there has been a rebirth in the use of bacteriophage therapy in treatment of resistant pulmonary disease (Nick) and in veterinary medicine (Appendix A-2).

Internal Protection Provided by the Immune System
Innate and Adaptive Immunity
The host is protected by two separate but interconnected immune systems. The innate system is common to all cellular life forms, is present throughout life (Figure 1.2), and discriminates between self and pathogenic microbes that can cause harm; it provides an early warning signal. Adaptive immunity is a feature of higher vertebrates and allows them to somatically improve the effectiveness of their immune response. These systems are described in Chapter 6 and in greater detail in Appendix A-1.

Vaccines Stimulate Innate and Adaptive Immunity
In Chapter 6 we describe the history of vaccination as a way to improve internal protection. Vaccination and vaccines rose to prominence in the battle against smallpox in 18th-century England, and the practice spread worldwide and is now common. In Chapter 6, we also note that the innate immune system must be stimulated in order to stimulate an adaptive immune response. The mechanisms responsible are somewhat complicated, and some are discussed in that chapter.

Passive Immunity
This natural physiological mechanism provides internal protection by providing antibodies arising through the adaptive immune system. This occurs naturally during development in the Critical Window but is also used therapeutically. In Chapter 2, we describe how maternal immunoglobin G (IgG) antibodies are naturally transferred to the developing fetus, and in Chapter 3 we describe how this protection continues for the newborn via suckling. **Therapeutic antibodies** may be familiar as injected immune serum globulin. This was historically used to protect against measles, rabies, snake venom, and so on. Older generations may remember immune globulin intramuscular injections as protection against diphtheria or tetanus. Historically, immune globulin was prepared in horses used by the New York police department. It was reasoned that if these horses were simply around Manhattan to carry policeman and consume lots of food, perhaps they could also be of benefit to human medicine. Serum produced by these horses fell out of favor because they were of heterologous origin and repeated doses caused a hypersensitivity reaction that could be fatal to the recipient (Chapter 6). This was replaced by therapeutic intravenous immunoglobulin (IVIG) prepared from pooled human plasma, with multiple safeguards against the transmission of infection. Currently "humanized" monoclonal antibodies (mAbs) are used for passive immunotherapy, often advertised on TV for treatment of certain autoimmune diseases. Readers may recognize pharmaceuticals like Humira, Skyrizi, Dupixent, Cosentyx, and many others. The principles and production of mAbs is described in Appendix A-1.

Oral therapeutic immune globulin dates to the immune milk episode of the 1950s and the late Professor Peterson at the University of Minnesota. He promoted the use of milk from immunized cows as a source of oral passive antibodies for treating a broad range of human maladies from arthritis to lethargy to chronic back pain. At the time, neither the cause of these maladies, nor the mechanism by which ingested bovine antibodies functioned, was known. The eventual rejection of the professor's views led to his suicide, but the concept has lived on in modified form (Marcotte; Appendices A-1 and A-4). Heterologous immune globulin (from from cattle, goats, etc.) can be given orally and offers a low risk of causing hypersensitivity reactions since the immune globulin is not absorbed but rather its protective action is directly within the GI tract, much like the natural passive immunity provided by secretory immunoglobulin A (SIgA) antibodies to infants through breast-feeding (Chapter 3).

Nutrition
Introduction
The survival of all life forms depends on adequate nutrition. During fetal development in mammals, it is provided through transfer across the placenta, while in fishes, amphibians, reptiles, and birds, nutrients are stored in eggs. In all cases this is critical during the Critical Window of Development.

Nutrition of Human Offspring
While invertebrates and lower vertebrates provide nutrients for the developing offspring stored in their eggs (a fact soon discovered by other birds and mammals who dine on them), mammals have taken nutrient supply to a more secure level. Mammalian offspring have a physical connection to the mother while in the womb, so they enjoy physical protection while receiving a continuous supply of nutrients and factors that regulate internal protection (Chapter 2). When womb protection ends at birth, the nutrient supply system shifts to the use of a modified secretory organ, the mammary gland (MG), the organ from which mammals take their name. While there are numerous variations in postpartum relationships between mother and child among mammals (Appendix A-2), the basic mechanisms and principles are the same. In kangaroos (and other marsupials like the opossum) the "joeys" are born premature and placed in a pouch where, unlike human infants, they become more or less permanently attached to nipples of the mammary gland. Human infants and those of rats, mice, and carnivores are also born comparatively premature, a condition referred to as **altricial**. Some are born blind and hairless and need the help of their mother to introduce them to the MG. In farm animals and many of their relatives, offspring are **precocial**. These are born with fur and open eyes. They are immediately mobile and programmed to seek out the MG. Anyone witnessing the birth of a foal or calf will recall how they are standing, walking, and seeking out the MG within minutes after birth. In Chapter 3 we describe how nutrients are provided after birth through suckling and in Chapter 4 we describe how, in developed cultures, these nutrients may come from surrogate milks supplied as industrially produced infant formulas.

The transfer of nutrients and protective factors *in utero* and through breast milk carries with it certain risks, because it also provides an avenue for deleterious substances and pathogens. In Chapter 2 we discuss congenital (present at birth) infections using rubella (German measles) and cytomegalovirus (CMV) as examples. Chapter 3 draws attention to pathogens that are transferred through breast milk. The extent to which prescription pharmaceuticals, illicit drugs, and environmental contaminants are transferred is also reviewed in Chapters 2 and 3.

Nutrient Transfer and the Role of the Microbiome

The expression "you are what you eat" owes its origin in part to well-known phenomena. Anyone growing up on a dairy farm learns that when milk cows eat certain weeds and grasses, the flavor of their milk is negatively altered, and "tainted milk" is of lower value. In countries like Switzerland, milk cows are deliberately pastured on specific grasses to improve the flavor of their milk and the cheese produced from their milk. Beekeepers know that the flavor of the honey produced depends on the source of the nectar and pollen retrieved by the worker bees, so beekeepers move their hives to areas where certain flowering plants abound, resulting in more marketable honey. *In utero* and MG transfer of nutrients mainly includes those that impact the health of the neonate. Studies in macaque monkeys, which have a strong social hierarchy, have shown that the offspring of the alpha female are bigger and healthier because their reigning mother gets first choice of the food available to the colony. Perhaps this also occurs in wolf packs and lion prides. Folklore suggests that infants born to garlic-eating mothers crave garlicky foods.

The expression "you are what you eat" also has its origin in the actions of the bacteria that comprise the GI tract microbiome (Chapter 5). In Chapter 3 we describe the third-most abundant constituent in human breast milk, human milk oligosaccharides (HMOs), but these do not provide direct nutrition to the suckling neonate. Rather, certain members of the GI tract microbiome can convert them to short-chain fatty acids (SCFA) needed to maintain the integrity of the GI tract mucosa as well as other nutrients. In mammals like cattle, sheep, deer, and camels, nutrition is largely dependent on nutrients generated by the gut microbiome from cellulose foodstuffs that cannot be digested by the animals themselves. In these ruminants, the composition of the GI tract microbiome is influenced and maintained by the nature of the food ingested (Appendix A-2). Members of the GI tract microbiome that provide a nutritional advantage to the host flourish at the expense of others. It is known that surrogate milks and formulas that replace or augment human breast milk alter the composition of the GI tract microbiome, so its composition differs between the 60% of infants in developed countries that are formula fed and infants in underdeveloped countries that are largely breastfed (Chapter 5). The symbiotic relationship of the microbiome and the GI tract is an example of life's interdependence, and this symbiosis can also help to exclude GI tract pathogens (known as **colonization resistance**; see earlier and Chapters 3 and 5). The microbiome of Indigenous populations in South America that subsist heavily on plants thrives with little medical intervention and their microbiome is far more diverse than that in individuals from developed countries. This and similar observations have led to the belief that there is a correlation between the constituency and diversity of the microbiome and health, which has implications in diseases like obesity, diabetes, asthma, food allergies, and IBD in developed countries (Chapter 5).

Genetics and Health in the Critical Window
Basic Principles

The "third rail" of the triad, **genetics**, has been recognized for 2 millennia. Life on planet Earth carries with it a blueprint, the genetic code, which provides complete instructions for development, repair, and reproduction and is encoded in what is called the genome (Appendix A-1). Genetics is about **genes**, and the word *gene* is derived from the German word *Pangen*, meaning all offspring or life. Herdsmen raising domesticated animals recognized that certain traits were passed on from parent to offspring, so that in the Middle Ages royalty recognized the potential danger of marrying your sister or your cousin and passing on a negative trait. In Muslim cultures, it was believed that genetic traits could also be transferred by suckling, so children were often nursed by surrogates or "wet nurses" who were not allowed to marry a relative of the wet nurses.

We mention elsewhere in the book that the response to a microbial pandemic rests on the concept of "survival of the fittest" due to natural immunity or vaccination. Overcoming a pandemic without either means the loss of many lives. Are survivors just lucky or can it be due to genetics? We mentioned that the ability of a virus to infect depends on recognition of a receptor on a eukaryotic cell and, for diseases like sickle cell, on the host genome. It has been known for some time that some individuals are not susceptible to HIV, and we are learning that some individuals that acquire SARS-CoV-2 are asymptomatic. In the case of HIV, the virus requires CD4 as an entrance receptor but also the chemokine receptor type 5 (CXC5; see Chapter 6). Individuals who lack expression of CXC5 never become infected. In the case of SARS-CoV-2, ACE2 is needed for viral entry (Appendix A-4). It is reasonable to hypothesize that the reason people exposed to SARS-CoV-2 are asymptomatic or suffer from long COVID could have to do with their individual genetics.

Gene Expression and Epigenetics

For many beginning healthcare students, their view of genetics likely relies on Mendelian genetics, learned in high school. It is named for the Gregor Mendel, a monk from Brno (Czech Republic). Since the days of Mendel, in the 20th century and even more so in the 21st century, molecular geneticists now also focus on gene expression. This means that it is not merely the presence of a particular inherited gene, but also how the gene is phenotypically expressed, that characterizes genetic differences. A familiar example is the more than 100 breeds of dogs, which differ very little in their genome but are phenotypically different. Consider the dachshund, shepherd dogs from all continents, Great Danes, toy poodles, greyhounds, retrievers of various types, and sled dogs. Recent reinforcement of this concept comes from the analysis of some 4,000 domestic, semiferal, and wild carnivores. Ten canine lineages were identified to show that behavior differences were driven by noncoding genetic variations (Dutrow). Recent studies in mice have shown that epigenetic changes resulting from methylation of DNA can be propagated across several generations (Cheng). Their differences are not due to major changes in their structural genes, but in how these genes are expressed. Sometimes the term *epigenetics* is used in connection with this concept.

In Chapter 2 we mention the possibility that environmental factors transferred *in utero* may alter gene expression and might explain some forms of autism spectrum disorder (ASD). Can gene expression also be responsible for the increase in inflammatory bowel disorders (IBD) and allergies in developed countries?

Rapid Genetic Changes in Pathogens Challenge Internal Immune Protections and Compromise Human Health

We describe in mathematical terms how microbial pathogens can more rapidly alter their genomes than can humans and other mammals (Chapter 6). Added to their ability for rapid genomic change through spontaneous mutation is their capability of undergoing horizontal transfer of genetic information (HGT; see Appendix A-1). These events allow the "microbial empire" (Chapter 6) to counter the somatic feature of internal protection provided by the adaptive immune system.

Correction of Genetic Defect Through Bioengineering

Human genetic disorders have been poorly amenable to mediation by routine medical practices, through parenting, or by nutritional adjustments. Apart from advising newly-weds and expectant parents about certain genetic dangers, currently only animal scientists are allowed to freely alter genes that are transferred during the reproductive process, and genetic manipulation is viewed by many with suspicion. Use of technologies that manipulate the human genetic blueprint that is transmitted to offspring crosses over into the areas of social and cultural mores and medical ethics. Readers may remember the negative reaction toward a Chinese scientist who modified a gene in human embryonic stem cells to block infection by HIV. While this unapproved treatment did not satisfy current ethical practice, it served as a precursor to practices that are ongoing. Appendix A-1 describes examples of genetic engineering such as gene editing and other measures that can be used to correct specific genetic defects in humans, such as sickle-cell anemia, leukemia, and other childhood malignancies.

We should not forget that there are also nongenetic treatments that can overcome genetic defects. For example, amniocentesis can show whether a fetus expresses red cell markers that will be attacked and destroyed by its mother's serum antibodies that are transferred *in utero*. This can be treated by blood transfusion at birth by replacing the infant's targeted red cells (Chapter 2). It has become popular to attribute 30% of human maladies to genetics and the remainder to environmental factors and lifestyle.

Students who are "rusty" on their understanding of genetics and molecular genetics should find Appendix A-1 useful. This will refresh their understanding of meiosis, HGT in bacteria, and the mechanisms involved in rapid genetic changes in lymphocytes because of their ability to somatically rearrange their genes and undergo somatic mutation.

The Place of Basic Science in Medicine
The "Go/No Go" Decision

It is important for students to understand how investigative science and clinical trials are applied in medical practice. Achieving the optimal outcome for issues dealing with **nutrition, protection,** and **genetics** depends on decisions made by parents and caregivers, so it is best that one understands how these decisions are made. The expression that introduces this section is adopted from aviation and is a reference to the decision of the pilot to fly or not fly based on reliable information on the weather, the capability of the aircraft, and the health of the pilot making the decision. In medicine this may be equivalent to deciding between the risk of intervention versus no intervention. Choices regarding breast-feeding, formula, the use and timing of vaccines, and antibiotic therapy fall within this category.

In Chapter 7, we discuss the difficult decisions faced by caregivers and review the steps in the scientific method, the meaning of "fact" in science, and the design of clinical trials for vaccines, pharmaceuticals, and other treatments. Nevertheless, some decisions in clinical medicine are based only on correlations, since rigorous experimental testing may not have established causation, but for the health of the patient a decision must still be made. Such decisions remain a conundrum that providers continually face. In all situations, providers rely on the "hierarchy of strength as evidence" in making their decision. This process rests on a mixture of hard science, correlations, and their best judgment. Providers also base their decisions on guidelines from medical organizations such as Dietary Guidelines for Americans (provided by the USDA), the WHO, the Maternal and Child Health Bureau, and those established by the Centers for Disease Control (CDC). Recommendations are also based on the most reliable information from peer-reviewed scientific literature. Since the primary literature is often difficult for the public and beginning students to access and understand, they typically accept on faith what they are taught or what they learn from the media, review articles, or from continuing education programs. There is the story of an aspiring PhD candidate who was asked what proportion of what he knew was based on personal observation versus what he learned in the classroom. The correct answer is less than 2%. Aspiring and current providers should remember this story.

The Role of Animal Models and Comparative Biology

Much of what we know about the immune system and nutrition is based on studies using rodents and other mammals as experimental models. What we have learned about passive immunity and the composition of milks and functions of milk components comes from studies with farm animals (Appendix A-2). Much of what we know about developmental immunology has been dependent on studies in piglets and rodents. Knowledge of the role of the microbiome grew from studies on the GI tracts of cattle and other ruminant mammals. Many nutritional studies continue to use piglets and rats as models. We believe it is important for students to appreciate mammalian diversity so they can better interpret data derived from animal models, as animals' physiology may differ from humans. Therefore, we provide Appendix A-2.

Controversies, Misconceptions, and the Critical Window

The anti-vaccine movement and vaccine hesitancy in the United States, and its perpetuation by social media, the Internet, and some politicians, has interfered with the delivery of healthcare in America. Especially damaging has been the assertion that autism is the result of childhood vaccinations, which has contributed to vaccine hesitancy. Among the African American community, there are individuals who remember when African Americans and prisoners were used as "guinea pigs," often without their consent. Anti-vax adherents and those with vaccine hesitancy also include religious groups, and in the case of COVID-19, the public's skepticism that a safe vaccine could be developed in such a short time. We address this with the inclusion of Appendix A-1, which discusses modern biotechnology, which has changed since the time of parents and especially grandparents. Re-education is not only important in combating the public **infodemic** surrounding the COVID-19 pandemic, but especially for educating the next generation of healthcare providers. Throughout this textbook, we remind readers about the limits of antibiotic therapy and emphasize that symbiotic bacteria are not all dangerous "germs"—rather, most are important for proper nutrition and internal protection against colonization by bacterial pathogens. We also address "allergy," which has become a societal umbrella term for phenomena having little to do with medically defined allergies. To address this and other issues related to the health of neonates, we have included Chapter 8, where we discuss a spectrum of social, behavioral, educational, and scientific issues that impact wellness and that aspiring practitioners need to consider.

Suggested Reading (SR)

Aboud FE, Yousafzai AK. Global health and development in early childhood. *Annu Rev Psychol*. 2015;66:433–457.

Blaser MJ. *Missing microbes*. New York: Picador; 2014.

Krupovic M, Prangishvilli D, Hendrix RM, Bamford DH. Genomics of bacterial and archaeal viruses: Dynamics within this prokaryotic virosphere. *Microbiol Mol Bio., Rev*. 2011;4:610–635. doi:10.1128/MMBR 00011-11.

Morens DM, Fauci AS. Emerging pandemic diseases: How we got to COVID-19. *Cell*. 2020;182(5):1077–1092.

Pace NR. A molecular view of microbial diversity and the biosphere. *Science*. 1997;276:734–740.

The importance that events in the Critical Window play in the health of infants is also provided in the webinar Maternal & Infant Health Initiative Webinar Series" https://www.medicaid.gov/medicaid/quality-of-care/downloads/mhi-webinar-052024.pdf

References

Ahn SH, Jung H-W, Lee E, et al. Decreased serum level of sclerostin in older adults with sarcopenia. *Endocrinol Metab* (Seoul). 2020;37(3):487–496. doi:10.3803/EnM.2022.1428.

American Lung Association. Asthma trends and burden. www.lung.org/research/trends-in-lung-disease/asthma-trends-brief/trends-and-burden.

Burr ML, Wat D, Evans C, Dunstan FDJ, Doull IJM. Asthma prevalence in 1973, 1988 and 2003. *Thorax*. 2006;61:296–299. doi:10.1136/thx.2005.045682.

Cheng S, Mayshar Y, Stelzer Y. Induced epigenetic changes memorized across generations in mice. *Cell*. 2023;186:683–685.

Davies J, Davies D. Origins and evolution of antibiotic resistance. *Microbiol and Mol Biol Rev*. 2010;74:417–433. doi:10.1128/MMBR.00016-10.

Dutrow EV, Serpell JA, Ostrander, EA. Domestic dog lineages reveal genetic drivers of behavioral diversification. *Cell*. 2022;185:4737–4755.

Fleming, TH, Geiselman C, Kress WJ. The evolution of bat pollination: A phylogenetic perspective. *An. Bot*. 2009;104:1017–1043.

Fryar CD, Carroll MD, Ogden CL. Prevalence of overweight, obesity, and severe obesity among adults aged 20 and over: United States, 1960–1962 through 2015–2016. National Center for Health Statistics; September 2018. https://www.cdc.gov/nchs/data/hestat/obesity_adult_15_16/obesity_adult_15_16.pdf.

Goldstein JL. The Spanish 1918 flu and the COVID-19 disease: The art of remembering and foreshadowing pandemics. *Cell*. 2020;183:285–288.

Kaplan, G. The global burden of IBD: From 2015 to 2025. *Nat Rev Gastroenterol Hepatol*. 2015;12:720–727. https://doi.org/10.1038/nrgastro.2015.150.

Lipp JS, Morono Y, Iwagaki F, Hinricks K-U. Significant contribution of Archea to extant biomass in marine subsurface sediments. *Letter*. 2008;454(7207):991–994.

Marcotte H, Hammarstrom L. Passive immunization: Toward magic bullets. In Mestecky J, Strober W, Russell MW, Kelsall BL, Cheroutre H, Lambrecht BN, eds. *Mucosal Immunology*. 4th ed. Cambridge, MA: Academic Press; 2015:1403–1434.

National Center for Chronic Disease Prevention and Health Promotion, Division of Diabetes Translation. Long-term trends in diabetes. April 2017. https://stacks.cdc.gov/view/cdc/46096.

Nick JA, Dedrick RM, Gray AL, et al. Host and pathogen response to bacteriophage engineered against *Mycobacterium absecessus* in lung infections. *Cell*. 2022;185:1860–1874.

Winkler HC, Suter M, Naegeli H. Critical review of the safety assessment of nano-structured silica additives in food. *J Nanobiotechnology*. 2016;14:44. https://jnanobiotechnology.biomedcentral.com/articles/10.1186/s12951-016-0189-6.

Zhao J, del Marmol J. Why are some people more attractive to mosquitoes than others? *Cell*. 2022;185:4040–4042.

Figure Credit

CHAPTER 2

The Prepartum Maternal-Fetal Connections

1. Describe the maternal-fetal interface in the placenta.

2. Describe the different mechanisms involved in the transfer of nutrients, antibodies, and other substances across the placenta.

3. Provide examples of pathogens and deleterious substances that can cross the placenta.

4. Provide reasons the fetus is not rejected by the maternal immune system.

5. Describe the impact of maternal nutrition (properly nourished, malnourished, or starving) on early life and on the long-term health of the child.

Conception and Establishment of the Maternal-Fetal Connection

A new diploid cell is created by fertilization of the ovum. As soon as the spermatozoon has penetrated the ovum, the latter is sealed off to further penetration and the two cells and nuclei merge to form the zygote. The respective genomes combine, but as recently reported, 50–70% of the time the zygote has an incorrect number of chromosomes, a condition known as *aneuploidy* (Cavazza). The zygotes with abnormal chromosomal numbers usually cannot develop to term, a frequent cause of early miscarriage. The successfully formed zygote undergoes rapid cell division to form a ball of 16 cells, the morula. As cell division continues, the cell mass transforms into a blastocyst, a hollow body of about 100 cells. The blastocyst is less than a millimeter in diameter, with a fluid-filled center. The blastocyst embeds (implants) itself in the endometrium (the uterine mucosa) 6 to 7 days after fertilization. Recent studies show that the first division of the zygote already begins the differentiation process in that one cell of the diploid will lead to the formation of the placenta and its intersection with the fetus while the other will contribute to the epiblast, that goes on to form the vast majority of the human fetus.

Successful implantation of the blastocyst and its subsequent growth depend on intercellular messengers called **cytokines** and **chemokines**, including interleukins IL-1 and IL-3, and colony-stimulating factor. Implantation is characterized by a local, low-grade inflammatory response that also involves IL-6, IL-8, and tumor necrosis factor (TNF)-α (Hanson). Cytokines are discussed in Chapter 6. The mild inflammatory state must be controlled for pregnancy to continue, as discussed later.

Figure 2.1 illustrates the relationship between the developing fetus and mother through the placenta. The small insert provides an overview showing the position of the fetus in the uterus. As the embryo grows, it is surrounded by a fluid-filled sac called the **amnion** that is delineated by the amniotic membrane derived from the trophoblast.

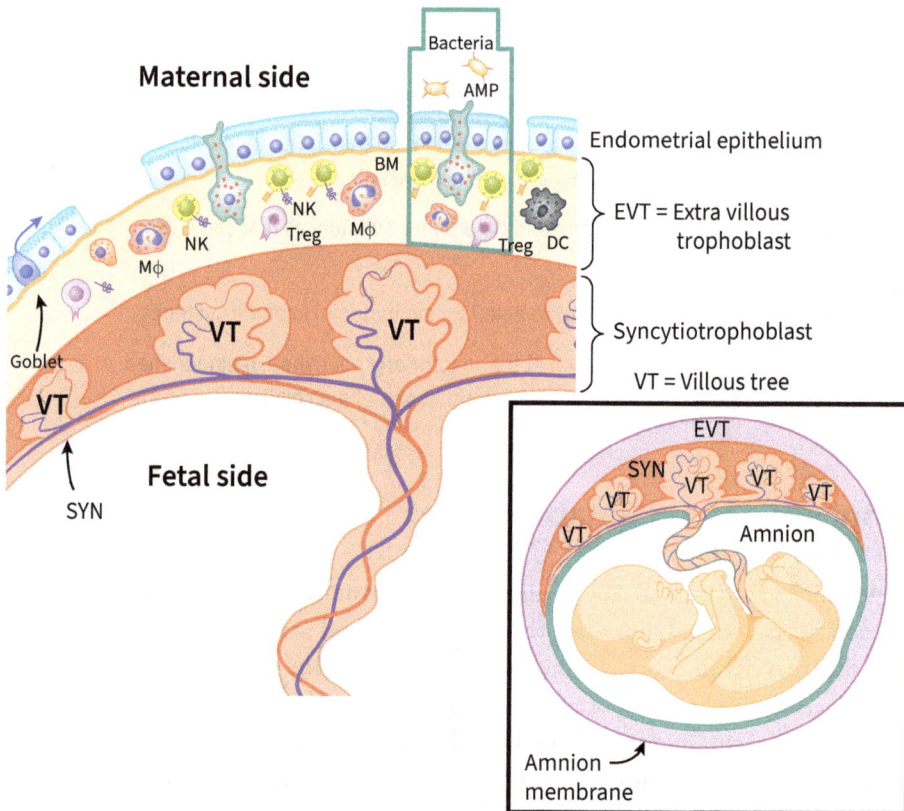

Figure 2.1 The anatomy of the maternal-fetal interface. The lower-right insert provides an overview while the main figure provides specific anatomical details that place emphasis on the development and function of the syncytiotrophoblast (SYN) and villous tree (VT) and their relationship to the extravascular trophoblast (EVT) and to the maternal side of the placenta. A rectangular "cutout" (green border) later becomes the basis for Figure 2.4. The icons used in this and other figures in this chapter are explained in Table 6.1.

Figure 2.1 provides an overview of the placenta and its relationship to the developing fetus and mother. The outer layer of the blastocyst is called the trophoblast; it provides nutrients to the developing embryo and later develops into several placental structures derived from trophoblast. After contact with the blastocyst, the uterine mucosa and maternal arteries in the uterus respond by developing the spiral arteries. Spaces (lacunae) develop within the trophoblast into which maternal blood is directed. Villi from the fetal tissues extend into these spaces. The villi contain capillaries from the fetal circulation. These fetal capillaries exit into larger vessels that lead to the umbilical vein (Figure 2.1). It is across these villi that the transfer of substances between the maternal blood and the fetal capillaries occurs. At no time are the two circulations (fetal and maternal) directly connected, as the maternal spiral arteries and the fetal capillaries keep them separated. As the embryo grows, so does the placenta, becoming a complex organ responsible for the transfer of oxygen and nutrients from mother to fetus and removal of metabolic waste from the fetus. The fetal red cells contain fetal hemoglobin that binds oxygen somewhat tighter than adult hemoglobin thus favoring transfer of oxygen from the maternal to fetal blood spaces. As the embryo grows, it is surrounded by a fluid filled sac called the amnion that is delineated by the amniotic membrane derived from the trophoblast. The fetus is able to swallow amniotic fluid beginning about halfway through pregnancy, exposing the GIT to the amniotic fluid, a rich source of chemokines and cytokines that affect its development. Additionally, the fetal GIT derives a portion of its nutrition from the amniotic fluid. The "water breaking" event known to mothers just before birth occurs when the protective amnion membrane ruptures.

The extravillous trophoblast (EVT) beneath the endometrium contains the spiral arteries and placental veins as well as numerous hematopoietic cells and, in a healthy pregnancy, regulatory T cells (Tregs) and natural killer (NK) cells (Figure 2.1). As with all epithelia, microvilli, tight junctions, and dendritic cells are present. Later in this chapter we will describe changes that can occur in unhealthy (dysbiotic) pregnancies and will expand on the cross-sectional insert of Figure 2.1 in doing so.

Nutrient Supply, Fetal Growth, and Postnatal Outcomes

During a healthy pregnancy, the fetus acquires all essential nutrients via the placenta, and thus a functional intestinal mucosa is not necessary *in utero* and does not develop (Figure 2.2A). Growth of the fetus is intrinsically regulated by the fetus. The maternal GI tract produces nutrients that enter the mother's bloodstream and are subsequently transferred via the placenta to the fetus. These nutrients include amino acids for protein building, lipids, minerals, carbohydrates, and vitamins. Nutrients are needed for both growth and maintenance of the infant's body, but during fetal development, most are used for growth. Glucose provided by the mother is the major source of energy. If the mother has diabetes mellitus, an oversupply of glucose to the fetus forces it to convert glucose to fat and to accumulate it in adipose tissue. Maternal glucose is transferred to the fetus, but insulin is not. Thus, the infant responds to the influx of glucose by producing insulin that drives fat accumulation.

Figure 2.2 The intestinal mucosa of the newborn.

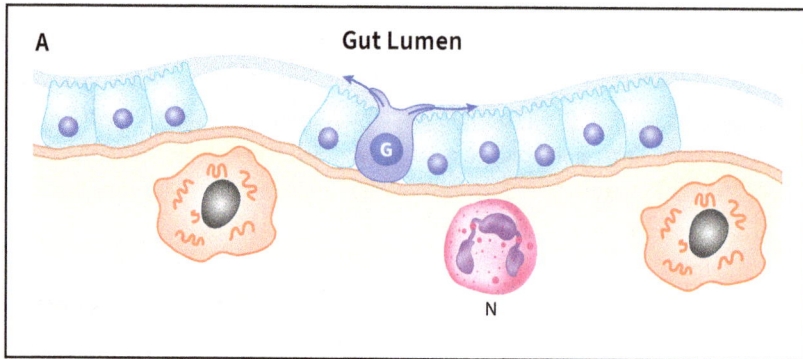

Figure 2.2A The fetal gut mucosa lacks development of villi but contains mucus-secreting Goblet (G) cells and dendritic cells (Figure 2.2B).

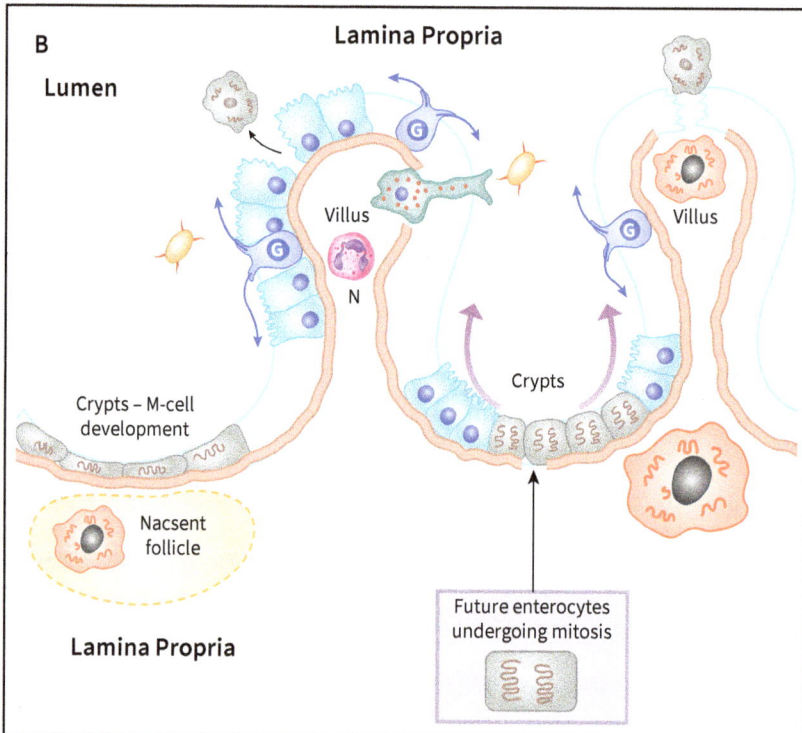

Figure 2.2B Development of the GI tract mucosa after initial encounter with nutrients and commensal bacteria. This is followed by convolution of the mucosal epithelium, which display "fingerlike" protrusions (villi) and "pockets" called crypts. Villi are maintained by continuous mitotic cell division in the crypts that move up (see arrows) to replace dead cells lost at the apex of the villi. Goblet cells (G) in the villi produce mucus which covers the enterocytes. Dendritic cells span the epithelium and capture bacteria. In the crypts region, some enterocytes are transformed into flattened cells called M cells that overlay follicles that will later develop into Peyer's patches (see Figure 6.6). The icons used for cell types are the same as those used in Figure 2.1.

After delivery, the infant may briefly have dangerous hypoglycemia (low blood glucose), until insulin production decreases. The excess fat resolves in the early months of life. The long-term implications of maternal type 1 diabetes or of gestational diabetes may differ, but these conditions have epidemiologic associations to obesity and metabolic syndrome in the offspring (Dabelea, SR; Clausen, SR).

Maternal intake of some nutrients, such as iron and folic acid, may be suboptimal and could fail to meet the needs of the fetus. To avoid insufficient intake of these nutrients by the mother, they can be provided as prenatal supplements, or more broadly be supplemented in foods, as is the case for folic acid. Outright deficiencies of minerals and vitamins in newborns are exceedingly rare because the fetus is a very effective in "pulling" nutrients from the mother, regardless of the size of the mother's reservoir of these essentials. In the case of healthy mothers (who have generally reasonable nutrition), small changes in the nutritional status of the mother do not change the transfer of nutrients to the fetus. It is known that the diet of the mother during pregnancy influences the maternal microbiome (Chapter 5), which can later influence the neonatal microbiome in a growth-dependent manner (Bardos).

If the mother is severely malnourished, the supply of nutrients to the fetus may be diminished, which is why malnourished mothers tend to have smaller babies. Malnutrition of pregnant women has been associated with alteration of metabolism later in the life of their unborn infants. This effect may have been first noted after epidemic malnutrition occurred late in World War II in the Netherlands. Infants born to the mothers who were malnourished in pregnancy were found to be prone to obesity, adult-onset diabetes, and cardiovascular disease as adults, a result sometimes referred to as fetal programming (Shulz).

Fetal malnutrition can occur even when the mother is well-nourished. The disorder of pregnancy called **preeclampsia** is due to placental malfunction and results in fetal malnutrition in the absence of maternal malnutrition. Preeclampsia is a major cause of pregnancy-related morbidity and mortality, endangering both the mother and baby. It causes maternal high blood pressure and proteinuria, impairs placental function, diminishes the transfer of nutrients to the fetus, and impairs fetal growth. There are several explanations for preeclampsia, including maternal-fetal genetic incompatibility (see the later section on allograft survival).

The Mechanisms of Transfer Across the Placenta
The Placenta: An Avenue From Mother to Fetus

Numerous substances pass from the mother's vascular system and are taken up by fetal capillaries in the villous tree (Figure 2.1) that have no direct connection with the maternal blood supply. Rather, during a healthy pregnancy, all substances must cross endothelial and epithelial barriers that act as filters but are also equipped with specialized molecular transport systems. The simplest border crossing is passive diffusion, but transport of many small molecules depends on their chemical nature. Small compounds with neutral charge, like lidocaine and warfarin, move across the placenta by simple passive diffusion. Lipophilic substances like cortisone and THC (tetrahydrocannabinol) that are small (less than 500Da) and have an affinity for the phospholipid bilayer of cells readily gain passage by dissolving into the lipid of the cell membrane. Many large molecules, like IgG, require energy-driven mechanisms and endocytosis. In addition to substances critical for the health and protection of the fetus, there are deleterious substances such as viral pathogens. In the following sub-sections, we describe the many substances known to cross the placenta and what is known about the mechanisms involved.

Transfer of Passive Antibodies

At birth, the infant's immune system has not yet fully developed **adaptive immune competence** to counter pathogens, so immune protection passively provided *in utero* by the mother is critical for wellness and survival. This includes passive antibodies but also regulatory factors (see below). Much of what has been learned about passive immunity was originally discovered in studies of farm animals and then lab rodents. To help students better understand the value and limitations of animal models, we provide Appendix A-2. Unlike in many farm animals and their close relatives, passive immunity in primates (including humans) depends on IgG antibodies delivered to the fetus *in utero*. In most farm animals, passive antibodies are only delivered postpartum through suckling (Figure 3.5). While there are several classes of antibodies (Table A3.1), only the class IgG is relevant to maternal-fetal transfer in humans. Others (such as immunoglobulin E [IgE], responsible for type I hypersensitivity or allergy) are not normally transported *in utero*, so that the mother's allergies are not passed to her fetus. While IgE is not transported, it is quite likely that small peptides derived from some food allergens are transported. The extreme rarity of food allergy immediately after birth suggests that the complete set of stimuli required to develop the immune response to food-derived peptides is not present *in utero* in most infants. Therefore, the higher incidence of food allergy in formula-fed infants (Chapters 4 and 8) is almost certainly a result of postpartum events.

Active transport of large molecules *in utero* depends on "molecular pumps" in the placenta that can work against a concentration gradient. Beginning in the second trimester of pregnancy, such a "placental pump" moves IgG from maternal blood to fetal blood (Roopenian, SA; Simister). This pump and other similar pumps are dependent on ATP-binding cassettes (ABC), transporters that control the activity of specific receptors and their transcellular movement. The transcellular transport of IgG depends on a membrane receptor structurally related to major histocompatibility complex class I (MHC-I; see Chapter 6 and Appendix A-1). The α-chain of the receptor is unique but the so-called "light chain" is β-microglobulin, the same used to form MHC-I. This receptor is called FcRn because it was originally described in enterocytes of the neonatal rat (Rn) and because it binds the Fc portion of rat IgG (Figure 2.3A; see also IgG structure, Appendix A-3). This receptor system allows neonatal rats to selectively absorb IgG from their mother's milk for 20 days postpartum (Chapter 3; Figure 3.4). The binding of IgG to FcRn occurs in the acidic (ie, 6.5 pH) micro-environment of the gut lumen (Simister). The IgG within acidic vesicles binds to FcRn and these vesicles move across the enterocytes until they encounter a neutral pH at the basal portion of the cell. Here IgG is released and then diffuses across the basement membrane (Figure 2.3A). Trafficking across enterocytes is bidirectional in some cases, which may explain the secretion of ruminant IgG1 into the mammary gland and the bovine GI tract (Figure 2.3B and Appendix A-2).

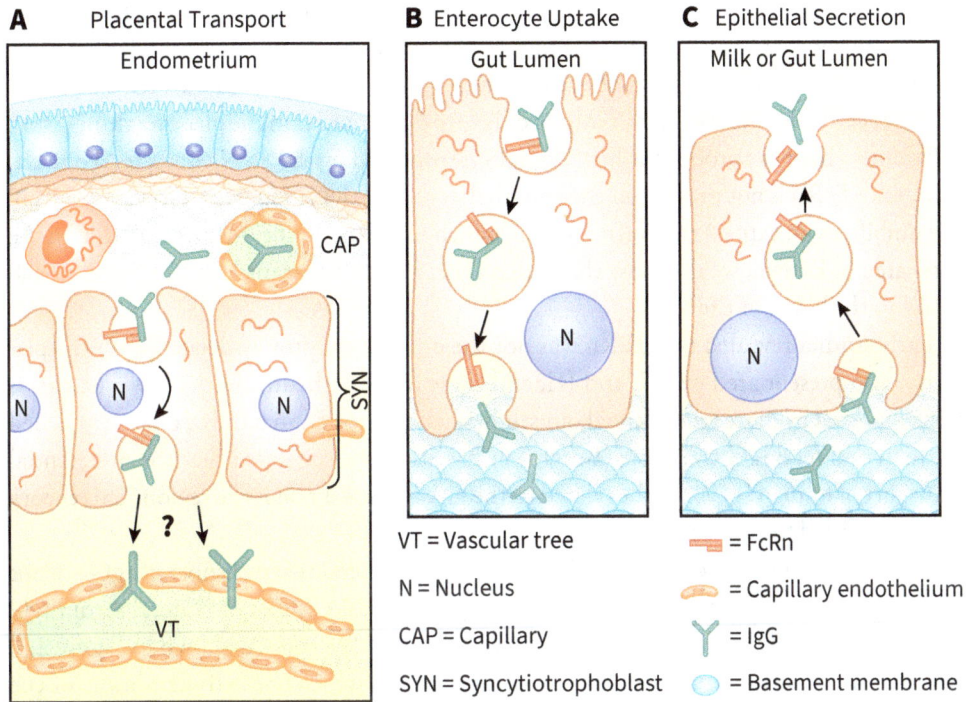

Figure 2.3   FcRn-mediated transport of IgG. (**A**) Transport of maternal IgG across the capillary endothelium is followed by subsequent uptake by FcRn-bearing cells of the syncytiotrophoblast (SYN) and the IgG is finally moved across the capillary endothelia of the fetal villus tree (VT). (**B**) Uptake (absorption) of IgG from the gut lumen of neonatal rats and certain other mammals. FcRn expressed on microvilli or in vacuoles binds IgG under acidic conditions and moves it across the cell for release into the neutral environment of the lamina propria interstitial space. (**C**) IgG present in the lamina propria of the GI tract or in interstitial spaces in the ruminant mammary gland (MG) is recognized by FcRn in vacuoles on the basal portion of the enterocytes or alveolar epithelial cells of the MG. A similar mechanism is presumably involved in moving IgG from blood across the capillary endothelium into interstitial spaces like the lamina propria of the GI tract or the spaces below the alveolar epithelial cells of the MG.

In the human placenta, FcRn is localized to the syncytiotrophoblast (SYN; Figure 2.1). However, moving human IgG from the interstitial space adjacent to the SYN is more complicated since it must first transit from maternal blood across the capillary endothelium. It is known that in mice and cattle IgG can also slip through tight junctions between the endothelial cells, especially during inflammation and edema. In any case, FcRn in healthy capillaries is important for transcellular transport in cattle, mice, and humans. This can partially explain differences in serum half-lives among IgG subclasses (Appendix A-3; Figure 2.1). The preferential endothelial transport of IgG1 in cattle can explain the longer serum half-life of IgG2 in this species (approximately 20 days versus 7 days for IgG1; see Appendix A-2). Overexpressing FcRn in rabbits allows serum IgG levels to dramatically increase since rabbit IgG, like bovine IgG2, is recycled back into blood.

The role of FcRn in the placenta still leaves some issues unresolved. Assuming that human IgG is transported or leaked into the interstitial space, this would not provide the acidic environment that favors binding of FcRn to the Fc portion of IgG. Therefore, the SYN must provide acidified vesicles to allow binding of IgG to FcRn, unless in the placenta things work differently. The next problem is how the IgG transported by the SYN enters fetal circulation, since FcRn is not present on the endothelial cells of the villous tree. However, cells in the umbilicus do express the FcRn α-chain, which may explain the dilemma. While all the facts are not known, we do know that FcRn is needed for the transfer of IgG in maternal blood to the blood of the fetus.

Early studies revealed that FcRn was not the only Fc receptor associated with the placenta; also present are FcγI, II, and III, and these may also be involved. However, this is not supported by more recent knockout studies, which showed that only FcRn was needed for maternal-fetal IgG transport (Borghi). It has also been suggested that the preferential transport of human IgG1 may be related to the glycans present on its Fc region. This theory has so far failed to gain support (Borghi).

While all of the molecular and cellular details of the selective transport of IgG are not known, we know the process is so efficient that, at 33 weeks of gestation, fetal serum IgG level equals that of the mother and then exceeds it after 40 weeks. As shown in Figure 2.3, transfer of IgG also requires endocytosis, a process in which the cell membrane of the transporting cell engulfs extracellular material into apparently acidified intracellular vesicles that are then transported through the cell and released on the opposite pole of the cell in a neutral environment. The control of this endocytosis lies beyond the scope of this textbook. Interested students will need to consult the primary literature.

Transferred IgG antibodies are protective against many pathogens, but they do not provide long-term or permanent protection after birth, as their postpartum concentration in the newborn's blood decreases with a half-life of about 3 weeks. Maternal antibodies are easily detected in the blood of newborns up to 5 months of life or beyond, and this influences the schedule of childhood vaccinations (Chapters 3, 6, and 8). In Chapter 6 we follow the processes leading to the production of protective IgG antibodies to the toxin of *Clostridium tetani*. Mothers who receive the tetanus toxoid vaccine during pregnancy to protect against *C. tetani*, and potentially fetal neonatal tetany, transfer their *C. tetani*-specific IgG antibodies, which decreases the incidence of newborn tetany by more than 75%. Similarly, mothers who have survived bouts with pathogens or who have received vaccines carry a reservoir of IgG antibodies of broad specificities that provide *in utero* and early postnatal protection. Hence, there is strong support for vaccination during or before pregnancy, keeping in mind that transferred IgG antibodies can interfere with the infant's response to early childhood vaccinations (Chu; Fouda). Passive immune protection can also depend on the health of the mother, as IgG transport is known to be impaired in HIV-infected mothers, those suffering from malaria, and those who have had a SARS-CoV-2 infection (Atyeo).

In Table A3.1 we describe four subclasses of human IgG. These differ in their Fc regions and their glycosylation, both of which influence IgG binding to the FcRn transport receptor (Jennewein). Placental transport in humans favors IgG1, which remains in the blood of the newborn longer and thus plays the major role in passive immunity *in utero*. As will be periodically mentioned throughout the book, monoclonal antibodies (mAbs) are now widely used therapeutically, especially in cases of autoimmunity, IBD, and cancer, and sometimes they are used during pregnancy. Transport of these therapeutic antibodies to the fetus appears to depend on how similar the molecules are to native IgG, and whether the Fc portion of these mAbs has been modified (Appendix A-1).

A historical comment regarding the transfer of maternal antibodies is the idiotypic network regulation concept of the 1970s and 80s. The concept rests on the observation that the 3-D structure of the antibody binding site (Appendix A-1) resembles the antigen itself. Thus, it was reasoned that a fetal response to the binding site of a transferred IgG antibody specific to polio becomes a means of immunization. This theory has largely been replaced by the current view that the fetus is unresponsive to any simple protein antigen delivered without a pathogen-associated molecular pattern (PAMP; see Chapter 6). PAMPs are recognized by a family of innate immune receptors on fetal hematopoietic cells. When not in the company of PAMPs, simple proteins, regardless of origin, are not seen as a danger and there is no response. *In utero* there is generally no exposure to PAMPs in healthy fetuses. However, a virus infecting the fetus may display PAMPs and prompt an adaptive immune response (see below and Table 2.1). If such transfer occurs in humans, it could establish some level of tolerance to those bacteria that will later colonize the GI tract after birth. Viruses encountered *in utero* present an additional danger, since in the education of developing T cells these viruses may be considered as "self" and are therefore not seen as "danger" (Chapter 6; Figure 6.5).

One more factor to be considered is whether IgG transferred *in utero* carries with it bacterial components that "piggyback" on and precondition the fetal immune system (Brodin, SR). This may have led some to believe they could explain how the fetus was colonized *in utero* (see Chapter 5).

Transfer of Regulatory Factors

In Chapter 3 we describe 18 cytokines and immunoregulators that can be transported through breast-feeding. Determining if these are transported *in utero* is technically challenging since radioactive tracers cannot be justified for such a purpose. Growth-promoting factors like glycan from natural killer (NK) cells located at the placental maternal-fetal interface appear to be transported to the fetus in humans and mice. Impairment of these NK cells in mice restricts fetal growth (Dogra). There is also evidence that preadipocyte factor is transported, but it seems unconnected to fetal growth.

TABLE 2.1   Congenital Fetal Infections in Humans

Infection	Organism	In Pregnant Mothers	In Fetuses of Infected Mothers[a]
CMV	Cytomegalovirus	1–3%	30–40%
Toxoplasmosis	Protozoan	Variable[b]	5–15%
Syphilis	Spirochete bacteria	Low	35%[b]
Rubella	Toga virus	Low	50–90%
Varicella	Herpes virus	Low	1%
Listeriosis	Intracellular bacteria	Low	>1%
Zika	Flavivirus	Variable[b]	10%
Herpes simplex	Herpes virus	Low	5%
Parvovirus B19	Parvovirus	Variable	30%

a/ Difficult to access, since most aborted fetuses are not tested for infection.
b/ Values are for developed countries, and values are lower in the Middle East, Africa, and in Indigenous populations in Australia and South America.

Cytokines are molecules that communicate between cells such as TNF-α, one of a group of pro-inflammatory cytokines that are important in innate immunity (Table 6.3). TNF release is triggered by infection and other events that cause inflammation, such as bee stings, poison ivy, tick bites, and open wounds. It is known that in the case of an infected mother, the levels of TNF-α and other pro-inflammatory cytokines rise in the blood of the fetus (Assadi). Whether the increase in the fetus is due to transfer from the mother or to production of cytokines by the placenta has not been firmly established, although evidence favors the latter, that is, that these cytokines are locally produced by the placenta and cells associated with it. This may be the case in preeclampsia, which causes mortality in newborns and their mothers (see later).

Other regulatory factors that are transferred include glucocorticoids that affect a broad spectrum of neuropsychiatric, metabolic, and cardiovascular functions. Their lipophilic nature helps in their transport. Transfer of the maternal glucocorticoids may have both negative and positive effects. From the negative point of view, maternal cortisol levels rise during stress and this stress factor is then transported to the fetus. Transfer of stress hormones may be another opportunity for fetal programming and a risk for postnatal neuropsychiatric and other disorders (Rakers). Psychosocial stress and low-level social support are associated with elevated levels of glucocorticoids as well as pro-inflammatory cytokines in the fetus. On the other hand, some level of cortisol is necessary for fetal development; if a deficiency of cortisol in the fetus occurs, cortisol can be supplied to the mother, as in the case of hypothalamic-pituitary-adrenal axis syndrome. Catecholamines such as epinephrine and norepinephrine can also affect fetal immune, metabolic, and neurologic function, but evidence that these are transferred to the fetus in significant amounts is not convincing.

Cellular Trafficking

The placental barrier blocks most cell traffic between mother and fetus in both directions. However, the placental barrier does not entirely restrict passage of fetal blood cells to the mother's circulation. A few fetal cells may enter the maternal circulation, especially near the end of some pregnancies, or during labor and delivery. An adverse result of such passage can occur if fetal red blood cells (RBCs) entering the maternal circulation are recognized as foreign, producing the disorder **hemolytic disease of the newborn** (see later). Some lymphocytes may pass from the fetus to the maternal circulation, an event which usually has no known effect. Evidence supporting this comes from mothers who have borne male children and have low numbers of circulating lymphocytes with a male (XY) genotype. While these transferred lymphocytes are usually of no known importance, this is not true in the uncommon severe combined immunodeficiency disorder (SCID; Chapter 6). Infants with this disorder lack T or B cells, and in a few cases they have experienced attacks (graft versus host disease) from the maternal lymphocytes that recognize the infant as non-self.

Transfer of Pathogens and Congenital Infections

At least eight pathogens are known to breech the human placental barrier, giving rise to congenital (present-at-birth) infections (Table 2.1). The majority are RNA viruses (ie, those that use their genomic RNA as a template for the translation and synthesis of proteins). As indicated, the frequency of new infections in pregnant women is low in developed countries. However, when infection does occur, the probability of transmission to the fetus is very high.

The outcome for fetuses infected with viral pathogens *in utero* can be severe, resulting in impaired neurological development, including microcephaly, a condition widely reported in the press in the case of the Zika virus. Zika is a flavivirus for which vaccines are still in clinical trials. The presence of infection of the fetus can be determined by using molecular biological methods such as the polymerase chain reaction (see Appendix A-1) to demonstrate the viral genome in the amniotic fluid. Sampling of the amniotic fluid is a minimally invasive procedure with a low probability of inducing abortion. Severe cases of fetal infection may be the basis for pregnancy termination.

Two long-studied examples of congenital infection are rubella (German measles) and cytomegalovirus (CMV). Rubella is a mild childhood illness associated with fever and rash first described in the 18th century by German physicians, thus its common name in English. However, if the virus infects the fetus during the first trimester of pregnancy, it can lead to a constellation of malformations, often called congenital rubella syndrome. Up to 80–90% of affected infants will have defects in hearing, eyesight, or cardiac development. The viral effects on the central nervous system (CNS), as with other congenital viral diseases such as Zika, can lead to microcephaly. Rubella is the leading vaccine-preventable cause of birth defects. Because of its devastating effect, the WHO is engaged in a global campaign to eliminate the disease using the measles, mumps, rubella (MMR) vaccine. In 102 countries, vaccination has reduced congenital rubella by 97%, which speaks volumes for the effectiveness of the vaccines. Despite such evidence, vaccine resistance is common in some areas of the world and among some groups. We discuss the issue of **vaccine hesitancy** in Chapter 8.

CMV is the most common congenital infection and can cause severe damage to the developing CNS (Table 2.1). In the United States, 0.5–1% of newborns are CMV-positive. This is in the same frequency range as trisomy 21 (Down syndrome) at 1.2%, and higher than cystic fibrosis at 0.3 % but only half the frequency of congenital heart malformation. Yearly, more than 20,000 infants in the United States are CMV-positive, but the number can exceed 250,000 in India. About 5% of CMV-infected infants will manifest disease at birth and approximately 15% of those infected will later develop disease symptoms. Hearing impairment is most common; it is estimated that 25% of all hearing defects in children can be attributed to CMV.

The nature of the virus explains why CMV is so often a problem for newborns. CMV is a member of the herpes virus family, the group of DNA viruses that includes the causes of oral and genital herpes (herpes simplex 1 and 2, respectively), chicken pox (varicella virus), and mononucleosis (Epstein-Barr virus). These viruses can become latent in at least one tissue of the body after a primary infection. The result can be recurring episodes of illness, as in recurrent herpetic cold sores (usually from herpes simplex 1), shingles from reactivation of varicella virus, or severe, multi-organ CMV disease complicating untreated HIV infection. In the United States, about 40–50% of women of reproductive age have had a prior CMV infection. Women who have a **primary** CMV infection while pregnant are at greatest risk of fetal infection; above 30% of their infants will be infected, and of these 10–15% will have symptoms. Women with **recurrent** CMV infection transmit the virus to the fetus at about a 1% rate, and less than 10% of these infants will have symptoms (National CMV Foundation, SR). The situation with CMV differs from rubella in that maternal immunity is no guarantee against transmission of the virus to the fetus. In parts of Asia, Africa, and South America, greater than 80% of child-bearing women have immunity to CMV, but congenital CMV infection rates are similar to those in areas with lower rates of maternal immunity to CMV (Manicklal).

There is no convincing evidence that SARS-CoV-2 is transmitted *in utero*. However, there is evidence that infection of the mother can interfere with placental transport of IgG and that children born to infected mothers are more vulnerable to other diseases than infants of noninfected mothers (Atyeo). A recent study showed that compared to the maternal-fetal transfer of IgG antibodies to influenza A and pertussis, the transfer of antibodies to the SARS-CoV-2 spike protein is significantly compromised during the third semester of pregnancy. The rapidly evolving knowledge on immunity to SARS-CoV-2 is covered in more detail in Appendix A-4. The current availability of COVID-19 vaccines raises the question of whether they or other vaccines can be safely used in pregnant women since these women were not specifically targeted in Phase 1–3 vaccine trials (Chapter 7). Some COVID-19 vaccines are composed of mRNA encoding the viral spike protein (Appendix A-1). Even if transmitted to the fetus, this mRNA cannot produce fetal infection with SARS-CoV-2. However, the transfer of the mRNA vaccine could allow the fetus to make the spike protein, which could theoretically trigger fetal immune tolerance proteins expressed by the fetus (ie, self-proteins, which can induce central immune tolerance; see Chapter 6; Figure 6.5). Nevertheless, the risk of not vaccinating pregnant women outweighs the theoretical risk of doing so (Esposito); however, this assessment might change as the virus changes and infection rates change.

A few other bacteria are particularly concerning to obstetric clinicians, as they can affect the placenta and fetus, presumably by spread from maternal blood: *Salmonella typhosa*, *Vibrio fetus*, and *Listeria monocytogenes*. The result of these infections can be spontaneous abortion.

Not all infections of the fetus are due to viruses or prokaryote bacteria. A major cause of pregnancy complications in equatorial regions is malaria, caused by several species of *Plasmodium*, a eukaryotic, obligate parasite that infects red blood cells. Some infants of infected mothers will also be infected prenatally, and may begin to have the cyclic illness, fever, and hemolysis that characterize malarial disease. Especially in sub-Saharan Africa where malaria is endemic, more than 1 million pregnancies annually occur in women with malaria (World Health Organization). Toxoplasmosis, also caused by a protozoan parasite, is discussed later.

The protective immune status of women planning a pregnancy should be determined by appropriate serological tests. As noted above, lack of maternal immunity can be corrected by immunization, though it is advised that pregnancy should be avoided for 4 weeks after recent vaccinations for rubella or varicella live virus vaccines. Pregnant mothers known to be infected can be treated with antiviral drugs like ganciclovir and acyclovir or, in the case of syphilis, with antibiotics.

The means by which pathogens pass from mother to child *in utero*, also called *vertical transmission*, is unclear. Figure 2.1 illustrates the cellular interface between mother and fetus that is a major barrier to almost all bacterial pathogens (with the exceptions described in Table 2.1). Several of the major pathogens that may pass vertically are sometimes referred to with the mnemonic TORCH (**T**oxoplasmosis, **O**ther, **R**ubella, **C**ytomegalovirus, and **H**erpes). *Toxoplasma gondii* is a protozoan parasite. The "others" in this mnemonic include syphilis (*Treponema pallidum*) and an organism responsible for some foodborne illnesses (*Listeria monocytogenes*), both of which are bacterial organisms that can potentially infect the fetus. Some suggest that because of the selective transport of IgG across the placenta, an infected mother could transport viral particles on virus-specific IgG (Figure 2.3). Others suggest that viruses might "grow their way across" the placenta by successively infecting one cell layer after another. This theory has support since virus transmission occurs in ruminant mammals that have a so-called seven-layered placenta that does not transport IgG antibodies (Appendix A-2). Along these same lines, RNA viruses like Zika are believed to replicate in the SYN or the extravillous trophoblast (Figure 2.1), which some believe is the "Achilles' heel" of the placenta. Of course, any damage to the placenta, such as collateral damage from an inflammatory immune response, could lead to the loss of integrity and compromise its barrier function. Appropriate precautions can reduce the risk of these infections to the fetus.

Placental Changes Associated With Infectious Disease

Maternal infections, whether or not they are transmitted to the fetus, can damage the placenta, which may also be damaged for other reasons; this can result in an unhealthy or dysbiotic placenta. The cross-sectional insert in Figure 2.1 has been expanded in Figure 2.4, which shows, in side-by-side illustrations, some of the features of an unhealthy placenta.

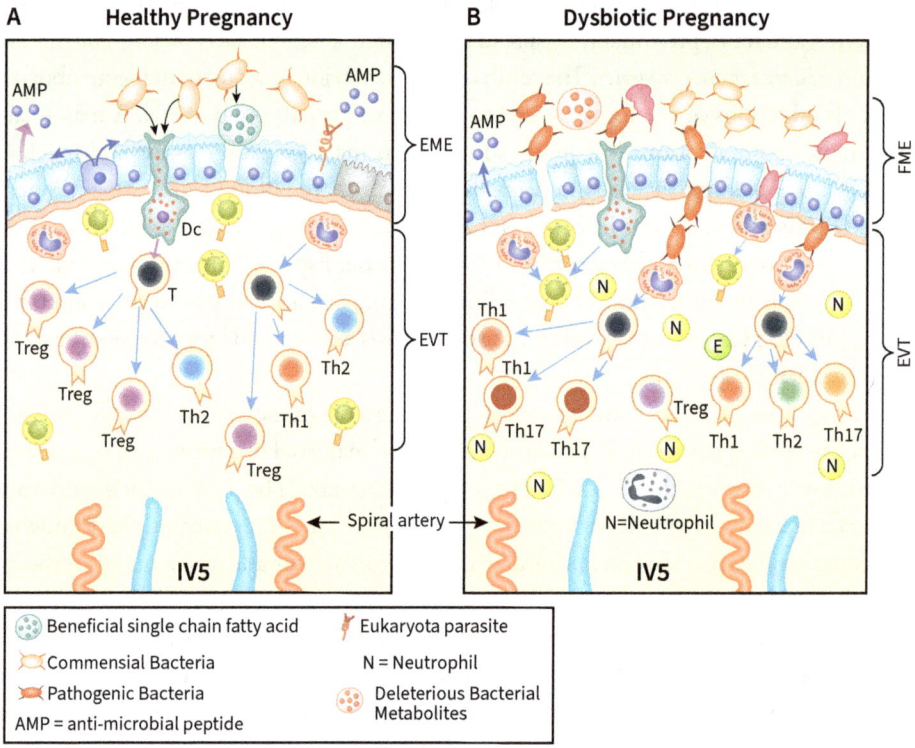

Figure 2.4   The healthy (left) and unhealthy (right) maternal-fetal interface. The micro-anatomical region depicted here was "cut" from the large placental model illustrated in Figure 2.1. (A) The cellular constituency of the extravillous trophoblast (EVT) region (see Figure 2.1) and the endometrium (EME) in a healthy pregnancy. This illustrates predominance of NK and Tregs cells in the healthy pregnancy. The abundance of NK cells (called uterine NK cells [uNK] by some) are believed to play a major role in preventing rejection of the fetal hemi-allograft (see text). (B) During an unhealthy pregnancy, DCs and macrophages present to uncommitted T cells (black nucleus), causing their differentiation into inflammatory Th1 and Th17 cells rather than Tregs. The inflammation is accompanied by an influx of neutrophils and, in parasitic infections, eosinophils. The action of these cells can potentially damage the placenta and result in abortion. Although not shown, the EME and SYN lack expression of MHC, so the histoincompatability of the fetal hemi-allograft is not easily detected by the mother, thus preventing fetal rejection. T cell subsets, their activities, and their icons are discussed in Table 6.1.

Figure 2.4A illustrates the extravillous trophoblast (EVT) region and shows that it is dominated by Tregs and NK cells that are presented antigens derived from commensal organisms, which in turn are believed to support the differentiation of Tregs and the expansion of NK cells. The epithelium of the healthy endometrium secretes antimicrobial peptides (AMP) and various useful short chain fatty acids (SCFA) produced by healthy commensal bacteria (Chapter 5). These help to maintain healthy tight junctions between the epithelial cells.

When pathogens or parasites are encountered by the mother and reach the endometrium or enter the EVT, healthy SCFA may be replaced by less healthy ones made by pathogens (Figure 2.4B). Loss of tight junction integrity allows pathogens to enter the EVT, where they are processed by APCs (macrophages and DCs) that present to uncommitted T cells and results in their differentiation to Th1 and Th17 inflammatory cells, typically accompanied by an increase in neutrophils. These changes reduce the proportion of protective Tregs and NK cells in the region. We shall discuss this further in the section on allograft survival.

Transfer of Drugs and Other Substances
Prescription Pharmaceuticals
A wake-up call for the medical community came from the drug thalidomide, which was marketed in 1958 in West Germany as a sedative or hypnotic and claimed to relieve "anxiety, insomnia, gastritis, and tension." Thalidomide was widely used, including by pregnant women, and was available over the counter (without prescription) in Germany from around 1960. Within a few years it was noted that about 6,000 infants in Germany had been born with a rare condition known as phocomelia. Phocomelia is marked by maldevelopment or absence of the limbs, which may be present only as small stumps. Other effects included deformation of the eyes, heart, or alimentary tract, and blindness and deafness. The epidemic of phocomelia was traced to the use of thalidomide. Throughout Europe and other countries where the drug was licensed, thousands more infants with phocomelia were seen, of which only 50% survived. The tragic malformations caused by thalidomide were a warning to the medical community of the risks of drug usage during pregnancy. The number of cases seen in the United States was much lower, as the drug was never licensed here, and mothers who obtained it had usually been in Europe when it was consumed. Recognition of fetal abnormalities due to thalidomide demonstrated that medicine needed a broader effort in teratology, the study of congenital abnormalities and malformations (from the ancient Greek *teras*, "monster" + *logia*, "study"). Academic and governmental investigators were also prompted to further investigate substances that could induce such abnormalities, correspondingly titled "teratogens."

Since humans cannot be used as experimental animals, much of what has been learned about the fetal transfer of prescription drugs and antibiotics comes from the use of animal models, from *in vitro* organ and tissue culture systems, and from examination of fetal tissues after birth. One method for measuring transfer has been to analyze fetal hair, which develops in the last 3 to 4 months of pregnancy. Nearly all antibiotics cross the placenta. Some, like ampicillin and methicillin, freely cross, while many others are more restricted, such as gentamicin and vancomycin. Several expert organizations maintain tabulations of antibiotics and other drugs and their transfer potential and safe dosage in pregnant women.

Immunosuppressive Drugs

These represent a special category of prescriptions that are now commonly used. These are not limited to small molecular agents but now include certain mAbs used widely for treatment of autoimmune diseases. The development and rationale for mAbs therapy is described in Appendix A-1. Most current mAbs have a human IgG framework and are likely to be actively moved from maternal to fetal circulation, just as with a mother's own IgG. Thus, their use in pregnancy raises concerns about the effect on the fetus. This transfer may be absent when modified mAbs are used such as certolizumab, which lacks the Fc portion of IgG that binds to FcRn in the placenta. Certolizumab is used to treat several autoimmune diseases including inflammatory bowel disorders (IBD). It recognizes TNF-α and suppresses its activity. Since TNF-α is a part of the innate immune defense system of the fetus, it is preferable that it not be suppressed in the fetus by anti-TNF mAbs given to the mother. However, another commonly used mAb, adalimumab, is an unmodified IgG that also blocks TNF-α; it is clearly transported by the placenta and the newborns of mothers treated with it have slightly higher blood levels of the drug than their mothers. There is inconclusive data as to whether it has adverse fetal effects, reflecting the near absence of ethical ways of investigating drug teratogenicity in humans (see Chapter 7 for issues on clinical research design).

Smoking, Alcohol, Dietary Supplements, and Nonprescription Drugs

While pharmaceuticals are tested prior to their use in humans, there is little or no regulation of herbal products sold in health food stores. Pregnant women can also be exposed to other categories of "drugs." For example, 16% of pregnant women are smokers, 10% drink alcohol, and 5% use illegal narcotics. Among the drugs recoverable from newborns are nicotine and its metabolite cotinine in infants of smokers, and methamphetamine, cannabinoids, cocaine, fentanyl, ketamine, and opiates in infants of illegal drug users. In one study of 3,000 babies born to users of illegal drugs, 44% tested positive for some drug, with methamphetamine being most common (Anderson). A correlation between autism spectrum disorder (ASD) and maternal use of alcohol and cocaine in pregnancy has been reported. There is considerable literature on the impact of these products on the developing fetus. Behavioral and neurologic signs are seen with several drugs (Vargish). Narcotic withdrawal symptoms can occur in babies of opiate-using mothers. Learning disabilities, depression, and other behavioral symptoms have been associated with babies of illegal drug users. Some of the strongest evidence links prenatal cocaine exposure to central nervous system abnormalities. The degree of impairment varies greatly and may depend on the mother's usage as well as the infant's genetic susceptibility.

Babies born to smokers have been reported to be more excitable, to experience CNS stress, and to have retarded learning and lower IQs. The mean birth weight of babies born to smoking mothers is diminished by 200 grams and the frequency of low birth weight is nearly doubled. Smoking increases the likelihood of malformations, shortens the duration of pregnancy, and increases the risk of chronic involuntary movement disorder and attention deficit disorder. Maternal smoking has also been linked to an increased likelihood of obesity later in life.

Alcohol ingested by the mother readily reaches the fetus. Small amounts of alcohol are probably safe, but since a "safe" level of consumption is not known, total abstinence is recommended during pregnancy. This recommendation is made by experts across the globe but may contradict traditional folk practices such as the German *Frauenbier* that has low levels of alcohol. Fetal exposure to alcohol can cause permanent damage (fetal alcohol syndrome). In its most severe form, fetal alcohol syndrome is manifested by small head size, hearing and vision problems, learning disabilities and mental retardation. Behavioral difficulties and some decrease in IQ are the most commonly associated symptoms. It is difficult to distinguish the direct impact of alcohol on the developing fetus from the social factors possibly present in the households of women who have elevated alcohol intake while pregnant. Other exposures with adverse impacts are often also present in these households, such as smoking, illegal drug use, and lifestyles and eating habits that may affect the child before and after birth.

Delta-9-Tetrahydrocannabinol (THC)

Marijuana usage is widespread in the United States and many other countries. In the United States usage has been legalized (or at least decriminalized) in many states and it is sold in retail establishments as medical marijuana. Medical marijuana has been a popular remedy in the treatment of chronic pain and epilepsy. Studies since the 1970s have consistently confirmed the *in utero* transfer of cannabinoids (Wu). THC and other cannabinoids can be recovered from the muscle tissues of human users. While THC may have short- or long-term problems, convincing data supporting the latter in human newborns is still lacking, although some *in vitro* studies indicate it may adversely affect trophoblast-endometrium crosstalk. Concern for human fetal effects is extrapolated from studies in rodents that show THC affects normal gonad development in males, apparently acting on the hypothalamus-pituitary-gonadal axis. Rodent studies also suggest that THC alters aspects of nervous system development that can modify respiration (resulting in apnea) and produce altered social behavior of the offspring (Vargish). Too little information is currently available from human studies to identify negative effects. In the next chapter we shall review the transfer of THC by nursing mothers who are regular users, in which we conclude that THC transferred in breast milk has minimal consequences for the suckling neonate.

Other Environmental Teratogens

Potential teratogens (for example, some pesticides) are transplacentally transferred and have been linked to perinatal mortality and intrauterine growth retardation in animal models. Some pesticides have been banned, but environmental residues may persist. Some hypothesize that such agents that are the product of developed, industrialized, or so-called chemical societies play a role in IBD, allergy, and ASD. The widespread use of pesticides and herbicides in modern societies raises the question of whether such chemicals in maternal blood are transported to the fetus. One of the organochlorine pesticides (OCP) is dichlorodiphenyl trichloroethane (DDT), which more than 60 years ago prompted Rachel Carlson to write *Silent Spring* to describe the catastrophic effects of DDT on birds like eagles and robins, and many other species (Yin). Concern over these effects and over probable human carcinogenicity led to the ban of DDT in the United States and most of the world. The WHO now supports the use of DDT only for indoor mosquito control in regions of sub-Saharan Africa where the risk of malaria is judged to outweigh the potential human risk of exposure. OCP, neonicotinoids, polychlorinated biphenyls (PCBs), and DDT can all be transmitted to the fetus (Table 2.2). OCP, PCBs, and DDT are currently banned worldwide but neonicotinoids are not. While current information on OCP effects on the fetus is limited to animal studies, studies in India of the OCP pesticides aldrin and dieldrin show that they are also transferred to the fetus and are associated with adverse effects on reproduction. What Table 2.2 reveals is how little we know about the effects of the substances that are transferred *in utero* on the health of the fetus and the offspring.

TABLE 2.2   Cytokines, Metabolic Regulators, and Environmental Agents Transferred In Utero

Category	Transfer	Comments
Cytokines		
TNF-α	+	Fetal origin[a]
CSF	?	In rodents
GPF (growth-promoting factor)	+	Growth promoter (mice)
Pref-1 (preadipocyte factor)	+	No fetal effect
IL-1b	+	Fetal origin[a]
IL-6	+	Fetal origin[a]
Metabolic Regulators		
Catecholamines	+	
Glucocorticoids	+	
Glucose	+	Normal, but excessive with maternal diabetes
Drugs and Narcotics		
Antibiotics	+	Most all forms[b]
Lidocaine	+	UD[d]
Warfarin	+	Hemolysis and UD[d]
THC	+	Neurological effects in rodents

TABLE 2.2   Cytokines, Metabolic Regulators, and Environmental Agents Transferred In Utero *(Continued)*

Category	Transfer	Comments
Cortisone	+	Could be of fetal origin[a]
Nicotine	+	CNS problems, retardation
Methamphetamine	+	
Cocaine	+	CNS abnormalities
Fentanyl	+	
Ketamine	+	
Alcohol	+	Fetal teratologies
Environmental Agents[d]		
Organochlorines (OCP)	+	
Neonicotinoids (NN)	+	
Polychlorinated biphenyls (PCBs)	+	
Dichlorodiphenyl trichloroethane (DDT)	+	
Hexachlorocyclohexanes (HCH)	+	
Aldrin and dieldrin	+	Reproductive failure
Arsenic (dimethylarsenic acid)	+	
Lead (Pb)	+	CNS damage in neonates
Mercury (Hg)	+	

a/ In humans, radiolabeled tracers cannot be used, so that cytokines found in cord blood (CB) could be of fetal origin.
b/ Follow safe dose recommendations of obstetricians and pediatrician.
c/ Data based on correlations between levels in CB and maternal blood (MB).
d/ UD = undefined in some or all cases.

Mercury, lead, and arsenic are well-known examples of environmental pollutants. As many as 50% of eagles dying of human-related causes succumb to the first two. In developed countries, the human fetus acquires only small amounts of arsenic and lead, as these agents are tightly regulated. However, lead readily crosses the placenta and, depending on the resultant exposure, can theoretically do significant damage to the CNS of the fetus. We know that childhood lead poisoning was a significant problem in the 1950s and 1960s, but it has become less common since lead has been removed from paint and gasoline and the use of lead pipes was discontinued. There is substantial evidence of damage to neonates and young children if the mother's drinking water contains elevated levels of lead. Exposure of the mother to lead in the workplace could be toxic to her fetus but is unlikely where regulation prevents high exposure. The impact on the fetus of low levels of maternal lead exposure is unclear (see American College of Obstetricians and Gynecologists in References).

Allograft Incompatibility and Other Consequences of Pregnancy

The Miracle of Fetal Survival

As a consequence of sexual reproduction, a topic mentioned in Chapter 1 and detailed in Appendix A-1, the human fetus will not be genetically identical to either parent, so the mother carries the fetus as an **organ allograft**, technically as a "hemi-allograft" since the fetus obtains half of its genes from its mother. *Allo* means genetically different while *auto* means genetically identical. A graft from child to parent would normally be rejected like any other genetically incompatible allograft. Given that the fetus and mother are not a perfect match the fetus should in theory be rejected like any other allograft or hemi-allograft. Discrimination of self and non-self depends on many factors, but in humans it largely depends on cell surface markers encoded by genes in the **major histocompatibility locus** (MHC; Chapter 6 and Appendix A-1). As most readers are aware, the successful transplantation of organs from one individual to another depends on finding an acceptable MHC match. However, the uterus belongs to a category of **immune-privileged sites**; within the uterus the mother recognizes the fetus as "temporary self" (Trowsdale, SR). An early hypothesis used to explain why the immune system does not reject the fetus was that the maternal immune system is systemically suppressed during pregnancy. This argument was used to explain why pregnant women were more severely affected by influenzas, hepatitis B, and herpes simplex and why pregnant mothers had lower resistance to cancer.

More recent studies suggest the concept of maternal immune suppression is incorrect, and that other mechanisms prevent rejection of the fetal allograft. First, during a healthy pregnancy, NK cells and immunosuppressive T cells dominate and antagonize the action of pro-inflammatory T cells and their cytokines, the actions of which can cause collateral damage that would damage the placenta (Table 6.3). Amniotic fluid contains a number of chemokines that are involved in trafficking of T cells, dendritic cells (DC), and NK cells (Table 6.1). The later comprise approximately 70% of leucocytes in a healthy pregnancy (Figure 2.4). An imbalance of these cells and other factors may be associated with fetal rejection (Figure 2.4B; Maymon). Second, macrophages and SYN cells of fetal origin (Figure 2.1) secrete cytokines, especially TGFβ at about 22 weeks, that favor the development of regulatory T cells (Tregs) that suppress the action of cells producing pro-inflammatory cytokines (Figure 2.4A; Altman). Loss of Tregs in mice results in failed implantation (Saito; Dogra). Second, at the same time, the mother downregulates inflammatory lymphocytes at the placental interface that would normally respond vigorously to the cells of an incompatible allotransplant, and replaces them with Tregs. While the exact role of NK cells, perhaps a special category called uterine NK cells (nNKs) remains unknown, knockout studies in mice (see Appendix A-1 for the meaning of knockout) indicate that their absence leads to abortion. Third, the fetal membranes of the placenta express very few of the MHC-encoded markers, making the maternal-fetal interface relatively "invisible" to the mother's immune surveillance system. Despite these actions, this "protective system" may break down in cases of bacterial infections that breech the barrier provided by the cervix, reproductive tract mucosa, and endometrium, resulting in release of pro-inflammatory cytokines that can damage the placental barrier (Figure 2.4B). The maternal decidua and EVT (Figure 2.1) are associated with many DCs that regulate the differentiation of other leukocytes that play a role in recruitment of NK cells, key elements of the innate immune system (Figure 2.4A; Chapter 6; Juretic). There is strong evidence that these NK cells (perhaps nNK cells) are required for the initial development of the maternal-fetal interface and a successful pregnancy. It appears that these NK cells use nanotubules to inject granulysin into the bacterial cell membrane, which clears the area of bacteria without damaging the trophoblast. By doing so, the NK cells at the interface greatly reduce the chance for infection, such as by *Listeria*, which would set off an inflammatory response and prevent successful implantation or lead to abortion. In several clinical situations discussed below, it is likely that the mechanisms that prevent immune attack on the fetal tissues are not adequate in all situations.

Complications That Threaten Hemi-Allograft Survival
Preeclampsia

As mentioned above, immune mechanisms may underlie the serious pregnancy complication of preeclampsia, which leads to maternal hypertension and placental dysfunction. In the first section of this chapter, we described how the chorionic villous tree develops within the maternal endometrium (Figure 2.1). This event can be associated with maladaptive tolerance between maternal and fetal tissues, resulting in loss of maternal tolerance to paternally derived antigens of the hemi-allograft. Another possibility involves the NK cells that are present at the maternal-fetal interface (Figure 2.3B). These innate immune cells come to the rescue of virus-infected cells that cannot "call for help" when their MHC expression is suppressed due to viral infection (see Chapter 6). Since suppression of MHC is a feature of the maternal-fetal interface, the NK cells may for some reason respond to the lack of expressed MHC as they would to a virus-infected cell and, in this case, attack the trophoblast. This could lead to incomplete development of the spiral arterioles (Figure 2.1), causing their restriction and impairing blood flow. As mentioned earlier, TGFβ from the SYN (Figure 2.1) promotes expansion of Tregs that downregulate inflammatory T cells at the maternal-fetal interface. Preeclampsia may be a consequence of a collective malfunction of these and other events.

Hemolytic Disease of the Newborn

Among the best-known consequences of maternal-fetal genetic incompatibility is **hemolytic disease of the newborn**, also called *erythroblastosis fetalis*. The blood group antigens on the surface of red blood cells (RBCs) are carbohydrate or protein structures that are inherited in simple Mendelian fashion. The blood group antigens determine the compatibility of RBCs between individuals. Successful transfusion of blood depends on matching the blood group antigens of the RBCs of the donor and recipient, so that recipients do not receive RBCs to which they have antibody. The number of blood groups is quite large, as many as 11 families, including the ABO system and the Rh system.

If the mother lacks the paternally inherited RhD protein antigen expressed on fetal RBCs, and the fetal RBCs enter her circulation, she may mount an antibody response to the RhD antigen. This exposure does not occur with every pregnancy but is thought to be an occasional birthing (peripartum) event, likely related to placental separation after delivery. The ensuing antibody production occurs after the infant is born, so that the antibody produced does not harm the infant of the current pregnancy. In subsequent pregnancies, if the mother has produced anti-Rh antibodies, maternal IgG transferred by the placenta beginning in the second trimester of pregnancy will include the anti-Rh IgG and can lead to hemolysis of the fetal RBCs, leading to hemolytic disease of the newborn. This incompatibility can be diagnosed during pregnancy; severely affected fetuses may be transfused *in utero* with red cells that will be tolerated by both mother and fetus. A better solution, and common obstetrical practice, is prevention. If a mother is known to lack the RhD antigen, and her infant's RBCs express it, an injection of pooled human immunoglobulin, selected to have high levels of anti-RhD antibody, is given in the immediate postpartum days. Additionally, Rh negative mothers can be given anti-Rh antibody at about 28 weeks of pregnancy to lower the propensity of their immune response to the possible transmission of some fetal cells to her in the third trimester. This antibody blocks recognition of the fetal Rh and reduces the maternal antibody response drastically. In contrast, significant hemolysis due to maternal antibodies to ABO blood group antigens on fetal RBCs is seldom seen. ABOs are carbohydrate antigens for which humans inherently produce antibodies of the IgM class; IgM class immunoglobulin does not cross the placenta, thus ABO differences between mother and baby do not generally cause hemolysis. This hemolytic disorder again demonstrates the complex nature of fetal survival in the face of potential maternal hemi-allograft rejection, the success of which has allowed approximately 200 million years of mammalian evolution.

Other Factors Affecting Fetal Health and Survival

In clinical medicine, poor fetal growth may be labelled **intrauterine growth restriction** (IGR), a common complication of pregnancy. There are many possible causes, including umbilical artery thrombosis, chronic vascular disease of the mother, and conditions such as maternal diabetes. Another factor that could lead to complications is an inflammatory response in the endometrium (Figure 2.1) caused by responses to pathogens that enter the microbiome. IGR also has non-immune precipitants; it has been linked to smoking and the use of opiates, alcohol, and cocaine. In each of these situations, there is transmission of these metabolites to the fetus (Table 2.2).

Non-Infectious Diseases in the Fetus, Newborn, and Child
Genetic-Based Congenital Disease

Pathogen-related congenital diseases can result in malformation or death of the fetus, while others that threaten survival and health have a genetic basis. Among these are **phenylketonuria** (PKU), galactosemia, and glycogen storage disorders. There are numerous other less common genetic disorders. Signs of these disorders appear very early in infancy and require prompt detection and the institution of lifelong treatment to minimize impairments. Some forms of ASD also appear to have genetic components.

Phenylketonuria

PKU is a defect in the metabolism of the amino acid phenylalanine, which accumulates in the form of the metabolite phenylketonuric acid that can be measured in blood and urine (hence the name of the condition). Untreated PKU leads to intellectual disability, seizures, behavioral problems, and mental disorders. The treatment is reduction (near elimination) of phenylalanine from the diet from early infancy. This is accomplished by feeding phenylalanine-free formula in addition to breast-feeding, if desired (Chapter 4). The diet must be instituted soon after birth (hence the need for newborn screening) and continued in some form for life. The fetus is protected from the effect of PKU *in utero*, as the accumulation of amino acid metabolites is reduced by transfer to the maternal circulation. As in other inborn errors of metabolism, the health of the infant is not threatened until after birth.

Galactosemia

Galactosemia involves the inability to metabolize galactose produced by the intestinal breakdown of lactose into glucose and galactose. Intestinal lactase cleaves lactose, but in those with galactosemia, galactose cannot be normally metabolized, so galactose conjugates accumulate in tissues. Since lactose is a main source of energy for infants from breast milk or cow's milk (Chapter 3), the treatment requires feeding with formula in which lactose is replaced by carbohydrates that do not contain galactose (eg, glucose polymers and/or sucrose; Chapter 4). Untreated infants may become very ill within days of birth; thus, tests for galactosemia are part of newborn screening. With a galactose-free diet, infants are not at immediate risk. As with PKU, the infant *in utero* remains "well" because of maternal metabolic compensation, and because the infant is not exposed to lactose. Exposure begins with milk or formula feeding (Rubio-Gozalbo).

Glycogen Storage Disease

Glycogen storage disease is an umbrella term for a group of disorders of glycogen metabolism. There are six types of glycogen storage disease, all resulting from defects in the ability to split glucose from glycogen (a polymer of glucose). These defects often result in the accumulation of excess glycogen in the liver and muscle tissue. Usually, these disorders become a concern in early life, as the inability to mobilize glucose from glycogen stores in the liver impairs maintenance of normal blood glucose levels between meals and necessitates measures to prevent dangerous hypoglycemia (low blood glucose). In distinction to many genetic metabolic disorders, one form of glycogen storage disease (type IV) may cause accumulation of glycogen prenatally, in the fetus. A few other rare but related disorders have been reported to be damaging to the fetus (Vianey-Saban).

Autism Spectrum Disorder

ASD, including Asperger syndrome on the milder end of the spectrum, affects an estimated 22 million people worldwide and is thought to affect about 1.5% of children in the United States. ASD is about 4 times more common in boys than girls (CDC). The reported prevalence has increased since the 1980s, perhaps because of changes in diagnostic definitions that expanded the spectrum to a broad range of intellectual and social disabilities, rather than restricting the diagnosis to certain profound disabilities described in the 1940s. ASD results in alteration of cognitive development and language use that creates problems in socialization. Affected children learn differently than others and attend to and react to visual and aural stimuli differently. A range of 60–80% of autistic individuals have poor muscle tone and motor skills. Some are gifted in some intellectual domains but have difficulty with social skills and interactions.

ASD is a group of syndromes of poorly understood etiology. In some cases, strong but heterogeneous genetic bases have been reported. These include single gene mutations, copy number variations, and/or the combined effect of many minor allelic changes. When a genetic basis is suspected/detected, about 30% of cases are *de novo* (not present in the parents) and may reflect abnormalities occurring during mitosis in sperm cells (Lafourche). Copy number variations have the effect of providing "variable gene dosage," resulting in heterogeneous outcomes. Genes associated with ASD are expressed during brain development in mid and late gestation. Events in uterine life have also been implicated in the disorder. For example, there is evidence that *in utero* infection with rubella or exposure to thalidomide or valproic acid (a seizure medication) may also cause ASD (Halsey). Collectively these observations indicate that ASD is largely an *in utero* genetic malady. As we discuss in Chapter 8, this would rule out most postpartum influences such as childhood vaccination as the basis for ASD (CDC). However, there is growing evidence that postpartum events are involved, such as the establishment of a healthy microbiome (see Chapter5).

Changes in the GI Tract at Birth

Prior to birth, a completely functional GI tract is not needed and therefore its absorptive capacity is little used. The fetus receives nutrition from the passage of maternal nutrients to the fetal blood via the placenta (see "Nutrient Supply, Fetal Growth, and Postnatal Outcomes"). In the fetal GI tract via the cells (enterocytes) that line the lumen, the fetus also obtains metabolites and nutrients from the swallowed amniotic fluid. After birth the GI tract must rapidly begin to both digest and absorb nutrients. The digestive and absorptive ability is immature in preterm infants because these functions have not had time to develop. In the very premature infant, enterocyte numbers are low, and villi are short or absent (Figure 2.2A). Birth is normally accompanied by (1) colonization of the gut and skin by bacteria, (2) exposure to major nutrients in breast milk or formula, and (3) exposure to various growth factors in colostrum and milk such as colony-stimulating factor, epithelial growth factor, and insulin-like growth factor (Chapter 3 and Chapter 6, Table 6.3). As we discuss in Chapter 5, there is controversial evidence that bacteria are present in the fetal gut as early as the second trimester that are not the result of exposure to the extrauterine world. When colonizing bacteria and colostrum-derived factors arrive, they collectively promote rapid mitosis of enterocyte precursors in the crypts and consequently the growth and lengthening of the villi (Figure 2.2B). These changes are accompanied by the later immigration of leucocytes of various types, some later becoming lymphoid follicles called Peyer's patches (Chapter 5).

Changes in the Immune System at Birth

The protective nature of intrauterine life also changes at birth. The amnion and placenta provide a protective barrier that limits the passage of substances or organisms that can be dangerous to the fetus. After birth, these physical barriers no longer shield the infant from harm. Protection will now depend heavily on the **adaptive immune system**; a system evolved for discrimination of self/non-self (Chapter 6). This system requires exposure to PAMP to become active and protective; thus, it offers little protection immediately after birth. In the period immediately after birth, much protection depends on the **innate immune system** and passive maternal antibody transferred to the fetus in the third trimester (Figure 1.1 and Chapter 6).

Lymphocytes that can discriminate between self and non-self begin to develop *in utero*. During the first trimester lymphocyte development begins in the fetal liver but moves to the bone marrow and the thymus; both of which are referred to as **primary lymphoid tissues**. As development continues, thymus-derived lymphocytes (T cells) and bone-marrow-derived lymphocytes (B cells) emerge from these organs after "learning to be tolerant to self." The fetal thymus is most important in the establishment of central **immunological tolerance** (Chapter 6, Figure 6.5). This educational process is needed to prevent the fledgling immune system from attacking tissues of the developing fetus (ie, attacking "self"). Maternal antibodies and regulatory factors crossing the placenta will be understood as "self" because exposure occurs when the developing immune system learns to become tolerant to antigens. Exposure at birth to bacteria, viruses, or other microbes that signal "danger" by their display of PAMPs allows for the development after birth of a fully competent adaptive immune system.

Summary

Placental nurturance of the next generation puts the embryo and fetus in a more protected environment than nonplacental embryos in an externally deposited egg. The success of this mode of nurture of the embryo has been the result of a multitude of adaptations of hormonal, immunologic, behavioral, and basic cellular systems. The fetus is not completely shut off from the world, however, and may be perturbed by several infectious or toxic agents, by adverse genetic inheritance, and by misadventures of the maternal immune system.

Suggested Readings (SR)

Al-Nasiry S, Maymon E, Romers R, et al. The interplay between reproductive tract microbiota and immunological system in human reproduction. *Front Immunol*. 2020;11:378. doi:10.3389/fimmu 2020.00378.

American Pregnancy Association. Cytomegalovirus (CMV) infection. www.americanpregnancy.org/healthy-pregnancy/pregnancy-complications/cytomegalovirus-infection/.

Brodin P. Immune-microbe interactions in early life: A determinant of health and disease long term. *Science*. 2022;376:945–950.

Clausen TD, Mathiesen ER, Hansen T, et al. Overweight and the metabolic syndrome in adult offspring of women with diet-treated gestational diabetes mellitus or type 1diabetes. *J Clin Endocrinol Metab*. 2009;94:2464–2470.

Dabelea D, Hanson RL, Lindsay RS, et al. Intrauterine exposure to diabetes conveys risks for type 2 diabetes and obesity: A study of discordant sibships. *Diabetes*. 2000;49(12):2208–2211.

National CMV Foundation. CMV & pregnancy. www.nationalcmv.org/overview/cmv-pregnancy.

Roopenian, DC, Akilesh S. FcRn: The neonatal Fc receptor comes of age. *Nat Rev Immunol*. 2007;7(9):715–725.

Trowsdale J, Betz AG. Mother's little helpers: Mechanisms of maternal-fetal tolerance. *Nat Immunol*. 2006;7(3):241–316.

References

Altman D.J, Schneider SL, Thompson DA, Cheng HL, Tomasi TB. A transforming growth factor beta 2 (TGF-beta 2)-like immune suppressive factor in amniotic fluid and localization of TGF-beta 2 in RNA in the pregnant uterus. *J Exp Med*. 1990;172(5):1391–1401.

American College of Obstetricians and Gynecologists. Lead screening during pregnancy and lactation. Committee opinion no. 533. https://www.acog.org/clinical/clinical-guidance/committee-opinion/articles/2012/08/lead-screening-during-pregnancy-and-lactation.

Anderson M, Choonara I. Drug misuse during pregnancy and fetal toxicity. *Arch Dis Child Fetal Neonatal Ed*. 2007;92:332–335.

Assadi F. Neonatal nephrotic syndrome associated with placental transmission of pro-inflammatory cytokines. *Pediatr Nephrol*. 2011;26:469–471.

Atyeo C, Pullen KM, Bordl EA, et al. Compromised SARS-Cov-2-specific placental antibody transfer. *Cell*. 2021;184: 628–642.

Ayatollahi M, Geramizadek B, Samsami A. Transforming growth factor beta-1 influence on fetal allografts during pregnancy. *Transplant Proc*. 2005;37:4603–4604.

Bardos J, Forentino D, Longman RE, Paidas M. Immunological role of the maternal uterine microbiome in pregnancy: Pregnancies, pathologies and altered microbiome. *Front in Immunol*. 2020;10:2823. doi:10.3389/fimmu.2019.02823.

Borghi S, Bournazos S, Thulin NK, et al. FcRn, but not FcγRs, drive maternal-fetal transplacental transport of human IgG antibodies. *Proc Natl Acad Sci*. 2020;117:12943–12951.

Cavazza T, Takeda Y, Politi AZ, et al. Parental genome unification is highly error-prone in mammalian embryos. *Cell*. 2021;184:2860–2877.

Centers for Disease Control (CDC). About autism spectrum disorder. https://www.cdc.gov/autism/about/.

Chu HY, Englund JA. Maternal immunization. *Clin Inf Dis*. 2014;59:560–568.

Dogra P, Farber DL. Stealth-killing NK cells for tolerance and tissue homeostasis. *Cell*. 2020;182:1074–1076.

Esposito S, Bosis S, Morlacchi L, Braggi E, Sabatini C, Principi N. Can infants be protected by means of maternal vaccination? *Clin Microbial Infect*. 2012;18(5):85–92.

Fouda GG, Martinez DR, Swamy GK, Permar SR. The impact of IgG transplacental transfer on early life immunity [published ahead of print February 14, 2018]. *ImmunoHorizons*. https://www.ncbi.nlm.nih.gov/pmc/articles/PMC5812294/.

Halsey NA, Hyman SL. Measles-mumps-rubella vaccine and autism spectrum disorder: Report from the New Challenges in Childhood Immunizations Conference convened in Oak Brook, Il. *Pediatrics*. 2001;107:E84. doi:10.1542/peds.107.5.e84.

Hanson LA, Dahlman-Höglund A, Karisson M, et al. Mother-infant interactions during fetal and neonatal life with special reference to atopy. *Ped Pulmonology Suppl*. 1997;16:8–9.

Jennewein MF, Goldfarb I, Dolatshadi S, et al. Fc glycan-mediated regulation of placental antibody transfer. *Cell*. 2019;178:202–215.

Juretic K, Strbo N, Bogovi Crneic T, Laskarin G, Rukavina D. An insight into the dendritic cells at the maternal fetal interface. *Am J Reprod Immunol*. 2004;52:350–355.

Lafourche LM, Muotri AR, Sebat J. Getting to the core of autism. *Cell*. 2019;178:1287–1298.

Manicklal S, Emery VC, Lazzarotto T, Boppana SB, Gupta RK. The "silent" global burden of congenital cytomegalovirus. *Clin Microbiol Rev*. 2013;26(1):86–102. doi:10.1128/CMR.00062-12.

Maymon E, Romero R, Bhalli G, et al. Chronic inflammatory lesions of the placenta are associated with an up-regulation of amniotic fluid CXCR3: A marker of allograft rejection. *J Perinat Med*. 2018;46:123–137.

Rakers F, Rupprecht S, Dreiling M, Bergmeier C, Witte OW, Schwab M. Transfer of maternal psychosocial stress to the fetus [published ahead of print February 22, 2017]. *Neurosci Biobehav Rev*. doi.org/10.1016/j. neubiorev.2017.02.019.

Rubio-Gozalbo ME, Haskovic M, Bosch AM, et al. The natural history of classic galactosemia: Lessons from the GalNet registry. *Orphanet J Rare Dis*. 2019;14:86. doi:10.1186/s13023-019-1047-z.

Saito S, Shima T, Nakashuma A, Inada K, Yostuno O. Role of paternal antigen-specific Treg Cells in successful implantation. *Am J Reprod Immunol*. 2016;75:310–316.

Shulz LC. The Dutch Hunger Winter and the developmental origins of health and disease. *PNAS* 2010;107:16757–16758.

Simister NE. Placental transport of immunoglobulin G. *Vaccine*. 2003;21:3365–3369.

Vargish GA, Pelkey KA, Yuan X, et al. Persistent inhibitory circuit defects and disrupted social behavior following in utero exogenous cannabinoid exposure. *Mol Psychiatry*. 2017;22:56–67.

Vianey-Saban C, Acquaviva C, Cheillan D, et al. Antenatal manifestations of inborn errors of metabolism: Biological diagnosis. *J Inher Metabol Dis*. 2016;39:611–624. doi:10.1007/s10545-016-9947-8.

World Health Organization. World malaria report 2021. December 6, 2021 (Section 3.10). https://www.who.int/teams/global-malaria-programme/reports/world-malaria-report-2021.

Wu F, Jensen TL, Memillin GA. Detection of in utero cannabis exposure in umbilical cord tissue by a sensitive liquid chromatography-tandem mass spectrometric method. *Methods Mol Biol*. 2019;1872:211–222.

Yin S, Zhang J, Guo F, Poma G, Covaci A, Liu W. Transplacental transfer mechanism of organochlorine pesticides: An *in vitro* transcellular study *Environ Intl*. 2020;135:105402. doi:10.1016/j.envint.2019.105402.

CHAPTER 3

The Role of Breast-Feeding in Infant Health

1. Describe the major health benefits of breast-feeding for infants.

2. Describe the major components, macro nutrients, and prebiotics in milk.

3. Discuss mammary gland structure and the physiology of milk production.

4. Discuss the role of the major protective components in human milk.

5. Define the role of passive antibodies and immune regulatory factors in breast milk.

6. Outline how pathogens, drugs, and environmental agents are transferred in breast milk.

Breast-Feeding and Alternatives

The Role of Breast Milk for Newborns

Milk is the defining feature of mammals. When umbilical support comes to an abrupt end at birth, the newborn turns to the mammary gland (MG) for sustenance and internal protection. Birth constitutes a transition from *in utero* nutrition and passive protection to **external nutrition** and initially **internal protection** through passive immunity. In this chapter we emphasize the importance of milk and regulatory factors provided by the mother through nursing. Unlike other exocrine secretions that serve the mother, the secretions of the MG have special significance since they benefit another individual, the suckling neonate. Milk directly nourishes the infant, provides passive immunity against pathogens, and guides the development of the infant's immune system (Butler, 1979).

The Importance of Breast-Feeding

The WHO and UNICEF recommend exclusively breast-feeding for the first 6 months of life, but societal changes in industrialized Western cultures are associated with shifts from breast-feeding to bottle-feeding, either using stored breast milk or formula. Recent studies show that only 25% of children in America meet the World Health Organization's recommendations on breast-feeding. Much evidence supports the value of breast-feeding, including strong evidence for lower incidence of childhood diarrhea, pneumonia, and chronic allergy in breastfed children. In less developed countries, death rates of non-breastfed infants are elevated, presumably due to the higher incidence of pathogens in their environment. The risk of dying of diarrheal diseases for a non-breastfed child in developing countries is 25 times greater than for a breastfed child. In Pakistan, breast-feeding for as little as the first week of life reduces mortality by more than 70%, and in Rwanda, for each additional month of breast-feeding, the infant mortality risk drops by 6.2 per 1,000. There are even claims in developed countries that breast-feeding reduces sudden infant death syndrome and childhood asthma. A recent editorial in the *Lancet* argues that, globally, breast-feeding could prevent over 800,000 child deaths and 20,000 maternal deaths per year; others estimate that 15 million child deaths could have been averted over a 10-year period if breast-feeding was the rule (Victora). If accurate, these observations suggest that exclusive early breast-feeding is very important for the survival and wellness of human offspring.

In pre-industrial societies, breast-feeding is the norm, whether by the infant's own mother or a surrogate nursing mother called a "wet nurse." In the past, if a wet nurse was not available, attempts to nourish the infant involved use of milk from cattle, goats, and related animals. Feeding newborns unmodified milk of other species was associated with high infant mortality, but wet nursing by a healthy woman was more successful. This suggests that fresh or stored animal milk lacks certain ingredients needed for infant health and/or growth. However, animal milk provides a base for the construction of modern formula (see Chapter 4).

Societal and Economic Issues and Breast-Feeding

Credible evidence shows that even under the most favorable circumstances in industrialized countries, only 90% of attempts to breastfeed full-term infants are successful. The reasons for lack of success are multiple and involve both the baby and the mother. One reason why many mothers cut short the duration of breast-feeding is that they must return to work and cannot or prefer not to nurse on the job. In most European countries and Canada new mothers are allowed to stay home for up to a year and even longer. Hence, breast-feeding duration is on average much longer in these countries than in the United States. Other social, behavioral, and societal factors also impact the duration of breast-feeding. For example, smoking mothers are known to breastfeed for shorter periods than nonsmoking mothers, for reasons that remain unknown. The complicated web of social, societal, emotional, and economic pressures that influence the decision to start or stop breast-feeding greatly complicates attempts to discern the relative importance of breast-feeding for infants.

Many cultures rely on folklore regarding foods that a nursing mother should avoid and foods that she should consume. In Germanic countries beverages include a diluted version of beer (*Frauenbier* or *Ammenbier*) for nursing mothers. Most cultures discourage lactating mothers from consuming alcoholic beverages. Consumption of some foods by the mother (eg, cabbage and related vegetables) is discouraged as they are alleged to cause flatulence in the infant, while consumption of certain foods may be promoted. This advice about the maternal diet is often only based on informal observations with a minimum of scientific credibility (see Chapter 8).

Prior to the availability of safe alternatives to breast milk, wet nursing, as noted previously, could be lifesaving for infants whose mothers had died or could not nurse. Attitudes toward wet nursing have varied widely over time and across cultures. In 17th- and 18th-century France, upper-class women frequently placed their infants with wet nurses. Some complained that this was not in the best interest of the infant, but the practice seems to have been common among the wealthy. Abuses occurred, for example, there were reports of wet nurses accepting multiple babies simultaneously, and mostly feeding them crude substitute diets. In some cultures, wet nursing was believed to transfer properties of the wet nurse to the nursling. Even today some cultures consider a special bond to exist between individuals nursed by the same mother, making them equivalent to siblings. While wet nursing is now uncommon, sharing milk through milk banks is common. Milk expressed and stored in milk banks can be very useful in the management of some infants, as in preterm infants. Unregulated sharing or selling of milk by a mother to others is discouraged by groups such as the American Academy of Pediatrics (AAP) because of the possibility of pathogen spread or of unsuspected drug or chemical contaminants.

Breast-Feeding and Later Health

Much evidence supports the value of breast-feeding for the health of the infant in early life and for its positive effects after the nursing period (Brodin, SR). The USDA recently sponsored a review and summary of the literature concerning the effects of breast-feeding during infancy on subsequent health outcomes. The project produced a series of systematic reviews of the scientific evidence for the effects of breast-feeding on health outcomes later in life. The absence of breast-feeding was associated with increased risk of asthma, but the evidence for an increase in the risk of food allergies, allergic rhinitis, and atopic dermatitis was weaker. Evidence for an association between the absence of breast-feeding and an increased risk of celiac disease remains controversial and is largely dependent on case studies. Some evidence indicated an association between the absence of breast-feeding and increased risk of type 1 diabetes. The review found limited evidence that lack of breast-feeding is associated with a slight increase in the risk of childhood leukemia (USDA, SR). All the studies analyzed in this review were observational; thus, the correlations seen may not indicate a causative role of breast-feeding in later outcomes (Chapter 7). In addition to a large set of such reviews, an older systematic review of data from nine studies involving 69,000 participants led to the conclusion that breast-feeding was associated with a small but consistent decrease in obesity in later childhood (Arenz), but the specific mechanisms involved remain unresolved. Collectively, these observations suggest that breast-feeding causes modifications of the infant's metabolism and immune system. Conclusions are confounded by unmeasured factors, issues of study design, and the strength of evidence, as discussed in Chapter 7.

When Breast-Feeding Is Not an Option

Breast-feeding may not be an option due to illness or death of the mother or when the mother receives drugs that may endanger the infant if transferred in her milk. In the 20th century, formulas based on modifications of cow's milk became available and provided nutrition that was largely free of short-term adverse effects, allowing a reasonable alternative to the wet nurse. In many developed countries, less than half of infants are now breastfed. Development, composition, and use of infant formulas is the subject of Chapter 4.

Milk banks and "pumped milk" provide additional options. Mothers who have given birth to preterm infants are initially prevented from breast-feeding because of the infant's inability to suck and swallow milk. However, these mothers can express or mechanically pump their milk, which can then be fed to the infant by appropriate methods that avoid the need to have the infant put to the breast. Because the quantity of milk produced by mothers of preterm infants is often inadequate, milk donated by other mothers may be substituted. For safety reasons, milk donated by another mother is generally pasteurized to avoid the transfer of pathogens, but pasteurization may have other consequences. Many large intensive care nurseries have substantial numbers of preterm babies in need of supplemental breast milk. These nurseries often establish milk banks to collect leftover milk (usually from mothers of full-term infants who produced more milk than their own infants needed). The collected milk is pooled, pasteurized, and stored at −20 °C for up to 1 year. However, pasteurization can lead to the loss of some protective properties of milk (to be discussed later), but it appears that enough substances survive pasteurization that these milks are sufficient to reduce the risk to preterm infants of illnesses such as necrotizing enterocolitis (NEC) and sepsis. Feeding donor breast milk is an important means of ensuring that all preterm infants enjoy at least some level of the protection offered by human milk obtained from the mother's own milk.

A condition that may prevent breast-feeding is **mastitis**, or inflammation/infection of the mammary gland characterized by the accumulation of neutrophils and other inflammatory cells. This condition can lead to breast abscess and sepsis. The incidence of mastitis ranges from 2–33% in lactating mothers (Angelopoulou). Milk stasis can occur when milk is not removed properly and may predispose the MG to mastitis. Stasis can be due to poor attachment of the infant, inadequate suckling, or blockage of ducts. Usual management aims to improve removal of milk from the ducts and maintain nursing if possible.

There are a few medical conditions that may be contraindications to breast-feeding. The breast-feeding statement of the AAP describes a few absolute contraindications to breast-feeding (Johnston, SR). In the rare genetic disorder of congenital lactase deficiency, nursing is prohibited, and lactose-free formula must be used. In this complete lactase deficiency, hydrolysis of nonabsorbable lactose to absorbable galactose and glucose does not occur, resulting in severe osmotic diarrhea. Infants with **galactosemia** cannot normally metabolize the galactose derived from digestion of lactose and become ill on exposure to lactose from milk (or formulas with lactose), because they accumulate galactose and abnormal metabolites. Breast-feeding is also contraindicated if mothers are using opioids (not prescribed), cocaine, or phencyclidine (commonly known as PCP or angel dust). Some mothers with prenatal opioid use can safely breastfeed if the infants are monitored for withdrawal symptoms. Mothers positive for human T cell lymphotropic virus types I or II or with untreated brucellosis should not breastfeed. If the mother has active tuberculosis or has herpes simplex lesions of the chest, she should not breastfeed, but the pumped milk she produces can be fed to the infant. Similarly, mothers who develop varicella (Chapter 6) from 5 days before birth to 2 days after should be temporarily separated from their infants. In this situation also, the mother's pumped milk may be fed to the infant. The issue of breast-feeding by HIV positive mothers is a bit more complicated. In wealthy countries, breast-feeding by the HIV positive mother is discouraged because the risk of HIV transmission from the milk is thought to be too high; however, in areas of low wealth where there is high risk of fatal infectious diseases in infancy, the calculation is reversed, and breast-feeding is encouraged as the infant is more at risk from non-HIV infection if not breastfed. A recent update from AAP discusses this issue and quantifies the risk (Abuogi 2024).

Physiology and Function of the Mammary Gland
The Basic Structure of Milk

Many authors refer to milk as a tissue (as it contains cells and other structures); therefore, it is reasonable to consider the structural components of milk. One way to look at milk "structure" is by observing how milk is "disassembled" by the dairy industry. In a dairy, milk is left to stand (usually under refrigeration) or processed by centrifugation to recover a cream layer, which contains the fat. Since fat is less dense, it floats to the top in storage or is easily separated by centrifugation. Many adults raised on dairy farms may recall sneaking a spoonful of this cream from the milk that had cooled overnight in the milk room. Removing the fat layer results in skimmed milk. Skimmed milk is rich in proteins and carbohydrates and contains a few leukocytes and shed MG epithelial cells. The cells found in milk are discussed in detail in the next section. In the dairy industry, the proteins of skimmed milk are further subdivided into **casein** and **whey**. The casein in milk forms protein micelles that cause cow's milk to appear white. The word *casein* is derived from the Latin for cheese (*caseum*). In the cheese-making industry, and in the stomachs of young ruminant mammals, the milk is acted upon by the enzyme rennin. Rennin causes casein to coagulate into curds that are then processed into various cheeses. The watery, bluish, and protein-rich solution left after the removal of casein and fat is termed **whey**. Whey contains carbohydrates (lactose and oligosaccharides) and many proteins. Casein, whey, and fat are present in all milks, but there is marked interspecies variation in the amounts of these components in different milks (Butler 2015, Table A2.3). In summary, milk is comprised of water, fat, casein, whey, and a few cells. The role and importance of the various proteins and other components is described in the next section.

Anatomy and Physiology of the Mammary Gland

The number and arrangement of MG vary widely among the eutherian mammals, as does the character of the milk that has evolved to best suit the needs of newborns of different mammals (Appendix A-2). The internal structure of the gland and the neural and hormonal control of milk production appears to be consistent across species. Milk arises from alveoli within the breast tissue, and many such alveoli empty into small ductules that converge on a smaller number of lactiferous ducts that join within the nipple to form the lactiferous sinus (Figure 3.2). The individual alveoli and smaller ducts are surrounded by a spider-like net of contractile cells termed *myoepithelial cells*. During pregnancy, prolactin, estrogens, and other hormonal factors induce proliferation and expansion of ducts and alveoli. After parturition, prolactin and oxytocin appear to be critical to maintenance of lactation (Figure 3.1).

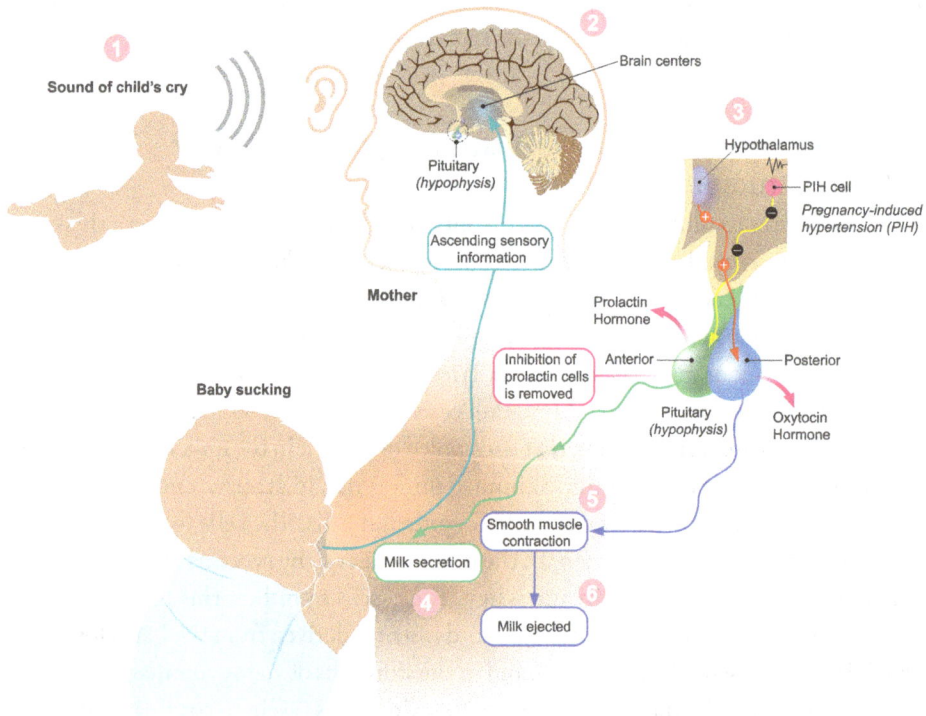

Figure 3.1   The pituitary gland control of milk secretion. The events in pregnancy and their regulation by pituitary hormones, prolactin, and oxytocin.

The alveolar cells of the lactating MG continuously produce milk that accumulates in the ductules. The ability of the infant to access this milk depends on the letdown reflex (sometimes referred to by physiologists as milk ejection). The myoepithelial cells contract in response to oxytocin, and their sensitivity to oxytocin increases markedly after childbirth (Figure 3.1). Skin-to-skin contact of mother and infant and stimulation of the nipple by the newborn induce the release of oxytocin from the pituitary gland; the oxytocin induces contraction of the myoepithelial cells, propelling milk from the alveoli and onward to the lactiferous sinus. The rapidly increasing sensitivity of the myoepithelial cells to oxytocin in the first 48 hours after birth correlates with the time frame in which the mother begins to be aware of milk letdown (Neville; Grattan). When the infant is first put to the breast, the cellular mechanisms to synthesize milk increase in activity and the composition of milk rapidly evolves over the following days. If the infant is not put to the breast, rudimentary MG function remains, but it persists only for a few days. If suckling is initiated and continues, the milk volume increases dramatically over a few days and the milk undergoes profound compositional changes. The details of the changes of milk volume and composition during lactation are covered in the next section.

Skin-to-skin contact soon after birth is beneficial for physiological stability of the infant and breast-feeding initiation. Early skin-to-skin contact facilitates the establishment of an emotional bond that likely increases breast-feeding success. There is evidence that the amount of physical contact may shape breast-feeding behavior and influence the frequency of breast-feeding sessions. Physical contact may also improve the mother's perception of infant signals of hunger.

The alveolar epithelium in the breast is responsible for milk production. Cells in the alveolar epithelium are rich in mitochondria and Golgi bodies consistent with the metabolic functions necessary to assemble and secrete milk components (McManaman, SR). Several pathways exist to secrete the individual components. Exocytosis is the mechanism by which the cells secrete lactose, calcium, phosphate, oligosaccharides, and most proteins into the alveolar fluid. The molecules to be secreted are gathered into vesicles by the Golgi; these vesicles then fuse membranes with the cell's membrane, discharging the contents into the fluid in the lumen of the alveolus.

Lipids are secreted by a very specialized process. Fatty acids are imported into the alveolar cell from maternal circulation. Triglycerides (TG) are then assembled in the endoplasmic reticulum and gathered into protein-coated structures called lipid bodies. The lipid bodies are transported to the cell membrane adjacent to the lumen; there they are secreted by budding off the lipid along with an enclosing envelope of cell membrane and sometimes a bit of cytoplasmic content (Figure 3.2). The secreted structures are called **milk fat globules** (MFG). More information on the MFG and its membrane and potential benefits are discussed in the next major section.

A number of membrane transport pathways exist to move water, ionic salts, and other small molecules from the circulation through the epithelial cells to the milk (transcellular transport). Small molecules and a few macromolecules may also pass between the cells of

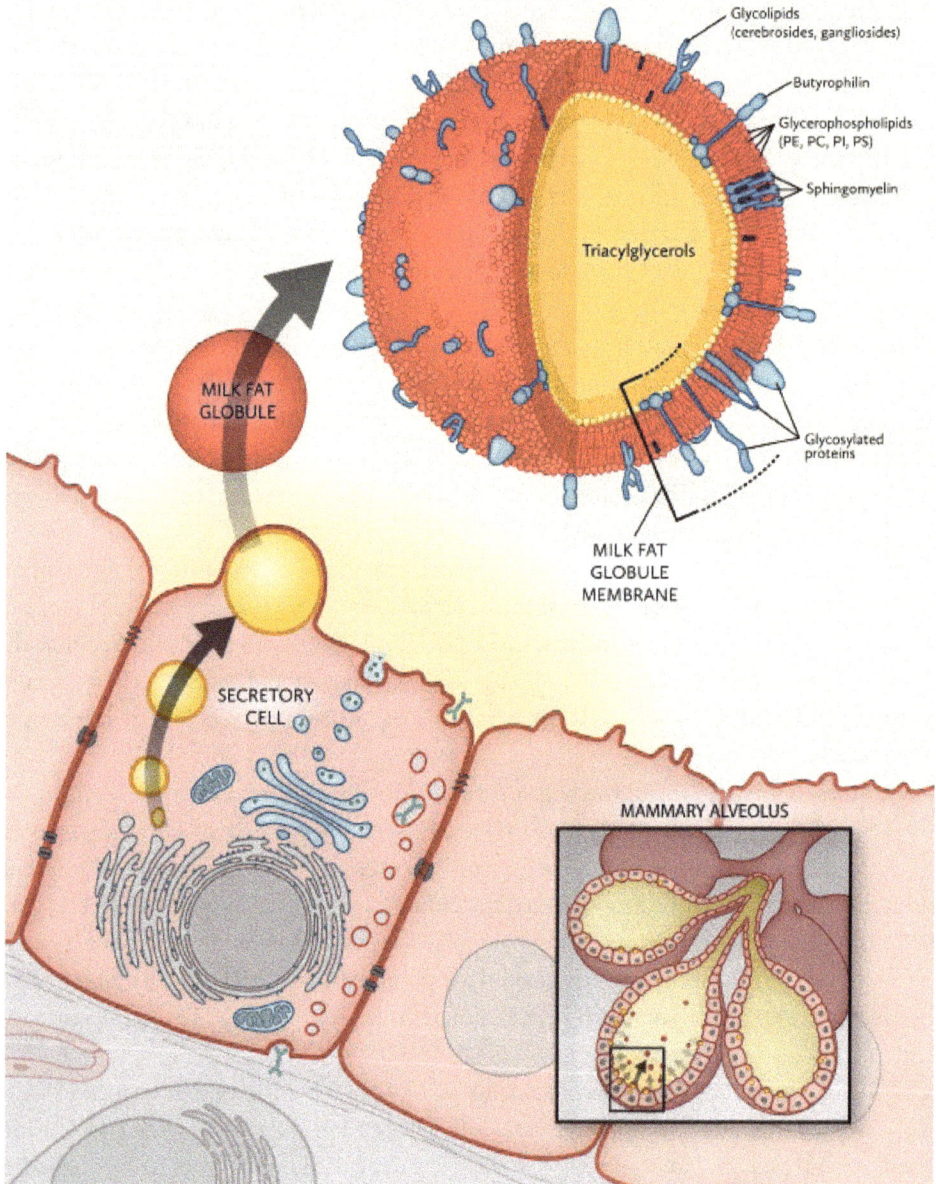

Figure 3.2   The secretion of the MFG and the structure of the MFG membrane.

the alveolar epithelium to enter the alveolar lumen. This sort of movement is called **paracellular** transport. This pathway functions prior to delivery and allows fluid accumulation in the ducts and alveoli in pregnancy, without excretion of much fluid. At delivery the paracellular path is closed by formation of tight junctions between the alveolar cells, so that during lactation only the pathways that are transcellular are active in moving substances into milk.

Proteins and other macromolecules in whey are derived from the blood plasma or secretory cells within the MG. These are taken up by endocytosis at the basal region of the MG epithelial cell, then moved intracellularly to the apical portion of the cell where active transport mechanisms move them into the alveolar lumen of the MG. For example, dimeric IgA is produced locally by plasma cells in the breast tissue, transported into the alveolar cell by endocytosis, and then secreted into the alveolar lumen as SIgA with the help of the polymeric immunoglobin transport receptor (Figure 6.6; Table A3.1).

Specific biochemical pathways in the breast produce the carbohydrates (lactose and human milk oligosaccharides; **HMOs**) found in milk. Lactose is a disaccharide synthesized in the breast by the covalent bonding of the precursors glucose and galactose. Lactose furnishes about half the energy in human milk and is secreted at high levels throughout lactation (Figure 3.3A). In human milk more than in ruminants, enzymatic pathways are strongly expressed that assemble multiple oligosaccharides into HMOs, largely from the precursors lactose, fucose, and sialic acid. The enzymes that promote fucosylation and sialylation of lactose are shared with some blood group antigen pathways (discussed later). Except for proteins drawn from the circulation and interstitial fluids, proteins in milk are assembled in the endoplasmic reticulum of the alveolar epithelial cells by translation of the appropriate mRNA. The triglycerides (TG) in milk are assembled using the same cellular machinery as in other cells and transferred as described earlier.

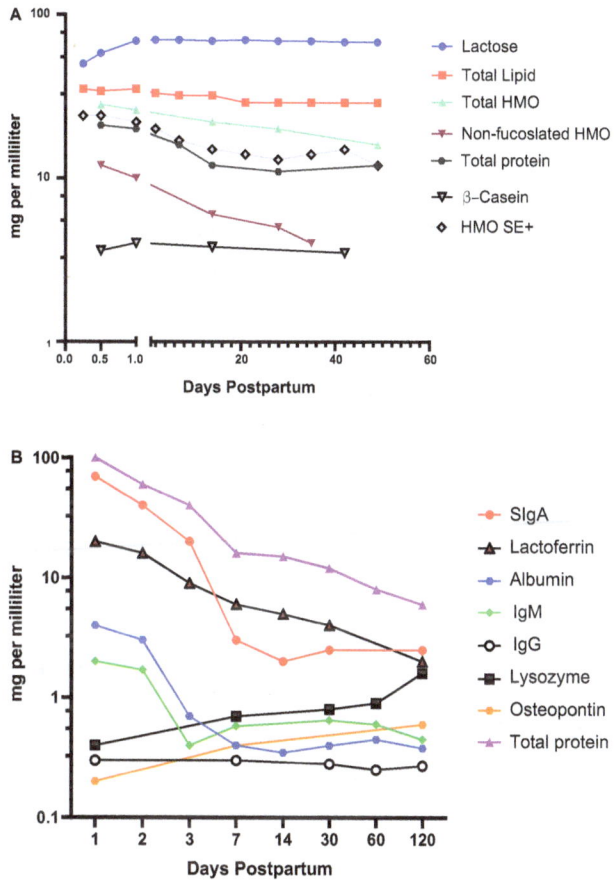

Figure 3.3   Trends and changes in the level of major nutrient (Figure 3.3A) and major proteins (Figure 3.3B) during human lactation. Actual values for SIgA vary from 30–80 mg/ml among individuals but the trend is the same.

Changes in Mammary Gland Function During Lactation

The first milk obtained by suckling was formed before delivery and is called **colostrum**. It is very high in protein, especially due to SIgA antibodies (Figure 3.3B). It appears bluish like whey because of the low level of casein compared to cow's milk (Table 3.1). The quantity produced is low, typically less than 20 ml per session of nursing. Over a few days, the nature of the milk produced rapidly evolves. For example, the amount of lactose synthesized by the breast steeply increases by postpartum day 2 (Fig. 3.3A), which is paralleled by a rapid increase in milk volume (Figure 3.4) and a decrease in the relative concentration of protein largely due to the decrease in SIgA secretion (Figure 3.3B). The milk secreted in the next few days is often called **transition milk**, and after 10 days it is considered **mature milk**. Protein content continues to decrease gradually until it levels out at about 2 months of lactation. Protein in human milk is mainly contributed by the **whey** fraction (~80%), whereas in cow's milk, casein makes up 80% of the protein (Table 4.1). Through the transition period, the energy delivered to the infant increases in line with increasing production (Figure 3.4) and increasing consumption by the infant. Energy is mostly provided by sugar (lactose) and by lipids, each providing about half of the energy (Figure 3.3A). Lactase, the lactose-digesting enzyme, is present in abundance in the infant's gastrointestinal tract, even for individuals who are destined to be lactose intolerant later in life.

As shown in Figures 3.3 and 3.4, both milk composition and volume change rapidly within the first week. In fact, milk composition even changes during the course of each feeding session. The first milk (foremilk) produced in a feeding session is lower in fat content than at

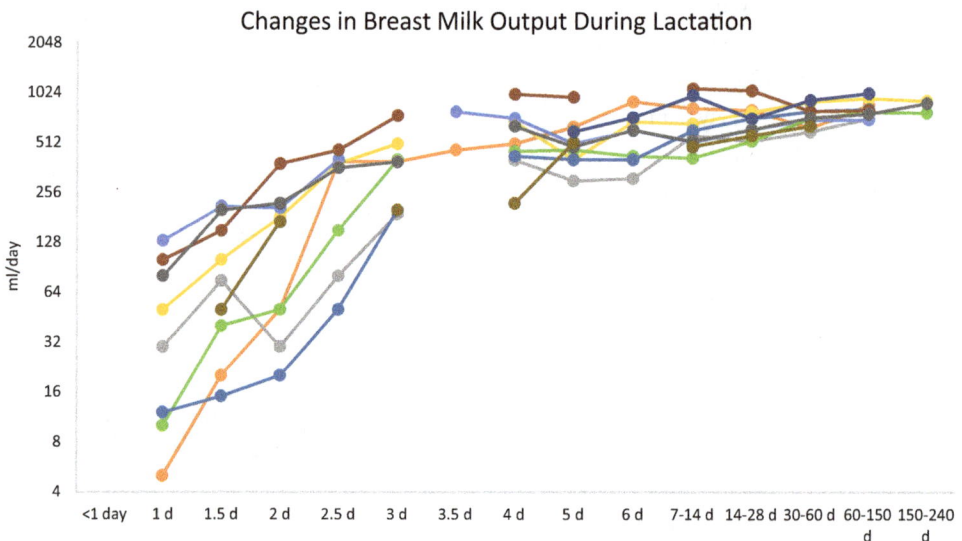

Figure 3.4 Daily output of milk (ml) from a dozen or more lactating mothers from day 1 to day 240 (8 months). The values connected by dots and lines of the same color are for samples collected from the same mother at various times.

TABLE 3.1   Concentration of Proteins and Regulatory Factors in Human Colostrum and Mature Milk

Values represent a consensus from data published by Chatterton et al., Zambruni et al., Vass et al., Dawood and Marshall, and Groer et al. Values for regulatory factors typically cover a broad range that may reflect the assay used or differences among individuals at the time of sampling. Data are presented as mg/ml or ng/ml (*) or pg/ml (**). For comparison, values in red in parentheses are for cow's milk. When credible values are not available for cow's milk, a "+" is used to indicate their presence.

Category	Colostrum	Mature Milk
Whey Protein		
α-lactalbumin	2.6–4 (2.0)	2.3–3.8 (~ 1.2)
β-lactoglobulin	none (14.3)	none (3.4)
Lysozyme	0.27–0.4 (0.14–0.7)	0.2–0.4 (0.07–0.6)
Lactoferrin	3–7 (1.5)	1–2 (> 0.1)
IgA	30–80 (~ 3)	0.6 (~ 3)
IgG	0.5 (50–80)	0.4 (~ 6)
IgM	1.3 (8–12)	0.45 (< 1)
β-defensin 1*	0.15	0.08
β-defensin 2*	0.8	0.2
β-defensin 5*	0.09	0.09
Casein		
αS1-casein	Trace (< 15)	Trace (13.7)
β-casein	2.6–3.8 (< 6)	2.2–4 (6.2)
κ-casein	0.4–1.2 (< 3)	n.d. (3.7)
Cytokines and Growth Factors		
EGF*	2.3–10 (18–320)	20–100 (+)
IGF-1*	29–49	3–6
IGF-2*	10	3.5
IGF-3*	3.5	2–3
CSF*	0.3	0.2 (+)
TGFβ**	300–6,000	> 4,000 (250)
INFγ**	20–700	0.7–170 (+)
IL-1β**	0.7–3	0.3–1.3 (+)
IL-2**	0.15–4	~ 0.1
IL-4**	0.9–170	0.15–600
IL-5**	6–80	6–140
IL-6**	7–80	0.2–150
IL-7**	250	232
IL-8** (CXCL8)	200–2,000	60–200 (+)
IL-10**	3–120	30–200
IL-12**	3–300	30–40 (+)
Chemokines		
MCP-1** (CCL-2)	1,500–3,000	300–700
MIP-1** (CCL-3)	10–300	6–100
RANTES** (CCL-3)	60–150	4–170

the end of the feed (hindmilk). Note that the terms *foremilk* and *hindmilk* as defined earlier are commonly used in the medical lactation community, but among animal physiologists, these terms may refer to milk from mammary glands nearer the head (foremilk) or the tail (hindmilk; see Appendix A-2). Whether the difference in composition during a single nursing session has any physiological effect (eg, induction of satiety) is not firmly known. Milk composition also changes over the course of the day (circadian changes) and can even differ between breasts. These changes are modest and usually smaller than the differences between lactating women. The decrease in protein content as lactation continues (Figure 3.3A and B) is not mimicked by formulas, which instead provide a constant and higher content of protein (see Chapter 4). The greater protein intake of formula-fed infants is believed to explain their more rapid growth. As shown in Table 3.1, the concentration of most regulatory factors decreases during lactation, which may impact events in the developing neonate (see later).

Energy From Milk Drives Infant Growth

The caloric requirement of warm-blooded vertebrates is 10 times greater than that of cold-blooded vertebrates, some of which can go weeks without eating, and may overwinter in a state of torpor, without eating. However, there are also certain mammals that shut down their metabolism and hibernate or go into torpor, greatly reducing their caloric needs (Appendix A-2). The continued high energy requirement of human infants is attributed by some developmental biologists to the rapid growth of the cerebral cortex, which is also disproportionally large in humans compared to many other mammals. In addition to meeting the energy need for growth of the brain and body, nutrition for infants must meet the requirements for maintenance of the body and replace ongoing losses. Due to the rapid growth of infants in early life, the energy required for growth exceeds the need for maintenance. As growth slows after early infancy, this relationship inverts, and the needs for maintenance then exceed the needs for growth. Clinicians monitor infant growth (mass and length) to judge the adequacy of an infant's nutrition (see Figure 8.3). In healthy mothers, breast milk is usually available in amounts that exceed the infant's needs; preterm infants are an exception. Healthy breastfed infants appear to self-regulate their intake to obtain sufficient, but not excessive, energy. In most mammalian species, milk is intended to be, at least temporarily, the sole or main source of nutrients for the suckling neonate and therefore provides all essential nutrients as well as energy in increasing amounts to meet the needs of the growing infant.

After birth several days elapse before the milk produced fully meets the demands of the infant and growth resumes. This is in contradistinction to formula-fed infants, who obtain more food in the first few days and regain birth weight sooner than breastfed infants (Chapter 4). Formula-fed infants may consume somewhat greater volumes than breastfed infants, perhaps because obtaining formula from a bottle requires less effort on the part of the infant than obtaining breast milk from the breast.

Of course, normal development and growth will require the introduction of complementary feeding at some point in infancy. The manner and timing of these feeds have varied greatly among human cultures. Currently most nutritional and medical bodies recommend exclusive breast-feeding for about 6 months. Prior to this age the infant's oral motor skills have not developed sufficiently to allow movement of even soft foods from the front to the back of the mouth for swallowing; and of course, the dentition is not yet sufficient to chew food that is not a puree. The details of complementary feeding are beyond the scope of this text, but those seeking further information might read resources at the WHO website on this topic (reference list as World Health Organization).

Although most infants grow satisfactorily while exclusively breastfed, after complementary feeds are added, in many low-wealth settings the percentage of infants who fail to grow normally rises. This increase in the percentage of children with **growth faltering** reflects the fact that many complementary foods fail to provide sufficient energy and an appropriate distribution of macronutrients. As little as a 5–6% shortfall in daily caloric intake can measurably impair the growth of the child. As noted earlier, WHO resources on the nature of adequate complementary feeding are available.

The Relationship Between Maternal Diet and Milk

One might expect a major influence of the mother's diet on milk composition. In fact, the gross nutrient content of breast milk is controlled by the breast, largely independent of the mother's nutritional status or of her diet, barring extremes of poor nutrition. The diet of the mother only has a minor effect on the composition of her milk and may be limited to the fatty acid distribution of the milk fat without influencing the total amount of fat in her milk. Maternal vitamin C levels may also influence the amount of vitamins in breast milk (Bravi). It seems that flavoring substances in the maternal diet are expressed in breast milk as tastes or aroma. Some intriguing research suggests that infants become acquainted with the mother's diet through flavoring substances and later show a preference, or at least acceptance, of complimentary foods with similar flavors to those encountered in the mother's diet (Spahn). The folklore around the preference for garlicky foods by infants of mother who eat garlic was mentioned in Chapter 2. It appears that spices consumed by the mother, along with various pharmacologic agents (including legal and illicit drugs and caffeine) are transferred. Alcohol from mothers who drink during the nursing period is excreted in milk. Infants are sensitive to low levels of alcohol and the main effect on the infant is the induction of sleep. However, severe effects of alcohol, as exemplified in the prenatal fetal alcohol syndrome, are not observed in breast-feeding infants.

The Role of Individual Milk Components

The Complexity of Milk

There are well over 100 identifiable components in milk. Most have nutritive or protective functions, consistent with the dual roles of milk in **nutrition** and **internal protection**. Some components may be less critical and are simply leftovers shed into the milk; the basis for the description by some that the MG is a "secondary excretory organ" (Butler 2015). Next we detail the role of individual components that have well-defined functions.

Caseins

Caseins, a family of calcium phosphoproteins found in eutherian milks, are the products of three to four genes; αS1-, αS2-, β, and κ. β-casein is the dominant isoform (Table 3.1) with a much lower contribution from κ-casein and αS1-casein. These are heavily glycosylated proteins and may be protective since their carbohydrate moieties serve as decoys for bacterial attachment, and some studies have shown they can reduce the frequency of *H. pylori* (Chapter 5). Within the MG, caseins act as molecular chaperones to prevent protein aggregation such as occurs when misfolded fibrils form amyloids, as happens in cataract formation in the lens of the eye or perhaps in Alzheimer's disease. In this manner, casein performs the same function as heat shock proteins, for readers who may be familiar with that process. Caseins assemble into micelles that appear to have three functions. First, they allow the safe export of calcium phosphate, preventing calcification of the mammary gland ducts. Second, they allow safe secretion of potentially dangerous fibrillogenic complexes. Third, their non-fibrillar structure allows them to be retained in the infant's stomach, allowing longer accessibility to proteases. In short, the casein micelle is a mechanism for supplying the neonate with a high concentration of protein and calcium phosphate without clogging the breast lacteals with fibrils that could otherwise form from high concentrations of proteins. Casein micelles are also the reason milk appears white.

Lactoferrin

Lactoferrin is a 77kD iron-binding glycoprotein that is a member of the transferrin family. It is abundant in human colostrum, at about 6 mg/ml, and decreases to less than 2 mg/ml in mature milk (Table 3.1; Figure 3.3B). By comparison, SIgA, an important protective factor, decreases from more than 30 mg/ml to less than 1 mg/ml over the same period. Their abundance in colostrum suggests that both play their most important roles early in lactation. A homologous protein to lactoferrin is found in the milk of almost all mammals, but in bovine and porcine colostrum and mature milk, concentrations are much lower than in human milk. Interestingly, rat milk lacks lactoferrin and instead uses transferrin as the iron-binding protein. Lactoferrin is quite resistant to intestinal proteases, so it largely arrives intact at its intestinal receptor. Lactoferrin has an extremely high affinity for iron, greater than transferrin. Separately from its iron-binding site, lactoferrin also binds to lysozyme, LPS (lipopolysaccharide), Igs, and DNA. The net positive charge of lactoferrin favors its binding to the LPS in the cell wall of Gram-negative bacteria such as *E. coli* (Chapter 5). This contact directly damages the bacteria and also sequesters iron from them, thus inhibiting their metabolism. A receptor for lactoferrin is found on the brush border of the enterocytes of the GI tract. The receptor facilitates the uptake of lactoferrin-bound iron from milk upon its internalization by the enterocytes. After uptake, intracellular lactoferrin triggers signaling pathways and affects gene transcription through DNA binding. By some mechanism, lactoferrin also affects the neonatal GI tract by increasing crypt depth and villus height in a concentration-dependent manner.

Many studies ascribe a role for lactoferrin in the early development of the newborn GI tract and the neonatal microbiome (Chapter 5). For example, lactoferrin reduces colonization by *Salmonella* and *E. coli* while promoting an increase in *Bifidobacteria* and *Lactobacilli*. Lactoferrin binds negatively charged bacterial membrane components like LPS and lipoteichoic acid, which could explain why it can block bacterial binding to adhesion receptors for pathogenic Proteobacteria. In studies using recombinant lactoferrin, a 1,000-fold decrease in *E. coli* adhesion was observed. Since it binds to LPS, it may also antagonize activation of Toll-like receptors (TLR) and perhaps block inflammatory cascades. As mentioned in earlier chapters, the risk of necrotizing enterocolitis (NEC) is greater in preterm infants reared on formula as compared to breast milk, leading some to believe that lactoferrin may play a role in the reduction of NEC in preterm infants.

α-Lactalbumin and β-Lactoglobulin

Human and bovine milks differ with respect to the presence of α-lactalbumin and β-lactoglobulin. β-lactoglobulin is not present in human milk (Table 3.1) and is therefore foreign to the human immune system; it would be recognized as a "non-self" and can be involved in allergy to cow's milk (see Chapter 8).

The α-lactalbumin in human milk is of ancient evolutionary lineage and has several functions. It binds the metallic ions Ca^{2+}, Mn^{2+}, and Mg^{2+}. Prior to its excretion into the milk, its major role in alveolar cells of the mammary gland is as an essential catalyst with β-1, 4 galactosyl transferase (GT) for the synthesis of milk sugar (lactose):

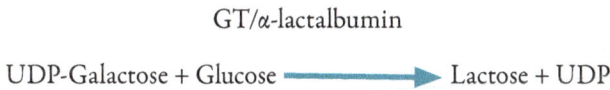

$$GT/\alpha\text{-lactalbumin}$$

$$UDP\text{-Galactose} + Glucose \longrightarrow Lactose + UDP$$

The expression of GT by the MG alveolar epithelial cells is tightly regulated by various hormones, including prolactin. Progesterone has a negative effect while EGF, estrogen, and glucocorticoids have variable effects. Those seeking greater detail are referred to a recent review by Sadovnikora et al. (2021).

Lysozyme and Defensins

Lysozyme is a prominent protective factor in milk that is noted for its ability to attack bacterial membranes. It lyses sugars in the peptidoglycans that constitute the cell walls of Gram-positive bacteria but may also be involved in intracellular destruction of Gram-negative bacteria. Lysozyme occurs at high levels in neutrophils. Serum lysozyme is considered an acute phase reactant and an indicator of inflammation and infection when present at less than 1 mg/ml. Milk levels are less than 200 ug/ml and remain constant throughout lactation (Figure 3.3B; Table 3.1). In addition to lysozyme, colostrum and milk contain a number of antimicrobial peptides. These include multiple members of the β-defensin family (Table 3.1). Defensins are small peptides made by alveolar epithelial cells of the breast and enterocytes of the GI tract. Defensins intercalate into bacterial membranes, causing bacteriolysis. In human milk, defensin levels remain relatively constant throughout lactation, resembling the pattern of lysozyme but at lower concentrations. This suggests they provide sustained protection for the MG and the infant.

Antibodies and Immunoregulatory Factors

Breast milk transmits passive antibodies, growth factors, cytokines, and chemokines that influence the development of important systems in the neonate. The role of these components is discussed in the section on "Passive Immunity and the Mammary Gland."

Milk Fat and Milk Fat Globules (MFG)

Milk fat levels vary greatly among mammals, but the majority of fats in all species are tri-acylglycerol (TG) that are built around a 3-carbon glycerol backbone with 3 ester-linked fatty acids. In addition to the TGs, the globule contains phospholipids, sphingolipids, and many cellular proteins including enzymes. Milk fat content is very high in bears, dolphins, elephants, seals, whales, and reindeer compared to humans and ruminant mammals. Milk fat content differs among dairy breeds due to selection by animal breeders for high-volume milk production (see Appendix A-2). Fat is a concentrated energy source and also a carrier for lipid-soluble molecules such as vitamins A, D, E, and K, plus LDL cholesterol, fatty acids, and various hydrophobic flavor compounds. Figure 3.3A shows that the level of total fat increases when lactation begins and thereafter remains constant. Milk TGs are primarily a mixture of saturated, monounsaturated, and polyunsaturated fatty acids. Cholesterol and phospholipids comprise less than 10% of the total lipids. The TG makeup is partially reflective of the mother's diet but is also influenced by the makeup of the maternal adipose tissue. As described above, milk fat is secreted from the alveolar epithelial cells of the MG as a milk fat globule (MFG) surrounded by a membrane, the MFG membrane (MFGM), that is derived in part from the plasma membrane (Figure 3.2). The MFGM contributes 1–4% of the total protein in mature milk (Figure 3.3A) and therefore contributes to milk's overall energy (Kcal/kg). MFGs remain stable in the stomach after ingestion but the associated membranes are gradually degraded by pepsin and other proteases in the intestine. The value of the MFGM for the infant is suggested by clinical trials of MFGM supplements in infant formulas that have reported reduction of bloody diarrhea and otitis media in addition to other benefits. Their use as supplements in infant formula is discussed in the next chapter.

The MFGM is very complex; it contains mostly glycophospholipids, sphingolipids, and glycosphingolipids but about 120 proteins are also present or associated with it (Brink, SR; Figure 3.2). Forty percent of the MFGM glycoproteins from cow's milk are accounted for by butyrophilin (function unknown), but lactadherin and mucin-1 (MUC1) are also present. In rat studies, MFGM have been shown to ameliorate NEC, an inflammatory condition of the GI tract of preterm infants (see above). Glycoproteins of the MFGM have been shown to inhibit the growth of *E. coli* and *Salmonella* (Proteobacteria; see Chapter 5) both *in vitro* and *in vivo*. Lactadherin levels are correlated with a lower incidence of rotavirus infections. MFGs also hamper adhesion of *E. coli* to enterocytes (Douëllou). In addition to proteins, the MFGM also supplies sialylated oligosaccharides, which are believed to be important for neurological development. In addition, their TGs are believed to be important in brain development. Studies in lab rodents support a correlation between neurological development and the MFGM (da Silva).

HMOs (Human Milk Oligosaccharides)

Human milk contains 10–15 mg/ml of **HMOs** (thus 10–15 g/L), which is higher than the typical milk protein concentration of human milk and much higher than the 1.1 mg/ml of milk oligosaccharides in bovine milk. HMOs are complicated sugars (saccharides) that cannot be digested by the intestinal enzymes of the human neonate and are not directly absorbed in appreciable amounts. They serve as **prebiotics** for the microbiome, especially *Bifidobacteria* and *Bacteroides* (Thomson, SR; Chapter 5). HMOs support those organisms in the microbiome that have the enzymatic ability to digest them. Microbial digestion of these prebiotics produces by-products including **short chain fatty acids** (SCFA; eg, butyric acid). These fatty acids are readily absorbed by the gut epithelium where they are an energy source for enterocytes. They support epithelial development and functions such as maintenance of the tight junctions between enterocytes. HMOs range in size from 3–15 monosaccharide units and about half are fucosylated or sialylated. The structure of HMOs is diverse; more than 150 of these oligosaccharides have been described. Data are available on around 30, but 10 have been the most studied (Austin). HMOs are built around a core of lactose and elongated by the addition of various oligosaccharides, sometimes including N-acetylneuraminic acid and typically containing fucose residues; 2-fucosyllactose (2-FL) and 3-fucosyllactose (3-FL) are the most abundant. Fucosylated HMOs comprise the bulk of those in human milk (Figure 3.3A). The levels and structures of milk oligosaccharides vary widely among species, but levels and structures like those in humans are seen among other higher primates (Appendix A-2). Their levels appear to depend on the presence and activities of several fucosyl transferases. The fucosyl transferases are the product of the same genes as the transferases responsible for the secretion of fucosylated blood group oligosaccharides (Siziba) and are highest in individuals called "secretors" (SE+; Figure 3.3A) and that are positive for the Lewis blood group (Le+).

Besides acting as a preferred substrate for these "good" bacteria, HMOs may also act as decoy molecules for pathogenic bacteria, blocking attachment to host enterocytes. This effect depends on the presence of structures resembling HMOs on many human cells that are targets for pathogenic bacteria. Experimental studies have shown that HMOs can competitively block such interactions, such as the binding of *Campylobacter* (a cause of childhood diarrheal disease) to intestinal epithelium. Fucosylated HMOs can block *Campylobacter* from binding to the MHC proteins on neonatal enterocytes. Additionally, epidemiologic data supports a decrease in *Campylobacter* disease in the infants of nursing mothers who are SE+ (secretor for fucosyl HMO). Sialylated HMOs can also prevent cellular adhesion of *E. coli*. For these reasons, HMOs are of increasing interest among pediatric nutritionists, infectious disease specialists, and developmental biologists. As we will see in Chapter 4, a few of the HMOs are now available for addition to infant formulas. We describe in

Chapter 5 how HMOs promote the expansion of *Bifidobacteria* and Bacteriodetes in the GI tract microbiome of suckling infants. Thus, the infant's microbiome differs in composition and diversity from that obtained through vertical transmission from the mother, so *Bifidobacterium infantis* is dominant in breastfed infants (Olin).

Maternal Cells in Colostrum and Milk

Cells in milk include shed mammary gland epithelial cells, macrophages, and neutrophils. A low level of neutrophils is normal, and their innate immune protective properties (see Chapter 6) keep the MG healthy, but a high number of neutrophils can occur with **mastitis**. Neutrophils are especially important since environmental bacteria normally enter through the nipple or teat during nursing. Neutrophils remain the major cell type in healthy mature milk except near the end of lactation, when epithelial cells are being shed from the involuting MG.

Extreme infection triggers recruitment of additional neutrophils to "clean up the mess." An influx of neutrophils may also signal a deficiency of other internal immune protective factors. In the dairy industry, the maternal cells are referred to as **somatic cells** and the somatic cell count (SCC) is one measure of milk quality in dairies. In an infected MG (ie, in mastitis), the SCC can reach high levels of which more than 90% are neutrophils, a measure of inflammation. A high SCC means the milk is not marketable.

Small numbers of lymphocytes are also present in breast milk. Their role is rather controversial. Studies in the 1970s in experimental animals suggested they may take up residence in tissues of the suckling neonate and thereby transfer some immune function. Theoretically this could be dangerous since their lack of histocompatibility may allow them to recognize the tissues of the neonate as foreign, with negative consequences (Chapters 2 and 6). In the rare disorder SCID (severe combined immunodeficiency), transferred maternal lymphocytes can attack the child's organs. Most instances of this phenomenon have been ascribed to *in utero* lymphocyte transfer via the placenta, possibly as a late peripartum event involving a damaged placenta. SCID is described in Chapter 6 and in Appendix A-1. Although controversial, some research has indicated that hematopoietic stem cells are also transferred in colostrum and milk and could influence lymphocyte development in the newborn (reviewed in Lokossou).

Natural killer cells (NK cells) are important players in the innate immune response. They represent approximately 0.5% of all colostrum-derived leucocytes and, together with transitional leucocytes, comprise approximately 2% of the leucocytes transferred in breast milk. We mentioned the role of NK cells in the placenta (Chapter 2) and detail their activity in Chapter 6.

Bacteria in Milk

Milk within the MG was traditionally considered to be sterile, a view that grew out of the dairy industry where any bacteria in the milk were considered contaminants and possibly the cause of mastitis. The MG is not sterile and human milk contains 10^3–10^4

colony-forming units per ml of bacteria; therefore, nursing infants ingest 10^5–10^7 bacteria daily, as well as HMOs, which only some bacteria can metabolize. In the past 20 years, data has led many biologists to shift from considering bacteria in milk and the breast as merely being pathogens or opportunistic commensals to viewing some as helpful symbionts (ie, bacteria in milk may act as probiotics). The concept of **probiotics** has a long history, dating to around 4000 BC when Abraham attributed his long life to drinking fermented milk (Genesis 18.8), which we now know contains live bacteria. Popular use and marketing of yogurts for their probiotics is common. Such products contain strains of lactic acid bacteria (phylum Actinobacteria; Chapter 5). This phylum contains more than 20 species of *Bifidobacteria*, named because of their Y-shaped (bifid) appearance. Other Actinobacteria such as *Lactobacillus* are found in sauerkraut and kimchi (sour fermented cabbage). Regular use of probiotic cultures for term infants has been proposed, and there are studies suggesting they would reduce sepsis and NEC (Panigrahi). Since *Bifidobacteria* and *Lactobacillus* are elevated in the GI tract of healthy, vaginally delivered breastfed infants, they are viewed as being a part of the healthy microbiome of infants (Underwood; Chapter 5). Species belonging to these genera are used in some nurseries as probiotics for preterm infants. Instead of a healthy or "good" microbiome, preterm infants are often colonized by Firmicutes like *Staphylococci*, *Streptococci*, and *Enterococci* and an abundance of Proteobacteria like *E. coli* that may include pathogenic variants. This condition is referred to as **dysbiosis** and it is associated with NEC, bacterial infections, and other inflammatory conditions (Chapter 5).

Passive Immunity and the Mammary Gland

Transfer of Maternal Antibody

Colostrum contains the major immunoglobulin classes: IgA, IgG, and IgM (see Table A3.1). IgG in milk is derived from the blood of the mother, and therefore represents the mother's **systemic immunologic experience** (Butler 1974). This results from her encounters with pathogens that become systemic so that antigen-specific immune cells primarily develop in lymph nodes and spleen and then release IgG antibodies into the bloodstream. During pregnancy these are subsequently transferred across the placenta, as described in Chapter 2. Except for the oral polio vaccine (Chapter 6), IgG antibodies account for the bulk of the antibodies that appear in response to childhood vaccinations, so their value is systemic protection.

    Mucosal immunologic experience refers to the response to pathogens detected at mucosal surfaces. Pathogens that colonize mucosal surfaces in the GI tract, upper airway, urogenital tract, and tracheobronchial tree trigger the production of IgA antibodies. B cells from these mucosal sites, especially the GI tract, are recruited to the mammary gland near the end of pregnancy through the action of chemokines and their receptors (Table 6.3). These migrant B cells produce IgA antibodies that are transported across the alveolar epithelium of the breast ducts into colostrum and milk using the mechanism illustrated in Figure 6.6, and are then called SIgA. This connection is often referred to as the gut-MG axis (Roux; Macpherson). This results in the transfer of the mucosal immune experience of the mother's gut to the GI tract of the suckling infant. SIgA antibodies account for 90% of passive antibodies in breast milk and reach concentrations of 30–80 mg/ml, while IgG antibodies account for less than 10% of passive antibodies. B cells arriving from the GI tract would typically be specific for pathogens encountered there and could provide the newborn with antibodies against gut pathogens. Studies emerging from the COVID pandemic reveal that the majority of nursing mothers that have received two doses of an mRNA COVID-19 vaccine (see Appendix A-4) transmit IgG- and SIgA-neutralizing antibodies to SARS-CoV-2 in their breast milk (Yeo), further supporting the value of breast-feeding.

SIgA in colostrum and milk also possesses some special properties, including its protease resistance in the gut lumen (Atyeo). Ingested SIgA antibodies act primarily within the lumen of the gut and on the surface of enterocytes that comprise the epithelial cells lining the gut. Enterocytes are a "soft" barrier that prevent environmental pathogens and undigested macromolecules from being absorbed while allowing absorption of nutrients. SIgA particularly binds and removes pathogenic gut bacteria and viruses, such as polio virus and rotavirus, that can infect enterocytes. Their specificity and effectiveness are demonstrated by the fact that approximately 60% of bacteria recovered in stool samples of breastfed infants have SIgA attached to them (Bunker). SIgA in colostrum and milk also appear to favor colonization with commensals that form attachment with the gut mucosa (Donaldson). In addition, SIgA complexes with receptors that have immunoregulatory properties, including DC-SIGN, a receptor on dendritic cells (DCs) that induces them to produce large amounts of IL-10 (suppressive) instead of inflammatory IL-12 (Table 6.3). IL-10 causes expansion of FOXP3 regulatory T cells (Tregs). These cells act along with TGFβ and certain other cytokines to downregulate inflammatory responses in the GI tract (Brenmoehl, SR; Zimmermann and Macpherson; Dawood).

Figure 3.5 illustrates the relative concentrations of various immunoglobulin classes and subclasses in milk of several representative species and emphasizes the special situation in humans that does not apply to all mammals. Figure 3.3B shows that immunoglobulin levels (the biochemical term for an *antibody*) are higher in human colostrum than in mature milk, and that SIgA is concentrated in colostrum (Table 3.1). Figure 3.5 illustrates that this pattern is not seen in all mammals. In human colostrum SIgA accounts for approximately 90% of total immunoglobulin, whereas in cattle and swine IgG comprises greater than 85% of total immunoglobulin (Figure A2.5). These large differences among species in the relative concentration of IgG and SIgA in colostrum reflect the mode of passive transfer of protective IgG antibodies to the young. Mammals in Group I include humans in which IgG is selectively transported to the fetus *in utero* (Chapter 2) that do not depend on breast-feeding for transfer of IgG. By contrast, the IgG concentration in colostrum of Group III mammals can exceed 100mg/ml and is the only means of transferring the mother's **systemic immunological experiences** to the newborn.

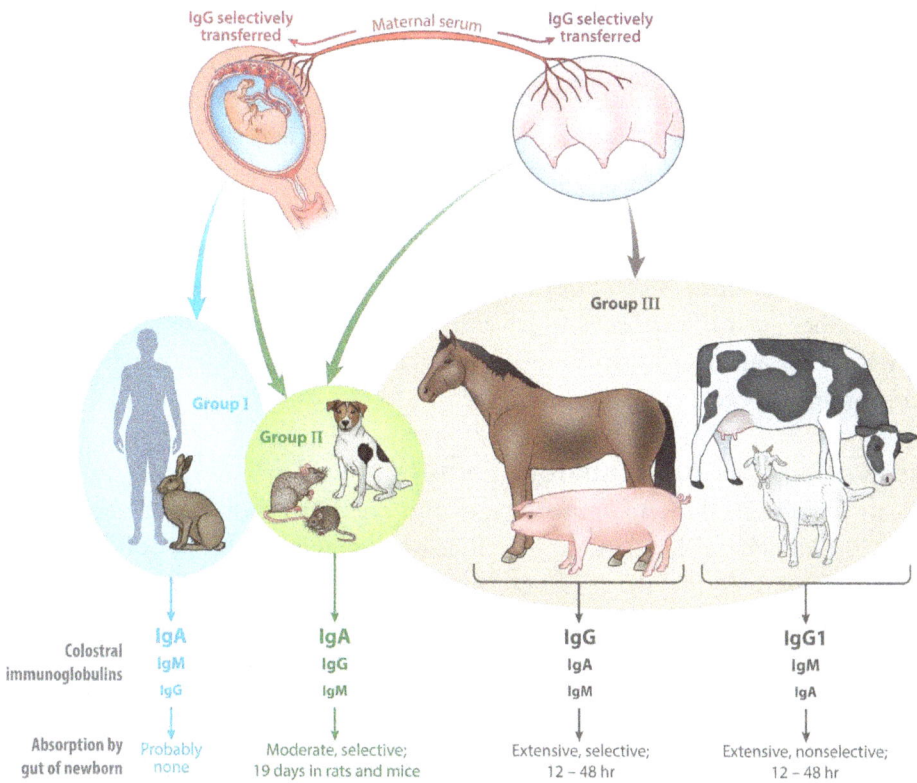

	Group I	Group II	Group III	
Colostral immunoglobulins	IgA IgM IgG	IgA IgG IgM	IgG IgA IgM	IgG1 IgM IgA
Absorption by gut of newborn	Probably none	Moderate, selective; 19 days in rats and mice	Extensive, selective; 12 – 48 hr	Extensive, nonselective; 12 – 48 hr

Figure 3.5   Transmission of passive antibody immunity from mother to young. Group I mammals, including humans, transfer IgG *in utero* before birth and SIgA in colostrum after birth. In Group III mammals, there is no *in utero* transfer of any antibody class, so colostrum in the first few days postpartum is needed to transfer IgG. After about 1 week, there is a transition to mature milk, in which SIgA is the major antibody class transferred, as in human colostrum (see Figure A2.5). Group II mammals depend on both *in utero* and breast milk transfer of IgG. Also shown is that absorption by the GI tract of the suckling differs greatly among groups. More details are available in Appendix A-2.

Differences in the mode of transfer of IgG from mother to young are correlated with the activity of the GI tract enterocytes. In humans, the infant GI tract is relatively "closed" at birth, meaning that only trace amounts of intact proteins are absorbed. In contrast, in the mammals of especially Group III, the gut remains "open" during the first 24 hours and nonselectively absorbs all macromolecules, even synthetic polymers (Figure 3.5 and Appendix A-2).

Passive Antibody and Childhood Vaccinations

Maternal IgG transferred *in utero* remains in the blood of the newborn and decreases with a half-life of about 3 weeks (Table A3.1; see also Figure 6.3). IgG antibodies transferred *in utero* are easily detectable for up to 4 to 6 months. If these IgG antibodies bind vaccine antigens, they could theoretically remove the vaccine before it stimulates the immune system of the newborn. The veterinary field has struggled with this dilemma for more than 50 years (Appendix A-2). The prenatally acquired maternal antibody may be partially responsible for the observation that infant antibody responses to vaccinations increase sequentially with repeat doses for babies at 2, 4, and 6 months of age, which may be related to the decay of potentially interfering passive maternal IgG. Studies in mice suggest polio-specific antibodies obtained *in utero* or via breast milk can interfere with the immune response to the polio vaccine. However, controversy still exists concerning interference by antibodies transferred from the mother, so that childhood vaccinations are delayed or given multiple times during infant life (Table 6.4). This issue may be most significant with live, attenuated virus vaccines, such as measles, in which a small amount of residual maternal antibody might block the initial replication of the virus that is necessary to adequately stimulate the infant's immune system.

Passive Transfer of Regulatory Factors

At least a dozen cytokine and growth regulators are transferred through breast milk (Table 3.1). Absolute levels differ among published data, presumably because the assays used, the time of sampling, and the condition of the mothers differed. Table 3.1 provides an overview of the levels of proteins and regulatory factors in colostrum and mature milk. Table 6.3 describes the function of the various cytokines and regulatory factors. In general, the concentration of most regulatory factors is lower in mature milk than colostrum. However, since breast milk output increases during lactation, the total amount ingested by the infant increases (Table 3.2). Before assigning functions to immune regulatory factors in colostrum and milk, we need to consider the alternative view that these factors are merely "leftovers" from maternal serum that entered the MG or are the result of activity within the MG. This might agree with some who regard the MG as a "secondary excretory organ."

TABLE 3.2 Nanograms (ng) of Regulatory Factors Ingested Daily by a Healthy Breastfed Infant

Values based on data in Figure 3.4 and Table 3.1.

Milk Volume (ml)	130	1,000	1,200
	Colostrum	At about third week of lactation	At about sixth week of lactation
Regulator			
EGF	780	5,000	7,000
MCP-1	325	500	840
RANTES	13	100	75
TGFβ 1-3	325	400	500
IL-4	5	10	15
IL-6	4.6	25	30
IL-10	5.2	10	12
INFγ	3.9	10	12
IL-8 (CXCL8)	156	85	192

Among these regulators are cytokines like TNFα, IFNγ, TGFβ, IL-4, IL-6, IL-8, IL-10, and others (Trend). Growth factors, especially EGF and insulin growth factor (IGF) are present at ng/ml levels throughout lactation (Table 3.1). Chemokine levels (eg, MCP-1), are also present at high levels as compared to most cytokines with the exceptions of TGFβ and IL-8; the latter is now regarded as a chemokine like MCP-1 (Table 6.3).

The level of TGFβ is 1–2 logs higher than other cytokines (Table 3.1), suggesting it may play a major role in the MG or in the suckling infant. In studies with rodents, TGFβ aids in the establishment of oral tolerance (Holvoet). The colostrum of preterm mothers contains very high levels of TGFβ (Trend), suggesting it is involved in preparing the MG or that it is needed to suppress inflammatory responses in the MG or the neonate. TGFβ, along with IL-10, dampens inflammatory T cell (Th1) activity by promoting the development of Tregs. TGFβ also promotes the switch to IgA production in the GI tract, the growth of the intestinal villi, and increases in production of tight junction proteins, and it is also involved in the preparation of the MG for secretion and later in its involution after nursing (Brenmoehl, SR).

Studies suggest infants lacking TGFβ may later experience severe skin and intestinal inflammatory reactions after GI tract colonization (Wildin). Among its various roles, TGFβ is involved in differentiations of FOXP3 Tregs, which play a major role in suppression of the inflammatory response and, some believe, in suppression of food allergy (Holvoet). Actual values differ among investigators, and some report an approximately 10-fold drop during transition to mature milk. Based on the daily consumption of approximately 130 ml of colostrum (Figure 3.4), infants could receive 300 ng of TGFβ daily and as much as 2 times more in lactation (Table 3.2). The reported concentration of TGFβ in bovine milk is 250 ng/ml, similar to swine milk, which has 125–260 ng/ml. TGFβ and certain other cytokines initially occur as inactive proteins, which become activated by factors in their environment that include pH. Hence, the level of active TGFβ and other regulators may differ.

Given the connection between TGFβ and Treg activity, it is interesting that in suckling mouse pups, SIgA and Treg levels are inversely related. Germ-free mice have very low Treg activity, and it has been speculated that this is because there are no bacteria in the GI tract to induce an immune response that needs to be suppressed (Zimmermann and Macpherson). It is speculated that immune suppression is needed since an immune response to the GI tract microbiome could negatively affect establishment of a healthy microbiome. That high SIgA levels are inversely correlated with Treg activity could be explained by the SIgA coating the bacteria (Bunker), thus reducing the need for the suppressive influence of TGFβ in the suckling neonate.

Bovine colostrum is reported to contain 18–320 ng/ml of EGF. EGF accelerates intestinal growth and increases jejunal lactase and sucrase activity when fed to piglets. Antigen sensing in the GI tract seems regulated by Goblet cells and EGF inhibits this function (Knoop). This may help explain why breastfed infants have a lower risk of allergy and other immune regulatory illnesses. Insulin-like growth factor (IGF) is present in human milk at less than

30 ng/ml while values range from 70–350 ng/ml in swine and cattle milks. While actual values may vary, administration of IGF at 100 ng/ml stimulates brush border enzymes and general GI tract development in various animals.

Many cytokines and other regulatory factors, unlike Igs in breast milk, are labile. This may explain their lower levels in banked donor milk (Groer). While their protein concentrations may remain stable, their bioactivity may deteriorate during storage (Ramirez-Santana). As previously mentioned, most cytokines need to be converted to an active form, either by pH changes or other environmental factors. This could be an important consideration when using stored or donor milks, especially for preterm infants (Figure 3.6). If the factors being discussed perform a function in the suckling neonate, this concern also applies to infant formula or processed animal milks (Chapter 4).

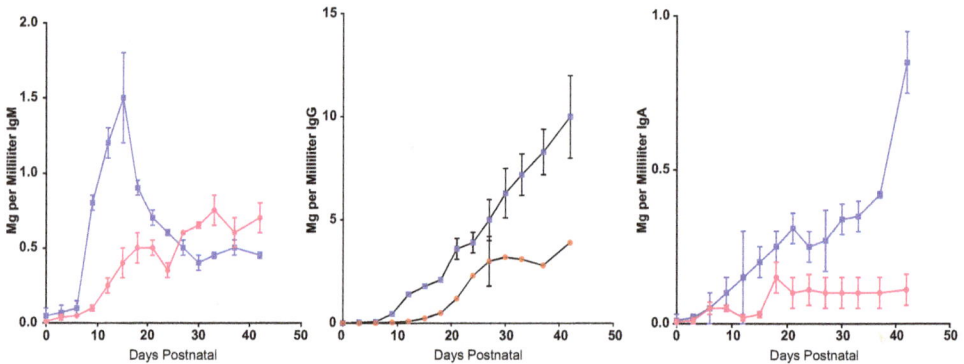

Figure 3.6 Labile factors in colostrum control immunoglobulin synthesis. The effect of fresh (red) or frozen (blue) colostrum on the *de novo* synthesis of IgM, IgG, and IgA in cesarian-derived piglets reared in an "autosow" feeding facility (Appendix A-2). Studies were done with colostrum frozen for 48 hours, 7 days, or 8 years. There was no difference between the length of storage, so only the values for colostrum stored for 48 hours are presented (Butler et al., 2019).

Evidence that regulatory factors in colostrum and milk have a regulatory role comes from a much older study using SPF piglets derived by C-section and reared in isolation units on fresh or stored bovine colostrum. Storage of colostrum at −20 °C (which does not affect immunoglobulin levels in colostrum) impacts the degree of *de novo* synthesis of IgM, IgA, and IgG synthesis in these piglets. Storage for 48 hours, 7 days, or 8 years gave identical results, indicating that freezing but not time caused this effect. At the time this study was performed, few cytokines had been described and no reagents were available for their measurement. Given what is currently known, there are numerous candidates, including TGFβ and IL-10. While the cytokine proteins may survive freezing or short-term storage, their bio-viability may be weak or lacking (Ramirez-Santana).

Transfer of Harmful Agents in Milk

Pathogens in Milk

Breast milk is a convenient conduit for the transfer of pathogens, including many viruses. One example is the transfer of CMV (cytomegalovirus) from seropositive mothers (those with serum antibodies to CMV) to preterm infants through breast milk. Due to immunologic immaturity, preterm infants have little protection and can become seriously ill. Research raises the possibility that, even in the absence of severe illness, infection of preterm infants with CMV could lead to measurable cognitive impairment later in life. Therefore, some neonatologists advocate the pasteurization of milk from seropositive mothers that is to be fed to premature infants, while others are opposed because of the adverse effects of pasteurization on labile regulatory factors in breast milk (see earlier). The percentage of neonatal ICUs practicing pasteurization of milk from seropositive mothers is not known but is assumed to be increasing.

In the absence of prophylactic intervention, approximately 30% of infants born to HIV-positive mothers acquire HIV, and it is primarily transferred *in utero* (Chapter 2). HIV can also be transmitted through breast-feeding, but as previously noted, in developing countries the benefit of prevention of diarrheal disease by breast-feeding outweighs the risk associated with HIV transfer. In the case of SARS-CoV-2, infants less than about 2 months of age are most susceptible to infection and hospitalization, possibly due to insufficient transfer of SARS-CoV-2 antibodies *in utero*. While SARS-CoV-2 is quite likely transferred through breast milk, the WHO recommends that mothers suspected to be COVID-19 positive should continue to nurse. Currently, administration of COVID-19 vaccines to pregnant or nursing mothers is also recommended, since the risk of infection is greater than any known consequence of using the vaccine. For details on COVID-19 and current vaccines, refer to Appendix A-4. Finally, Epstein-Barr virus (EBV), a cause of infectious mononucleosis, and which is associated with a variety of lymphomas and autoimmune diseases, is also transferred in breast milk (see Chapter 6 for further details on EBV).

Drugs and Environmental Contaminants in Milk

As previously mentioned, some physiologists and milk chemists have described the breast as a "secondary excretory organ," implying that left-over metabolites in the blood of the mother are transferred to the breast, secreted into milk, and may affect the suckling neonate. The term *drug* has various meanings. In the broad context used here, it includes prescribed pharmaceuticals, over-the-counter pain medication, narcotics, antidepressants, substance abuse cessation products, and circulating compounds resulting from smoking. The AAP periodically publishes information on the transfer of such drugs (Sachs, SR). We summarize some major issues here. Women planning to become pregnant and to breastfeed should consult their pediatrician/gynecologist since knowledge evolves over time. The LactMed Drugs and Lactation Database, available online, regularly updates information on the subject (National Library of Medicine).

In considering the impact of a drug on the nursing mother and infant, a number of variables should be kept in mind: (a) age of the nursling, (b) the infant's metabolic and immunologic health, (c) the retention time (half-life) of the drug or substance, (d) the availability or absorption of the drug by the infant's GI tract, and (e) the relative risk to the mother of withholding or using the drug. Antibiotics in particular fall into the last category. In many cases, only the short-term effects of drugs are published, so decisions regarding the effect of continual use rest on "strength of evidence" (Chapter 7). Lactating mothers receiving iodine-131 (^{131}I) radiation treatment for cancer are a special category. Although the iodine primarily becomes concentrated in the thyroid gland, breast-feeding should be interrupted during such treatment.

Over-the-counter pain medications like ibuprofen, acetaminophen, aspirin, and naproxen are considered compatible with breast-feeding when moderate doses are used. While low doses of aspirin (75–162 mg/day) are acceptable, excessive use can result in rash, platelet abnormality, and bleeding in the neonate. Extra caution and consultation with a pediatrician is necessary when codeine, morphine, or related narcotics are used. Central nervous system depression has been reported in 20% of infants exposed to oxycodone during breast-feeding. Antidepressants or psychoactive drugs may have long-term effects that are currently unknown; therefore, decisions regarding their use might involve the infant's pediatrician. In general, maternal smoking is not associated with immediate infant problems, but it is known that nicotine passes freely into human milk and is absorbed by the neonate. The same is likely for metabolites of recreational drugs. Lactating women are generally advised to refrain from smoking, alcohol consumption, and use of recreational drugs. Agents used to facilitate cessation of drug abuse or alcohol dependence warrant discussion since the use of methadone and buprenorphine (opioids) can present a risk to the suckling. Reports suggest that maternal consumption of opioids is associated with lethargy, respiratory difficulties, and poor weight gain by the suckling. Maternal use of such agents can also lead to a "neonatal withdrawal" syndrome if the mother stops using them during lactation.

Substances usually considered part of alternative medicine include herbal products that are sold as dietary supplements and are not regulated as drugs by the FDA. Some have reported adverse effects, such at St. John's Wort, which can lead to colic, drowsiness, and lethargy of the nursing infant. A major danger signal regarding all herbal medications comes from studies showing that 16 of 40 dietary supplements contain pesticide residues, which fall into the category of environmental contaminants.

The potential effects of *in utero* transfer of environmental contaminants were touched on in the previous chapter. Biphenyl compounds, dioxins, furans, and particularly organochlorines have been detected (at low levels) in 9% of maternal adipose tissue samples and in 62% of breast milk samples. There are currently little data on the effect of these contaminants, but students and parents should remain vigilant of the possible effects. In the absence of firmer data on the danger from low-level environmental chemicals in breast milk, breast-feeding is still the feeding strategy preferred by most practitioners.

Breast Milk Supplementation

Supplementation During Breast-Feeding

There are a few nutrients for which breast milk does not completely meet the needs of the full-term infant. The exceptions include vitamin D and the trace minerals iron, zinc, and copper. Since evolutionary pressure did not select for the addition of these to milk, other sources must have sufficed in the pre-industrial world, such as sunlight for vitamin D and dirt for minerals. Infants draw on prenatally acquired stores of minerals to avoid deficiency prior to the addition of complementary feedings that include minerals. In today's world of low sun exposure for many in North America, vitamin D supplementation is recommended for breastfed infants.

The energy and protein requirements for tissue maintenance and growth of preterm infants are far higher than for term infants. Breast milk alone does not meet their optimal needs, as more energy, protein, and minerals are needed. Supplements for breast milk are available that help fill these needs. Specially designed infant formulas can provide appropriate proteins and micronutrients for preterm infants (Chapter 4) when breast milk is not available.

A number of breast milk components have been used in management of either non-breastfed infants or infants and children with illnesses. Common examples are the use of prebiotics and probiotics. Prebiotics like HMOs are a major constituent in breast milk (Figure 3.3), and emerging evidence points to the presence of bacterial strains in breast milk that can metabolize HMOs (ie, act as probiotics). In recent years, HMOs and MFGM have been added to some infant formulas for healthy infants who are not breastfed. The use of prebiotics and probiotics in the care of premature infants varies widely around the world but each has strong advocates.

Preterm Birth Presents a Special Situation

The physiology and challenges facing the mother and infant after preterm birth deserve separate mention, especially considering that preterm births account for 10% or more of all births in many countries. Gestational age at birth is correlated with the frequency of late onset sepsis and necrotizing enterocolitis (NEC; Ramani); the risk of both is reduced by feeding breast milk. The prevalence of NEC is quite variable, both between nurseries and over time at individual nurseries. The rate may vary from below 5% in infants with birth weights under 1,500 grams, to as high as 20% in outbreaks in individual nurseries. Animal studies (Appendix A-2) suggest that sepsis and NEC are associated with immaturity of the preterm GI tract. Studies have shown that colostrum from mothers who delivered preterm had different levels of regulatory factors in colostrum than at the time of full-term delivery. TGFβ (suppressor of inflammatory T cells, see earlier) and antibacterial peptides are elevated in the milk of preterm mothers (Hennet). This may be interpreted to suggest that the MG in late gestation is prepared to deliver protective and regulatory factors to the GI tract at the time of birth. Evidence that breast milk reduces the risk of NEC is in line with the hypothesis that protective and regulatory factors present in breast milk are important. As we illustrated (Figure 3.6), freezing colostrum destroyed its ability to normally suppress *de novo* immunoglobulin synthesis by suckling piglets. Such suppression may be important in reducing the neonate's ability to mount an antibody response to self/maternal proteins and eubiotic commensal bacteria. Preterm infants that typically lack access to fresh colostrum are about 3.6 times more likely to become asthmatic and suffer from other immune-related diseases (Trønnes). Mothers of preterm infants can only provide milk by manual expression or use of a breast pump, but production may be low, leading to the use of banked milk that has been pasteurized and stored at low temperatures. The best means to provide a sufficient supply of breast milk appears to be frequent and thorough emptying of the breasts during infant suckling or pumping. Some health practitioners have employed so-called galactogogue supplements in attempts to increase milk production. Galactogogues may be pharmaceutical or herbal. This practice is not supported by a large body of research and discussion of this topic goes beyond the scope of this book (Brodribb).

Even when breast milk is available, administering it to preterm infants can be challenging. Even late preterm infants (34–36 weeks) are unlikely to latch onto the breast well enough to adequately suckle. Furthermore, preterm infants of less than about 32 weeks of gestation may not coordinate swallowing.

Summary

Evolution over more than 150 million years has equipped mammals with the powerful tool of milk to provide nutrition and protection to newborns and infants. The multiple and overlapping protective and immunoregulatory attributes of milk attest to the eons of responses to evolutionary pressure. From the deepest time of human history, a key to the species' survival has been the survival of an adequate number of infants. Humans are now the only mammalian species to use any alternative to feeding the young with milk from their mothers (Chapter 4). Even in our most advanced societies, it would be overconfident to think that we could replace all functions of breast milk with a substitute. In developing societies, the risk of substitutes for breast milk is evident in rates of infection and infant mortality. In advanced countries, the risk associated with absence of breast-feeding is low but still present, though it may not be apparent to the individual parent.

Suggested Readings (SR)

Brenmoehl J, Ohde D, Wirthgen E, Hoeflich A. Cytokines in milk and the role of TGF-beta. *Best Pract & Res Clin Endocrinol & Metabol*. 2018;32:47–56.

Brink LR, Lonnerdal B. Milk fat globule membrane: The role of various components in infant health and development. *J Nutri Biochem*. 2020;85:108465. doi:10.1016/j.jnutbio.2020.108465.

Brodin P. Immune-microbe interactions in early life: A determinant of health and diseases long term. *Science*. 2022;376:945–950.

Johnston M, Landers S, Noble L, Szucs K, Viehmann L. Breast feeding and the use of human milk. *Pediatrics*. 2012;129:e827-41. doi:10.1542/peds.2011-3552.

McManaman JL, Neville MC. Mammary physiology and milk secretion. *Adv Drug Deliv Rev*. 2003;55:629–41.

Sachs HC. The transfer of drugs and therapeutics into human breast milk: An update on selected topics. *Pediatrics*. 2013;132:e796. doi:10.1542/peds.2013-1985.

Thomson P, Medina DA, Garrido D. Human milk oligosaccharides and infant gut *Bifidobacteria*: Molecular strategies for their utilization. *Food Microbio*. 2018;75:37-48.

US Department of Agriculture (USDA). Pregnancy and birth to 24 months systematic review: Infant milk-feeding practices technical expert collaborative. https://nesr.usda.gov/infant-milk-feeding-practices-technical-expert-collaborative.

References

Abuogi L, Noble L, Smith C, et al; American Academy of Pediatrics Committee on Pediatric and Adolescent HIV, Section on Breastfeeding. Infant feeding for persons living with and at risk for HIV in the United States: Clinical report. *Pediatrics*. 2024;153(6):e2024066843 DOI: https://doi.org/10.1542/peds.2024-066843

Angelopoulou A, Field D, Ryan CA, et al. The microbiology and treatment of human mastitis. *Med Microbiol & Immunol*. 2018;207:83–94.

Arenz S, Rückerl R, Koletzko B, et al. Breast-feeding and childhood obesity—a systematic review. *Int J Obes*. 2004;28:1247–1256. doi:10/1038/sj.ijo.0802758.

Atyeo C, Alter G. The multifaceted roles of breast milk antibodies. *Cell*. 2021;184:1486–1499.

Austin S, Casto CA, Bebet T, et al. Temporal changes of the content of 10 oligosaccharides in milk of Chinese urban mothers. *Nutrients*. 2016;8:346–368.

Bravi F. Impact of maternal nutrition on breast-milk composition: A systematic review. *Am J Clin Nutr*. 2016;104:646–662.

Brodribb W. ABM Clinical Protocol #9: Use of galactogogues in initiating or augmenting maternal milk production, second revision. *Breastfeed Med*. 2018;13(5):307–314. doi:10.1089/bfm.2018.29092.wjb.

Bunker JJ, Flynn TM, Koval JC, et al. Innate and adaptive humoral responses coat distinct commensal bacteria with immunoglobulin. *A Immunity*. 2015;43:541–553.

Butler JE. Immunoglobulins of the mammary secretions. In: Larson BL, Smith V, eds. *Lactation: A Comprehensive Treatise*. New York: Academic Press; 1974:217–255.

Butler JE. Immunologic aspects of breast feeding, anti-infectious activity of breast milk. *Semin Perinatol*. 1979;3(3):255–270.

Butler JE, Rainard P, Lippolis J, Salmon H, Kacskovics I. The mammary gland in mucosal and regional immunity. In: Mestecky J, Strober W, Russell MW, Kelsall BL, eds. *Mucosal Immunology*. 4th ed. Cambridge, MA: Academic Press; 2015:2269–2306.

Butler JE, Sinkora M, Wang G, Stepanova K, Li Y, Cai X. Perturbation of thymocyte development underlies the PRRS pandemic: A testable hypothesis. *Front Immunol*. 2019;10:1077. doi:10.3389/fimmu.2019.01077.

Chatterton DEW, Nguyen DN, Brandt Bering S, Torp Sangild P. Anti-inflammatory mechanisms of bioactive milk proteins in the intestine of newborns. *Int J Biochem Cell Biol*. 2013;45:1730–1747.

da Silva RC, Colleran HL, Irahim SA. Milk fat globule membrane in infant nutrition: A dairy industry perspective. *J Dairy Sci*. 2021;88:105–116.

Dawood B, Marshall JS. Cytokines and soluble receptors in breast milk as enhancers of oral tolerance development. *Front Immunol*. 2019;10:16. doi:10.3389/fimmu.2019.00016.

Donaldson GP, Ladinsky MS, Yu KB, et al. Gut microbiota use immunoglobulin A for mucosal colonization. *Science*. 2018;360:795–800.

Douëllou T, Galia W, Kerangart S, et al. Milk fat globules hamper adhesion of enterohemor-rhagic *Escherichia coli* to enterocytes: *In vitro* and *in vivo* evidence. *Front Microbio*. 2018;9:947. doi:10.3389/fmich.2018.00947.

Grattan DR. Sixty years of neuroendocrinology: The hypothalamo-prolactin axis. *J Endocrinol*. 2015;226:T101-22. doi:10.1530/JOE-15-0213.

Groer M, Duffy A, Morse S, et al. Cytokines, chemokines and growth factors in banked human donor milk for preterm infants. *J Human Lact*. 2014;30:317–323.

Hennet T, Borsig L. Breastfed at Tiffany's. *Trends Biochem Sci*. 2016;41:508–519.

Holvoet S, Perrot M, de Groot N, et al. Oral tolerance induction to newly introduced allergens is favored by a transforming growth factor β-enriched formulas. *Nutrients*. 2019; 11(9):2210. doi:10.3390/nu11092210.

Knoop KA, Gustafsson JK, McDonald KG, et al. Microbial antigen encounter during preweaning intervals is critical for tolerance to gut bacteria. *Sci. Immunol*. 2017;2(18):eaao1314. doi:10.1126/sciimmunol.aao1324.

Lokossou GAG, Kouakanou L, Schumacher A, Zonclussen ZG. Human breast milk: Food to active immune responses with disease protection in infants and mothers. *Front Immunol*. 2022;13:849012. doi:10.3389/fimmu.2022.849012.

Macpherson AJ, Uhr T. Induction of protective IgA by intestinal dendritic cells carrying commensal bacteria. *Science*. 2004;303:1662–1665.

National Library of Medicine. LactMed Database, Drugs and Lactation Database. National Institute of Child Health and Human Development. https://www.ncbi.nlm.nih.gov/books/NBK501922/.

Neville, MC, Neifert MR. *Lactation: Physiology, Nutrition, and Breast Feeding*. New York: Plenum Press; 1983.

Olin MR, Dahan D, Carter MM, et al. Robust variation in infant gut microbiome assembly across a spectrum of lifestyles. *Science*. 2022;376:1220–1223.

Panigrahi P, Parida S, Nanda NC, et al. A randomized symbiotic trial to prevent sepsis among infants in rural India. *Nature*. 2017;548:407–412. doi:10.1038/nature 23480.

Ramani M, Ambalavanan N. Feeding practices and NEC. *Clin Perinatal*. 2013;40:1–10. doi:10.1016/j.clp.2012.12.001.

Ramirez-Santana C, Oerez-Cano FJ, Audi C, et al. Effect of cooling and freezing storage on the stability of bioactive factors in human colostrum. *J Dairy Sci*. 2012;95:2319–2315.

Roux ME, McWilliams M, Phillips-Quagliata JM, et al. Origin of IgA secreting plasma cells in the mammary gland. *J Exp Med*. 1977;146:1311–1322.

Sadovnikova A, Garcia SC, Hovey RC. A comparative review of the extrinsic and intrinsic factors regulating lactose synthesis. *J M Gland Bio & Neopl*. 2021;26:197–215.

Siziba LP, Mank M, Stahl B, et al. Human milk oligosaccharides profile over 12 months of lactation. *Ulm SPATZ Hlth Stdy Nutri*. 2021;13:1973. doi:org/10.3390/nu13061973.

Spahn JM, Callahan EH, Spill MK, et al. Influence of maternal diet on flavor transfer to amniotic fluid and breast milk and children's responses: A systematic review. *Am J Clin Nutr*. 2019;109 (Suppl. 7):1003S–1026S.

Trend S, Strunk T, Lloyd ML, et al. Levels of innate immune factors in preterm and term mother's breast milk during the 1st month postpartum. *Brit J Nutr*. 2016;115:1178–1193.

Trønnes H, Wilcox AJ, Lie RV, Markestad T, Moster D. The association of preterm birth with severe asthmas and atopic dermatitis: A national cohort study. *Pediatr Allergy Immunol*. 2013;24:782–787.

Underwood MA, German JB, Lebrilla CB, Mills DA. *Bifidobacteria longum subspecies infantis*: Champion colonizer of the infant gut. *Ped Res*. 2015;77:229–235.

Vass RA, Kemeny A, Dergez T, Ertl T, Jungling A, Tarnes A. Distribution of bioactive factors in human milk samples. *Int Breastfeed J*. 2019;14:9. https://internationalbreastfeedingjournal.biomedcentral.com/articles/10.1186/s13006-019-0203-3.

Victora CG, Bahl R, Barros AJD, et al. Breast feeding in the 21st century: Epidemiology, mechanisms, and lifelong effect. *Lancet* 2016;387:475–90.

Wildin RS, Ramsdell F, Peake J, et al. X-linked neonatoal diabetes mellitus, enteropathy and endocrinopathy syndrome is the human equivalent of mouse scrufy._*Nat. Genetics*. 2001;27:18–20.

World Health Organization. WHO Guideline for complementary feeding of infants and young children 6–23 months of age. Geneva: World Health Organization; 2023. Licence: CC BY-NC-SA 3.0 IGO.

Yeo KT, Chia WN, Tan CW, et al. Neutralizing activity and SARS-CoV-2 vaccine mRNA persistence in serum and breast milk after BNT162b2 vaccination in lactating women. *Front Immunol*. 2021;12:783975. doi:10.3389/fimmu 202 783975.

Zambruni M, Villalobos A, Somasunderam A, et al. Maternal and pregnancy-related factors affecting human milk cytokines among Peruvian mothers bearing low-birth-weight neonates. *J Reproductive Immunol*. 2017;120:20–26

Zimmermann J, Macpherson AJ. Breast milk modulates transgenerational immune inheritance. *Cell*. 2020;187:1202–1204.

Figure Credits

CHAPTER 4

Infant Formulas as Breast Milk Alternatives

LEARNING OBJECTIVES

1. Describe the history and development of human milk alternatives.

2. Discuss the areas of knowledge required to construct nutritionally adequate infant formulas.

3. Learn what modifications of macronutrients are required to make ruminant milks acceptable for human infants.

4. Learn what human milk components are proposed as additives to infant formulas and the rationale for their use.

5. Learn what national and international organizations regulate or recommend the composition of infant formulas.

The History of Surrogate Milks and Infant Formulas

Maternal production of milk for nutrition of the nursing infant defines mammals, but only humans have successfully provided alternatives for the infant that does not have access to its mother's milk. The lobby of the office of the American Academy of Pediatrics (AAP) for many years held a display of ancient (and not so ancient) devices to allow liquid foods to be administered to infants. These devices and the use of unmodified milks from other species, or even non-milk substitutes, clash with modern sensibilities about infant feeding. The outcome of feeding alternatives to the nursling were known to be poor, but the practice continued through necessity or callousness. Safe alternative infant formulas could not be developed until there was an adequate understanding of the chemical components of human and animal milk, microbiology, food chemistry, packaging safety, safe cow's milk production and handling, and refrigeration. One of the major thrusts of pediatric medicine in the early 20th century was to improve the quality of the milk substitutes offered for these infants, as an alternative to wet nurses or unmodified animal milks.

For millennia multiple cultures solved the problem of milk substitution by use of wet nurses paid to assume feeding of the infant. In some societies, the upper-class viewed the use of wet nurses as very appropriate behavior that freed the wealthy mother from breast-feeding, which was viewed as humble and crude. Europe in the 17th and 18th centuries offers an example of such a system. For the first 2 to 3 years of life, infants of well-heeled parents were often housed with and completely reared by the wet nurse in her home. Sentiment against wet nursing has also periodically been strong, with some societies encouraging mothers to nurse their own infants as a moral or religious obligation. Feedings other than human milk have long been known to be inferior; wet nursing avoided such feedings. However, even infants fed by wet nursing had poorer outcomes than those fed by their own mothers. Survival of infants in the first 5 to 10 years of life in pre-industrial Europe and early in the industrial age was appallingly low by today's lights. A discussion of this history is in Stevens (SR).

Alternatives to breast-feeding were limited both by the availability and safety of liquids for feeding and by the absence of safe methods of administering the feeding. Existing examples of ancient feeding spoons and "pap boats" demonstrate that feeding was given by dripping into the infant's mouth; no artificial substitute for the nipple yet existed. Advances in the understanding and use of latex rubber allowed the production in the late 1800s of rubber nipples that could be cleaned.

The shift of society in the 19th and 20th centuries from largely rural to mostly urban also complicated the provision of cow's milk for infants. Removal of the infant from the vicinity of the cow meant that the milk, even if appropriate for older infants, was more likely to be contaminated by overgrowth of bacteria. The first technology that helped bridge this gap was production of canned foods. Concentrated (evaporated or condensed) milk was available in cans by the 1860s. The heat and pressure used in the production process usually rendered the contents sterile until opened. Condensed milk brands with or without added sugar were first marketed, and later modified milk products specifically intended for infants came on the market. By 1900 a number of canned milk products intended for infant feeding were available, but the caloric content and distribution of fat, carbohydrates, and protein varied widely. The mineral and vitamin content of human milk was not understood, and none of the early formulas included appropriate mineral alterations or vitamin additions. In fact, vitamins had not been discovered as late as 1910. At the turn of the 20th century these products had limited acceptance by physicians or mothers and were too expensive for general use.

In the late 19th and early 20th centuries the chemical compositions of animal milks and human milk were defined, giving insight into the modifications of the proteins and fat needed to make animal milks suitable for use by human infants (Wargo, SR). The available animal milks (usually cow, sheep, and goat milk) contain more protein than human milk, and the extra protein consists largely of casein (Table 4.1). When exposed to gastric acid, bovine casein forms a tough curd that is poorly digested and absorbed by human infants. Dilution of cow milk to a protein concentration similar to human milk partly solves this problem because fewer and smaller curds are produced with an equivalent volume fed. Heat and pressure used in production of canned milks (evaporated or condensed milk) further reduces the size and negative impact of these curds. Eventually many commercially available formulas began to use semi-purified bovine milk protein components (such as whey powder and caseinates) that allowed formulations with a whey-to-casein ratio that more closely resembled that of human milk. However, today some infant formulas continue to use cow's milk protein without modification of the whey/casein ratio with no adverse effect.

TABLE 4.1   Content (per 100 ml) of Some Major Nutrients in Bovine Milk, Human Milk, and Formulas

Typical formulas from around 1970 and more recently are shown and compared to human and bovine milk. The full range of formula content is not reflected in the table, but the allowed ranges are discussed in the text.

	Human Milk	Cow's Milk	Typical Formulas, 1970	Typical Formulas, 2018
Total protein (g)	0.89	3.30	1.6	1.2
Casein (g)	0.25	2.60	1.26	0–0.6
Whey proteins (g)	0.70	0.67	0.34	0.6–1.2
α-Lactalbumin	0.26	0.12	0.06	0.21
β-Lactoglobulin	—	0.30	0.15	0.54
Lactoferrin	0.17	tr	tr	tr
Lysozyme	0.05	tr	tr	tr
Immunoglobulins	0.105	0.15	0.07	0.27
Iron (mg)	0.032	0.5	1.2	1.2
Vitamin D (IU)	22	14	40	40

tr = trace amounts

Butterfat, the fat in cow's milk, is poorly digested by human infants. Removal of butterfat from cow's milk (leaving skimmed milk) left the milk with roughly half its caloric content. Replacement of fat was initially not technologically feasible, but replacement of the missing calories by carbohydrates exceeded the capacity of the infant to digest and absorb carbohydrates. Eventually manufacturing techniques were developed to use emulsified vegetable oils to replace butterfat. Today formulas typically include lactose as the source of carbohydrate calories, vegetable oils for fat calories, and varying ratios of cow's milk whey and casein. As currently manufactured, these nutrient components are well-digested and absorbed by normal infants. The addition of multiple micronutrients to commercially produced formulas further improved nutritional quality.

Before commercial formulas were widely used, homemade formulas were prepared by mixing evaporated milk (which contains butter fat) with corn syrup and water. This preparation was less expensive than commercially prepared formula, thus it appealed to many families. If care to maintain hygiene and the correct measures of the components was taken, the product was adequate for infant growth; however, appropriate vitamins were also required in the diet. Until the 1970s, instruction in preparation of such formula was routinely taught to pediatric and dietetic trainees, as many parents used this method and would need instruction.

As use of early formulas spread, survival of formula-fed infants in highly developed countries improved; by the mid-20th century survival rates of formula-fed infants approached those of breast-fed infants. Widespread adoption of formula feeding then occurred, perhaps aided by an unstated assumption that it was "science-based," and nutritionally superior to breast feeding. Furthermore, formula feeding allowed mothers to know the volume of formula consumed by the infant and, if desired, to control the volume consumed. In terms of growth, formula-fed infants tended to outperform breast-fed infants in early months of life. Whether this is the result of higher nutrient content of formulas or that formula is easier to obtain by the infant than human milk (less vigorous suckling required) remains unresolved. Whether due to the convenience of formula feeding or the lack of information about the value of breast feeding, it took decades to convince mothers and healthcare providers that "nature's way" of breast feeding provides superior health benefits to the infant (Fomon, SR).

Formulas using soy protein isolates as the source of protein were first developed to meet the need for formulas free of cow's milk. Soy-based formulas also usually contain no lactose and thus are useful whenever intolerance to lactose is suspected. As soy-based formulas fully meet nutrient needs and are well-tolerated by infants, they found wide acceptance even when there was no specific need for them. Some vegan families prefer soy formula to avoid the feeding of animal products.

Milks and Formulas in Special Medical Situations
Premature Infants (Preterms)
In the early 20th century, pulmonary immaturity and poor thermoregulation were the immediate threats to the survival of premature infants. As progress was made in supportive care, including use of oxygen, ventilators, and incubators, attention could shift to the nutritional needs of the infants. The unique nutrient requirements of preterm infants are complicated by immaturity of the gastrointestinal tract, with variable digestive and absorptive function depending on the degree of prematurity (see Figure 2.2). Immaturity of the gastrointestinal tract includes impaired ability to suck and swallow, reduced gut motility, malabsorption, and susceptibility to necrotizing enterocolitis (NEC) and septicemia. Special feeding techniques that address these concerns include the temporary use of parenteral nutrition (feeding of nutrient solutions directly into the circulating blood, usually by a vein),

enteral feedings (feeding into the stomach or upper intestine via a tube) and non-nutritive sucking to support development of sucking and swallowing skills.

Composition of feedings provided via enteral feedings or bottles must meet the high nutrient needs of premature infants for energy, protein, and micronutrients. Breast milk is the feeding of choice for preterm infants. Compared to infant formulas, human milk is protective against NEC and septicemia. When milk from the infant's mother is not available or insufficient in amount, donated milk can be used. Large nurseries may set up milk banks that pool milk from multiple donors and pasteurize it, thus producing human milk for infants lacking their mothers' own milk. Where such systems are set up, few preterm infants are deprived of the benefits provided by human milk.

Unfortunately, unmodified human milk, whether the mother's own or donated milk, is inadequate to meet the increased nutrient needs of small, rapidly growing preterm infants. Fortifiers to be added to human milk have been developed and are commercially available. Breast milk fortifiers add the additional protein, energy, minerals, and vitamins required for healthy growth of small preterm infants. They are available in powder or liquid form.

Historically, the increased nutrient needs of preterm infants were recognized before the special immunologic needs, leading to the development of formulas specially designed to meet nutrient needs of preterm infants. When human milk is not available, preterm formulas are fed rather than formula designed for term infants. Preterm formulas have increased protein, energy, and minerals compared to formulas for term infants. Use of these formulas supported adequate growth of these infants; however, they did not protect infants from septicemia and NEC.

Formulas for Infants With Metabolic Diseases

Metabolic diseases were discussed in Chapter 2; here we describe formulas to treat them. It is now possible to manufacture milks that contain no intact proteins but instead are based on protein hydrolysates or on free amino acids. Formulas based on free amino acids can also be manufactured to omit one or more amino acids. Thus, formulas devoid of phenylalanine were developed for infants born with the metabolic defect phenylketonuria (PKU), because these infants cannot metabolize the amino acid phenylalanine. The availability of these formulas revolutionized the management of infants and children with PKU. Formulas devoid of other amino acids have been designed specifically for other metabolic diseases. Suppliers of such formulas typically produce 12–15 variants to fit the needs of the wide range of deficits in metabolism. Formula with no lactose is critical for management of galactosemia; this need is often met with soy-based formulas that contain glucose polymers or sucrose instead of lactose.

Formulas for Gastrointestinal Illnesses

Several disorders of the gut can impair the infant's ability to use the nutrients in standard feedings including breast milk. Severe infectious gastroenteritis, especially in the setting of preexisting malnutrition, can damage the absorptive surface of the intestine, reducing the ability to absorb carbohydrates and fats. Disorders of the pancreas also can decrease production of enzymes necessary for fat and protein digestion, with resulting malabsorption. Formulas containing only medium-chain triglycerides (MCTs) as fat are useful in the management of infants lacking pancreatic lipases because the MCTs can be directly absorbed without digestion by lipase. Other specialized formulas were developed for infants with obvious malabsorptive states, even before the pathophysiologic basis was fully understood. Some examples of formulas commercially produced in the past include meat-based and banana-based formulas, which are now medical curiosities. In some areas of the world, however, meat-based formulas have at least some continued use as a way of providing a more affordable formula for infants with severe allergy or intolerance to cow's milk proteins.

Historically, much of the attention paid to malabsorption was particularly related to infectious gastroenteritis. The development of formulas with carbohydrates other than lactose allowed feeding of these infants when lactase deficiency from mucosal injury was significant. Medical opinion on the need for such feedings has varied over the decades, with some physicians still routinely recommending temporary use of a lactose-free formula during and after gastroenteritis; however, analyses of other experts have concluded routine avoidance of lactose is not necessary (Brown).

Formulas for Allergy to Milk

Disorders with intolerance to cow's milk and other foods are well known and can have multiple causes (see Chapter 8). Among these are true allergy to cow's milk in some infants and children. Prior to the development of commercial formula that had no cow's milk, only inadequate homemade substitutes might be created, generally with inadequate protein. Early commercial formulas were sold that employed either meat proteins, as noted above, or vegetable sources of protein, such as wheat, oats, or soy. Soy flour was used to produce commercial formulas for this purpose by the 1930s; however, these early products contained nondigestible, complex carbohydrates in soy flour that impair calcium absorption. By the 1960s soy formula had been reformulated using isolated soy protein, producing a formula that was not expensive, was generally well-tolerated, and supported growth. Not all infants with milk allergy can tolerate soy formula. In particular, infants with isolated gut symptoms related to milk allergy are less likely to tolerate soy protein. Methods were standardized in the 1940s to hydrolyze (digest) bovine casein, producing a mixture of small fragments and free amino acids that a great majority of milk-allergic infants will tolerate. As mentioned in a previous section, formulas with only free amino acids and no intact protein have also been used to treat cow's milk allergy.

Not all approaches to nutrition for milk-allergic infants have been successful. For several common food allergies, there has been interest in genetic modification of the responsible protein to reduce or eliminate the amino acid sequences within the protein that are recognized by the immune system. A large number of plants and animals have now been bioengineered to eliminate or modify proteins that are known food allergens, with the possible use for management of food allergy (Jutel). One example is the bioengineering of cows that produce no β-lactoglobulin, a protein absent from human milk and a frequent allergen (Chapter 8 and Appendix A-2). Unfortunately, almost all allergenic food proteins induce antibodies or T cell responses to multiple regions (epitopes) of the molecule. For several food allergens, such as milk proteins and peanut proteins, the allergic immune reaction usually reflects recognition by the immune system of more than one protein, and more than one epitope on several proteins. Thus, the genetic modifications might need to address an unmanageable number of proteins and epitopes to be non-allergenic in nearly all people. Some attempted modifications have also been incompatible with normal growth of modified plants.

Consequences of Using Infant Formulas
Short-Term Versus Long-Term Issues
In the short term, the feeding of formula produces differences in stool consistency and increases flatulence, both of which fall into the category of nuisance. One clear advantage of formula use is the ease by which third parties, such as other family members, can take over feeding if the mother is temporarily or permanently unable to breastfeed. Also in the short term, formula feeding usually leads to more rapid weight gain than breast-feeding. The difference in weight gain is not marked but has been seen in numerous studies. The slightly lower weight gain in breastfed infants is not associated with any adverse consequences but instead is hypothesized to be beneficially related to positive health outcomes later in childhood (Dewey).

As noted in Chapter 3, there are multiple lines of evidence suggesting short- and long-term advantages to breast-feeding instead of formula feeding. We will not repeat that information here but only note that good data supports the protective effect of breast-feeding against multiple infectious diseases in the first 3 to 5 years of life, and data also suggests a decrease of allergic disease and asthma. There continues to be debate in the field as the data are usually observational, an issue discussed in Chapters 7 and 8.

Why Might Immune-Related Maladies Be Associated With Formula Feeding?
As described earlier, the substitution of formula feeding for breast-feeding is correlated with several disorders, all of which seem to have an immunological component. Most immunological disorders are a consequence of immune dysregulation, such as lupus, rheumatoid arthritis, myasthenia gravis, and certain forms of diabetes (Chapter 5 and Chapter 6). Inflammatory bowel disease (IBD) is a multifactorial illness involving the immune system (Chapter 6) and the microbiome (Chapter 5). Here we speculate on the mechanisms that might connect immune disorders to replacement of breast-feeding by formula feeding.

We first focus on immune regulators in colostrum, since infants exclusively reared on formula would be denied access to these immune and growth regulators. At least 30 cytokines and chemokines are active in the mammary gland and 18 of these are found in the whey of human, pig, and cow milk (Dawod; Ramirez-Santana). As we describe in Chapter 6, these are chemical messengers that act between cells. Especially noteworthy is TGFβ, which is present at high levels in human colostrum, so that with a daily consumption of 700 ml, about 125 mg of active TGFβ goes to the infant's gastrointestinal (GI) tract. The GI tract bears receptors for this cytokine, which promotes development of the intestinal mucosa. TGFβ also modulates the activities of T cells, converting them from inflammatory T cells to so-called suppressor T cells (Tregs) that dampen local immune responsiveness. Cytokines, unlike immunoglobulins, can be inactivated by pasteurization and storage, although their concentrations may not be altered. (Ramirez-Santana). Although the cytokines involved were not identified, bovine colostrum frozen for 48 hours at −20 °C (normal freezer temp) lost its ability to suppress the synthesis of IgM, IgA, and IgG in cesarean-derived piglets reared in isolator units (Figure 3.6). Compared to inflammatory cytokines, the level of TGFβ as well as IL-10 (both immunosuppressive cytokines) significantly decreases in mature milk compared to colostrum (Trend). This might explain why breast-feeding with fresh colostrum may dampen the infant's ability to mount an immune response to foreign proteins (in the experiment described, bovine milk proteins). While not documented in the piglet study, it is reasonable to hypothesize that synthesis of IgE, the antibody responsible for type I allergy, would also be suppressed. About 3% of infants have type I allergy to milk proteins.

In addition to immune regulators, colostrum also contains epithelial growth factor (EGF); it is present at greater than 1500 ng/ml in porcine and human colostrum. EGF is necessary for the proper development of the GI tract epithelium and increases lactase and sucrase activity. Insulin-like growth factor (IGF) stimulates enzyme activity and growth of enterocytes. Colony-stimulating factor (CSF) also contributes to proper development of the GI tract epithelium (Figure 2.2). In Chapter 3 we described human milk oligosaccharides (HMOs), the third-most abundant ingredient in human milk. These complex carbohydrates are metabolized by certain bacteria of the microbiome (Chapter 5), generating short-chain fatty acids (SCFA) that are needed for development of the tight junctions between enterocytes. Tight junction integrity prevents the unrestricted passage of intact food protein and bacteria. It seems that all four of these substances aid the natural development of the GI tract. It is the disturbance of this barrier that is a feature of IBD and NEC. Combine this damage with the loss or suppression of inflammatory T cells and antibody synthesis, and you have something of a "perfect storm." In certain types of IBD, members of the microbiome are also involved, because of the disturbed epithelial barrier (Chapter 5). NEC is almost entirely limited to preterm infants and is much less frequent in breastfed infants.

Another factor that can contribute to maladies correlated with formula feeding is the absence of protective SIgA antibodies. Analyses of infant stool samples show that approximately 60% of bacteria recovered have SIgA bound to their surface (Figure 6.6). Levels are higher in the small intestine than in the colon (Bunker). While some may be SIgA specific to epitopes of the bacteria, the majority appear attached through glycan moieties, which are present on the secretory component (Perrier; Chapter 3; Table A3.1; Figure 6.6). Regardless of the mechanism of attachment, bacteria are removed from the GI tract. If those removed are predominately disease associated (eg, Proteobacteria; Chapter 5) this might reduce the level of enteric infection, which in turn would reduce damage to the gut epithelium that could be the cause of the enterocolitis and sepsis associated with NEC.

In Chapter 6, we review the so-called hygiene hypothesis, which posits that infants and children exposed early in life to many microorganisms and potential allergens have a lower frequency of allergy later in life. The evidence from actual clinical trials of early peanut feeding is so compelling that the AAP has recommended early exposure of infants to peanut allergens to reduce the frequency and severity of peanut allergy later in life. This observation suggests that other mechanisms are also at play that are independent of breast-feeding. The only way to bridge these two observations is to observe that newborns benefit from the regulatory factors provided through breast milk in the same window of time that exposure to potential allergens occurs.

Parents and students in the medical professions should be aware of the complexity of events that occur within the Critical Window and appreciate their multifactorial elements. The direct study of human infants is unlikely to resolve all the problems associated with neonatal development since ethical constraints prevent many studies and the genetics of human populations are too varied for focused studies even if ethical. For that reason we include Appendix A-2, which describes the use of other mammals as experimental models to address such issues.

Infant Formula Changes Over Time
Composition and Regulation

Infant formulas have evolved considerably in the 100 years of their commercial availability. Over the last 50 years, intense interest at national and global levels has led to multiple guidelines from specialty societies and regulations from national governments concerning the composition of infant formulas. Table 4.2 outlines the current formula requirements for macronutrients from the European Union Commission (EU Commission), the US Food and Drug Administration (FDA), and Codex Alimentarius (CODEX, the food standards developer for the World Health Organization and the Food and Agriculture Organization of the United Nations). Most countries either directly adopt one of these schemes or heavily draw upon them to set national guidelines. As you can see, these independent organizations have generally similar guidelines for formula for term infants. There are differences in the precise amounts of nutrients allowed, and in the distribution of calories among fat, carbohydrate, and protein, but all three are in similar ranges. Protein

TABLE 4.2 Macronutrient Compositional Requirements for Formula for Healthy Infants as Specified by Regulation (US FDA and the EU Commission) and the Recommendations of CODEX

The US regulation applies to formulas sold for infants age 0–12 months. The EU and CODEX listings are for formulas intended for age 0–6 months. All values are quantity per 100 kcal of prepared formula, except energy, which is kcal per 100 ml.

		US FDA Regulation		EU Commission Regulation		CODEX	
		min	max	min	max	min	max
Energy (per 100 ml)		not specified[2]		60 kcal	70 kcal	60 kcal	70 kcal
Protein		1.8 g	4.5 g	1.8 g	2.5 g	1.8 g	3.0 g
Fat	Total fat	3.3 g[1]	6 g[1]	4.4 g	6.0 g	4.4 g	6.0 g
	Linoleic acid	300 mg		500 mg	1,200 mg	300 mg	1,400 mg
	Alpha-linolenic acid	not specified		50 mg	100 mg	50 mg	not specified
	DHA	not specified		20 mg	50 mg		
Carbohydrate		not specified		9 g	14 g	9 g	14 g

[1] US regulations require fat to be at least 30% but not more than 54% of total calories.
[2] US law supporting the regulations does not specify energy range; the FDA allows roughly 60–70 kcal/100mL.

content may be the most variable of the mandated components, for reasons discussed next. Table 4.3 similarly shows the standards for micronutrients (vitamins and minerals). For those seeking more detailed information, the US and EU regulations are available online (FDA, SR; EU, SR).

Globally, most infant formulas are manufactured by multinational corporations (Nestlé, Mead Johnson, Danone, Abbott Nutrition, Friesland Campina, Kraft Heinz, HiPP, Arla, and a few others). All manufacturers must rigorously follow the regulations for formula in the countries in which they intend to sell it. Table 4.4 shows the content of some representative infant formulas intended for the first 6 months of life (or beyond). Some countries also have many smaller national or subnational (regional) manufacturers (eg, China and India). Vigilance by regulators is generally high, perhaps driven by memories of adverse events within the last few decades. An example of such an event is the production of a chloride-deficient formula in the United States in the 1970s, with resultant injury to some infants, that led to legislation that defines formula composition in the United States. In China in 2008, the falsification of protein content in a few formulas by the addition of melamine was responsible for severe injury to affected infants. The Chinese experience also led to closer regulatory scrutiny of manufacturing practices and quality, particularly for the several hundred small-scale companies. A recent recall of formula in the United States because of possible bacterial contamination (see Chapter 7) demonstrates that the appropriate means

TABLE 4.3 Micronutrient Compositional Requirements for Formula for Healthy Infants as Specified by Regulation (US FDA and the EU Commission) and the Recommendations of CODEX

The US regulation defines formulas sold for infants aged 0–12 months. The EU and CODEX listings are for formulas intended for 0–6 months. The listings vary for form of folate and units for Vitamins A and D, as shown in the table footnotes.

	US FDA Regulation		EU Commission Regulation		CODEX	
	min	max	min	max	min	max
Vitamins						
Vitamin A[1]	250 IU	750 IU	70 mcg	114 mcg	60 mcg RE	180 mcg RE
Vitamin D[2]	40 I.U.	100 IU	2 mcg	3 mcg	1 mcg	2.5 mcg
Vitamin E	0.7 mcg		0.6 mg	5 mg	0.5 mg	5 mg
Vitamin K	4 mcg		1 mcg	25 mcg	4 mcg	27 mcg
Thiamine	40 mcg		40 mcg	300 mcg	60 mcg	300 mcg
Riboflavin	60 mcg		60 mcg	400 mcg	80 mcg	500 mcg
Vitamin B6	35 mcg		20 mcg	175 mcg	35 mcg	175 mcg
Vitamin B12	0.12 mcg		0.1 mcg	1.5 mcg	0.1 mcg	1.5 mcg
Niacin	250 mcg		400 mcg	1,500 mcg	300 mcg	1500 mcg
Folic Acid[3]	4 mcg		15 mcg	47.6 mcg	10 mcg	50 mcg
Minerals						
Sodium	20 mg	60 mg	25 mg	60 mg	20 mg	60 mg
Potassium	80 mg	100 mg	80 mg	160 mg	60 mg	180 mg
Chloride	80 mg	200 mg	60 mg	160 mg	50 mg	160 mg
Calcium	60 mg		50 mg	140 mg	50 mg	140 mg
Phosphorus	30 mg		25 mg	90 mg	25 mg	100 mg
Magnesium	6 mg		5 mg	15 mg	5 mg	15 mg
Iron	0.15 mg	3.0 mg	0.6 mg	2 mg	0.45 mg	
Zinc	0.5 mg		0.5 mg	1 mg	0.5 mg	1.5 mg

[1] Vitamin A: 1 IU = 1 mcg retinol equivalent (RE) = 0.3 mcg
[2] Vitamin D: 1 IU = 0.025 mcg
[3] FDA and CODEX specify folic acid in micrograms (mcg). The EU folic acid requirement is specified as dietary folate equivalent (DFE): 1 µg DFE = 1 µg food folate = 0.6 µg folic acid from formula.

of maintaining bacteriologic safety of the formula is not always self-evident, especially for powdered formulas, as they cannot be manufactured with guaranteed sterility.

The nutrient needs of the infant are not constant but instead change over time, with protein and mineral needs (per unit body weight) slowly decreasing as the growth rate of the infant slows. It is difficult for formulas to mimic these changes in nutrient needs. Hence,

TABLE 4.4 Composition of Some Infant Formulas in the United States, Europe, and Asia, Illustrating the Application of the Guidelines

Inclusion here does not imply endorsement by the authors. Units noted are for 100 kcal of prepared formula, except for the Energy row, which shows kcal for 100 ml of prepared formula. Data reflects online sources or labels as of 2021.

		Holle Stage 1 Organic (EU)	Similac Advance (US)	Enfamil Neuro-Pro Infant (US)	Good Start Gentle (US)	Mamil 1 (Singapore)	Nan Optipro (UK)
Energy	kcal per 100 ml	67 kcal	67 kcal	67 kcal	67 kcal	67 kcal	67 kcal
	Nutrient concentration	per 100 kcal	per 100 kcal	per 100 kcal	per 100 kcal	per 100 kcal	per 100 kcal
Protein	g	2.09	2.07	2	2.1	2.1	2.03
Total Fat	g	5.07	5.6	5.3	5.1	5.2	5.6
Carbohydrate	g	11.47	10.7	11.3	11.4	10.4	11.5
Vitamins							
Vitamin A	mcg	87.76	90	90	90	86	106
Vitamin D	mcg	2.08	1.88	1.88	1.63	1	1.4
Vitamin E	mcg	2.53	1.07	1.34	1.34	2.8	1.7
Vitamin K	mcg	9.39	8	9	8	8.3	8.7
Thiamine	mcg	96.6	100	80	100	77	117
Riboflavin	mcg	268.2	160	140	140	200	214
Vitamin B6	mcg	83	63	60	75	73	81
Vitamin B12	mcg	0.3	0.26	0.3	0.33	0.45	0.3
Niacin	mcg	671	1100	1000	1050	717	936
Minerals							
Sodium	mg	42	25	27	27	27	27
Potassium	mg	117	110	108	108	88	106
Chloride	mg	78	68	63	65	57	73
Calcium	mg	83	82	78	67	58	67
Phosphorus	mg	49	44	43	38	36	37
Magnesium	mg	8	6	8	7	6.9	8.9
Iron	mg	0.8	1.9	1.8	1.5	0.9	1.1
Zinc	mg	0.66	0.79	1	0.8	0.75	1.1

nutrients are provided in excess of actual needs. Until recently formulas provided protein at approximately 2.3 g/100 kcal, which covered the needs of the very young infant, when the needs are highest, plus an excess to make up for presumed lower quality of formula protein. With the quality of formula protein now similar to that of human milk, the protein content of typical formulas has recently been lowered to the range of 1.92–2.0 g/100 kcal. That change still provides an excess of protein intake for infants older than 2 months, but the excess is certainly less than with earlier formulas. Follow-up studies have provided evidence that an excess of protein intake during infancy is associated with obesity in childhood and in later life, again supporting minimizing excess protein intake from formula (Arenz).

Recently Proposed Additions to Infant Formula

Nutrition investigators have produced evidence for (and against) the importance of several other components now sometimes added to infant formula. Among these are the following: the long-chain polyunsaturated fatty acids DHA (docosahexaenoic acid) and arachidonic acid; oligosaccharides identical to some of the more than 150 known HMOs; milk fat globule membranes; and lactoferrin (see Chapter 3). Formulas designed for preterm infants provide an example of this practice. For most of these components, there is not a consensus among nutrition experts on the necessity of their inclusion in formula. The published studies on these potential components of formula often have limitations that prevent enthusiastic adoption. The limitations include small study size, confounding by multiple variables, lack of confirmatory trials, and uncertainty as to whether the reported outcomes were indeed declared *a priori*, or determined after the fact. In Chapter 7 we will discuss issues of study design and strength. A number of other nutrients are often added to formulas, subject to upper limits by several regulatory and advisory bodies such as the EU Commission and CODEX. These nutrients are generally added because they are present in breast milk, but some do not have strong evidence of harm if omitted. Examples include inositol, choline, taurine, selenium, copper, manganese, iodine, and nucleotides. A full discussion of all these is beyond the scope of this book, but discussions can easily be found at pubmed.gov.

Among the components cited earlier, DHA is the longest studied and used. A few polyunsaturated fatty acids have long been known to be essential in the human diet; that is, they cannot be produced in the body from precursors but must be consumed by humans to avoid deficiency. Thus, content of the essential fatty acids alpha-linolenic acid (ALA) and linoleic acid are specified by the EU Commission and Codex. US law only specifies a minimum content for linoleic acid. Some regulatory and advisory bodies mandate inclusion of DHA in formula, but not all do so. ALA is a precursor for the synthesis of DHA. Opinion is divided within the nutrition community as to whether term infants synthesize adequate DHA if their diet has sufficient ALA. DHA intake may be more critical for preterm infants, as their rapid growth gives rise to a need for DHA that appears to exceed the synthetic ability to provide it, for neural tissue in particular. Thus, most authorities advise adding DHA to formula intended for preterm infants. Data to establish the optimum concentrations of DHA and arachidonic acid in preterm feeding remain to be developed.

HMOs, described in Chapter 3, are the third-most prevalent by weight of the non-water components of human milk, which is quite different from the composition of most other species' milk, including bovine milk. The evolutionary pressure that produced this difference is not obvious, but the value of these compounds is strongly supported by epidemiologic studies by several groups. Five HMO compounds have been introduced into a few formulas around the world: 2'-FL (2'-fucosyllactose), LNnT (lacto-N-neotetraose), 3-FL (3-fucosyllactose), 3'-SL (3'-sialyllactose), and 6'-SL (6'-sialyllactose). Since available ruminant milks lack appreciable quantities of such oligosaccharides, these compounds are made by proprietary fermentation technology or chemical synthesis, and thus are not as readily available as many other formula components. Expert panels have not yet recommended routine inclusion of these oligosaccharides in infant formula, but some epidemiologic studies suggest that HMOs in breast milk benefit human immune function; limited human trials also support their addition to infant formula. In human milk, the total quantity of HMOs is in the range of 12–14 g/L, but due to the cost of the components, the level in formula is generally less than 1 g/L.

Fat in human and ruminant milks is provided as microscopic structures called milk fat globules (MFG, Figure 3.2). MFG are surrounded by the MFG membrane (MFGM), which contains components derived from mammary cell membranes. The MFGM also transports protein components to the infant. In human milk MFGM may deliver 1–4% of the total protein in the milk, with greater than 100 maternal proteins identified within them (Chapter 3). The MFG are viewed mainly as carriers of the milkfat, allowing micelles of fat to remain suspended in the aqueous milk rather than rapidly separating even before nursing removes the milk from the breast. In addition, MFG carry specialized lipid compounds that are not present in vegetable oils, including phospholipids, sphingolipids, and cholesterol (Chapter 3). Although there are some marketed formulas with bovine MFGM, there is not yet broad use in the industry.

Lactoferrin is a protein component present in higher concentration in human milk than bovine milk (Chapter 3). Its name reflects one of its earliest known attributes, that it binds and carries iron. It has multiple known functions in assorted biologic settings: as an anti-inflammatory, antioxidant, antimicrobial, iron binding, iron transfer, anticarcinogenic, and others. The multiple functions have led to multiple hypotheses of its importance in the growth and survival of human infants. The use of bovine lactoferrin in infant formulas is complicated by several factors. Firstly, sourcing is limiting as the concentration in bovine milk is on the order of 1–2% of that in human milk. Recombinant human lactoferrin expressed in plant systems has been produced but is likely to present cost hurdles. Secondly, lactoferrin is denatured at temperatures commonly used in the production of sterile liquid products and may be denatured at temperatures used in the spray-drying process used to produce powdered infant formula. Thirdly, clinical trials of its effect in infants have often been complicated by the presence of confounding factors, such as trials with multiple novel components compared to formula lacking the same multiple components. Clinical trials in premature infants suggest a preventive effect against sepsis and NEC. The trials, however, have been generally small and sometimes included confounding factors. A large, pharmaceutical grade, definitive trial has not been performed. For full-term infants, proof of the importance of lactoferrin is less compelling, but suggestive trials do exist.

Conclusions

Infant formulas have evolved markedly in the hundred years of their commercial existence. Manufacturers continue to compete to deliver the formula best suited to meet the needs of the infant and to approach the outcomes of breast-feeding. It should be obvious that all components of human milk cannot be added to formula, but marginal improvements are still possible. Formula manufactured in accordance with high global standards and reconstituted with clean, safe water is of low risk, but especially in settings of the developing world, it is not equivalent to human milk in outcomes.

Suggested Readings (SR)

EU formula regulation (annexes at end contain formulation requirements): www.legislation.gov.uk/eur/2016/127/contents

FDA regulations for formula: CFR-2021-title21-vol2-part107.pdf

Fomon SJ. Infant feeding in the 20th century: Formula and beikost. *J Nutr.* 2002;131:409S–420S. doi:10.1093/jn/131.2.409S.

Stevens EE. A history of infant feeding. *J Perinat Educ.* 2009;18:32-39. doi: 10.1624/105812409X426314.

USDA formula feeding analysis: https://nesr.usda.gov/infant-milk-feeding-practices-technical-expert-collaborative

Wargo WF. A history of infant formula; quality, safety and standard methods. *Jour AOAC International* 99. 2016;99:7-11. doi:10.5740/jaoacint.15-0244.

References

Arenz S, Rückerl R, Koletzko B, et al. Breast-feeding and childhood obesity—a systematic review. *Int J Obes.* 2004;28:1247–1256. doi:10.1038/sj.ijo.0802758.

Brown KH. Dietary management of acute diarrheal disease: Contemporary scientific issues. *J Nutr.* 1994;124:1455S-1460S. doi.org/10.1093/jn/124.suppl_8.1455S.

Bunker JJ, Flynn TM, Koval JC, et al. Innate and adaptive humoral responses coat distinct commensal bacteria with immunoglobulin A. *Immunity.* 2015;43:541–553.

Dawod B, Marshall JS. Cytokines and soluble receptors in breast milk as enhancers of oral tolerance development. *Front Immunol.* 2019;10:16. doi:10:3389/fimmu.2019.00016.

Dewey, KG. Growth characteristics of breast-fed compared to formula-fed infants. *Biol Neonate.* 1998;74:94–105.

Jutel M, Solarewicz-Madejek K, Smolinska S. Recombinant allergens. *Hum Vaccin Immunother.* 2012;8:1534–1543. doi:10.4161/hv.22064.

Perrier C, Sprenger N, Corthesy B. Glycans on secretory component participate in innate protection against mucosal pathogens. *J Biol Chem.* 2006; 81:14280–14287.

Ramirez-Santana C, Pérez-Cano FJ, Audí C, et al. Effect of cooling and freezing storage on the stability of bioactive factors in human colostrum. *J Dairy Sci.* 2012;95:2319–2325.

Trend S, Strunk T, Lloyd ML, et al. Level of innate immune factors in preterm and term mothers breast milk during the 1st month postpartum. *Br J Nutr.* 2016;115:1178–1193.

"A Little Help From Our Little Friends"

Establishment of the Microbiome and Constituency in Health and Disease

LEARNING OBJECTIVES (SECTION I)

1. Describe the different ways that the GI tract microbiome contributes to human health.

2. Review features of bacteria (phyla or species) that constitute a healthy GI tract microbiome.

3. Explore how cultural behavior and ethnic differences influence the gut microbiome.

4. Describe changes to the gut microbiome when vaginally born neonates transition to adults.

5. What factors contribute to dysbiosis, and how can these negative influences be controlled?

The Microbiome: Posterchild of Life's Interdependence

The study of infectious diseases in the 20th century taught the public to avoid bacteria because of their connection to illness. However, especially the last 2 decades, the millions of bacteria found everywhere in the human body are being viewed as essential symbionts, needed for healthy nutrition and at the same time providing a barrier to disease-causing microbes. Global health and proper nutrition is dependent on the microbiome (Gordon). The interdependence of bacteria and eukaryotes is one of the best examples of symbiosis on planet Earth. Termites, cockroaches, many other invertebrates, and ruminant mammals are totally dependent on symbiotic bacteria in their gut for nutrition and survival. The rumen, one of the "four stomachs" of cattle and other ruminant mammals, is a bacterial fermentation center for converting cellulose and other plant fibers into nutrients for their mobile hosts. Such bacteria are referred to as *symbionts* or *mutualists*, since both the host and the bacteria benefit. Bacteria that cause no harm that reside in the gastrointestinal tract (GI tract) are referred to as *commensals*, but they are also mutualists. The relationship between mammals and their microbiome is a co-evolutionary event that has led to a situation in which humans harbor more than 10^{12} bacteria, which amounts to more than 10 bacteria for each cell in the body. A much higher ratio is seen in the GI tract. These comprise > 1,000 species with at least 160 species per individual. Two phyla, Firmicutes and Bacteriodetes, account for approximately 90% of the healthy GI tract microbiome (Table 5.1; Powers, SR). It is understandable that such complexity has hindered studies on this complex ecosystem, but in the last 2 decades this has been aided by 16S mRNA sequencing (Milani, SR; Appendix A-1). Given ethnic, geographic, and dietary differences among humans, discrepancies among studies should not be surprising. In this chapter, we present a summary of major findings to arrive at several concepts regarding the role and establishment of the microbiome. The role of the microbiome in the health of the neonate is discussed by Brodin (SR).

Important to know is that while bacteria-free mouse pups and piglets can grow and remain healthy in germ-free isolators, their weight gain is 50% less than conventional pups and piglets. Furthermore, these animals die if moved to a conventional environment. A similar outcome occurs with cesarean-derived piglets reared in so-called autosows on bovine

TABLE 5.1   Distribution of Major Phyla in Healthy and Non-Healthy Individuals

Healthy (Eubiotic): A population of 10^{12} bacteria of at least 1,000 species and belonging to four major phyla, the majority (90%) of which are obligate or facultative anaerobes (eg, Bacteriodetes and Firmicutes). A number of bacteria from the genus *Clostridium* are strict anaerobes.

Unhealthy (Dysbiotic): A low diversity (ie, less than 300 species) and an increase in the Proteobacteria and in the Firmicutes to Bacteriodete ratio (from 0.5 to 1.6). Some Firmicutes like *Clostridium* and *Strepococci* can become pathogens.

Phylum	Metabolism	Principal Genera	Mouth	Proportion (%) Healthy GI Tract	Unhealthy GI Tract
Actinobacteria	Facultative anaerobes	*Bifidobacteria* *Actinomyces*	> 10	1	5
Firmicutes	Facultative anaerobes	*Clostridium* *Enterococcus* *Streptococcus* *Lactobacillus*	40	30	40
Proteobacteria	Facultative anaerobes	*E. coli* *Salmonella* *Yersinia* *Shigella*	25	6	30
Bacteriodetes	Gram-negative anaerobes	*Bacteriodes* *Prevotella* *Fusobacterium* *Ruminococcus* *Faecalibacteria*	25	63	25

colostrum (Appendix A-2) then transferred to enclosures containing naturally reared piglets. Natural vaginal birthing combined with breast-feeding (VgBF; Figure 5.2) permits newborn mammals to obtain their mother's bacterial flora or microbiome, which is necessary for their healthy survival and proper weight gain. In developed countries, this natural pattern can be disrupted by an alteration in the uterine microbiome, C-section delivery, induced preterm delivery, the switch to infant formulas, and antibiotic therapy. The core GI tract microbiome that develops in VgBF infants is exclusively obtained from the mother, but it changes with age and development (Figure 5.1). Especially relevant are changes that occur with aging; the aged portion of the population has increased and is more vulnerable to disease (Biagi).

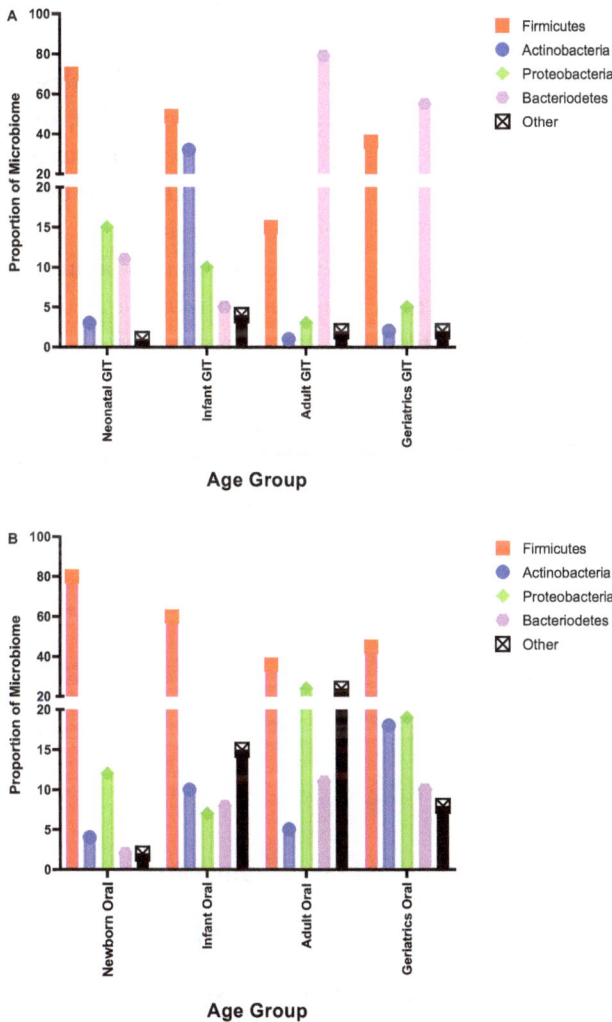

Figure 5.1   A. The constituency of the GI tract microbiome at various stages of life. B. Comparison of the oral microbiome at different stages of life.

Actinobacteria represented by *Bifidobacterium* (see next section and Table 5.1) are highly represented in breastfed infants but become a minor genus in adults, whose GI tract is primarily comprised of Bacteriodetes and Firmicutes. The constituency of the microbiome in the oral cavity differs (Figure 5.1B), notably because of the persistence of Actinobacteria and the higher frequency of Proteobacteria and miscellaneous others combined with the lower contribution by anaerobic Bacteriodetes. The maternal origin of the infant's microbiome suggests that the health of the VgBF newborn's microbiome is likely to reflect that of its mother. Resilience is a feature of the microbiome unless it is perturbed by disease or use of antibiotics. The exact GI tract microbiome is unique to each individual and remains stable for at least 65 years (Jost) but may change during the geriatric period (Figure 5.1). A second feature is that its constituency is linked to long-term dietary patterns, which, as we describe later, differ among countries and cultures. Later described is the major rise in inflammatory diseases, such as various forms of IBD, which is correlated with industrialization and the change to a so-called Western diet that contains less fiber, grains, and fermented foods (kimchi, yogurt, etc.). Some report that healthy Africans who migrate to the United States often develop these inflammatory diseases upon dietary change. It is important that neonates establish a healthy microbiome and diets that maintain this microbiome be promoted. Pregnant mothers suffering from IBD or other conditions associated with an unhealthy microbiome can pass them on to their infants at birth. IBD is an umbrella syndrome of disorders. Altered microbiomes frequently harbor less mutualistic and more pathogenic

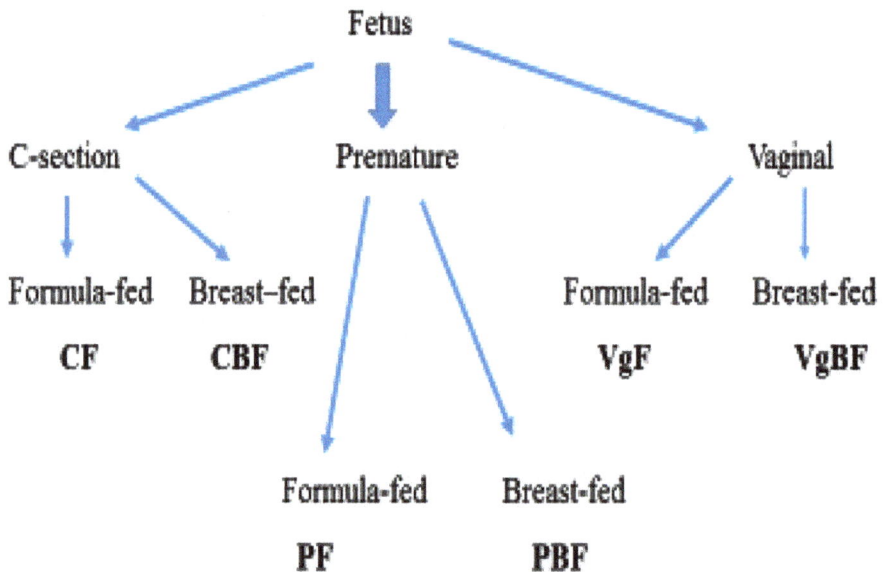

CBF includes those breastfed and those receiving stored of milk bank milk

Figure 5.2   Variations in birthing and infant feeding that affect the establishment of the microbiome. VgBF = vaginally born and breastfed, VgF = vaginally born and formula fed, CF = cesarian-derived and formula fed, CBF = cesarian-derived and fed stored human milk or milk bank milk, PF = preterm formula fed, PBF = preterm breastfed.

forms, a condition known as **dysbiosis**, which often correlates with disease. It is common to refer to "healthy/good" (**eubiotic**) and "unhealthy/bad" (**dysbiotic**) microbiomes. In this chapter the GI tract and vaginal microbiomes will be featured since they are major contributors to the infant's microbiome. Over 15,000 scientific articles on the microbiome appeared in 2019 alone, and the news, social media, TV, and Internet are anxious to link human health to features of the microbiome. However, these are often based on testimonials and correlation without causation (see Chapter 7). Nevertheless, we cite correlation studies, such as with autism spectrum disorder (ASD) but little information about the causative mechanisms is available. Considering the size and complexity of the microbiome, it is not surprising that medical science is only now beginning to learn about the importance of the microbial ecosystem to human health. A significant portion of what is known has been obtained using animal models, including germ-free rodents colonized with healthy and dysbiotic microbiomes. Information has also been gained using fecal microbial transplants (FMT). This chapter is not a substitute for a comprehensive undergraduate or graduate microbiology course. Our focus is primarily on teaching concepts involving microbes that establish and comprise the GI tract microbiome and are important for healthy neonatal growth and nutrition and contribute to internal protection.

A major focus of this book has been the maternal-fetal and maternal-neonatal connection and the transfer of passive immunity, immune regulators, pathogens, and nutrients. Because of this, we have emphasized the role of the gut microbiome in the process. However, microbiomes outside of the GI tract also play important roles in health and disease. Many wonder why certain individuals are more likely to attract female mosquitos seeking a blood meal to support their reproduction. This attraction extends beyond personal discomfort, since nearly half of the world is susceptible to mosquito-borne disease; malaria alone is responsible for 241 million infections and over 600,000 deaths each year worldwide. Mosquitos are attracted to a number of volatile amines and carboxylic acids (Benton; Obaldia). Some may arise from the skin microbiome, especially in the case of flaviviruses like Dengue and Zika, which infect approximately 400 million people each year. These viruses also alter the skin microbiome to favor *Bacilli* that release acetophenone-attracting substance (Guli).

Short Course in Bacteriology

Throughout this book, but especially in this chapter, we use terms common to the medical science community that may be foreign to the public and healthcare students with no previous training in microbiology. A number of these concern bacteria, including their classification and their family, generic, and species names. In Chapter 1, we described the three major life forms on planet Earth: Archaea, Eubacteria (or true bacteria), and the eukaryotes. We also mentioned the small noncellular forms such as viruses, viroids, and prions, which exist as cellular parasites on other life forms. These subcellular forms impact the GI tract microbiome. We mention diverse forms of true bacteria, the names of which often reflect their microscopic appearance in shape, colony structure, and constituency of their cell walls; oxygen dependence; and metabolism. Their diversity is illustrated by the fact that while all vertebrates from fish to primates belong to just one phylum (phylum Chordata) there are as many as 92 phyla of bacteria alone. Throughout this book less than half a dozen will be mentioned, and in discussing the GI tract microbiome we will primarily discuss only four phyla.

The many shapes taken by bacteria are often the reason for their names. Some occur as single small spheres called cocci, in pairs called diplococci, or in clusters called staphylococci. Others like bacilli (called rods) resemble bullets; those that are "curved rods" are called vibrios. Bacteria that grow in corkscrew form are called spirochetes. Some, like Actinobacteria, grow in a tangled web that resembles the mycelium of fungi. Thus, one such phylum is called Actinomyces (*myces* is the word for fungus). In the next chapter we describe the role that Actinomyces played in antibiotic therapy.

Early life forms existed in an oxygen-free Earth that favored the Archaea and some Eubacteria (Chapter 1). Some of their modern descendants, especially many that comprise the mature GI tract microbiome, do not require oxygen or are killed by it (obligate anaerobes). Certain others can "take it or leave it" (facultative anaerobes) while still others require oxygen (obligate aerobes). These different dependencies are important in understanding the establishment and maintenance of the GI tract microbiome and life's pyramid (Chapter 1).

We focus primarily on bacteria in phyla Proteobacteria, Firmicutes, Actinobacteria, and Bacteriodetes (Table 5.1). Phylum Proteobacteria includes a number of Gram-negative bacterial families that include pathogens that cause enteric diseases. The term *Gram* refers to a staining procedure developed by Christian Gram, which distinguishes bacterial groups based on the chemistry of their cell walls. Many Gram-negative bacteria belong to the family *Enterobacteriaceae* of phylum Proteobacteria that include genera like *Escherichia*, *Salmonella*, *Klebsiella*, *Shigella*, and *Yersinia*. The latter genus contains species responsible for the bubonic plague of the Middle Ages. Genus *Salmonella*, often mentioned in relation to food poisoning, is also the cause of typhoid fever, while *Shigella* causes dysentery and *Klebsiella* causes urinary and respiratory infection. Hence, high levels of Proteobacteria are associated with an "unhealthy" or dysbiotic microbiome (Table 5.1). However, a phylum or generic name may not always mean that every member of the phylum, family, or genus is a pathogen or a member of a dysbiotic community. Many *Escherichia coli* (*E. coli*) are harmless commensals. Some perform essential functions like making vitamin K and B12 and blocking colonization by pathogens and they have been used as probiotics in humans (Wassenaar). However, benign bacteria like commensal *E. coli* are well-known for their ability to receive new genetic information through horizontal gene transfer (HGT) using plasmids and other means that can transform a harmless *E. coli* into a pathogen (Appendix A-1). Examples include EHEC (enterohemorrhagic *E. coli*) and ETEC (enterotoxigenic *E. coli*). We collectively refer to the different forms of bacteria as taxa, which refer to differences in phylum, family, genus, and even species without needing a complete phylogenetic breakdown.

The distribution and diversity of human the human microbiome changes along the digestive tract in part due to the changing levels of oxygen and pH which favors/disfavors growth of certain bacteria (Table 5.2; Ritter). Highest oxygen levels are found in the mouth, which

TABLE 5.2

Organ	pH	pO2(%)	CFU/ml	SD	Percentage of Microbiome					
					Firmi	Fusob	Bacti	Actino	Proteo	Other
Mouth	6.5	100	log 3	log 1	32	16	27	7	16	tr
Esophagus	5.5	90	log 2	log 0.6	NA	NA	NA	NA	NA	NA
Stomach	2.0	60	log 2	log 0.4	42	7	9	8	30	—
Duodenum	4.0	15	log 3.5	log 1.5	45	10	15	5	24	1
Jejunum	6.2	8	log 5.5	log 1.8	NA	NA	NA	NA	NA	—
Ileum	7.0	10	log 6	log 2.5	50	3	29	2	14	—
Colon	6-7	12	log 11.5	log 2	55	4	31	1	8	2

Phylum abbreviations:
Firmi = Firmicutes; Fusob = Fusobacteria; Bacti = Bacteriodetes; Actino = Actinobacteria; Proteo =
Proteobacteria
Sources of Data: Vasapolli R, Schutte K, Schulz C, Vital M, Schomburg D, Pieper D H, Vilchez-Vargas
R, Malfertheiner P. Analysus if transcriptionally active bacteria throughout the gastrointestinal tract
of healthy individuals. Gastroenterology *2018; 1081–1092*
Ritter P, Kohler C, von Ah U. Evaluation of the passage of Lactobacillus gasseri K7 and bifidobacteria
from the stomach to intestine using a single reactor model. BMC Microbiology *2009;9:87–96*

also displays the greatest microbial diversity in part because it offers an aerobic environment while anaerobic bacteria are favored by low oxygen levels in the bowel (Vasapolli). Bacterial concentrations are highest in the colon and 6–8 logs higher than in the ileum and duodenum (Table 5.2). Actinobacteria, especially important in establishment of a healthy infant microbiome (see later) are reduced to near trace amounts in the anaerobic environment of the lower GI tract (Table 5.2). The low pH in stomach is least favorable for colonization but occasionally harbor *Helicobacter pylori*, an organism associated with stomach ulcers (Raghavan). One can also distinguish between bacteria free in the gut lumen (the so-called digesta) and those attached to the gut mucosal epithelium, which some refer to as "border-dwellers." We may occasionally refer to such categories.

Role of the Bacteriophage

A sub-cellular life form that must be considered when discussing the GI tract microbiome are bacteriophages. Bacteriophages were described in Chapter 1 as viruses that infect bacteria. Because of the size of the GI tract microbiome, it should not be surprising that it harbors over 140,000 discrete phages (Camarillo-Guerrero). These play a role in regulating the activities of the GI tract microbiome. Bacteriophages are differently distributed among phyla and species and are associated with the geographical location/culture of the host. Bacteriophages play a role in shaping the constituency of the microbiome. They form different associations within the microbiome. *Prevotella* is associated with rural/traditional lifestyles, while *Bacteriodes* is associated with urban and Western lifestyles. Each is associated with separate bacteriophage clusters. The number of bacteriophage clusters in *Prevotella* in Africa, South America, and

Fiji is 10 times higher than in North America, Asia, Europe, and Australia, whereas the number of bacteriophage clusters found in *Bacteriodes* is 40 times higher in North America, Asia, Europe, and Australia. While much remains to be learned about how bacteriophages determine the constituency and activities of bacteria that comprise the microbiome, correlative data suggest that bacteriophages may influence the distribution of "good" bacteria (see next section) that in turn seem related to human lifestyle and diet. In the 1920s and 1930s, bacteriophage therapy was used to treat for various bacterial infections (see Chapter 6).

Bacteriophages are a major vehicle for what is called horizontal gene transfer (HGT). This often occurs among members of Proteobacteria like *E. coli* and *Salmonella*, which are responsible for several enteritic diseases. The mechanisms of HGT are described in Appendix A-1, and its relationship to antibiotic therapy is discussed in Chapter 6.

Role of Mucosal Fungi

The human GI tract is also colonized by fungi including 260 species (Yan). Mucosal associated fungi, called the mycobiome, can protect against bacterial colonization but also exacerbate IBD (Yan).

The GI Tract Microbiome: The Good, the Bad and the Ugly

The GI tract microbiome is the best studied and its constituent bacteria have been classified as "good/healthy" versus "bad/unhealthy," or **eubiosis** versus **dysbiosis**; this has been used as a benchmark for pathobiological studies. The human GI tract microbiome has approximately 10^{12} (1 trillion) members, but the role of most nonpathogenic members remains unknown. This is exacerbated since many of its members cannot be cultured and studied *in vitro* and are known only by their 16S mRNA profiles (Milani, SR). Accepting these limitations, some generalizations can be drawn, such as that members of the phylum Proteobacteria are considered "bad," or even ugly, because it includes families and genera that are pathogens of the GI tract (see next section). The dominant phylum in the healthy GI tract microbiome are the "good" Bacteriodetes, which includes the genera *Bacteriodes*, *Prevotella*, and *Fusobacteria*, and the Firmicutes, which include the genera *Lactobacillus* and *Ruminococcus* (Table 5.1). *Bifidobacteria*, phylum Actinobacteria, has a major presence in establishing the microbiome in newborns, and although "good," it comprises only a tiny portion of the mature healthy GI tract microbiome. Phylum Actinobacteria also includes *Actinomyces*, which is a pathogen of the oral cavity associated with dental caries and is considered unhealthy when it becomes part of the GI tract microbiome. As we cautioned above, classifying bacteria according to family or genus as "good" or "bad" can be misleading. Most *E. coli* are harmless commensals but some we describe in the next section are "bad actors." While the many species of *Clostridium* (phylum Firmicutes) account for a large portion of the healthy microbiome, some strains of *C. difficile* are dangerous pathogens often transmitted in a hospital setting, and in adults often following antibiotic therapy. Carriage is especially high in preterm and C-section infants, but inflammatory illness of the colon occurs less commonly than in adults. While never found in the GI tract microbiome, another "bad actor" is *Clostridium tetani*, a deadly pathogen for which an effective vaccine exists (Chapter 6). There are also C. *perfringens*, an organism responsible for gangrene, and *C. botulinum*, which produces a toxin that causes botulism, a major cause of food poisoning. Among the numerous commensals are *Streptococci* and *Enterococci*, but *S. pneumoniae* causes otitis media and pneumonia while *E. faecalis* is responsible for urinary infections, endocarditis, and other serious diseases.

There is an adage "The enemy cannot always be detected by the coat they wear or the color of their skin." Skin has its own unique microbiome, which includes one of the world's best-known bacteria, *Staphylococcus aureus*. It is a ubiquitous member of a group of skin commensals that also includes *Pseudomonas*. Both are examples of commensals that remain commensals if they "stay home"! However, any skin lesions allow these organisms to gain access to deeper tissues where they can produce serious infections. *S. aureus* levels are therefore elevated at sites of skin inflammation and also play a role in eczema, a common form of childhood allergy. *Pseudomonas* infections characterize burn patients and *S. aureus* infections are common in untreated abrasions and wounds. Some forms of *S. aureus* such as MRSA (methicillin-resistant *S. aureus*) are serious antibiotic-resistant pathogens that belong to the category some call the *resistome*, the name used for that portion of the microbiome that contains bacteria resistant to antibiotic therapy. The genes providing resistance are called *AR genes*, meaning antibiotic resistance.

While generic names have their limitations, Table 5.1 provides a useful guide for discussion of the GI tract microbiome, although both the oral and GI tract microbiome change with age, both in constituency and diversity (Figure 5.1). While Firmicutes dominate in newborns and infants, Bacteriodetes become dominant in the GI tract during adult life. *Bifidobacteria* (phylum Actinobacteria) is at a higher level in the GI tract of VgBF infants and Proteobacteria comprise a larger proportion of the GI tract in infants than in adults. Proteobacteria may be the second-most-abundant phylum of bacteria in newborns, but these typically give way to *Bifidobacteria* in VgBF infants (Figure 5.1A). Firmicutes dominate the oral cavity not only in infancy, but at all life stages, due to the presence of *Streptococcus mutans*, a potential cause of dental caries, and in the GI tract by beneficial species of the *Clostridium*.

Ethnic and Cultural Influences on Diet and Microbiome Diversity

The constituency of the GI tract microbiome differs among countries and cultures, suggesting it may be influenced by diet, behavior, the level of endemic pathogens, or even host genetics (Figure 5.3). Some studies indicate that Firmicutes are less well represented in the United States and India, whereas Bacteriodetes are prominent. Firmicutes are highly represented in Italy, Russia, Papua New Guinea, Tanzania, Venezuela, Malawi, and China. The elevated levels of Firmicutes could reflect a higher levels of endemic pathogens like certain *Streptococci* and *Staphylococci*, but it is more likely due to an expanded population of commensal *Enterococci*, *Clostridium*, Lactobacillus, and genera encouraged by a plant-based diet. Diets also influence the predominant Bacteriodetes genera. Individuals on vegan diets have a greater abundance of *Bacteriodes* and lower levels of *Prevotella*. In Papua New Guinea and several other countries, but not in India, the GI tract microbiome of adults resembles that of human infants in the United States, in which Firmicutes dominate. The GI tract microbiome of children in Burkina Faso resembles the healthy GI tract microbiome of adults in America and Europe but is low in *Bifidobacteria* (Figure 5.3). While this may reflect infants' early high-fiber diet, their microbiome may also be affected by access to breast milk. The level of *Bifidobacteria* in infants of different ethnic groups may also be related to the level and nature of human milk oligosaccharides (HMOs) in breast milk (Chapter 3). In Bangladesh and parts of India, where infants are almost exclusively breastfed, *Bifidobacteria* are dominant in suckling infants (Olin).

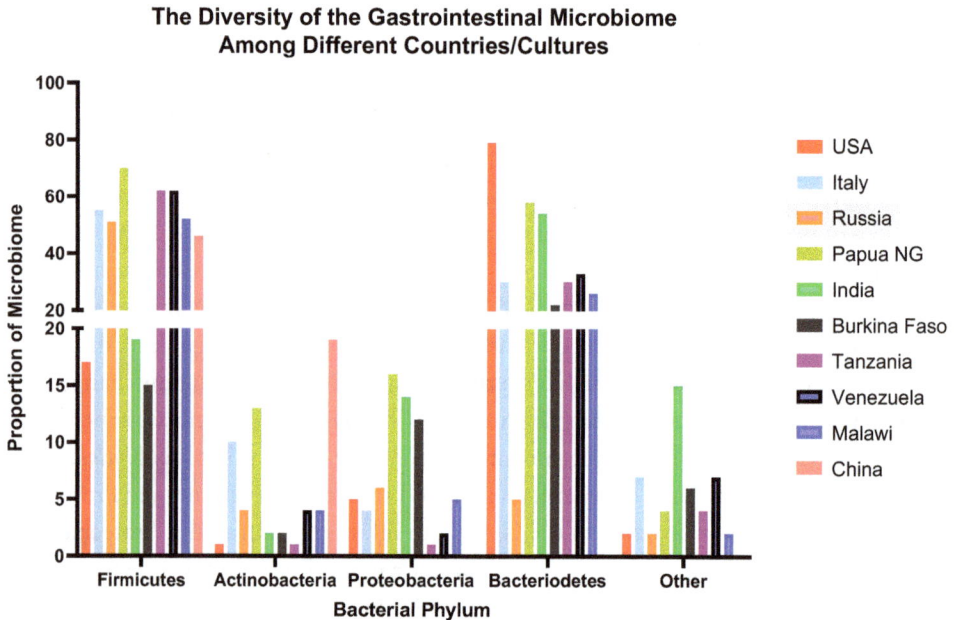

The Diversity of the Gastrointestinal Microbiome Among Different Countries/Cultures

Legend: USA, Italy, Russia, Papua NG, India, Burkina Faso, Tanzania, Venezuela, Malawi, China

Figure 5.3 Differences in the relative distribution of major phyla in the GI tract among a sampling of countries. The large standard deviations are not depicted.

Culture and ethnicity also affect diversity. An interesting study compared Indigenous groups from Venezuela and people in Malawi and the United States (St. Louis, Philadelphia, and Boulder, Colorado). While gut maturation in infants was similar in all three groups, the Indigenous people of Venezuela and residents of Malawi had hundreds more taxa in their GI tract microbiome (ie, higher diversity) than US residents. This difference was attributed to improved hygiene and sanitation in industrialized societies. However, the Indigenous Venezuelans survive without modern medicine on diets heavily dependent on plants, leading to the concept that species diversity means good health and low-level diversity correlates with disease (Yatsunenko). Short-term studies compared two different healthy diets, one high in fiber and the other high in fermented food (yogurt, kimchi, kombucha). The fermented food diet significantly increased the diversity of the microbiome and especially decreased immunological markers of inflammatory disease (Wastyk). Readers should remember that use of fermented foods, the persistence of "wet markets," or the making of hard sausage and salami originated during a period when refrigeration did not exist. Other studies indicate that diversity is not the sole criterion of health and may be an indicator of other factors such as diet. In a study of the Indigenous Tsimome people from Bolivia who live a subsistence lifestyle on a high-fiber and low-sugar diet, 85% of more than 700 individuals (mostly over age 60) had no coronary atherosclerosis, yet they carried a high inflammatory burden (Irima). Animal studies suggest that the inflammation that initiates the innate and adaptive response remodels the GI tract immune system, leading to protection from "the ugly" through **colonization resistance** (Gomez de Agüero).

LEARNING OBJECTIVES (SECTION II)

1. Identify mechanisms used by pathogenic gut microbes that explain their virulence.

2. Contrast the nature and origin of the microbiome of vaginally born and preterm infants.

The "Ugly" Challenge the GI Tract Epithelial Barrier

The wellness of the GI tract is dependent on how the bacteria of the GI tract microbiome interact with the enterocytes, sometimes called mucosal epithelial cells. The "good" members, like Bacteriodetes and most Firmicutes (Table 5.1), convert carbohydrates to short chain fatty acids (SCFA) that strengthen the tight junction between the enterocytes that are an essential barrier against invasion by the "ugly" Proteobacteria. "Good" bacteria also regulate healthy turnover and are involved in the maturation of GI tract epithelium and stimulate the production of mucus. Mucus aids in producing a barrier and butyrate (a SCFA) and up-regulates defensins (antimicrobial peptides). Enterocytes are armed with pattern recognition receptors (PRR; Chapter 6) that provide a "danger signal" to the host. Invading pathogens also face a gauntlet of innate factors like lysozyme, proteases, bile, and defensins. Newly introduced bacteria, like those in probiotics and pathogens, face obstacles collectively called **colonization resistance**; which, simply considered, is a "settler dispute" between these new entrants and bacteria already extant in the microbiome.

Colonization resistance is considered an important bulwark against pathogens that could violate the GI tract enterocyte barrier. Most members of the GI tract microbiome are harmless commensals that are not crucial for nutrition conversion but could be considered mutualists since their abundance and diversity plays a blocking role in colonization resistance.

Diversity is considered a feature of a healthy microbiome, which may explain the health of Indigenous people in Venezuela, while the lack of it in newborns, germ-free animals, and the geriatric population increases the risk of pathogens gaining a foothold (Figure 5.1A). Above and in other chapters, we have mentioned that there are ten bacteria for each human cell, but in the GI tract the ratio is higher and there are 10^{11} bacteria per millimeter in the large intestine or colon. Within this massive population pathogens are a small subset, which includes mostly Proteobacteria that possess tools to damage or breech the enterocyte barrier and displace commensals. At least three mechanisms explain their pathogenicity: (a) non-invasion mediated by toxins, (b) non-invasive bacteria that adhere to the enterocytes, and (c) truly invasive forms (Hurwitz). Examples of the first category are enterotoxigenic *E. coli* (ETEC) and *Vibrio cholera*, which first attach themselves to "receptors" on the enterocytes, often called **adhesion molecules**. Like mammals lacking a specific virus receptor, some mammals lack the appropriate adhesion molecules. Certain swine lack adhesion molecules, so ETEC is not pathogenic (Baker; Bosworth). This is a common theme for many microbial pathogens: no receptor means no infection. Enterohemorrhagic *E. coli* (EHEC), of which the 0157:H7 strain has caused several meat and produce recalls, adheres to adhesion receptors by a biochemically complex pilus. This adherence activates what microbiologists call the Type III secretion system that has numerous negative consequences, all of which cause diarrhea. The process also damages the enterocytes and allows release of what are called "Shiga-like toxins," the name derived from the enteric infection caused by *Shigella*, the cause of bloody dysentery. The second example is *V. cholerae*, which release cholera toxin, some of which is internalized by the enterocytes. The toxin causes voluminous secretion of liquid by the enterocytes, which results in dehydration and diarrhea and then allows the vibrio to contaminate the environment and increase the spread of the infection.

Another example of an enterocyte-pathogen interaction that violates the healthy GI tract epithelial barrier involves invasive pathogens that penetrate the enterocytes and gain access to deeper tissues of the host. This allows them to travel to many areas outside of the GI tract, a condition that can lead to septicemia. While some may be able to gain access through the tight junctions, others gain their entrance though M cells. These are cells that normally sample antigens from the gut lumen and are part of the mucosal immune system (Figure 6.6). These pathogens hijack the system and use it to breach the GI tract epithelial barrier. Typically, those entering in this manner are delivered to antigen-presenting cells (APCs), which stimulates an adaptive mucosal immune response (Chapter 6), but in the case of *Shigella*, pathogens trigger APCs to undergo apoptosis, thus thwarting the host's ability to mount an adaptive or innate immune response against the invader. Another feature exemplified by *Shigella* is called "cytoplasmic expulsion," which refers to the phenomenon in which *Shigella* becomes enclosed in endocytic vacuoles that are transferred and infect other cells. *Listeria* relies on a similar tactic, as does *Yersinia*, famous for the catastrophic Black Death of the Middle Ages.

We provide one more example of an invasive Proteobacteria. *Salmonella* are a diverse group of Gram-negative enteric pathogens that are also responsible for many foodborne illnesses. These include those responsible for typhoid fever (*S. typhi*). Like *Shigella*, *Salmonella* crosses the enterocyte barrier by inducing endocytosis. Once internalized, *Salmonella* stays within the APC and, rather than causing their apoptosis, uses the travelling APC (ie, macrophage), to distribute the bacteria from the site of entrance, which leads to septicemia.

In summary, while the commensal or "good" (eubiotic) members of the microbiome perform many activities that maintain a healthy and diverse microbiome, "bad" (dysbiotic) members, often belonging to phylum Proteobacteria, can exploit cracks in the armor of the GI tract enterocyte barrier.

The Microbiome of the Reproductive Tract

We do not discuss the constituency of the microbiome at all sites but instead focus on (a) those of the mother that contribute to the establishment of the microbiome of the neonate and (b) those sites in the newborn that are the recipients. We have concentrated on the GI tract since it is affected by the type of birth and the subsequent source of nourishment. It is likely that differences in both affect the nature of the established microbiome. One contributor to the infant's microbiome is the female reproductive tract, in which pregnancy is accompanied by a shift in the bacterial structure of the vagina to favor *Lactobacillus* (MacIntyre).

Reproductive complications are a worldwide health concern. Some research suggests that there are over 40 million couples worldwide that are infertile. Add to this the approximately 15% that lose pregnancies and the approximately 10% that experience preterm births. This raises the question as to whether the microbiome of the reproductive tract plays a role in reproductive problems. In the section entitled "Origin of the Early Settlers," we note that the source of the newborn's microbiome depends on the birthing method. In the vaginally born (Vg; Figure 5.2), the reproductive tract is a major source of colonizers. While the vagina has been well-studied, the once popular myth that the mammary gland was sterile was at one time applied to the uterus. It was known that the uterine microbiome contains many of the same phyla as the GI tract, but with a distribution that heavily favors *Lactobacillus*. *Lactobacilli* normally comprise 90% of the bacteria in the vagina, which explains the origin of *Lactobacilli* in the uterus. The secretion of lactic acid by *Lactobacillus*, which occurs at levels as high as 10^7 to 10^9 per gram of vaginal fluid, leads to a low pH that may be protective against colonization by Proteobacteria pathogens and *Staphylococcus*, which prefer a more alkaline environment. *Lactobacillus* levels in the vagina are also related to hormones of the estrus cycle and have been linked to the use of oral contraceptives.

The success of *in vitro* fertilization can depend on the microbiome of the reproductive tract; lower levels are associated with better outcomes. While *Lactobacilli* are abundant, markers for dysbiosis like *E. coli*, *Staphylococcus*, *Enterococcus faecalis*, and *Chlamydia* are a feature of chronic endometritis. This dysbiosis is frequently secondary to anatomic issues or prior sexually transmitted diseases like gonococcus or human papilloma virus.

As with the GI tract microbiome (Figure 5.1) there are also ethnic variations in the constituency of the vaginal microbiome. Less diverse microbiomes dominated by *Lactobacillus* occur in Asian and white women while more diverse microbiomes occur in African American and Hispanic populations. The latter have less *Lactobacillus*, but more *Prevotella* and various *Clostridia* species associated with bacterial vaginosis. An interesting feature of the vaginal microbiome is that a major change in composition occurs during the first 6 weeks of postpartum. Levels of *Lactobacilli* fall 100 to 1,000-fold at parturition, so that the proportion of *Lactobacillus* drops from 90% to 35% while that for *Clostridia* rises to 6% and *Bacteriodes* rises to 20%. The dominance of *Lactobacilli* during pregnancy has been linked to estrogen-driven maturation of the vaginal epithelium and accumulation of glycogen, the breakdown of which provides a rich source of sugars for *Lactobacilli*. A comprehensive discussion of the microbiome of the reproductive tract, its relationship to the GI tract microbiome, and its clinical implications are provided by Al-Nasiry (SR).

Establishment of the GI Tract Microbiome

The microbiome established early in life remains stable until age 65 unless it is disrupted by courses of disease and antibiotic therapy. The established microbiome reflects the environmental exposure of the neonate and can have long-term health effects (Walker, SR). Initial colonization of the GI tract has multiple effects. As described, it impacts the anatomy of the gut epithelium, resulting in thickening of the mucosa, deepening of the crypts, and lengthening the villi (Figure 2.2). In Chapter 6 we describe how mucosal development through bacterial colonization stimulates the development of the adaptive immune system, including establishment of oral tolerance to dietary antigens. Colonization also (a) increases the turnover rate of epithelial cells, (b) increases the secretion of antimicrobial factors by Paneth cells, (c) increases mucus secretion by Goblet cells, and (d) triggers peristalsis. Studies using mouse pups indicate that the microbiome that is initially established tends to be unique for each pup and is maintained for life (Chen; Faith). This also is the case in humans (Chen; Jost). This suggests that in newborn infants, the mode of delivery and the diet received thereafter (Figure 5.2) may have a long-lasting effect on the population structure of their core GI tract microbiome, which can have both short-term and long-term effects on health.

The newborn mammal (or the offspring of any multicellular eukaryote) is an "uninhabited island," which may give early settlers (eg, the "sooners," a reference to the first settlers in Oklahoma) an advantage. Early settlers create conditions for later immigrants, which affect those who later colonize and may heavily influence the eventual makeup of the mature microbiome. Early Oklahomans who ploughed the prairie ("the sod busters") were settlers who subsisted on the crops they raised for themselves and their animals, as opposed to ranchers who used only what existed on the native prairie. Using the pioneer analogy, cultivating the prairie disturbed the natural ecosystem, just like disease, medical treatment, and unnatural birthing and feeding practices are likely to disturb the ecosystem of the healthy GI tract microbiome (Figure 5.2).

The establishment of the mature GI tract microbiome involves the expansion of some bacterial taxa and decline of others, typically based on the availability of food and oxygen and the chemical microenvironment. Earlier in this chapter we mentioned the different nutrients and oxygen needs of bacteria. It is not surprising that bacteria that can thrive in the presence of oxygen may be dominant among early settlers (Jost; Adlerberth). These include the Proteobacteria but also *Lactobacillus* and *Bifidobacteria* (an Actinobacteria). These comprise 10^{10} CFU/g of feces (ten billion) compared to 10^7 CFU/g of feces in adults with a healthy microbiome, a 1,000-fold advantage. As these aerobes and facultative anaerobes consume the initial oxygen, they gradually create an environment favorable to facultative anaerobes (eg, Firmicutes) and eventually obligate anaerobes (Bacteriodetes). Thus, aerobic organisms decline until they become outnumbered 1,000-fold by anaerobes. This pattern is well-documented in studies on microbiome development in agricultural species (Appendix A-2). Therefore, as a healthy mature GI tract microbiome develops, there is a transition from Proteobacteria to Firmicutes (*Clostridium*, *Enterococcus*, *Streptococcus*, and *Lactobacillus*) and eventually to the obligate anaerobes of the phylum Bacteriodetes such as *Prevotella* and *Ruminococcus* (Table 5.1). Some use the analogy of the progressive ecological development of a mature forest, in which pioneer species like aspen are gradually replaced by so-called climax forest species (eg, Douglas fir, pines, and oaks), which is influenced by the nutrient supply.

As mentioned in an earlier section, the enterocyte barrier, together with a healthy microbiome, can provide colonization resistance, making it difficult for the "ugly" (dysbiotic) gut pathogens of phylum Proteobacteria to find "living space." This is like the eventual dominance of Firmicutes and Bacteriodetes in an oxygen-deprived environment and how *Lactobacilli* creates a pH unfavorable for the growth of Proteobacteria. Thus, the number of "ugly" Enterobacteria like *E. coli* that can attach to adhesion receptors on enterocytes and *Salmonella* that invades the enterocytes is reduced.

Studies have shown that colonization resistance is lowest in neonates with an immature microbiome, which may explain the higher proportion of Proteobacteria in neonates (Figure 5.1). Colonization resistance tends to parallel development, so "early settlers" resist colonization by those that appear later. One animal study ascribes this to remodeling of bile acid metabolism, which favors taxa that utilize taurine, a sulfonic acid that can inhibit aerobic cellular respiration used by pathogenic Proteobacteria and is sometimes used as a diet therapeutic in human and veterinary medicine (Appendix A-2). Taurine shifts growth to anaerobic Bacteriodetes that are a feature of a healthy microbiome. The low biodiversity associated with dysbiosis is often encountered after antibiotic therapy, which can result in increased levels of *C. difficile*. Supplementation with Firmicutes can convert bile salts and can inhibit the growth of *C. difficile* up to 1,000-fold.

Colonization resistance is not limited to pathogenic bacteria but also involves viruses, since both viral infection and colonizing bacteria modulate the host immune system through cytokine signaling. Specifically, the release of the interferon–α (IFN-α) and interferon-β (IFN-β) features of innate immunity (Chapter 6); both signal through a common receptor, and are stimulated by colonization with the healthy commensal microbiome (Gomez de Agüero). Cytokines are described and discussed in Chapter 6. The Bacteriodete *B. fragilis*, utilizes the outer membrane of this Gram-negative member of the healthy GI tract microbiome to stimulate release of alkaline phosphatase and heat shock proteins (Lallès). Induction of IFN-β by early colonizers also enhances resistance to the vesicular stomatitis virus infection and influenza A.

Origin of the Early Settlers

Where do the early settlers come from? Until recently, it was believed that the womb was sterile and infants acquire colonizing bacteria during birth as they slide through the birth canal. Alternatively, several studies have reported that a low mass (less than 2ng per gram of placenta) of bacteria are present in the meconium and the amniotic fluid. Therefore, some have suggested the placenta is a source of the bacteria that initially colonizes the GI tract of the newborn but also the oral cavity; the issue remains controversial (Leiby; Perez-Muñoz; Aagaard). Interestingly, the placental microbiomes that have been described most resemble those of the oral cavity of the mother, leading some to suggest that the bacteria are trafficked by dendritic cells from mouth to placenta; a similar system connects the gut to the mammary gland (MG; Chapters 3 and 6). Support for *in utero* colonization comes from studies based on 16S mRNA technology (Appendix A-1) showing evidence of bacteria in the fetal gut during the second trimester. This is supported by electron microscopic identification of bacteria and evidence that T cells in the placenta have been diversifying and responding. Detractors of the *in utero* colonization theory suggest that (1) the samples may have been contaminated during collection, (2) the bacteria-positive placenta samples came from complicated pregnancies that involved long-term labor or cesarian recovery and during this process became contaminated, and (3) the DNA may have come from non-living bacteria. Support for detractors is that the diversity of the placental samples does not resemble the microbiome first established in the newborn GI tract. Animal researchers argue that if the placenta had been colonized it would not be possible to deliver germ-free mice and piglets for over 70 years and for these to remain bacteria-free. It is easier to accept that womb sterility is lost during complicated parturitions than to accept that colonization by bacteria from the placenta is the major source for establishing the GI tract microbiome in newborn infants. Bacterial infection of the placenta has been known for decades and *Brucella abortus* and *Listeria* can cause abortion. However, these organisms are not recovered during healthy deliveries. In this chapter we shall consider the "womb" concept as not yet proven and will focus on the various forms of birth and feeding that can explain the initial colonizers from non-womb sources. One argument for placental/fetal colonization has been the presence of activated/memory T cells in the fetus. Their activation could be explained by piggyback transfer of bacterial components on IgG transferred *in utero* (Chapter 2).

Figure 5.2 summarizes the various birthing and feeding processes that play a role in the establishment of the infant microbiome. It does not distinguish exclusively breastfed infants from those receiving a mixture of formula and breast milk and does not consider differences in the duration of breast-feeding. The same concerns apply to infants recovered by cesarian or who were born prematurely. Vaginal birth (Vg) followed by breast-feeding (VgBF) is the natural process that serves all mammals, but vaginal birth followed by formula feeding (VgF) is common in industrialized countries. Vaginal delivery involves contact with the maternal microbiota of the vagina and the GI tract microbiome of the feces. Normally, the vaginal flora is dominated by *Lactobacilli* while Bacteriodetes like *Prevotella* are dominant in feces.

After birth, breast-feeding offers an additional source of bacteria for colonization as well as nutrients that can give advantages to certain early settlers (Zimmermann). Once considered sterile, breast milk provides a continuous supply of commensal and probiotic bacteria (Fernandez; SR). At least 58 different phyla and many classes and families of bacteria are found in breast milk. The most common genera are *Lactobacillus*, *Staphylococcus*, *Enterococcus*, and

Bifidobacteria. Most of the milk microbiome are not contaminants, but their composition is influenced by the experience of the mother. Some appear to be translocated from the GI tract, something like the gut-mammary gland axis described in Chapter 3 (Fernandez, SR). Examining the stools of VgBF infants shows a high relative abundance of *Bifidobacteria* but also *Staphylococci, Streptococci,* and *Enterobacteriaceae.* By contrast, VgF infants have an abundance of *Bacteriodes, Clostridia, Enterobacteriaceae* and *Enterococcus* (Proteobacteria), and *Lachnospiraceae.* These studies leave no doubt that breast milk influences the establishment of the infant's microbiome and can be beneficial for preterm infants (Gregory). In fact, bacteria like *S. salivarius* in breast milk can inhibit colonization of the suckling infant by pathogenic *S. aureus* (Heikkila). However, the microbiome in milk varies geographically and changes during lactation and observation, which is supported by studies in swine during lactation (Wang; Appendix A-2). Best documented and considered most important in the infant GI tract is the early prevalence of *Bifidobacteria,* which depend on certain HMOs provided in breast milk (Chapter 3) that allow them to thrive; this is believed to be why their levels increase in breastfed infants (Figure 5.1A). Diversity is initially low in VgBF infants but stools from infants in this group contain high counts of *Lactobacilli* and *Bifidobacteria* but few Proteobacteria. In the VgBF group, the most dramatic change is seen at weaning and features a major increase in diversity. Since the HMOs in breast milk are no longer available, there is a reduction in *Bifidobacteria* that thrive on these HMOs. The high protein content that characterizes infant formulas (Chapter 3), and the addition of fiber resulting from the shift to solid food, results in an increase in Bacteriodetes like *Prevotella* and *Faecalibacteria.* Both are features of a healthy adult GI tract microbiome (Table 5.1). Bacteriodetes can utilize plant-derived polysaccharides, which they convert to SCFAs like acetate, propionate, and butyrate that contribute to the development of healthy tight junctions between enterocytes, increasing the length of villi and the depth of the crypts. Among the SCFA, butyrate has the best correlation with a healthy microbiome.

Figure 5.4A illustrates a healthy mucosa that involves regular growth of villi through replacement of enterocytes from precursors in the crypt and proper maintenance of tight junctions using SCFA produced by commensal Bacteriodetes. The underlying lamina propria is rich in Tregs and dendritic cells that sample the bacteria of other environments of the gut lumen. The Peyer's patches (PP) are well-developed with macrophages and M cells that sample the environment. The right villus shown in Figure 5.4A demonstrates that stimulation in the PP results in plasma cells that migrate into the villi and secrete dimeric IgA, which is then transferred across the epithelium to become SIgA, which subsequently removes bacteria and other antigens (see Chapter 6, Figure 6.6). Stimulated T cells mostly differentiate into Tregs, and the Th2 cells generated engage B cells in germinal center reactions (GCRx; Chapter 6). Goblet cells lay down protective mucus that is important for trapping certain bacteria and food antigens.

In the next chapter we describe the major α/β T cell subsets and emphasize a proper balance among those that help in the production of specific antibodies, those that facilitate inflammatory responses that control pathogens, and those that keep the action of inflammatory

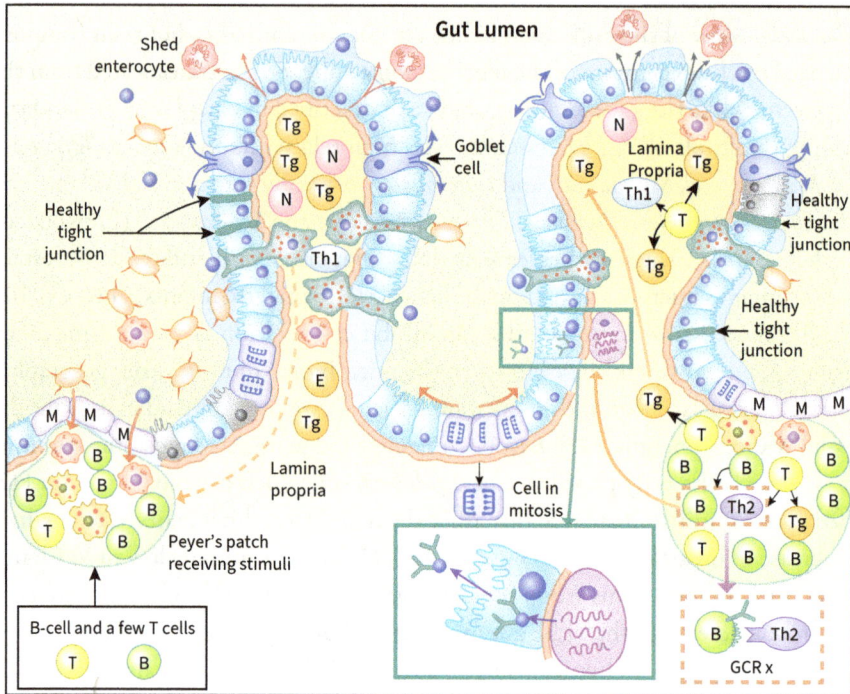

Figure 5.4A   The lamina propria contains neutrophils but also an abundance of Tregs (Tg) and plasma cells producing dimeric IgA, which is transported into the lumen as SIgA. Its role is discussed and illustrated in Figure 6.6. These plasma cells originate from B cells stimulated in the Peyer's patches (PP) in response to antigens transported there by dendritic cells or by macrophages that underlie the M cell and sample the healthy environment. Healthy villi are maintained by mitotic events in the crypt region, which replaces enterocytes lost from the villi. Events in the PP involve germinal center reactions (GCRx), which are discussed in Chapter 6.

T cells in check (so-called regulatory α/β T cells or Tregs; Chapter 6). There is evidence that metabolic products like certain SCFAs promote expansion of Tregs, which are abundant in the healthy GI tract (Figure 5.4A; Tg). SCFAs are secreted by colonizers referred to as "border dwellers" and are part of the mucosa-associated microbiome as opposed to bacteria living free in the digesta. However, Proteobacteria pathogens may displace border-dwelling Firmicutes and Bacteriodetes (see next section). This reduces the output of SCFA and correspondingly the proportion of Tregs, allowing the return of inflammatory T cell subsets that aid in elimination of the pathogens but can also cause damage through "friendly fire." Inflammatory T cells are also involved in IBD. In a later section dealing with prebiotics and HMOs in infants, we mention their importance as nutrients for the Actinobacteria Bifidobacteria, Firmicutes like Lactobacillus and Bacteriodetes. These eubiotic flora generate SCFA that are absorbed by the GI tract and which then promote the release of enteroendocrine peptides like GLP-1 that act in health and disease.

Vaginally born infants that are formula fed (VgF) have a significantly more diverse microbiome than VgBF infants that is characterized by more Firmicutes that include *Staphylococci* and certain pathogenic *Clostridia* species, but also various Proteobacteria like Enterobacteria

Loss of microvilli

(Dysbiosis)

Weak tight junctions

IgG

SIgA

Blow-up

Mesenteric Lymph Node

Commensial Bacteria   N = Neutrophil
Pathogenic Bacteria

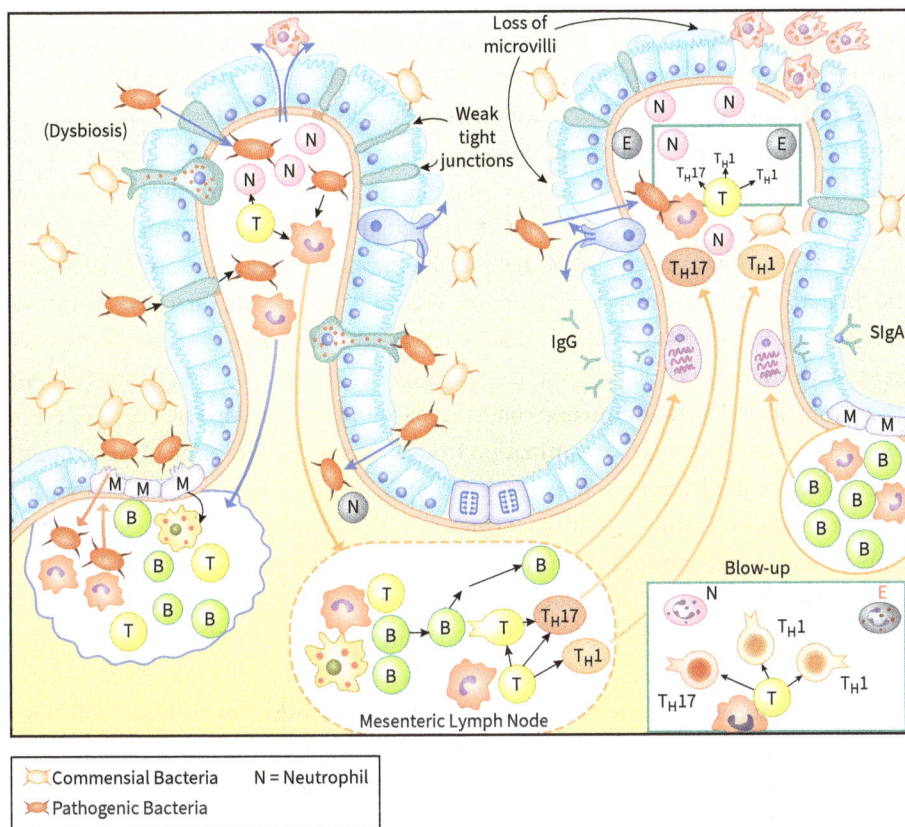

Figure 5.4B   The unhealthy or dysbiotic mucosa is characterized by the weakening of tight junctions, which allows the mucosa to be breeched by members of the microbiome and un-degraded macromolecules normally blocked from entry. Certain pathogens also gain access through M cells because they recognize certain receptors on M cells. Pathogenic bacteria and other environmental antigens that have breached the barrier are transported by antigen-pre-senting cells (APCs) to the PP, as well as to the mesenteric lymph nodes. This allows for the differentiation of T cells into inflammatory subsets and for the stimulation of B cells producing IgG antibodies that can exacerbate local inflammatory conditions. This may be accompanied by replacement of Tregs by inflammatory T cells (see Chapter 6).

and *Endococci*. For example, there is a higher incidence of *C. difficile* in VgF than in VgBF infants. This suggests that in formula-fed infants, the microbiome progresses more rapidly toward an adult-like GI tract microbiome. However, the absence of HMOs that are normally provided by breast milk means that some members of the microbiome (like *Bifidobacteria*) that utilize these HMOs proportionally decline. The microbiome of the mother also changes throughout pregnancy. In the vagina, there is an overall decrease in diversity but a shift toward *Lactobacillus*, which is considered protective since lactic acid lowers the pH of the vagina and discourages colonization by many pathogenic bacteria.

The remaining categories of delivery that influence the type of first settlers are preterm and C-section infants (Figure 5.2). In both groups the vertical transfer of the maternal microbiome seen in vaginally born infants does not occur. Studies show the mode of preterm delivery does not appear to affect the initial colonizing community, which is surprising since during C-section delivery the amnion is not ruptured so the newborn should not encounter bacteria from the vagina. Preterm infants born vaginally have a less well-developed GI tract and respiratory tract and often endure long hospital stays that potentially expose them to pathogens found in hospital environments that can result in nosocomial (hospital) infections. Therefore, preterm infants have a lower colonization rate and lower ratio of anaerobe to facultative anaerobe than vaginally born infants, which translates to lower counts of *Bifidobacteria* and *Bacteriodes fragilis* and greater counts of *C. difficile* and *E. coli*. In both C-section and preterm infants, this could result from their delayed exposure to breast milk. Proteobacteria like Enterobacteria and *Enterococci* are typically recovered together with environmental bacteria like *S. aureus*, *S. epidermidis*, and various *Clostridia*. The last group includes environmental commensals found on skin and elsewhere. These may colonize the infants through contamination from the medical staff or medical equipment. By comparison, colonization by *S. aureus* is rare in VgBF infants, but may account for 10^8 CFU/g of feces in CF and CBF infants (Figure 5.2). Colonization in C-section infants resembles that of preterm infants in that they have fewer *Bifidobacteria* and *Bacteriodes*. These infants may also acquire nosocomial infections, which may include *C. difficile* and Proteobacteria. In healthy VgBF infants, there is a large increase in *Bifidobacteria* and *Bacteriodes* by 6 months, but by 2 years the microbiome resembles that of adults as the diet shifts away from dependence on lactose and HMOs with the introduction of solid food (Figure 5.1A). Again, there are ethnic and cultural influences on the constituency of the microbiome (Figure 5.3), and not surprisingly these differences are also seen among infants. For example, for neonates in Luxembourg, Proteobacteria may be more dominant than Bacteriodetes.

Recent studies show that the diversity and constituency of the microbiome of VgBF infants is distinct from that of their mothers. This is expected since HMOs and lactose provided through suckling give competitive advantage to *Bifidobacterium* and certain *Bacteroides*, which alters the infants' microbiome from the one they obtained from their mother through vertical transmission at birth. This difference is especially apparent in Bangladesh, where all infants are breastfed for 6 months and many for 2 years and where a distinct clade of *Bifidobacterium* thrives during weaning (Vatanen, Yan Ang, et al.). Conversely, this pattern of neonatal development is not followed in industrialized countries in North America and Western Europe where cesarian birth, formula feeding, and early cessation of breast-feeding are common practices. The pattern in industrialized countries is correlated with a higher incidence of allergy and autoimmunity (Vatanen, Plichia, et al.). However, correlation is not causation (see later). Other factors can also account for differences between the microbiome of VgBF infants and their mothers. In Chapter 1 we introduced the concept of horizontal gene transfer (HGT), and in Appendix A-1 we describe some of the mechanisms involved. Some differences between the infant and maternal microbiome can result from the transfer of mobile elements (eg, plasmids and phages; Vatanen, Jabbar, et al.). This includes HGT of genes for glycoside hydrolases needed for the metabolism of HMOs. This may explain the unexpected proportional increases in *B. fragilis* and *B. ovatus* and the decrease in the proportion of other Bacteriodetes that were obtained through vertical transmission.

1. Describe how the diet and condition around the of a nursing mother influences the microbiome of her child.

2. Explore arguments connecting the constituency of the microbiome to maladies like inflammatory bowel disorders, allergy, ASD, and diseases of the newborn like NEC.

3. Describe therapeutic measures that can be used to correct the microbiome in infants and adults.

The Maternal Diet and Other Influences on the Microbiome During Pregnancy

Pediatricians refer to nutrition in the first 1,000 days as pivotal for adequate neonatal growth and development, and this involves establishing a heathy microbiome. Since the neonate obtains its initial microbiome from the mother by various routes, it is important that a healthy eubiotic microbiome is transferred. It is known that dysbiosis during pregnancy increases the risk of preeclampsia, diabetes, and childhood atopy (Sohn, SR). The major contributors to the newborn microbiome are the vaginal and GI tract microbiome. The vaginal microbiome changes during pregnancy and favors an abundance of *Lactobacilli* at birth, which are believed to be protective against pathogenic Proteobacteria that do poorly at low pH.

The placenta also has a microbiome that appears most similar to that in the oral cavity, where Firmicutes are in abundance (Figure 5.1B). However, the placental microbiome of preterm infants may differ and levels of Proteobacteria are elevated.

Dysbiosis of the GI tract microbiome is known from data from overweight mothers, in which *Bifidobacteria* are less abundant and *Staphylococci* and Enterobacteria, (eg, *E. coli*) abundance is higher. Decreased levels of colonization by *Lactobacillus* and *Bifidobacteria* in the newborn have been correlated with an increase in childhood allergy, maternal periodontal disease, preterm labor, and low birth rates.

The diet of the pregnant mother can alter her GI tract microbiome and maternal obesity and diabetes are known to negatively affect the constituency of the mother's microbiome (Voreades). One study correlated the maternal diet of pregnant mothers to clusters of bacterial species, by which mothers can be divided into either a *Prevotella* or the *Ruminococcus* group; one is a Bacteriodes and the other a Firmicutes (García-Mantrana; Table 5.1). A higher intake of omega-3 fatty acids and total fibers favors the *Ruminococcus* group, which was correlated with a healthy BMI for their offspring. The intake of omega-3 fatty acids also correlated with the reduced risk of preeclampsia and preterm birth (see Chapter 2). C-section infants fell into the *Prevotella* group and had higher BMI scores and a higher risk of being overweight. *Prevotella copri* favors glycogen storage and can also be linked to glucose intolerance. Besides *Ruminococcus*, the higher fiber intake group was associated with *Faecalibacterium prauznitzii*. These correlation studies do not always fit nicely with healthy versus disease categories. For example, high fiber intake is also correlated with the incidence of periodontal disease. The sheer size of the GI tract microbiome and the fact that so much relies only on correlation (Chapter 7 and next) is a warning that the field of microbiome research is still in its infancy and that some conclusions drawn at this stage of knowledge should be reviewed with caution (Chapter 8).

Factors other than diet may also affect the pregnant mother's microbiome. The Strachan **hygiene hypothesis** or "dirt hypothesis," introduced in 1989, attained considerable attention, especially the correlation between early childhood exposure to potential allergens and the later incidence of asthma and allergy (Chapter 6). More recently there have been efforts to link the hygiene hypothesis with perturbation of the microbiome, including that of the mother, and extend it to childhood obesity and type 2 diabetes. In highly developed countries of North American and Europe, the increase in food allergy, eczema, and asthma has doubled in the last 20 years; those affected represent a quarter of the world's population. Studies have shown that low microbial diversity is a feature of children experiencing atopic eczema before 2 years of age. Eczema favors high levels of *Clostridia* and a lack of *Bifidobacteria* (see below). In Chapter 6 we review the Amish-Hutterite study and others showing a correlation between reduced risk of allergy and asthma and the simple Amish lifestyle. It is reasonable that the hygiene hypothesis should be extended to exposure to allergies during pregnancy, not just those impacting the newborn. In breastfed infants in Bangladesh and Malawi, *B. infantis* and B. longum are dominant (Vatanen, Yan Ang, et al.), but it is not the case in Europe and North America. Thus, cultural differences (ie, reliance on formula feeding in Europe and the United States) provide an interesting contrast in that type 1 diabetes and other immune-related maladies, are more frequent in America and Western countries than in less-developed countries.

Prevotella is one of the Bacteriodetes that comprise the healthy (eubiotic) GI tract microbiome (Table 5.1). Prevotella is under-represented in the microbiome of individuals in developed Western cultures, the same individuals that suffer from a high incidence of allergy, asthma, eczema, psoriasis, and IBD (Chapter 6 and below). *Prevotella* levels are directly correlated with a high-fiber diet, production of SCFAs, and development of regulatory T cells (Tregs). *Prevotella* links together diet and the constituency of the microbiome and favors conversion of T cells to Tregs.

In the case of asthma, the microbiome of the lungs and bronchi should be more relevant. *Prevotella* is an important member of the bronchial microbiome and suppresses IL-8 and TNF-α production in the lungs but could protect against dysbiosis caused by Proteobacteria like *Haemophilus influenza* that promote an inflammatory response. However, high levels of *Prevotella* have also been linked to inflammatory disorders, suggesting that a balance among the constituency of the microbiome is also important.

Childhood Allergy and the Microbiome

Like IBD, the incidence of childhood allergy has been increasing in North America and Western Europe (Figure 5.5). As discussed previously and in Chapter 6, the Strachan hygiene hypothesis suggests that early childhood exposure to potential allergens reduces the probability of type I IgE-mediated allergy later in life, and various studies have linked this to the constituency of the microbiome (Greer, SR; Penders, SR; Rachid). The GI tract microbiome is established early in life and is correlated with type of birth and feeding regiment (Figure 5.2). VgBF infants have high levels of *Bifidobacteria* while preterm infants have a higher incidence of allergy and those that were not colonized by vaginal birth have higher levels of Proteobacteria. As mentioned earlier, VgBF infants also differ because breast milk contains approximately 15 mg/ml of HMOs (Chapter 3), which encourages the expansion of *Bifidobacteria* and may encourage colonization of the newborn by other "good" bacteria in breast milk. To compensate for the denial of natural colonization, preterm infants are routinely given probiotics rich in various strain of *Lactobacillus* and *Bifidobacteria*. However, a meta-analysis indicated that probiotics do not appear to diminish the propensity to develop childhood eczema (Rachid). *Clostridia* species (Firmicutes) favor the development of Tregs, and the release of TGFβ and other cytokine can dampen the infant's immune response to allergens, especially those in food (Table 6.3). In contrast to VgBF infants, the microbiome of cesarian-delivered formula-fed infants (CF; Figure 5.2) may have richness but lacks diversity, which some believe is a feature of a healthy GI tract microbiome (Yatsunenko). This has led to the metamorphosis of the Strachan hypothesis (Chapter 6) into the biodiversity hypothesis, the assertion that lower diversity is dysbiotic.

The propensity for infants to develop allergic disease, eczema, and asthma has been linked to the dysbiotic nature of the GI tract microbiome. An abundance of *Faecalibacterium prausnitzii* and reduced levels of butyrate (an SCFA generated by *Bacteriodes*) is associated with eczema (Sjödin). A lower abundance of *Ruminococcus* seems to be associated with food allergy and eczema, and eczema is correlated with lower diversity of the microbiome and higher abundance of Proteobacteria, *C. difficile*, and lower levels of Bacteriodetes. The intestinal inflammation of newborns is silenced when colonized by strains of *B. infantis* that carry genes needed for metabolism of HMOs in breastfed infants (VgBF; Figure 5.2; Henrick). This promotes polarization of T cells to Tregs (such as Th2 and Th17, which are a feature of inflammation; see Gelfen), and production of IFNβ. *B. infantis* is common in Bangladesh, where immune-medicated diseases are low compared to Europe and North America, where *B. infantis* levels are low and immune-mediated diseases are common.

In the case of VgBF infants, the microbiome they obtain is transferred from their mother, so the propensity of infants in this group to develop eczema and other forms of allergy might be linked to the dietary behavior of their birth mothers (see earlier section). Pregnant mothers living on a high-fat and low-fiber diet, which favors lower diversity and low abundance of *Faecalibacterium prausnitzii*, can be considered dysbiotic, and this microbiome can be transferred to the VgBF infant. The dietary habits of the mother influence the constituency of her microbiome, so it would not be surprising if this is linked to the propensity of allergy in her offspring (García-Mantrana).

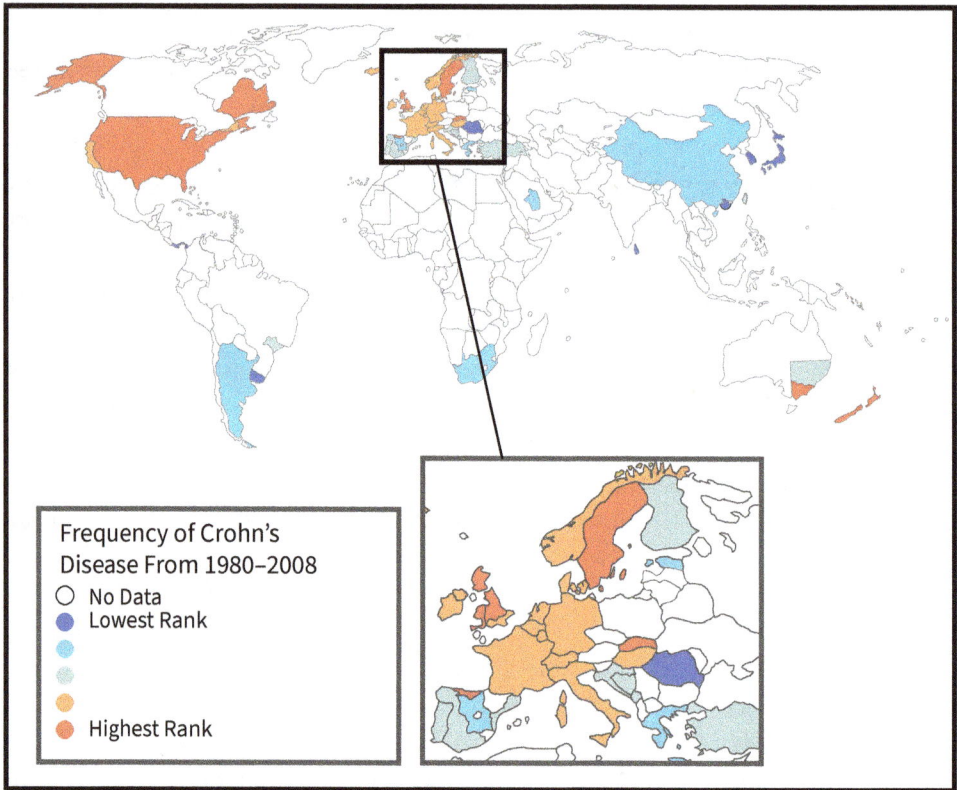

Figure 5.5A   The geographical distribution of IBD.

Disease and the Microbiome
Correlation and Causation

There has been a "tsunami" of reports correlating various diseases to certain features of the microbiome; we review and cite a number of these. However, the sheer size (10^{12}) and diversity (thousands of species) of the microbiome, which can differ among cultures (Figure 5.3), makes it extremely difficult to link correlation with causation; a subject addressed in Chapter 7. Studies linking a particular bacterial species or subspecies to a specific member of the microbiome are few. There is irrefutable evidence linking *H. pylori* to peptic ulcers, *C. difficile* to diarrhea, *V. cholera* to cholera, and strains of *Salmonella* and *E. coli* to many foodborne illnesses that result in diarrhea. However, caution is needed when following the "bandwagon" that links so many human illnesses to the make-up of the microbiome when the mechanism connecting the disease to a particular bacterium has not been described. Correlations with dysbiosis have been described for allergy, obesity, IBD, Parkinson's disease, depression, ASD and colorectal cancer. Rodent models (dubbed human microbiota associated, HMA) that depend on transfer of the dysbiotic microbiome from individuals to germ-free

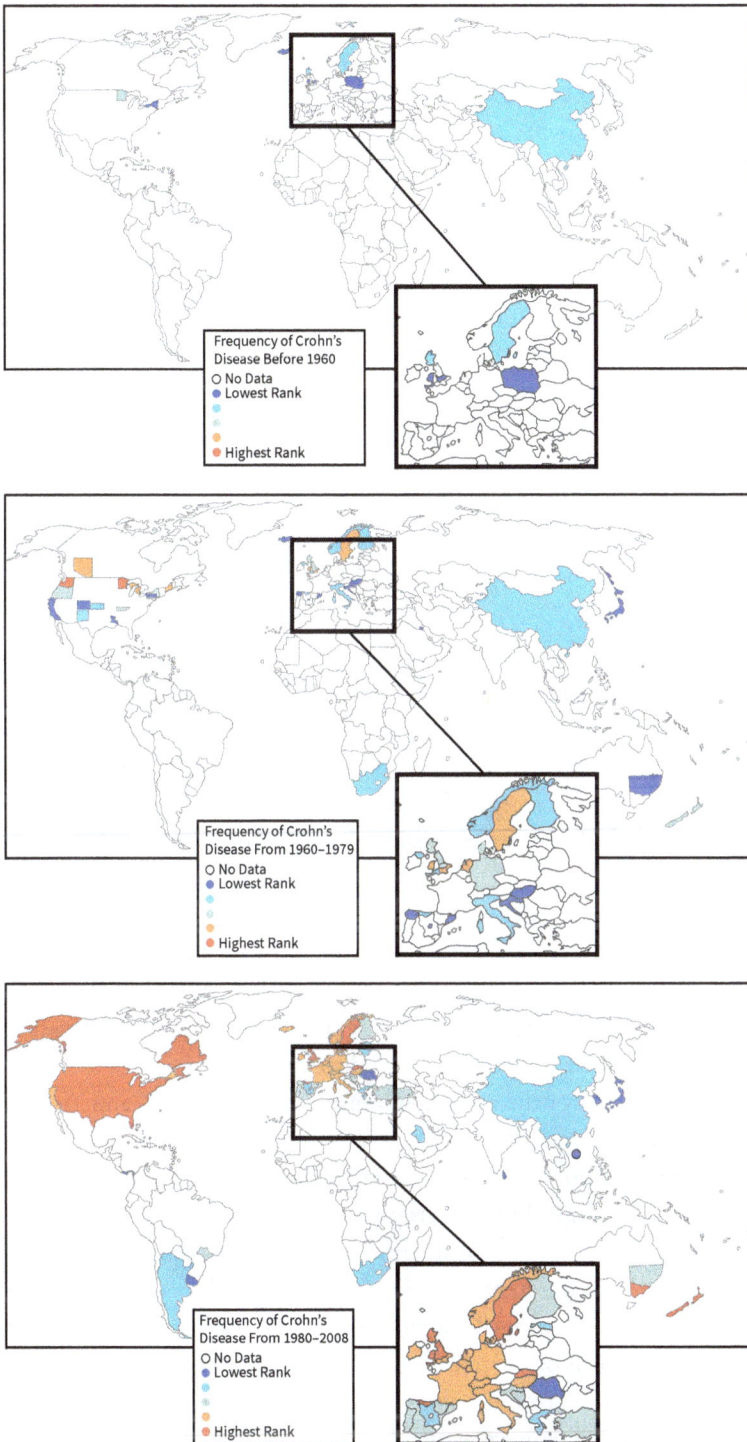

Frequency of Crohn's Disease Before 1960
- ○ No Data
- ● Lowest Rank
- ● Highest Rank

Frequency of Crohn's Disease From 1960–1979
- ○ No Data
- ● Lowest Rank
- ● Highest Rank

Frequency of Crohn's Disease From 1980–2008
- ○ No Data
- ● Lowest Rank
- ● Highest Rank

Figure 5.5B   Increase in the frequency of IBD.

rats and mice have been used to convert correlation to cause (Walter). One of the tenets of the Koch postulates for establishing the cause of disease is its successful transfer. In the case of HMA, transfer is not to another human but to a rodent, in which less than 20% of the rodents develop the disease, which weakens the model (Chapter 7). Not all animal models are applicable to humans (Appendix A-2). There are many reasons for the failure of animal models when addressing the issue. One is that some members of the human microbiome poorly colonize rodents and, when they do colonize them, produce no disease because the necessary receptors are not present. As we have mentioned, viral infection depends on the presence of specific host receptors, and some enteric bacterial pathogens, like ETEC, depend on adhesion receptors (see earlier). This explains why many viruses are species specific and certain mammals, including certain pigs, resist enteric bacterial pathogens. This does not negate using models but rather means that better models are needed. The best model is always the species itself, but this raises many ethical issues that are justified by more than a century of misuse. Given the density of the microbiome and the populations enrolled in studies, readers and students should use caution in forming conclusions regarding the role of the microbiome in diseases that are based only on correlations.

Disease Dysbiosis

Proteobacteria abundance, especially Enterobacteria, are often a cause of dysbiosis (Table 5.1), such as illness outbreaks caused by *Salmonella* and *E. coli*. These pathogens act in different ways, but all stimulate resident dendritic cells to release IL-1 and IL-2, causing differentiation of resident T cells to become inflammatory Th17 cells that secrete inflammatory cytokines that disturb the "peaceful coexistence" within the GI tract microbiome and the intestinal epithelium.

Figure 5.4B illustrates several features and events that occur during dysbiosis that is most often caused by an enteric bacterial pathogen. These include the weakening of tight junctions, allowing pathogens to breech the enteric mucosal defense. Some pathogens may damage the enterocytes, resulting in their loss or the loss of their microvilli and function. Goblet cells may be impaired and less able to produce protective mucus. Tregs in the healthy mucosa are replaced by many neutrophils, inflammatory T cells (Th1 and Th17), and macrophages battling the pathogens. In the healthy mucosa (Figure 5.4A), B cells stimulated in the PP develop into plasma cells and secrete dimeric IgA. However, during disease, antigen-presenting cells (APCs) like macrophages and dendritic cells also migrate to the mesenteric lymph nodes, resulting in the differentiation of T cells into inflammatory T cells and causing B cells to differentiate into IgG instead of dimeric IgA-producing cells. Damage to the mucosa (Figure 5.4B, right villus) allows bacteria greater access. Certain pathogens also use receptors on M cells to gain access. The overall result is inflammation with an accumulation of neutrophils and eosinophils (depending on the intruder) all of which can lead to bystander damage, which is seen in some forms of IBD and nosocomial "hospital illnesses" such as those caused by *C. difficile*.

An interesting correlation is that between multiple sclerosis (MS) and the microbiome, which may be an indicator of dietary habits in developed countries with "Western diets."

These countries have a high incidence of MS. Patients with MS are dysbiotic because of reduced levels of Firmicutes (Table 5.1) that convert fiber to SCFAs in the GI tract. Both IBD and MS are correlated with Enterobacteria, while age- and gender-matched control patients show a correlation with *Ruminococcus* (Table 5.1). *Prevotella* and *Faecalbacterium prauznitzii* are reduced in IBD patients (Mangalam). In one study of MS, propionate was significantly reduced in the serum and stools of MS patients and was correlated with a high level of Th1 and Th17 cells (Figure 5.4B) and with depleted levels of *Butyricimonas* and a higher level of Proteobacteria (Duscha). Therapeutic treatment with propionic acid reduced the annual relapse rate, reduced disease progression, and significantly elevated the levels of Tregs and lowered the proportion of inflammatory Th1 and Th17 cells (see Chapter 6, Table 6.1). In a mouse model of autoimmune encephalomyelitis, colonization with *Prevotella* decreased the level of pro-inflammatory Th1 and Th17 cells while simultaneously increasing the frequency of Tregs (Mangalam).

Obese patients have a high risk of type 2 diabetes. However, in many of these individuals, the ratios of good versus bad members of the microbiome (Table 5.1) is skewed in the "extra good" direction (ie, there is a higher proportion of Firmicutes and Bacteriodetes). This may reflect a much better conversion of food intake to fat storage. This is supported by studies in mice showing that colonization of germ-free mice with the microbiome from obese mice results in the accumulation increase body fat, indicating that the dominance of certain phyla does not always assure health. The correct balance is as yet unknown and may differ among species and individuals (Appendix A-2).

The differences in the constituencies of the earliest microbiomes of vaginally delivered infants (VgBF, VgF; Figure 5.2) and C-section and preterm infants have been associated with various short-term and long-term maladies. For example, there are reports that *E. coli* levels are correlated with eczema in children and that *C. difficile* colonization is associated with dermatitis. Correlation studies show that breast-feeding lowers the risk of infection with pathogenic Proteobacteria and the development of obesity, allergy, and type 2 diabetes. The literature is ripe with such reports and statistically sound, but as indicated above, operative mechanisms are conjecture in a field with so many variables.

Necrotizing enterocolitis (NEC) is associated with *E. coli*, *C. difficile*, and a high proportion of Proteobacteria. Since these disorders are less frequent in VgBF infants and such infants have a lower proportion of Proteobacteria and pathogenic Firmicutes, the nature of their microbiome reduces the level of GI tract inflammation. It has been shown that *Bifidobacteria*, as well as *Lactobacillus* and *B. fragilis*, thrive in breastfed infants because of the HMOs provided (Chapter 3). It is possible that the expansion of these "good" bacteria causes *colonization resistance* that excludes Proteobacteria and *C. difficile*. If HMOs are considered a major factor, then finding the optimal HMOs to add to infant formulas should be a priority (see Chapter 4).

Inflammatory Bowel Disease (IBD)

The role of the microbiome goes beyond short-term diseases like NEC to long-term illnesses like IBD, MS, psoriatic arthritis, and systemic lupus erythematosus (SLE). IBD is an umbrella term for Crohn's disease (CD), ulcerative colitis (UC), celiac disease (CD), and certain other intestinal maladies like irritable bowel syndrome (IBS). All are characterized by inflammation and damage to the intestinal mucosa (Figure 5.4B) and involve changes in the microbiome (Powers, SR; Leone).

There has been a rapid rise in the frequency of IBD in the last 40 years, particularly in North America and Western Europe (Molodecky; Figure 5.5). All forms of IBD are multifactorial and characterized by a pro-inflammatory cytokine profile and by Th1 and Th17 cells, INFγ, and IL-17 (Figure 5.4B; Figure 6.1). IBD is also correlated with a high fat and high carbohydrate diet that we and others have referred to as a "Western diet." IBD fails to develop in animals colonized with a healthy gut flora and germ-free mice and piglets never develop IBD. This suggests that IBD depends on the microbiome of the GI tract. The most extreme situation is seen in America, where one-third of the population is obese (Arroyo-Johnson) and 1.4 million adults suffer from IBD. There is a contingent who believes that changes in the human microbiome are due to the expansion of factory animal production and agriculture that shifted *Homo sapiens* to a meat diet rich in saturated fatty acids but deficient in plant fibers. This may also be abetted by a genetic component, since 20% of IBD patients follow a familial path, being very high among monozygotic twins. The remainder of cases point to life-type issues, diet, and the influence of the microbiome. There is also evidence that pancreatic cancer may belong in the same category. In Appendix A-1 we discuss the issues and mechanisms of HGT among the members of the GI tract microbiome that allow "bad" members of the microbiome to persist. There is now evidence that this may be more frequent in industrialized countries that have a high frequency of IBD. The frequency of IBD is also associated with other maladies like celiac disease, psoriasis, rheumatoid arthritis, and type 1 diabetes. Their connection to the microbiome remains unresolved.

One treatment for patients with various forms of IBD is fecal microbiota transplantation (FMT). Healthy donors can contribute stool samples to an FMT bank, a process humorously referred to as "giving a crap." FMT has claimed more than 30% remission rates. Recipients that received an FMT from a donor with a high level of *Ruminococcus* experienced approximately 40% remission. While the mechanism for success has not been fully established, it is reasonable to speculate that FMT increases the proportion of Bacteriodetes, thus lowering the proportion of Proteobacteria and increasing the level of Tregs that suppress the actions of Th17 T cells and reducing "friendly fire." The infant's microbiome is unstable (Voreades) and without vertical transfer of the maternal microbiome, C-section infants are more likely to be at increased risk for short-term and long-term health risks. These include chronic inflammatory diseases covered under the umbrella of IBD, rheumatoid arthritis, and type I diabetes. In a recent study of 17 mother-infant pairs in Finland, oral FMT was successful in establishing the mother's microbiome in these C-section infants. However, the sample is too small and the time too short to determine if oral FMT improves the long-term health of C-section infants. An interesting study showed that while FMT was very effective in restoring the healthy microbiome in adults, its effectiveness was hindered when probiotics were also used (Suez).

Microbiome-Gut-Brain-Axis (MGBA)

In the next chapter we describe the **internal protection** provided by the immune system and the role of the various T cell subsets and the mucosal immune system that oversees the GI tract. Increasing evidence suggests that the latter and the microbiome communicate with the central nervous system through the enteric nervous system (ENS). An increasing volume of research provides strong evidence for the MGBA (Longo S). This involves the production of SCFA by eubiotic members of the microbiome which are then absorbed by the enterocytes and can activate L-cells (sometimes called Els or enteroendocrine cells, EEC). These SCFA also stimulate the release of antibacterial peptides (AMP which orchestrate the mucosal barrier through the action of IL-18 and the ENS (Jaret; see Chapter 6). These cells release peptides called "enteroglucagons". Best known is GLP-1, a synthetic form that was initially used in treatment of diabetes with such pharmaceuticals like Wegovy and Ozempic, but have now become popular weight loss drugs. These peptides from so-called EL cells, message through the ENS which then leads to the vagus nerve and eventually to the hypothalamus and brainstem (Longo S). Thus, SCFA play an important role in the MGBA (Zeng; Everard). These enteroendocrine peptides transmits the feeling of hunger and satiation, and the so-called "gut feeling." Neurons in this system also display toll-like receptors (TLRs) that can respond to the PAMPs of the GI tract microbiome. Thus, the GI tract microbiome acts on both the ENS and the mucosal immune system (Lenfestey). ASD is a neurological disorder and has been speculated to involved the MGBA. ASD is associated with dysbiosis although the actual mechanism remains speculative. (Chernikova; Altharthi; Taniya). ASD is correlated with early colonization of the GI tract, mode of delivery (Figure 5.2) and antibiotic usage. Some have suggested that the dysbiotic microbiome may also act through epigenesis.

Other Diseases

The last 2 decades have witnessed a resurgence in studies on the microbiome that has led to a plethora of reports linking the microbiome to a broad range of diseases. These go beyond the examples provided above. An additional example involves cardiovascular disease, a major cause of death that is linked to atherosclerosis and its connection with the consumption of red meat, eggs, and high-fat dairy products (Koeth; Wang; Ettinger). Red meat consumption results in the release of carnitine and phosphotidyl choline; the latter is converted to trimethylamine by colonic microbes and its production ceases after long-term antibiotic treatment that destroys the GI tract microbiome.

The relationship between proper diet, longevity, and disease resistance is a common theme. Some now believe that the connection between ingestion of certain foods and health may be linked by the MGBA (Longo VD). This axis may explain why moderation of protein, sugar, and fat intake are related to health and longevity. In many cases, the nutritional value of ingested food depends in part on processing by the GI tract microbiome. As we described in Chapter 3 and above, the processing of HMOs by the microbiome of the suckling is necessary for their nutritive value to be realized. This is especially true for vegetable fibers, on which ruminant artiodactyls totally depend (see earlier and Appendix A-2). In humans, studies connecting the diversity and constituency of the gut microbiome to health through neuroendocrine connections will continue to fascinate nutritionists.

Multiple sclerosis (MS) is an autoimmune disease of the CNS that leads to progressive neurological disability. A recent study has shown that MS is associated with a change in the GI tract microbiome, especially a reduction in *F. preausnitzil*, one of the "good" members of the GI tract microbiome that converts ingested nutrients to SCFA (iMSMS Consortium). It remains to determine if MS causes the change in the microbiome or if it is vice versa. This is another example of correlation involving the connection between the microbiome and human health, and the reason we include Chapter 7.

Pre-, Pro-, and Synbiotics and the Newborn

The terms pre- and probiotics were described in Chapter 3. Prebiotics are best described as a source of complex carbohydrates that provide food for certain members of the microbiome but cannot be metabolized by the host. Human colostrum/milk provides prebiotics in the form of HMOs (Chapter 3). Fructo-oligosaccharides and galacto-oligosaccharides are some of the HMOs added to infant formulas (Chapter 4). The role of prebiotics is to expand the growth of *Bifidobacteria*, *Lactobacillus*, and also Bacteriodetes and Firmicutes that can convert prebiotics to nutrients for the infant and that collectively favor "good" members of the microbiome (Table 5.1). Prebiotics are finding increasing use in pediatric practice.

Probiotics are live organisms and when given together with a prebiotic are called *synbiotics*. Probiotics are widely advertised on TV for adults, but they are most valuable for preterm and C-section infants. They have been used in the prevention of NEC in preterm infants, and for a variety of inflammatory bowel diseases in adults and for recovery from *C. difficile* infection and periodic diarrhea. They have even been used in the treatment of ASD (Lenfestey). At this juncture, the use of probiotics and synbiotics (de Vrese) falls into at least three categories: (a) use in preterm and C-section infants, (b) use in adults whose normal GI tract microbiome was lost/reduced by oral antibiotic treatment, and (c) use in healthy adults. There is accumulating evidence for use in groups (a) and (b), while their value in healthy adults is controversial (Chapter 8).

Probiotics are not FDA approved pharmaceuticals but are classified as food supplements like fish oil and many other products sold by health food stores. Many brands of yogurt also advertise their probiotic content. The European Union has restrictions on the labeling of food as probiotics. *Yogurt*, a term recognized since 1925, is milk fermented with *S. thermophilus* and *Lactobacillus* and has a well-accepted safety record and a long history (McFarland). It is recommended in all countries that their content of live organism be indicated. However, this is not universal in the United States and many other countries. Yogurts, like Activia, claim to provide about 10^{10} bacteria per serving. One serving would then represent one-thousandth of the microbiome already present. This has raised the question as to whether probiotics are only a psychological supplement for the already healthy population (see next section). Some believe probiotics should be regulated in the same manner as pharmaceuticals, but this is a difficult proposition since even the most used probiotics, like *Lactobacillus rhamnosus* and

Saccharomyces boullardii, potentially produce many different metabolic/pharmaceutical agents that would complicate labelling. Until the action of these metabolites or other factors produced by these organisms can be defined, the process of FDA approval as pharmaceuticals is unlikely. The value attributed to probiotics, when used in otherwise healthy adults, is often based on user testimonials touted on the Internet and TV (Chapter 8).

The proven value of probiotics and synbiotics is for C-section infants (CF), especially those administered perinatal antibiotics (see below). Even for formula-fed infants (VgF; Chapter 4) their value is well-documented and is current practice. Infants in these categories either lack a microbiome or possess an altered microbiome. Some authors have labeled procedures used for CF, CBF, and VgF infants (Figure 5.2) as disrupters of eubiotic colonization (Mueller). C-section infants do not often encounter the *Lactobacillus* and *Bifidobacteria* obtained through vaginal birth. Such infants remain in pediatric care centers in isolators, where their primary exposure is to bacteria in the environment, sadly Proteobacteria like *E. coli, C. difficile*, and others obtained during surgical recovery or from the environment in the ICU facility. Thus, preterm and C-section infants (Figure 5.2) are those most likely to benefit from some form of probiotics or synbiotics. Probiotic therapy improves gastric motility and stimulates development of the adaptive immune system, leading to increases in IgA synthesis and SIgA secretion. There is some evidence that such treatments have been successfully employed to reduce the propensity for such newborns to later develop atopic eczema and food allergy (Rachid).

Especially relevant to events in the Critical Window (Chapter 1) is the previously mentioned NEC. NEC is a major problem for preterm infants and has a complex etiology/pathology. It can persist as inflammation and is fatal in some situations. Various studies have been conducted to determine if administration of probiotics could resolve NEC. Studies using probiotics therapy have mixed views (Slattery; McFarland). However, one study using *Lactobacillus* and *Bifidobacteria* in very low birthweight preterms was shown to reduce NEC, which could be due to banked milk or formulas enriched with HMOs. The host response to early colonization is not equal, especially when Proteobacteria are involved. Responding to *Lactobacilli* and *Bifidobacteria* rather than Proteobacteria is less likely to cause inflammation.

Probiotic Mediation in Selected Adult Maladies

The value of probiotics for adults often relies on folklore and testimonials. However, there are demonstrable situations in which their use has therapeutic benefits. A well-known application is in patients recovering from long-term antibiotic treatment, such as use of vancomycin in treatment of *C. difficile* and antibiotic cocktails used to eliminate *H. pylori*. Such individuals suffer serious loss of their GI tract microbiome through such treatment and have little microbiome to provide colonization resistance, so the newly acquired probiotic culture has a good chance to survive and become established. This in many ways parallels the routine administration of probiotics (and synbiotics) to preterms that were denied the opportunity to naturally acquire a microbiome through vaginal birth and breast-feeding (Figure 5.2).

IBD in adults causes collateral damage to the GI tract and occurs in 68% of adults with mild ulcerative colitis (a type of IBD). Remission may begin after 4 weeks of treatment with the yeast *Saccharomyces boulardi*. In the case of irritable bowel syndrome, often lumped together with IBD and which affects 10–20% of adolescents, results are mixed.

ASD (mentioned earlier) is an umbrella syndrome that includes Asperger syndrome, that has caught world attention in the last 3 decades. Many forms of ASD are a genetic disorder that can be traced to events *in utero*, and which may be due to gene regulatory factors triggered by environmental agents transferred during pregnancy (Chapter 2). In many cases, ASD is linked to a dysbiotic microbiome, which is a postpartum issue. ASD has drawn further attention to the MGBA (see above section) which sends messages to the vagusnerve when then sends signals to the brain. This connection has led some to believe that the GI tract microbiome indirectly signals the central nervous system and therefore might control neurological behavior in some ASD patients and other illnesses that involve the GI tract (Lenfestey).

Postnatal Feeding and the Microbiome

Figure 5.2 distinguishes among birthing methods and, for each group, the subsequent feeding regiments. The source of nourishment also determines the infant's exposure to regulatory factors that affect their development and health. Chapter 3 described factors like HMOs that would be denied to preterm and C-section infants not nourished on human milk. Even if infants in these groups are nourished on human milk from the mother or from milk banks, studies in animals have shown that these milks lose their regulatory effect when frozen (Figure 3.6). Equivalent studies comparing fresh colostrum with milk bank colostrum have not been reported.

Studies show the switch to formula feeding (VgF; Figure 5.2) causes perturbations in the establishment of the infant's microbiome that may have long-term consequences (Mueller). VgBF infants have a lower frequency of long-term morbidity with evidence for lower risk of obesity, type 2 diabetes, chronic intestinal inflammation, autoimmune disorders, and allergy (summarized in Chapter 3). A short-term effect is the lower incidence of NEC in breastfed infants that receive HMOs and higher levels of *Bifidobacteria*, such as *B. infantis* in Bangladesh and Malawi. Some believe that long-term risk factors are also due to the nature of the microbiome. Studies testing this hypothesis face numerous logistic challenges, for example controlling variations in consumption, the size of available stool samples, and differences among breast milks. It would be very difficult to test this in preterm infants since they cannot be exclusively fed breast milk. Therefore, most correlation studies have been done after 3 to 5 months. The results of such correlation studies indicate that (1) the microbiome of breastfed infants has significantly greater diversity or "richness" of taxa than that of infants fed on formula, (2) mixing breast milk with formula only partially restores microbiome diversity, and (3) formula-fed infants have a higher proportion of Enterobacteria like *E. coli* and *Enterococcus*, along with *B. fragilis* and *C. difficile*, while breastfed infants have more *Bifidobacteria*, *Faecalibacteria*, and *Lactobacillus*. While there are also a higher number of

Clostridia in VgBF infants, these do not include *C. difficile*. In addition to obtaining a source of HMOs, VgBF infants have access to various immune modulators (Chapter 3). Feeding mothers' milk to hospitalized preterm infants alters their microbiome, which then favors *Clostridia*, *Lactobacillus*, and *Bacteriodes* and increases microbiome diversity (Gregory).

Antibiotic Therapy and the Developing Neonatal Microbiome

Globally, antibiotic resistant (MDR) bacteria kill over 700,000 people per year and this is expected to continue to be a major cause of worldwide mortality (UN Interagency Coordination Group). Some suggest we live in the post-antibiotic age, so that infections once cured with antibiotics have become life-threatening. Antibiotics appear to select against/for certain taxa within the developing microbiome. Some have suggested antibiotics therapy in adults can cause a 10,000-fold reduction in the size of the healthy microbiome. Antibiotic therapy can eliminate certain taxa from the microbiome and enrich the number of MDR bacteria and the size of the **resistome** (see later). The various classes of antibiotics, their chemistry, and mechanisms of action are reviewed in Appendix A-3.

The healthy mature microbiome of adults is relatively stable, and recovers after disruption by antibiotic treatment, but incompletely (Dethlefsen). The developing microbiome of the neonate can be more easily altered by external factors like antibiotics. These are administered in the first year of life and their use has been linked to an increased risk for obesity, hypersensitivity pneumonitis, asthma, atopic allergy, NEC, and sepsis (Penders, SR; Tamburni; Gibson). Children aged 0–18 account for over 50% of antibiotics prescribed to individuals and 25% of all prescriptions. Preterm and very low birthweight infants are at highest risk for antibiotic disruption since they routinely receive antibiotics at birth. There are perturbations of the microbiome resulting in a decrease of the proportion of Bacteroides to Firmicutes, while the proportion of Proteobacteria increases. Bacterial resistance to antibiotics is increasing in the human population, whether or not individuals have ever experienced antibiotic therapy, because of the overall increase in the size of the **resistome** in all developed countries Early exposure to antibiotics appears to shape the maturing microbiome by increasing the number of MDR bacteria that are resistant to antibiotic therapy, that is, the **resistome.** The genetic basis for the expansion of the **resistome** and the related topic of HGT are discussed in Appendix A-1.

Exposure of infants to antibiotics occurs through three pathways. In Chapter 2 we described the pathway in which antibiotics given to the mother are transferred *in utero* to the fetus. Most agree the fetus has no microbiome, so *in utero* transfer seems inconsequential. However, antibiotics and other medications are transferred in breast milk, so a decision needs to be made before treating nursing mothers (Chapters 3 and 7). Formerly the "pump and dump" method was employed in situations in which a mother was receiving extensive antibiotic therapy. Since the effect on the suckling infant was unknown, mothers chose to err on the side of caution.

The third pathway is the current practice of direct administration of antibiotics to preterm and term infants and later to children and is based on the judgment of the attending pediatrician (Chapter 7). Direct administration of antibiotics is highest during the first years of life. In the United States they are the most prescribed medication in the neonatal period and within the pediatrics population and amoxicillin given to infants during the first month decreases the number of *Bifidobacteria* and *B. fragilis*, both considered important to the infant microbiome. Preterm infants appear most susceptible to the negative effects of antibiotics, and those given ampicillin and gentamicin have lower microbiome diversity and an increasing proportion of Proteobacteria like Enterobacteria, both features of dysbiosis. Fortunately, perturbations of the microbiome do not appear to be sustained after cessation of antibiotic therapy. The use of β-lactam antibiotics (penicillin family; Table A3.3) can increase the risk of NEC. In studies with mice, antibiotic-induced changes in the microbiome caused an increase in the inflammatory cytokine IL-17 (Chapter 6), which increases susceptibility to sepsis. Because NEC is a multifactorial disease without a clear microbial signature, it is difficult to connect it to a single factor like the microbiome. What does rest on solid evidence and was stated earlier is that NEC is reduced in VgBF infants suckling their own moms (Mueller). Since NEC is especially frequent in extremely preterm infants, developmental age may be a susceptibility factor. Results differ as to whether pasteurized donor milk can substitute for fresh mother's milk. Given the labile cytokines and other growth factors found in fresh mother's milk, loss of these immune and growth modulators by pasteurization or freezing may affect their efficacy in preventing NEC (see Chapter 3).

Suggested Readings (SRs)

Al-Nasiry S, Ambrosino E, Schlaepfer M, et al. The interplay between reproductive tract microbiota and immunological systems in human reproduction. *Front Immunol*. 2020;11:378. doi:10.3389/fimmu.2020.00378.

Brodin P. Immune-microbe interactions early in life: A determinant of health and disease long term. *Science*. 2022;376:945–950.

Fernandez L, Lanaga S, Martin V, et al. The human milk microbiota: Origin and potential roles in health and disease. *Pharmacol Res*. 2013;69:1–10.

Greer FR, Sichever SH, Burks AW. Effects of early nutritional interventions on the development of atopic disease in infants and children: The role of maternal dietary restriction, breast-feeding, timing of introduction of complementary foods and hydrolyzed formulas. *Pediatrics*. 2008;121:183–191.

Milani C, Durante S, Bottacini F, et al. The first microbial colonization of the human gut: Composition, activities and health implications of the infant gut microbiota. *Microbiol Molec Bio Rev*. 2017;81:1–51.

Penders J, Thiji C, Vink C, et al. Factors influencing the composition of the intestinal microbiota early in life. *Pediatrics*. 2015;118:511–521.

Powers SE, Otoole PW, Stanton C, Ross RP, Fitzgerald GF. Intestinal microbiota, diet and health. *Br J of Nutr*. 2015;111:387–402.

Sohn K, Underwood MA. Prenatal and postnatal administration of prebiotics and probiotics. *Semin Fetal Neonatal Med*. 2017 22:284–289.

Walker WA. The importance of appropriate bacterial colonization of the intestine in newborn, children, and adult health. *Pedatr Res*. 2017;82:387–395

References

Aagaard K, Ma J, Antony KM, Ganu R, Petrosino J, Versalovic J. The placenta harbors a unique microbiome *Sci Transl Med*. 2014;6:237ra65. doi:10.1126/scitrans/med.3008599.

Adlerberth I, Wold AE. Establishment of the gut microbiota in Western infants. *Acta Paediatrica*. 2009;98:229–238.

Alharthi A, Alhazmi S, Alburae N, Bahieldin A. The human gut microbiome as a potential fctors in autism spectrum disorder. *Int. J. Med Sci* 2002;25:1363. doi 10.3390/fjms 23031

Arroyo-Johnson C, Mincey KD. Obesity epidemiology worldwide. *Gastroenterol Clin North Am*. 2016;45:571–579.

Baker DR, Billey LO, Francis DH. Distribution of K88 *Escherichia coli*-adhesive and nonadhesivwe phenotypes among pigs of four breed. *Vet Microbiol*. 1997;54:123–132.

Benton R, Vannice KS, Gomez-Diaz C, Vosshall LB. Variant ionotropic glutamate receptors as chemosensory receptors in *Drosophila*. *Cell*. 2009;136:149–162.

Biagi E, Nylund L, Candela M, et al. Trough aging and beyond: Gut microbiota and inflammatory status in seniors and centenarians. *Plos One*. 2010;5:e10667. doi:0.1371/journal.pone.0010667.

Bosworth BT, Vogeli P. Compositions to identify swine genetically resistant to F18 *E. coli* associated diseases. USPTO No. 6965022 B2. November 15, 2005. https://patents.google.com/patent/US6965022B2/en.

Camarillo-Guerrevo LF, Almeidak A, Rangel-Pineros G, Finn RD, Lawley TD. Massive expansion of human gut bacteriophage diversity. *Cell*. 2021;184:1098–1109.

Chen L, Wang D, Garnaeva S, et al. The long-term genetic stability and individual specificity of the human gut microbiome. *Cell*. 2012;184:2303–2315.

Chernikova, M.A, Flores GD, Kilroy E, Labus JS, Mayer EA, Aziz-Zadeh LThe brain-gut-microbiome system: Pathways and implications for autism spectrum disorder. Nutrients 2021; 13: 4497. doi 10.3390/nu 13124497

Dethlefsen L, Relman DA. Incomplete recovery and individualized response of the human distal gut microbiota to repeated antibiotic perturbation *Proc Nat'l Acad Sci*. 2011;108(Supp. 1):4554–4561.

de Vrese M, Schrezenmeir J. Probiotics, prebotics and synbiotics. *Adv Biochem Engin Biotechol*. 2008;111:1–66.

Duscha A, Gisevius B, Hirschberg S, et al. Propionic acid shapes the multiple sclerosis disease course by an immunomodulatory mechanism. *Cell*. 2020;190:1067–1080.e16. doi:10.1016/j.cell.2020.02.035.

Ettinger G, MacDonald K, Reid G, Burton JP. The influence of the human microbiome and probiotics on cardiovascular health. *Gut*. 2014;56:719–728.

Everard A, Canai A D Gut microbiota and GLP-1 *Rev Endocr Metab Discord* 2014;15:189–196

Faith JJ, Guruge JL, Carbonneau MC, Subramanian S, Seedorf H, Goodman AL et al The long-term stability of the human gut microbiota *Science* 2013;5:341 doi:10.1126/science.1237439

García-Mantrana I, Selma-Royo M, Gonzáles S, et al. Distinct maternal microbiota clusters are associated with diet during pregnancy: Impact on neonatal microbiota and infant growth during the first 18 months of life. *Gut Microbes.* 2020;11:962–978. doi:10.1080/19490976.2020.1730294.

Gelfen T, Geva-Zatorsky N. What came first: The microbiota of the Tr(eg) cells? *Immunity.* 2018;48:1072–1078.

Gibson MK, Crofts TS, Dantas G. Antibiotics and the developing infant gut microbiota and resistome. *Curr Opin Microbiol.* 2015;27:51–56.

Gomez de Agüero M, Ganal-Vonarburg SC, Fuhrer T, et al. The maternal microbiota drives early postnatal innate immune development. *Science.* 2016;351:1296–1302.

Gordon JI, Dewey KG, Mills DA, Medzhitov RM. The human gut microbiota and undernutrition. Sci Transl Med 2012; 4:137 doi. 10.1126/scitranslmed. 3004347

Gregory KE, Samuel BS, Houghteling P, et al. Influence of maternal breast milk ingestion on acquisition of the intestinal microbiome in preterm infants. *Microbiome.* 2016;4:68. doi:10.1186/s40168-016-0214-x.

Guli L, Korosmaros T, Hall N. Flaviviruses hijack the host microbiota to facilitate their transmission. *Cell.* 2022;185:2395–2397.

Heikkila MP, Saris PEJ. Inhibition of *Staphylocoocus aureus* by commensal bacteria of human milk. *J Appl Microbiol.* 2003;95:471–478.

Henrick BM, Rodriguez L, Lakshmikanth T, et al. *Bifidobacteria*-mediated immune system imprinting early in life. *Cell.* 2021;184: 3884–3898.

Hurwitz JL, Orihuela C, DiRita VJ, Tuomann E. Bacterial interaction with mucosal epithelial cells. In: Mastecky J, Strober W, Russell MW, Kelsall BL, eds. *Mucosal Immunology.* Cambridge, MA: Academic Press; 2015:955–973.

iMSMS Consortium. Gut microbiome of multiple sclerosis patients and paired household healthy controls reveal association with disease risk and course. *Cell.* 2022;185:3467–3486.

Irima A, Chaudhari NN, Robles DJ, et al. The Indigenous South American Tsimane exhibit relatively modest decrease in brain volume with age despite high systemic inflation. *J of Gerontol: Series A.* 2021;76:2147–2155.

Jaret A, Jackson R, Duizer C, Healy ME, Zhao J, Rone JM, Bielecki P. et al Enteric nervous system-derived IL-18 orchestrates mucosal barrier immunity. *Cell* 2020; 180:50–63.

Jost T, Lacroix C, Braegger CP, Chassard C. New insights in gut microbiota establishment in healthy breast-fed neonates. *Plos One.* 2012;7:e44595. doi:10.1371/journal.pone.0044595.

Koeth R., Wang Z, Levison BS, et al. Intestinal microbiota metabolism of L-carntine, a nutrient in red meat, promotes atherosclerosis. *Nat. Med.* 2013;19:576–586.

Lallès J-P. Microbiota-host interplay at the gut epithelial level, health and nutrition *J An Sci Biotechn.* 2016;7:66–74. doi:10.1186/s40104-016-0123-7.

Leiby JS, McCormick K, Sherrill-Mix S, et al. Lack of detection of a human placenta microbiome in samples from preterm and term deliveries. *Microbiome.* 2018;6:196. https://microbiomejournal.biomedcentral.com/articles/10.1186/s40168-018-0575-4.

Lenfestey MW, Neu J. Probiotics in newborns and children. *Pediatr Clin North Amer.* 2017;64:1271–1289.

Leonardi I, Gao IH, Lin W-Y, et al. Mucosal fungi promote barrier function and social behavior via Type 17 immunity. *Cell.* 2022;186:831–846.

Leone V, Chang EB, Devkota S. Diet, microbes, and host genetics: The perfect storm in inflammatory bowel diseases. *J Gastrointerol.* 2013;48: 315–321.

Longo S, Rizza S, Federici M. Microbiota-gut-brain axis: relationships among the vagus nerve, gut microbiota, obesity and diabetes. *Acta Diabeto* 2023; 60: 1007–1017

Longo VD, Anderson RM. Nutrition longevity and disease: From molecular mechanisms to intervention. *Cell.* 2022;185:1455–1470.

MacIntyre DA, Chandiramani M, Lee YS, et al. The vaginal microbiome during pregnancy and the postpartum period in a European population. *Scien Rep.* 2015;5:8988. https://www.nature.com/articles/srep08988.

Mangalam A, Shahi SK, Luckey D, et al. Human gut-derived commensal bacteria suppress CNS inflammatory and demyelinating disease. *Cell Rep.* 2017;20:1269–1277.

McFarland LV. From yaks to yogurt: The history, development and current use of probiotics. *Clin Inf Disease.* 2015;60(S2):585–590.

Molodecky NA, Shian Soon I, Rabi DM, et al. Increasing incidence and prevalence of the inflammatory bowel diseases with time, based on systematic review. *Gastroenterology.* 2012;142:46–54. e42. doi:10.1053/j.gastro.2011.10.001.

Mueller NT, Bakacz E, Combellick J, Grigoryan Z, Dominquez-Bello MG. The infant microbiome development: mom matters. *Trends Mol Med.* 2015;21:109–117.

Obaldia ME, Mortia t, Dedmon LC, et al. Differential mosquito attraction to humans is associated with skin-derived carboxylic acid levels. *Cell.* 2022;185:4099–4116.

Olin MR, Dahan D, Carter MM, et al. Robust variation in infant gut microbiome assembly across a spectrum of lifestyles. *Science.* 2022;376:1220–1223.

Perez-Muñoz ME, Arrieta M-C, Ramer-Tait AE, Walter J. A critical assessment of the "sterile womb" and "in utero colonization" hypothesis: Implications for research on the pioneer infant microbiome. *Microbiome.* 2017;5:48–67.

Rachid R, Chatila TA. The role of gut microbiota in food allergy. *Curr Opin Pediatr.* 2016;28:748–753.

Raghavan S, Holmgren J, Svennerholm A-M. *Helicobacter pylori* infection of the gastric mucosa. In: Mestecky J, Strober W, Russell MW, Kelsall BL, Cheroutre H., Lambrecht BN, eds. *Mucosal Immunology.* Cambridge, MA: Academic Press; 2015:985–1001.

Sjödin KS, Vidman L, Rydén P, West CE. Emerging evidence of the role of gut microbiota in the improvement of allergic disease. *Curr Opin Allergy Clin Immunol.* 2016;16:390–395.

Slattery J, Mac Fabe DF, Frye RE. The significance of the enteric microbiome on the development of childhood disease: A review of prebiotic and probiotic therapies in disorder of childhood. *Pediatrics.* 2016;10:91–107.

Suez J, Zmora N, Zilberman-Schapira G, et al. Post-antibiotic gut mucosal microbiome reconstitution is impaired by probiotics and improved by autologous FMT. *Cell.* 2018;174:1406–1423.

Tamburni SN, Shen H, Chih Wu H, Clemente JC. The microbiome in early life: Implications for health outcomes. *Nat Med*. 2016;22:713–717.

Taniya M.A Chung H-J Al Mamun A, Alam S Abdul Aziz Md, Uddin Emon N et al. Role of gut microbiome on autism spectrum disorder and its therapeutic regulation. *Frontiers Cell Infect Microbiol*. 2022; 22:12.915701 doi 10.3387/fcimb

United Nations Interagency Coordination Group on Antimicrobial Resistance. No time to wait: Securing the future from drug-resistant infections. April 2019. www.who.int/antimicrobial-resistance/interagency-coordination-group.

Vatanen T, Jabbar KS, Ruohtula T, et al. Mobile genetic elements from the maternal microbiome shape infant gut microbial assembly and metabolism. *Cell*. 2022;185:4921–4936.

Vatanen T, Plichia DR, Somari J, et al. Genomic variation and strain-specific functional adaption in the human gut-microbiome during life. *Nat Microbiol*. 2018;4: 470–479.

Vatanen T, Yan Ang Q, Slegwald L, et al. A distinct clade of *Bifidobacterium longum* in the gut of Bangladeshi children thrives during weaning. *Cell*. 2022;185:4280–4297.

Voreades N, Kozil A, Weir TL. Diet and the development of the human intestinal microbiome. *Front Microbiol*. 2014;5:494. doi:10.3389/fmicb.2014.00494.

Walter J, Armet AM, Finlay BB, Shanahan F. Establishing or exaggerating causality for the gut microbiome: Lessons for human microbiota-associated rodents. *Cell*. 2020;180:221–232.

Wang Z, Roberts AB, Buffa JA, et al. Non-lethal inhibition of gut microbial trimethylamine production for the treatment of atherosclerosis. *Cell*. 2015;163:1585–1595.

Wassenaar TM. Insights from 100 years of research with probiotic *E.coli*. *Eur J Microbiol Immunol*. 2016;6:147–161.

Wastyk HG, Fragiadakis GK, Perelam D, et al. Gut-microbiota-targeted diets modulate human immune status. *Cell*. 2021;184:4137–4153.

Yan Q, Li S, Yan Q, Huo X, Wang C, et al. A genomic compendium of cultivated human gut fungi characterizes the gut myobiome and its relevance to common diseases. *Cell*. 2024;187(14):2969–2989.

Yatsunenko T, Rey FE, Manary MJ, et al. Human gut microbiome viewed across age and geography. *Nature*. 2012;486:222–227.

Zeng Y, Wu Y, Zhang Q, Xiao X. Crosstalk between glucagon-like peptides 1 and gut microbiota in metabolic diseases. 2024 *mBio* 16; 15 (1) e0203223 doi 1128/mbio. 02032-23

Zimmermann P, Curtis N. Breast milk microbiota: A review of the factors that influence composition. *J Infect*. 2020;81:17–47.

Chapter Reviewers

David Elliott Head of gastroenterology, Carver College of Medicine, University of Iowa

Michael Apicella Emeritus head of microbiology, Carver College of Medicine, University of Iowa

David Ashton Former head of microbiology for Hunt-Wesson Foods

Aloysius Klingelhutz Professor of microbiology/immunology, Carver College of Medicine, University of Iowa

CHAPTER 6

Internal Protection

Immune Systems, Vaccination, and Antimicrobials

Protection is a critical factor in the health and survival of offspring and, therefore, of species. In mammals, the developing fetus is protected in the womb of the mother, and after delivery by the guarding behavior of the parents. All life forms have erected protective external barriers; bacteria have cell walls, skin protects vertebrates, insects and crustaceans have an exoskeleton and turtles have carapaces. In mammals, skin protects against invading pathogens and the rays of the sun, and in marine mammals, against the near-freezing waters in which they live. The internal mucosal epithelia, like in the respiratory and GI tract, protect against pathogens but must simultaneously allow for gas exchange and nutrient uptake. Protection is, however, more than just skin-deep, and in this lengthy chapter we describe the immune systems that have evolved to provide internal protection, the antimicrobial drugs used to control bacteria (antibiotics), and vaccines used to counter viruses. While this chapter could be divided into several, we choose to unite these issues under the concept of internal protection and divide it into sections: (I) Basic concepts governing immune systems, (II) immunological tolerance and immunological injury, (III) vaccines and antimicrobials, and (IV) protection through use of antimicrobials.

Section I: Basic Concepts Governing Immune Systems

LEARNING OBJECTIVES

1. Describe the principles of self-/non-self-recognition and the mechanisms used to achieve it.

2. Discuss the importance of protection provided by the innate immune system versus protection provided by the adaptive immune system.

3. Learn why an adaptive immune system is needed to deal with microbial pathogens.

4. Discuss the role of intercellular messengers in innate and adaptive immunity.

5. Distinguish between mucosal, systemic, and passive immunity.

Immunology: "The Science of Self-/Non-Self-Discrimination"

The ability of life to discriminate self from non-self became the task of complicated immune systems in multicellular eukaryotes. In vertebrates there are two separate systems that work together to protect the host: the **innate** and the **adaptive** immune systems. Both evolved primarily to protect against microbial pathogens. Innate immunity is found in all multicellular eukaryotes, including vertebrate, invertebrates like insects and crustaceans, worms, and even plants. Many unicellular life forms also have primitive forms of **innate immunity**. However, invertebrates lack a well-developed adaptive immune system like that of warm-blooded vertebrates. Why such a system did not develop in invertebrates like insects is at most speculative. One possibility is that it is not required when the life of the adult is only weeks to months and most pathogens die with the host. This explanation would not work for nymphs of cicadas and dragonflies that live for many years. Perhaps the potent antimicrobial peptides, antibiotics, and other poisons found in a broad spectrum of invertebrates is alone adequate to control microbial pathogens.

Self-/non-self-discrimination is a property of the cells of all eukaryotic life forms, including unicellular protozoans that display surface molecules that are species-specific. In Chapter 1 we described the mixing of cells disrupted from two different species of sponges and then incubating them in a Petri dish to observe that the cells reorganized according to species. In higher vertebrates like humans, self-/non-self-discrimination extends to individuals within the same species. Most readers know that with certain exceptions, tissues and organs cannot be transplanted among just any individuals; success depends on their genetic relationship and their genetically determined cell surface molecules, making identical twins the best donors for each other. In humans, the cell surface markers that are most important in distinguishing individuals are known as the major histocompatibility complex (MHC), which is present in two different molecular configurations: MHC I and MHC II. MHC was briefly mentioned in Chapter 2 in regard to fetal-maternal tissue compatibility. However, MHC contains more than just surface recognition markers; it plays a critical role in adaptive immunity, which depends on the interactions of cells called the lymphocytes and various monocytes that act as antigen-presenting cells (APCs; Table 6.1) that present peptides bound to the MHC. Prior to the evolutionary appearance of lymphocytes and adaptive immunity, life forms depended on a range of receptors that evolved to recognize pathogens and thus danger, officially known as the innate immune system.

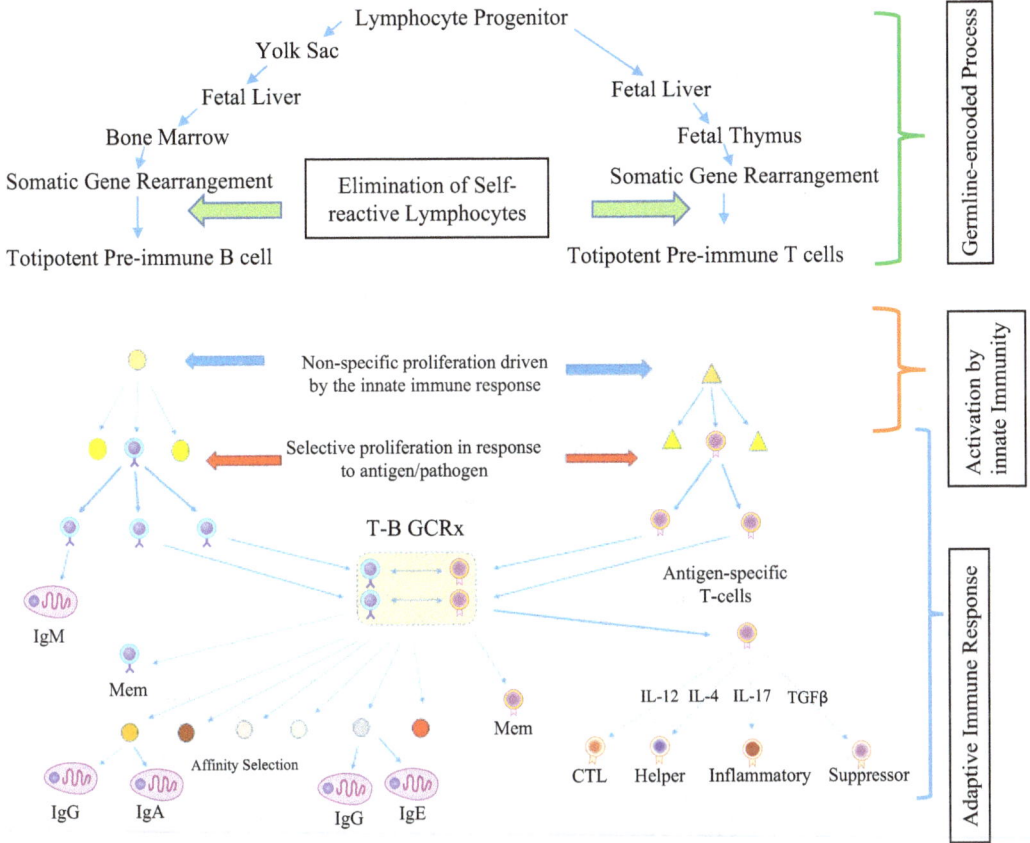

Figure 6.1 Lymphogenesis and lymphocyte diversification. The pathways of T and B cell lymphopoiesis from a common precursor are illustrated. Major events in lymphopoiesis are indicated on the right vertical axis. Major pathways, and lymphocyte selection and their differentiation, including cytokine-driven differentiation into T cell subsets, is shown. The central yellow box surrounded by an interrupted boundary represents a germinal center (GCRx) where T and B cells interact and where further contact with APCs occurs. Affinity selected B cells differentiate to antibody producing plasma cells. Mem = memory B cells or memory T cells. Icons described in Table 6.1.

Before proceeding to describe these systems, we warn that immunology can be difficult for some students, a situation made worse by an unfamiliar vocabulary that uses many abbreviations. Biologists have a reputation for naming things, sometimes even creating a new language, and immunologists may top the list. Terms like IL-5 and TNF-α (cytokines); TLR 2 and TLR 5 (toll-like receptors); and the names of different types of hematopoietic cells are summarized in Tables 6.1–6.3. Immunologists also often refer to CD markers like

TABLE 6.1 Leukocytes and Hematopoietic Cells

Name	Description	Icon Used in Book
Hematopoietic Stem Cell	An umbrella category for cells in the bone marrow that are the progenitors of leukocytes and erythrocytes.	NA
Thymocyte	Hematopoietic cells that have migrated to the thymus where they undergo differentiation and "education" before they emerge and circulate as mobile T cells. Appearance is similar to a plasmablast but they express CD3 associated with their TCRs.	
Erythrocyte or Red Blood Cell (RBC) 99% of blood cells	Spherical blood cells that appear red due to oxygen-carrying hemoglobin. In mature form they lack a nucleus. Immature forms called normoblast are nucleated. Appearance of the latter in blood reflects a stressed hematopoietic system.	
Leukocyte or White Blood Cell (WBC) 1% of blood cells	Umbrella term for mobile blood cells that appear translucent/white (*leuko*) and include granulocytes, monocytes, and lymphocytes (see later).	NA
Granulocyte	A category of leukocytes with tri-lobed nuclei and with cytoplasm filled with many granules that take different staining patterns, accounting for their names.	See variants later.
Neutrophil 60% of WBCs	Phagocytic granulocytes that take up a neutral pH stain (*neutro*). Their presence is a primary indicator of inflammation, and they secrete cytokines like TGF-α (see Table 6.3).	
Eosinophil Approximately 3% of WBCs	Granulocytes whose granules stain red with acidic stains (*eosin*). They are a feature of atopic allergy or parasitic disease and release numerous inflammatory cytokines.	
Basophil Approximately 1% of WBCs	Granulocytes with granules that stain purple with alkaline stains (*baso*). Especially important in atopic allergy because of their secretion of many vasoactive amines (see Figure 6.7).	

TABLE 6.1   Leukocytes and Hematopoietic Cells *(Continued)*

Name	Description	Icon Used in Book
Monocyte Less than 1% of blood cells	Leukocytes with a single nucleus surrounded by a moderate degree of cytoplasm containing various organelles. These circulate widely in blood and include plasmacytoid dendritic cells (pDCs).	
Macrophage	Monocyte that can assume an ameboid form and act as a major phagocytic and antigen-presenting cells (APCs). Found in lymphoid tissues in association with lymphocytes and at sites of inflammation, where they secrete IL-1, IL-6, and TNF-α (see Table 6.3).	
Dendritic Cell (DC)	Amoeboid-like cells with pseudopods that in mucosal tissue can extend between epithelial cells to capture antigens and pathogens. Some have other names such as Langerhans cells, which are found in association with dermal epithelial cells. DCs serve as major APCs.	
Lymphocyte Approximately 33% of WBCs	Small circulating or resident mononuclear cells in lymphoid tissue that appear to have little cytoplasm. These cells are responsible for the adaptive immune system. These types originate from a common progenitor, which then differentiates into many subsets (see Figure 6.1). Can only be distinguished based on biochemical or CD markers on their membranes. Different icons designate different subsets.	T-cell B-cell NK-cell
Th1 Helper and Cytotoxic T Cells (CTL)	T cells that secrete cytokine that promote inflammation and are directed to destroy other cells, such as those that are virus-infected (orange nucleus). CD8 is a diagnostic surface marker.	
Th2 Helper T Cells	T cells that secrete cytokines that promote B cells to become plasma cells and secrete antibodies (green nucleus). CD4 is a diagnostic surface marker.	
Regulatory T Cells (Treg)	These secrete cytokines like TGF-ß that especially suppresses inflammatory Th1 and Th2 helper T cells and thereby maintain homeostasis (purple nucleus). CD25 and FOXP3 are diagnostic markers.	

(Continued)

TABLE 6.1   Leukocytes and Hematopoietic Cells *(Continued)*

Name	Description	Icon Used in Book
Th17 T Cell	T cells that secrete IL-17, which can provide protection against pathogens but can also cause inflammation in the case of inflammatory bowel disease (IBD) and other autoimmune disorders.	
Plasmablast	Antigen-selected B cells with expanded cytoplasmic machinery for synthesizing of antibodies. These migrate in blood and lymph to sites where they become plasma cells.	
Plasma cell	Fully differentiated B cells with limited mobility that are "factories" for the secretion of antibodies, often illustrated by emerging/secreting antibodies.	

TABLE 6.2   Toll-Like Receptors (TLRs) and Their Specificity

TLR	Location	Ligand	Common Target Microbe
TLR1	PM	Triacyl lipopeptides	Mycobacteria
TLR2	PM	Peptidoglycans	Gram-positive bacteria
		Lipoproteins	Mycobacteria
		Zymosan	Yeast and fungi
TLR3	Endosome	Double-strandeded RNA	Viruses
TLR4	PM	Lipopolysaccharide (LPS)	Gram-negative bacteria
		F protein	Respiratory syncytial virus (RSV)
TLR5	PM	Flagellin	Bacteria
TLR6	PM	Diacyl lipopeptides	Mycobacteria
TLR7	Endosome	Single-stranded RNA	Viruses
TLR8	Endosome	Single-stranded RNA	Viruses
TLR9	Endosome	CpG oligonucleotides	Bacterial DNA
		Herpes infection	Some herpes viruses

PM = plasma membrane
Endosome = spherical intracellular organelles with a simple membrane

TABLE 6.3   Cytokines, Chemokines, and Growth Factors

Cytokine	Source	Role in Immune System
IL-1	Macrophages, DCs, and others	Feature of the innate immune response
IL-2	T cells	Overall stimulator of growth and proliferation of lymphocytes and NK cells
IL-4	T cells, mast cells	B cell activation, IgE class switch, and induction of Th2 helper cells
IL-5	Mast cells, T cells, eosinophils	Induces eosinophil differentiation
IL-6	Lymphocytes, inflammatory cells	Regulates T and B cell growth and differentiation
IL-7	Bone marrow, spleen, and thymus	Growth factor for T and B cells from stromal cells in primary lymphoid tissues
IL-10	Activated T cells and others	Suppresses macrophage function and cooperates with TFG-β in suppression of inflammatory (Th1) T cells
IL-12	Macrophages and DCs	Enhances IFNγ production and Type IV hypersensitivity
IL-17	Th17 T cells	Initiates inflammatory responses that can be either beneficial or, in autoimmunity, cause immunological bystander damage
IL-18	DCs, Goblet cells, and ENS neurons	Promotes inflammation in the GI tract
IFN-α	Almost all leukocytes	Mediator of inflammation that induces resistance to viral infection
IFN-β	Fibroblasts	Initiates antiviral response, increases MHC-I expression
IFN-γ	T cells and NK cells	Activates especially inflammatory (Th 1) T cells and suppresses (Th2) helper T cells
TGF-β	Most nucleated cells	Suppresses inflammatory lymphocytes, promotes switch to IgA and mucosal development
TNF-α	Macrophages, NKs, and T cells	Causes local inflammatory response

Chemokine	Cells Attracted	Receptor
CC 2 (MCP-1)	Effector T cells, NK, M/DC granulocytes	CCR2
CCL3 (MIP-1)	Th1 cells, NK, M/D, eosinophils	CCR1,5
CCL5 (RANTES)	Effector T cells, NK, M/D, eosinophils, basophils	CCR1,2,3
CCL11 (Eotaxin)	Effector T cells, eosinophils, basophils	CCR3,5
XCL1 (Lymphotactin)	Effector T cells, B cells, NK, neutrophils	XCR1
CXCL8 (IL-8)	Neutrophils	CXCR1,2
CXCL13 (BCA-1)	Homing of B cells	CXCR1,2

NK = natural killer cells; M/D = macrophages and dendritic cells

(Continued)

TABLE 6.3   Cytokines, Chemokines, and Growth Factors *(Continued)*

Growth Factor	Source	Role in Immune System
Epithelial growth factor (EGF)	Many sources, especially salivary glands	Receptor (EGFR) is widespread. Promotes cell differentiation and proliferation.
Insulin-like growth factor family (IGF)	Liver and elsewhere under stimulation of growth hormones	Cell proliferation and inhibition of apoptosis
Colony-stimulating factor (G-CSF; GM-CSF)	Bone marrow stomal cells and macrophages	Essential for growth and differentiation of neutrophils and other leukocytes
Colony-stimulating factor (C-CSF; M-CSF)	Endothelial cells, fibroblasts, and macrophages	Stimulates proliferation of granulocytes, osteoclasts, and macrophages.
IL-3	T cells or macrophages	Cell growth of stem cells of myeloid progenitors
IL-5, IL-6, IL-7	See cytokines.	See cytokines.

Cytokines. Intracellular messengers, especially among hematopoietic cells. Many are called interleukins (IL) because they message cross-talk among leukocytes. There are dozens and they belong to a number of families; individual members aredesignated by Greek suffixes such as in TNF-α, IFN-β, TGF-β.

Chemokines. Intercellular messengers that stimulate or aid in the migration of many types of leukocytes. More than 40 are known. They are designated as CCLs, CXCLs, or XCLs. Prior to efforts to standardize nomenclature, the literature used other names like RANTES (CCL5) or MCP-1 (CCL1) and MIP-1 (CCL2). Receptors for chemokines belong to 7 or more multidomain transmembrane molecules found on hematopoietic cells. Binding of a chemokine activates the cells, often resulting in stimulus to migrate in some fashion. Chemokines may have multiple receptors, some of which are shared and some of which are more specific.

Growth factors. This is a very broad category of factors that stimulate the differentiation and development of many cell lineages. The names typically designate a family of factors, the individual members quite often designated by Greek suffixes.

Category confusion. In addition to having dual names, some may have changed categories. IL-8 was originally considered a cytokine, but is now known as the chemokine CSCL8. IL-3 was once listed as a cytokine but is now in the growth factor category. IL-5, IL-6, and IL-7 (listed as cytokines) are also considered growth factors.

CD4, CD8, and so on, to identify different subtypes of hematopoietic cells. While more than 300 are known, we distill the number down to about a dozen of the more frequently used (Table A3.2). In this chapter, to focus on basic concepts and not cause confusion by providing too much detail, we have moved many molecular and cellular details and their associated genetics to Appendix A-1.

First Responders: The Innate Immune System

Innate immune receptors can be described as "what you inherited is what you get," whereas receptors for adaptive immunity are somatically generated in each individual and then selected to generate more highly specific receptors within the life span of the individual. Adaptive immunity is critical for the survival of higher vertebrates, but its activation depends on first activating the **pattern recognition receptors (PRR)** of the more primitive innate immune system that recognizes threats posed by pathogens as "danger." These are widespread among eukaryotes, dating back circa 600 million years to sponges. When a higher eukaryote encounters an infectious agent or foreign substance, a condition called **inflammation** develops, which is characterized in vertebrates by the accumulation of **inflammatory cells** such as neutrophils and macrophages (Table 6.1). These release many factors involved in resolving the infection and their intracellular accumulation are often called **inflammasomes**. When the intruder is a bacterium or a virus, the accumulation of inflammatory cells and their active factors depends on their ability to recognize features not found on cells of eukaryotic life forms (Chapter 1). In eukaryotes the best-known **PRRs** are the **toll-like receptors (TLRs)**. These take their name from the "beautiful receptors" first described in the common fruit fly (*Drosophila*) that enables the fly to recognize microbial pathogens. *Toll* is a German word for beauty. In addition to TLRs, there are a number of other PRRs, some of which we describe in Appendix A-1. TLRs and other PRRs recognize biochemical features unique to bacteria and viruses (Table 6.2). These biochemical features are referred to as **PAMPs**, short for **pathogen-associated molecular patterns**. We will later mention **damage-associated molecular patterns (DAMPs)**, which are also recognized by PRRs that are found in the cytosol. These include NOD-like receptors (NLRs), retinoic acid receptors, and the cGAS-STING system. These are very important in viral and intracellular bacterial infections and in responding to cytosolic DAMPs. These and their signaling pathways are described in more detail in Appendix A-1.

TLRs are widespread and share a common molecular structure (Appendix A-1). Some are found on the plasma membrane while others are intracellular on endosomes (Table 6.2). TLRs have an ancient history ranging in occurrence from coral to humans. TLRs are found on many cells but especially on macrophages and dendritic cells (DC; Table 6.2) that play the role of sentinels and detect "danger" for the host. Recognition of PAMPs by TLRs on a macrophage triggers a series of cellular events such as (1) engulfing bacteria, other microbes, and acting as APCs that present the degraded product of the microbes they have engulfed to lymphocytes of the adaptive immune system, and (2) releasing substances called **cytokines** and **chemokines**, which results in inflammation and cell migration (next section and Table 6.3). Stimulation of the innate immune system typically results in the release of cytokines like TNF-α, IL-1, and IL-6 (Table 6.3). Together with other functions, they activate certain T lymphocytes (T cells) of the adaptive immune system. The breakdown products of pathogens also serve as "adjuvants," a term discussed further in Section III.

Another ingredient of the innate immune system is the **complement system**, which draws its name from the observation that it "complements" the actions of antibodies of the adaptive immune system. Historically the components that comprise this system were characterized in studies in which they formed complexes with antibodies that caused lysis of red blood cells (hemolysis). Later studies revealed that the complement system carries out many activities that are independent of antibodies and cell lysis, so that the system is now regarded as part of the innate immune system.

The complement system is comprised of a cascade of up to nine "pro-enzymes" referred to as zymogens. Zymogens are inactive proteases that remain so until triggered by some inflammatory event. Once activated, they become active proteases that attack other zymogens, causing their activation and ultimately creating an amplification chain reaction, the endstage ov which could be lysis of some target cell or the killing of an invading pathogen. In the process, secondary products released by cleavage of certain zymogens have separate actions, such as cleavage products C3a and C5a that can recruit inflammatory cells and C3b that can bind special receptors on phagocytic cells and prepares them to become phagocytic, a process called opsonization. The actions of the complement system in the innate immune system can be summarized as (1) recruitment of phagocytic cells to a site of infection, (2) activation of phagocytic cells (opsonization), and (3) association with antibodies that target cells and bacteria, resulting in their lysis or damage to their cell membranes.

In the not-too-distant past the role of innate immunity in host protection was overshadowed since adaptive immunity held the spotlight. If adaptive immunity was the only "real" form of protection, how could transgenic mice that lack an adaptive immune system ward off various infections? It has been known for some time that the tuberculosis vaccine (BCG) not only decreases childhood mortality to severe disseminated forms of tuberculosis and sepsis, but through stimulating innate immunity also decreases the incidence of disease caused by completely unrelated respiratory pathogens for up to 3 months. This protective innate response is through the secretion of TNF-α, IL-1 and IL-6 (Table 6.3). The effectiveness of the innate immune response to substances like BCG appears to increases with age, and some have speculated that it can explain why in countries like the United States, Italy, the Netherlands, Spain, and Ecuador, which do not have a policy for universal BCG vaccination, the incidence of COVID-19 mortality is higher, especially among the elderly, than in countries that still regularly use BCG. Innate immunity may also explain why bats and certain other mammals survive SARS, Ebola, and other viral diseases (Appendix A-2). Some suggest that 80% or more of protection against pathogens depends on innate immunity.

Later we shall describe **immunologic memory** as being a key feature of **adaptive immunity**, which raises the question of whether the innate immune system also has memory. When macrophages of the innate immune system are stimulated by re-encounter with the initial or even an unrelated pathogen, they often act as if "trained" in that they more quickly release the cytokines that characterize their responses. This does not involve the type of somatic genetic change in lymphocytes that can modify gene expression without modifying the genes responsible (Appendix A-1). While cells of the innate immune system lack memory of a specific pathogen, they do retain "memory" of having previously activated and are able to mount a more vigorous innate response. This may be equivalent to the response of the neighborhood dog that was mistreated by one person but thereafter views all humans as a threat. This is now termed **trained immunity**, which is a feature of the innate immune system and should not be confused with **immunologic memory**, which is a feature of the adaptive immune system. Using the dog analogy, immunologic memory limits the dog's aggression only to the person that mistreated it.

Natural killer cells (NK cells) are another arm of the innate immune system. These are T cell-like, but they do not bear a T cell receptor (TCR; see later); instead, they recognize PAMPs with a variety of phosphorylated receptors. NK cells can provide protection before the adaptive immune system can respond. They bear both killer inhibitory receptors (KIRS) and killer activation receptors (KARS). KARS remain inactive when KIRS remain in contact with MHC I on any cell. Under healthy conditions, MHC I epitope presentation on the cell surface is used to display the degraded peptide of viruses that infect it, thus alerting APCs and signaling the need for help (see later). However, suppression of MHC I is common in infections with cytomegalovirus (CMV) and herpes viruses and is described in the section entitled "The Microbial Empire Strikes Back." With the loss of MHC- I expression by an infected cell, KARS become activated, and the NK cell now acts like a cytotoxic T cell to destroy the infected cell (Figure A1.7). An NK variant is known as NKt because it possesses an invariant TCR (NK cells lack a TCR). Some consider NKt cells to be T cell contaminants or "ghost cells." NK and NKt cells are further described in Figure A1.7. As mentioned in Chapter 2, NK or NKt cells appear to be important in helping to protect the fetal hemi-allograft.

Cancers of all kinds continue to plague humans, and it has been known for some time that induction of apoptosis of cancer cells is important for tumor reduction. This depends on triggering certain mitochondrial activities. As described in Chapter 1, mitochondria are cell organelles that possess a mini-genome distinct from the chromosomal genome of the cell. Tumor cell apoptosis can be triggered by mAb-like anti-CD20 and mAb to EGRF (epithelial growth factor; see Appendix A-3). However, activation of NK cells can also lead to pro-mitochondrial apoptosis. Hence there is renewed interest in the activity of NK cells (Nami-Mancinelli).

Critical Messengers: Cytokines and Chemokines

Both innate and adaptive immune systems depend on intercellular communication through direct contact or by using chemical messengers. A century ago biologists observed that when the media in which certain cells had been cultured was added to a culture containing different cells, these cells became "activated" and moved in the direction where the media had been added. Cells like macrophages, the cousins of free-living amoeba and found in all multicellular eukaryotes (Table 6.1), are highly mobile and will "crawl" toward an infected epithelial cell when activated. Observations like these led to the characterization of many intercellular mediators, which are called **cytokines** and **chemokines**. Their actions are not restricted to cells exclusively associated with immune systems; they are also involved in many other intercellular communications. All require specific chemokine and cytokine receptors. The system is complex, with over 40 known chemokines. Table 6.3 describes a number that are periodically mentioned in this book. Chemokines are classified into two subgroups: CC and CXC, based on the location of cysteines that are important to their structure. In brief, chemokines deliver the message that cells need to migrate while cytokines signal cells to make certain internal metabolic changes, to activate certain genes, or to secrete certain substances. It can be imagined that when large amounts of these are simultaneously released due to an inflammatory or infectious event, chaos may result, and this is sometimes referred to as a "cytokine storm." Such storms can cause "bystander" damage, such as the response to DAMPs (see Section II), as can occur with COVID-19 and many other infections (Venereau, SR). Such storms may also play a role in inflammatory bowel disorders (IBD), discussed in Chapter 5.

Several cytokines were mentioned in Chapters 2 and 3 because they regulate the activity of lymphocytes in passive immunity, such as chemokine CXCL13, which is involved in the migration of IgA-producing cells from the GI tract to the mammary gland; TGF-β, which promotes the switch from IgM to IgA at mucosal sites; and IL-4, which promotes the switch from IgM to other isotypes after a GCRx (Figure 6.1). When secreted in milk, TGF-β also suppresses development of inflammatory T cells associated with IBD in the GI tract (Chapters 3 and 5). IL-2 controls proliferation and activation of lymphocytes, and in viral infections, interferons (INF) α, β, and γ are released by the innate immune system and they activate inflammatory T cells and NK cells.

Antimicrobial Peptides (AMPs)

AMP comprise another arm of innate immunity. In Chapter 3 we mentioned that β-defensins (one type of AMP) are transferred through breast-feeding, and in Chapter 5 we mentioned them in their relationship to the microbiome of the GI tract. AMP are comprised of 10–100 amino acids and are divided into many families; 4,000 have been reported (Zhang). Nicin was the first AMP recovered from a bacterium; it is cytotoxic for other bacteria and is now used in food preservation. Defensins occur in three subtypes, but only α-defensins and β-defensins occur in humans. Defensins are made by various leukocytes and epithelial cells. These AMP occur in both anionic and cationic forms. Negatively charged LPS in Gram-negative bacteria (eg, Proteobacteria; see Chapter 5), and lipoteichoic acid in the cell walls of Gram-positive bacteria, are targeted by cationic AMPs. It is believed that the reason they do not target the plasma membranes of eukaryotic cells is because the phosphotidyl choline and phosphotidyl ethanolamine that comprise them bear a neutral charge. AMPs along with certain lipids form an epidermal barrier, in the oral environment as well as in protection against atopic dermatitis (Brogden; Imokawa; Dale).

Why Adaptive Immunity Is Needed

The adaptive immune system emerged with the evolutionary appearance of a special cell type, the **lymphocyte** (Table 6.1), that can somatically alter the genes encoding the specificity of its receptors; thus the origin of the term "adaptive." Star Wars fans may consider lymphocytes the Jedi Knights that enter the scene to do battle with the Microbial Empire. The need for this evolutionary adaption can be realized since the rate of spontaneous mutation is more rapid for viruses than bacteria and Eukaryotes (Figure 6.2) and that the human genome or that of other Eukaryotes is very large compared to microbes. Microbes also have a much faster rate of reproduction (ie, minutes for viruses and bacteria versus up to 13 years in humans; see Figure 6.2). Realizing that nearly all spontaneous gene mutations occur during replication of DNA (ie, during reproduction; Appendix A-1), the huge disparity in genome size, mutation rate and rate of reproduction allows the generation of the small table presented with Figure 6.2. This shows that bacteria can change their genome thousands of times faster than humans, and some viruses can do this a million times faster. Thus, higher vertebrates cannot alter their genomes fast enough to compete with genomic changes made by microbial pathogens. Enter the "Jedi lymphocytes," with their ability to perform somatic gene rearrangement and somatic hypermutation (SHM) during an individuals lifetime (see Appendix A-1 for details on the molecular genetics involved).

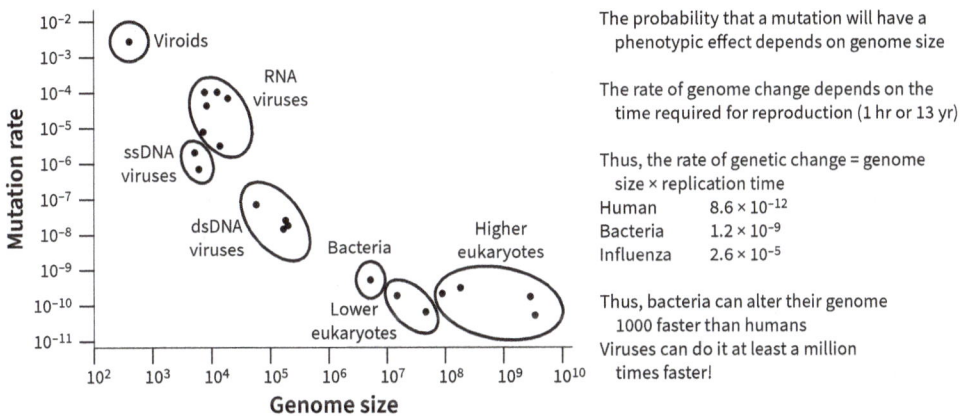

Figure 6.2   Genome size and reproductive rate determine the frequency of species diversification. Compared to eukaryotes, particularly higher vertebrates with large genomes, microbes dodge elimination by the host immune system through rapid genomic/phenotypic changes, regularly rendering them "invisible." Microbes reproduce in hours while vertebrates require years. This matters because the spontaneous mutations that lead to phenotypic change occur during DNA replication, and reproduction rates vary from minutes to hours to years. Genome size will affect whether a mutation will have a significant phenotypic effect.

Lymphocytes are the flagships of adaptive immunity and like other leukocytes develop from hematopoietic cells and come in several forms (Table 6.1). **T cells** are named because they mature in the thymus gland and there are both α/β and γ/δ variants. **B cells** are named because they mature in the bone marrow; both sites are referred to as **primary lymphoid tissues** (Figure 6.1). Lymphocyte development also requires help from cytokines; specifically, in the bone marrow and thymus they need help from IL-7 (Table 6.3). Differing developmental pathways generate T and B lymphocytes, each of which have different functions. Among the variants are memory B cells, plasma cells, and numerous α/β T cell variants, some referred to as inflammatory (Th1 and Th17) and other referred to as Th2 helpers and regulatory T cells (Treg) as well as cytotoxic T cells (CTL; Table 6.1). The differentiation of T cells into subsets depends on the influence of certain cytokines (Figure 6.1; Table 6.3). γ/δ T cells in mice and humans are largely confined to mucosal sites and represent a tiny portion of circulating T cells. This pattern differs from that in certain other mammals where they can be the dominant T cells (Appendix A-2).

Lymphocytes are small cells with little cytoplasm, unless a B cell differentiates into a **plasma cell** (PC; Figure 6.1; Table 6.1). Lymphocytes have membrane receptors that recognize non-self biochemical features and are not restricted to recognizing whether the invader is a bacterium or a virus, as is the case with the TLR "danger receptors" of the innate immune system (Table 6.2). The **B cell receptor** (BCR) is a complete membrane-bound antibody (Figure 6.1; Appendix A-1). BCRs and the monomeric version of all antibodies possess two identical binding sites. The **T cell receptor** (TCR) can be thought of as homologous to one binding site of the BCR (Figure 6.6; Appendix A-1). The TCR of α/β T cells evolved to recognize linear peptides degraded from foreign antigens presented to them on MHC I and II by APCs, while the BCR recognizes conformational or 3D patterns/epitopes on proteins and carbohydrates. However, the TCRs on γ/δ cells behave more like the BCRs and recognize non-peptides, proteins, and other intact molecules. While all lymphocytes can somatically alter the genes that encode their BCR and TCR receptors during the lifetime of the organism, these changes in lymphocytes are not passed on via egg or sperm, so that each generation must start again to somatically generate their own unique BCR or TCR repertoires. Hence antibody specificity is not inherited, only the mechanism for somatic change.

The initial response of naïve lymphocytes, often called "pre-immune" lymphocytes, is to proliferate. Some B lymphocytes can become IgM-secreting plasma cells in about 3 days, after antigen encounter without T cell help (Figure 6.1). The structure of the major types of antibodies is illustrated in Figure A1.7A and their major functions are summarized in Table A3.1. Secreted IgM constitutes the **early phase primary antibody response** (Figures 6.1 and 6.3). The genes encoding their antigen-binding site remain in near germline configuration and they are sometimes called "natural antibodies" (Panda). We addressed this question using a germ-free piglet model. As described earlier in the section titled "First Responders," PAMPs are recognized by PRRs; eg, lipopolysaccharide (LPS) is recognized by TLR-2, and MDP by TLR-6 (Table 6.2). Germ-free piglets have not previously been exposed to PAMPs or received passive antibodies *in utero* as have human infants and lab mice (Figure 3.3); they provide a *tabula rasa* but still produce "natural" antibodies. Figure A2.3 shows the serum IgM, IgG, and IgA response to a panel of bacteria after (a) infection with enterohemorrhagic *E. coli* 933D or (b) exposure to a combination of LPS and MDP. Germ-free piglets receiving only PAMPs produced IgM antibodies to the entire panel of bacteria and IgA antibodies to three members of the panel, but not 933D. There was no IgG response to bacteria in the panel. After infection with 933D, piglets mounted IgM, IgG, and IgA responses to 933D and two other bacteria in the panel, indicating these were **adaptive immune responses**. This study supports the view that the initial early IgM response (Figures 6.1 and 6.3) represents a type of innate or "natural" antibody response that can provide a first-responder protection. The IgA response following stimulation with PAMPs supports the view of Bunker (SR) that some IgA responses are also "natural" or innate.

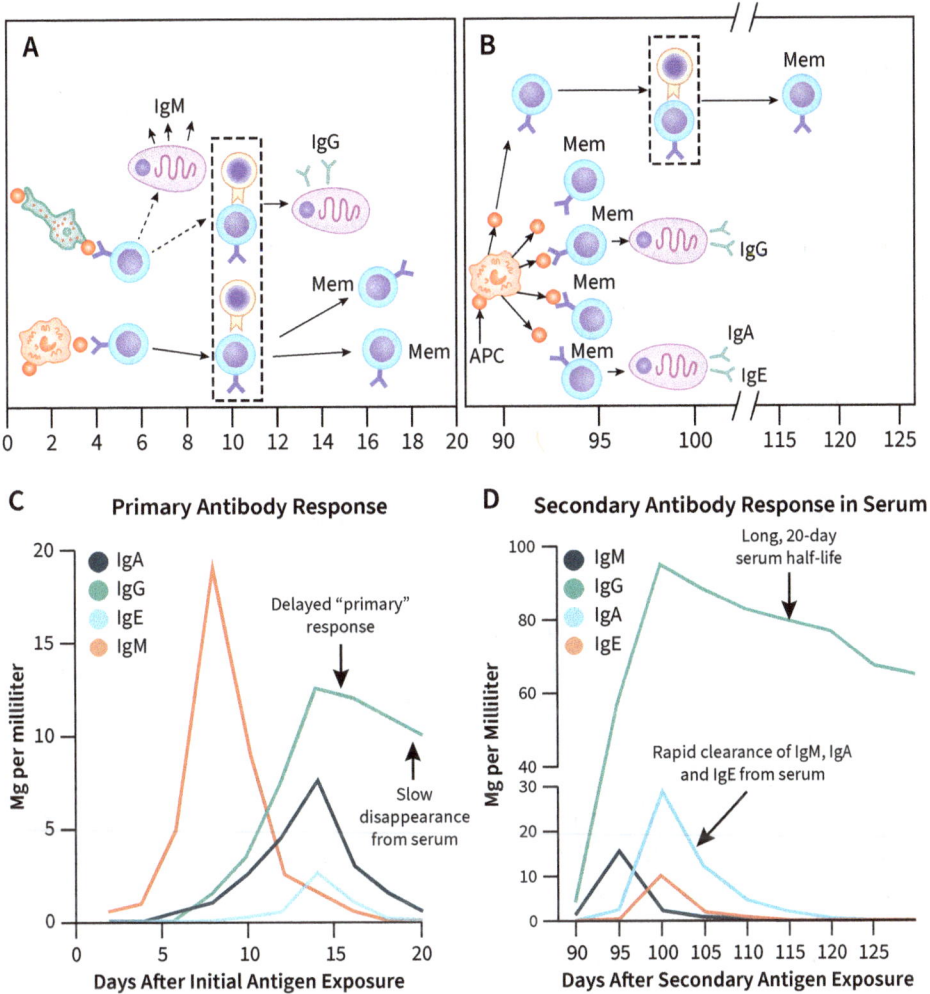

Figure 6.3   Events and kinetics of the primary and secondary antibody response.
Figures 6.3A and 6.3B illustrate the cellular events, while Figures 6.3C and 6.3D illustrate the serum antibody responses. The time scale used in Figure 6.3B has been interrupted so that the various cellular events could be illustrated. In Figure 6.3A APCs (DCs and macrophages) present a new antigen (red dot) to B cells, some of which respond without T cell help (thymus-independent antigens), which immediately results in plasma cells secreting IgM, which appears within 7 days in serum (Figure 6.3C). Those that require T cell help (thymus dependent) follow a delayed pathway and appear in serum after 2 weeks. The rectangular dotted boxes are where germinal center reactions (GCRx) occur (see text and Figure 6.1). Some B cells become memory cells (Mem). Figure 6.3B. Cellular events during the secondary immune response to an antigen previously encountered. A spectrum of memory B cells generated during the primary response becomes part of the memory cell pool. Those with BCRs with high affinity for the antigen presented to them by APCs become plasma cells that primarily secrete IgG, IgA, and IgE but seldom IgM. Others may enter a second GCRx and become the next generation of memory B cells. Continued exposure to the same antigen leads to progressive selection of B cells that then leads to plasma cells secreting antibodies of improved specificity. The kinetics of the secondary serum antibody response resulting from the cellular events illustrated in Figure 6.3B are shown in Figure 6.3D.

Although innate or "natural" IgM antibodies bind weakly to many antigens, they are still effective since secreted IgM is a polymer with 10 binding sites, so that its "stickiness" (like an octopus) makes up for the weak affinity of a single binding site. However, the foreign antigen that triggered the release of primary IgM antibodies also triggers B-cells that recognized the antigen to interact with antigen-specific T cell (Figure 6.3 and next section) to differentiate into plasma cells producing especially "better" IgG and IgA antiboides with a range of affinities for the original antigen (see also Appendix A-1, Figure A1.7A) The early appearance and broad specificity of these "first-responder" IgM antibodies amounts to "putting a finger in the dike" and providing temporary protection until reenforcements arrive that possess more refined specificity that can more efficiently deal with the invading foreign antigen. As we discuss in Appendix A-2, some also consider IgG3 and some IgA antibodies to be "natural antibodies" (Bunker,SR).

Lymphocyte Interactions, MHC, and Making "Better Antibodies"

While the previous sections described the components of innate and adaptive immunity, here we describe how they work together to produce an immune response. Adaptive immunity builds on the early action of the innate immune system and the early phase primary antibody response (Figure 6.3) to build a higher level of specific protection. Using the neighborhood dog analogy (see earlier), the adaptive immune system is like a dog that can distinguish the individual that mistreated him/her from all other humans.

We can use the example of the bacterial pathogen *Clostridium tetani* to explain how the system works. *C. tetani* is a soil bacterium that can enter a skin wound like one obtained while gardening. A toxin from *C. tetani* causes muscle tetany, and if it reaches the heart muscle the event can be fatal. Initially, certain TLRs of the innate immune system on macrophages or DCs recognize *C. tetani* (Table 6.2), which sets off "alarm bells," causing release of cytokines (Table 6.3) and resulting in recruitment of inflammatory neutrophils and more macrophages. Both the bacteria and its toxin can be referred to as foreign **antigens**. The term *antigen* is derived from the French/German words *antigène/Antigen*, in turn coined from the Greek *anti-* (against) and *-genes* (born or produced); it represents a bacterial toxin that is "anti-life." The responding macrophages act as APCs by engulfing and degrading the bacteria and its toxin and proceeding to present the breakdown products as small peptides in the grasp of the MHC molecules displayed on their surface as they interact with B cells (Figure 6.3A). α/β T cells have TCRs that can recognize the linear details of the peptide (sometimes called T cell epitopes) in the molecular context of the MHC that was used for the presentation of peptides. This results in the activation of the T cells. T cells from another individual, unless from an identical twin, will not be able to engage because their MHC is not recognized by the T cell as "self." This is an example of the self-/non-self-discrimination that is a hallmark of **adaptive immunity** while also serving as a fail-safe mechanism. Activated α/β T cells can transform into an array of what are called "T cell subsets" (see above and Table 6.1). Each subset performs different functions; some T cells become highly inflammatory Th17 cells, others become Th2 helper T cells that allow B cells to make better antibodies as shown in Figure 6.3. Th1 T cells increase inflammation while CTLs attack and kill tumors and virus-infected cells. These differentiate into subsets under the direction of different cytokines (Figures 6.1 and 6.4). It should be noted that it is common in the immunological literature to categorize the response of T cells as Th1 or Th2; the former is associated with inflammation while the latter is associated with the promotion of antibody production (Figure 6.3A & B) or some form of immune regulation.

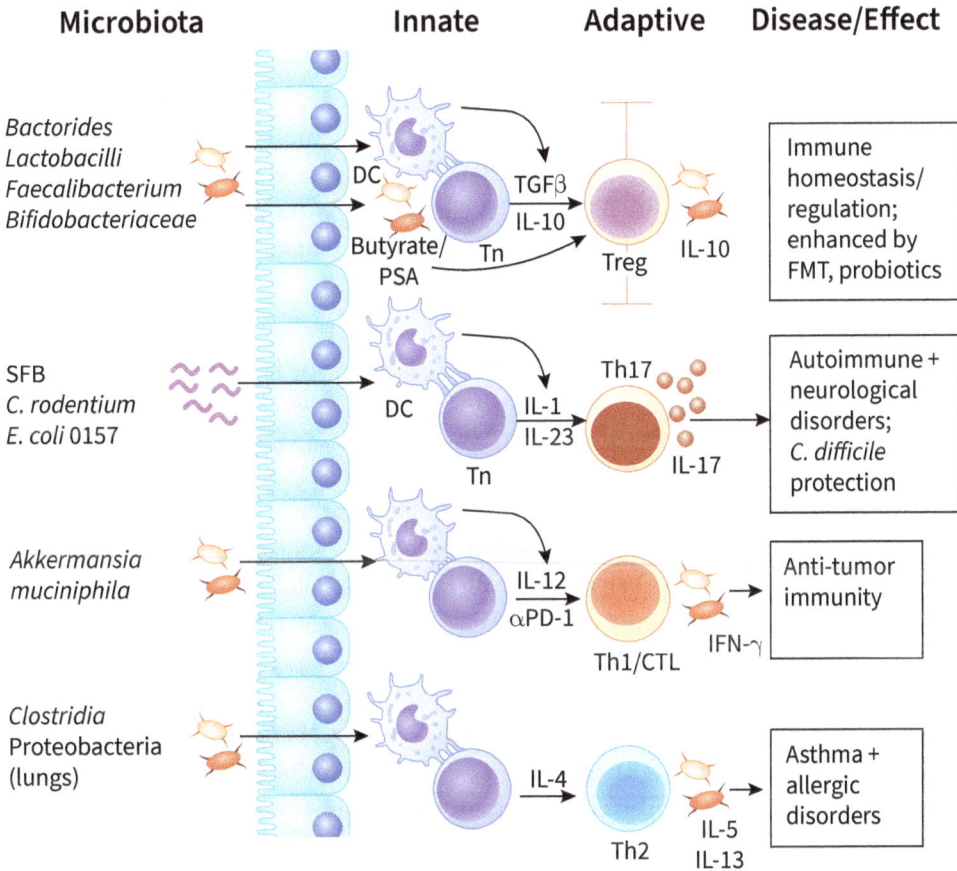

Figure 6.4   The differentiation of T cells into subsets with different functions are stimulated by different members of the microbiome (see Chapter 5). DCs acting as APCs, along with the influence of certain cytokines, results in differentiation into four categories of T cell subsets and physiological outcomes. The purple nucleus Treg creates immune homeostasis can block the actions of inflammatory Th17 cells. Butyrate is a SCFA produced by metabolic breakdown of foodstuffs, especially by Bacteriodetes that are members of the healthy GI tract microbiome. Their presence can improve the health of tight junctions between enterocytes (see Figures 5.4 and 6.6). SFB = segmented filamentous bacteria used in experimental studies, which like *E. coli* and *C. Rodentia* are also Proteobacteria (see Chapter 5).

The making of a better antibody requires an interaction between the activated Th2 helper α/β T cell and a B cell that has recognized the original antigen with its BCR. This

T-B cell interaction (Figures 6.1 and 6.3A) initiates a pathway of differentiation that involve a series of somatic events in the B cell that leads to the production of antibodies of greater specificity. These are primarily IgG, IgA, and IgE antibodies and comprise the late primary response (Figure 6.3B). During the T-B interaction, B cells are given a short burst of "lymphocyte adrenalin" (ie, IL-2; Table 6.2) that is mediated by an interaction between the CD40 ligand on the T cell and CD40 on the B cell. This causes the B cells to divide and make more of themselves; at the same time they begin somatically modifying their BCRs. T-B interactions occur in **germinal centers (GCs)** where somatic changes occur (see Figure 6.3A and B). These are found in what are called **secondary lymphoid tissues**. These include the spleen, peripheral lymph nodes, and the Peyer's patch follicles. At these sites, APCs again present the antigen to B cells, which now display a variety of somatically modified BCRs, some with higher affinity, allowing them to be selected. Selected B cells are then directed to differentiate to "endstage" B cells called **plasma cells (PCs)** that become factories for making large quantities of better antibodies (Table 6.1; Figures 6.1 and 6.3B). Immunologists often refer to this refinement process in GCs and the process of making better antibodies as "affinity maturation." Selection events that occur in the GC are called the **germinal center reaction (GCRx)**. In our *C. tetani* example, this leads to production of antibodies that can more tightly bind the *Clostridia* toxin and neutralize its physiological effects. The molecular genetic details underlying the somatic events in lymphocytes that improve antibody specificity are described in Appendix A-1.

The GCRx that leads to the production of a better antibody also involves a process called "class switch," which is first manifested by changes in the isotype of surface BCRs on memory B cells (Figures 6.1 and 6.3), which can later develop into PCs producing IgG, IgE, and IgA class antibodies instead of only IgM (Figure 6.3A; Table A3.1). The early IgM response may come in two forms. Some responses to antigens require help from T cells (called T-dependent antigens), while those that carry their own PAMP (eg, LPS, which is recognized by TLR4; see Table 6.2) are called T-independent antigens. **Early primary IgM immune responses** that do not require T cell help or the GCRx can appear in serum in less than 3 days, ie, "natural" antibodies. **Late phase primary responses** dominated by IgG class antibodies, but also IgM responses to T-dependent antigens, are delayed since they require a GCRx (Figure 6.3B). In the *C. tetani* example, class switch has positive consequences in protection against the bacteria and its toxin since the more specific and abundant IgG class antibodies are more effective at neutralizing and removing the deadly toxin from circulation than "finger in the dike" natural IgM antibodies (Panda). This same mechanism is used to generate antibodies that can neutralize a circulating virus, such as COVID-19. Continuing with our example, such antibodies also bind the *C. tetani* bacteria and, with the help of macrophages and neutrophils, destroy it, thereby eliminating the source of the dangerous *Clostridia* toxin. While IgM and IgA antibodies can directly neutralize the circulating toxins, IgE and IgA class antibodies are also the product of the GCRx. The effector function of the former will be discussed in relationship to allergy and that for the latter will be discussed in the subsection on mucosal immunity.

Immunologic Memory

In describing the innate immune system, we mentioned the term **trained immunity**, which involves the "learned" behavior of inflammatory cells. Figure 6.1 shows that not all B cells generated during the GCRx differentiate into PCs; some remain as "memory B cells" (Figure 6.1). **Immunological memory** means reencounter with the same antigen/pathogen quickly results in PCs secreting more effective, IgG and other antibodies (Figure 6.3). These have higher affinity for the foreign antigen or pathogens but are also "better" because they typically produce only IgG, IgA, and IgE class antibodies, each of which possesses special effector activities (Appendix A-3, Table A3.1). Because of the existence of memory B cells, there is no delay after a second encounter with the antigen/pathogens, so these "better" antibodies can appear in serum within 48 hours of re-exposure (Figure 6.3B). While some go directly to PCs, which secrete antibodies, others may enter another GCRx event, resulting in a new wave of memory cells, perhaps encoding BCRs with even higher specificity (Figure 6.3), although this is controversial (Guthmiller).

While mature α/β T cells do not engage in GCRx that alters their TCRs, they are nevertheless subject to selection for different functions (Figure 6.4) while some become **memory T cells**. These are very important in protection against viral infections such as SARS-CoV-2 (Appendix A-4).

The development of immunologic memory and the resulting protection it affords may not be automatic for all infections and should not be assumed. For example, the first encounter with Beta coronaviruses responsible for approximately 30% of common colds may not produce strong immunologic memory, which may explain why humans continually get the common cold. We know from animal studies that certain viral infections result in poor neutralizing antibodies, rendering the host susceptible to repeated infection. Early studies suggested durable immunity did not develop with Beta coronaviruses, and that neutralizing antibodies possessed near germline sequences, perhaps precluding the formation of long-term memory B cells. These conclusions have now been debunked, and recent studies show that memory B cells specific to SARS-CoV-2 persist for at least 8 months (Cohen) and that anti-SARS-CoV-2 antibodies show the same types of somatic mutations in their variable regions that are found in B cells that have been processed through a GCRx (Sokal). T cell memory may endure longer (Appendix A-4). It is still unresolved as to how long these SARS-CoV-2-specific memory cells remain, but studies show that protection following vaccination is good for at least 6 months, but booster immunization (see Section III) is needed, not only because antibody levels wane but because of the continuous emergence of new SARS-CoV-2 variants (Appendix A-4).

The Microbial Empire Strikes Back

We used the Star Wars Jedi Knight analogy to describe the role of lymphocytes in adaptive immunity. Not surprisingly, microbial pathogens, particularly viral pathogens, have evolved mechanisms to escape these Jedi Knights. As shown in Figure 6.2, viruses in particular can "change their coats" up to a million times faster than humans. It is not surprising that, based on the number of publications, PubMed shows that viral infections are currently the major focus of infectious disease research. Childhood diseases like smallpox, measles, rubella (German measles), polio, influenza, and the "common cold" are the consequence of infection by viruses. As we described in Chapter 1, viruses are cell parasites, and unlike bacteria they cannot be grown in the lab without providing them with a cell source to infect. Viruses most often infect and live in epithelial cells where they multiply and then release their offspring, called **virions**. A virion is an infectious sub-cellular particle that contains either viral RNA or DNA, a complement of enzymes needed for cell entry or for viral nucleic acid replication that are typically surrounded by an envelope containing virus-specific glycoproteins, sometimes called "spikes," like those illustrated in the media in connection to SARS-CoV-2. Epithelial cells have intracellular TLRs that recognize the intruders (Table 6.2) and can call for help by displaying peptides derived from the virus on their surface MHC. As with *C. tetani*, α/β T cells recognize the linear non-self-peptides derived from proteins produced by the infecting virus, while B cells recognize conformational epitopes expressed on the virus envelope. T-B interactions and the GCRx then result in the production of more specific antibodies that can neutralize the free virions, just as they neutralized the toxin from *C. tetani*. However, in the case of a virus, antibodies have no way to enter the infected cell and neutralize the virus. This job is left to CTLs (Table 6.1; Figures 6.1 and 6.4) that attack and kill cells infected by the virus that display peptide-MHC complexes on their surface. Although this comes at the expense of some epithelial cells, it ends their ability to produce more viruses and thus restores the health of the host. It is best to think of antibodies as weapons to prevent viral entry and CTLs as cells that close existing "virus factories."

Viruses are good examples of pathogens that have evolved systems to defeat or hinder the ability of the immune system to eliminate them. They use various means and below we describe three mechanisms and how the host can overcome these. First, the elimination of virus-infected cells by CTLs depends on the ability of the infected cell to signal it is infected, which it does by displaying virus or virus-derived peptides on its surface in the context of MHC I. However, the virus can avoid immune elimination by CTLs by inhibiting the ability of the infected cell to express MHC I. This denies the cell the ability to "call for help." This is the tactic of cytomegalovirus (CMV), mentioned in Chapter 2, as well as herpes viruses, some of which are responsible for genital infections or the familiar "cold sore." Fortunately, infected cells have another means to call for help. They can express unique surface molecules, a kind of SOS recognized by lymphocyte-like cells called natural killer or NK cells (see section on innate immunity; Table 6.1; Figure A1.7B). These cells express a unique set of receptors and can recognize infected cells that have lost their ability to call for help. Also, like CTLs, NK cells can kill the virus-infected cells.

A second escape mechanism used by some viruses involves killing the "helper" T cells (Figures 6.1 and 6.3A) that are needed to drive the adaptive antibody responses to produce "better antibodies" that can neutralize the virus. For example, HIV uses CD4 on helper T cells along with the chemokine receptor CXC5 to gain cell entry. These infected CD4 T cells are killed, and because of their loss, virus-specific viral neutralizing antibodies are also lost, which allows for further spread of the virus. There is no natural host response, but therapeutic measures can reduce replication of the virus.

A third mechanism involves interference with T cell development in the thymus. In Chapter 2, we mentioned **central immunological tolerance.** We describe in the next section and Figure 6.5 how this works and illustrate that newborns infected *in utero* now possess fewer peripheral T cells that can recognize the virus as foreign.

Figure 6.5   T cell development and establishment of central tolerance in the thymus.

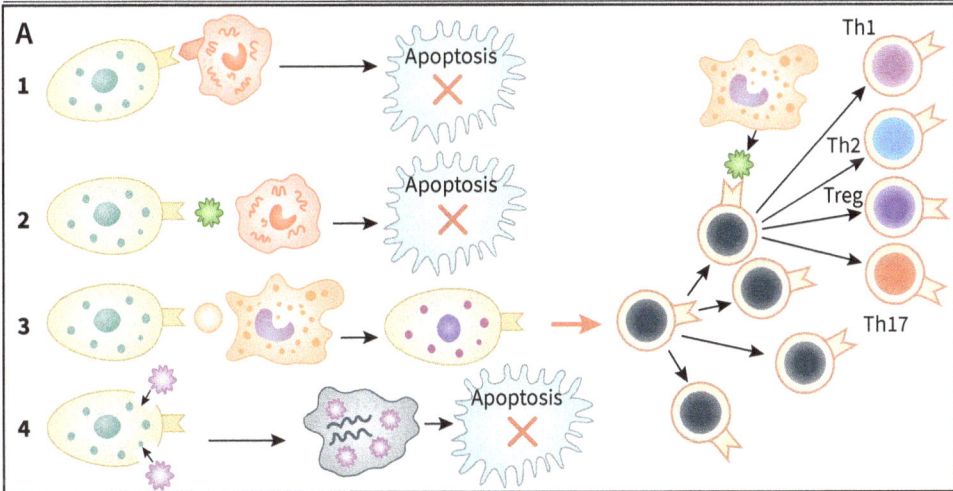

Figure 6.5A   On the left side are four examples that influence T cell development from thymocytes: (1) Presentation of a self-antigen by an APC to a developing thymocyte results in apoptosis (programmed cell death). (2) Fetal viral infection, resulting in the presentation of a viral antigen that is now recognized as self, and which leads to apoptosis which eliminates the emergence of peripheral T cells that can recognize the pathogen as foreign. (3) Presentation by an APC of a non-self-antigen, which allows further thymocyte development and the emergence in the periphery of a mature T cell. (4) Viral infection of the thymus by a virus such as PRRSV (porcine reproductive and respiratory syndrome virus), causing death of the infected thymocyte. On the right, thymocytes surviving elimination emerge as mature T cells can expand by mitosis or may be stimulated by APCs resulting in their differentiation into various T cell subsets. (See Figures 6.1 and 6.4).

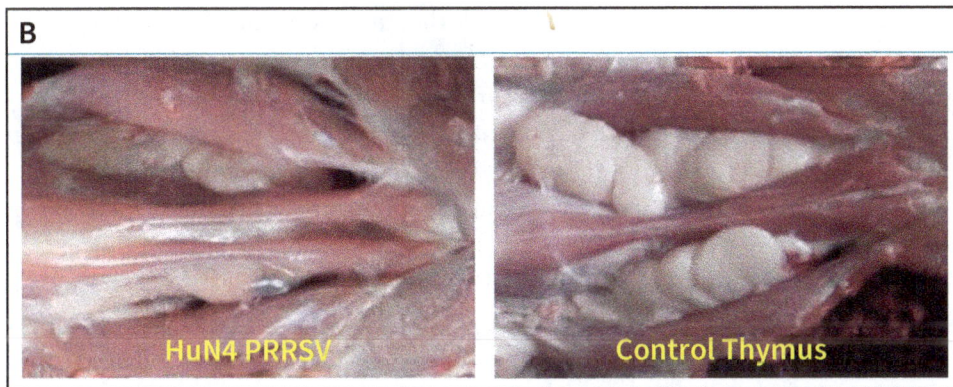

Figure 6.5B   Thymic atrophy in piglets infected with PRRSV (left) compared to the thymus in an uninfected piglet (right).

There are also mechanisms that allow viruses to establish peaceful co-existence with the host. A danger faced by all pathogenic bacteria and viruses is that they may be so virulent that they kill the host, which threatens their own existence. Remember the adage that "good parasites don't kill their host." HIV pushes that limit, as does Ebola, CMV, herpes viruses, and porcine respiratory and reproductive syndrome virus (PRRSV) in swine, which delays their expulsion by the host (see Appendix A-2). This allows more time for reproduction of offspring (virions) that can result in new infections without killing the host allowing spread to other individuals. Beta coronaviruses like SARS-CoV-2, which can jump to an unprepared new host, are especially virulent since the new hosts lack immunity, which allows the virus to rapidly reproduce and, through spontaneous mutation, generate new variants. With time, the surviving individuals gradually develop immune resistance. When this occurs, the originally highly virulent variants tend to be replaced by those that are less virulent, but which may be more contagious but allow a larger number of the host species to survive. The microbial-vertebrate ecosystem is a delicate balance that optimally allows both host and parasite to survive.

Mucosal Immunity: Anatomical Distribution and Function

The **mucosal immune system** is associated with all internal surfaces that have a mucosa, defined as a layer of "soft" columnar epithelial cells covered with mucus (Figure 6.6). They form a barrier against the outside world while allowing rapid gas exchange in the respiratory tract and allowing for nutrient uptake by the GI tract. Compared to the cornified epithelium of external mammalian surfaces, like skin, this internal "soft" barrier is more vulnerable to damage and pathogen entrance. Similar mucosae are found in the oral cavity, nasal passages, and elsewhere. In earlier chapters we mentioned Peyer's patches, which represent the **secondary lymphoid tissue** of the mucosal immune system of the GI tract (Figure 6.6). Similar structures are found in the upper respiratory tract. These sites are dominated by the presence of B cells committed to the later production of dimeric IgA (dIgA) antibodies (Table A3.1). At these sites, cytokines like TGF-β (Table 6.3) promote the switch from the initial production of IgM antibodies to IgA. That approximately 80% of all human PCs produce dIgA speaks to the important role that the mucosal immune system plays in internal protection. Pioneer investigators referred to IgA as "antiseptic paint" for mucosal surfaces, making them critical in defense against pathogen entry in the GI tract, respiratory tract, and at other mucosal sites. As illustrated in Figure 6.6, dIgA is produced by PCs in the GI tract and is transported through enterocytes, carrying with it part of the transport receptor (called secretory component) and emerging as secretory IgA (SIgA) in the lumen of the GI tract.

In Chapter 3, we indicated that SIgA antibodies comprise approximately 90% of all antibodies passively transferred in human colostrum. This SIgA is not absorbed in the GI tract of the newborn but acts within the gut lumen, like SIgA produced by the host and transported into the GI tract lumen. Passive SIgA in colostrum supplies the "first coat" of "antiseptic paint" until the newborn can produce its own SIgA. We also described in

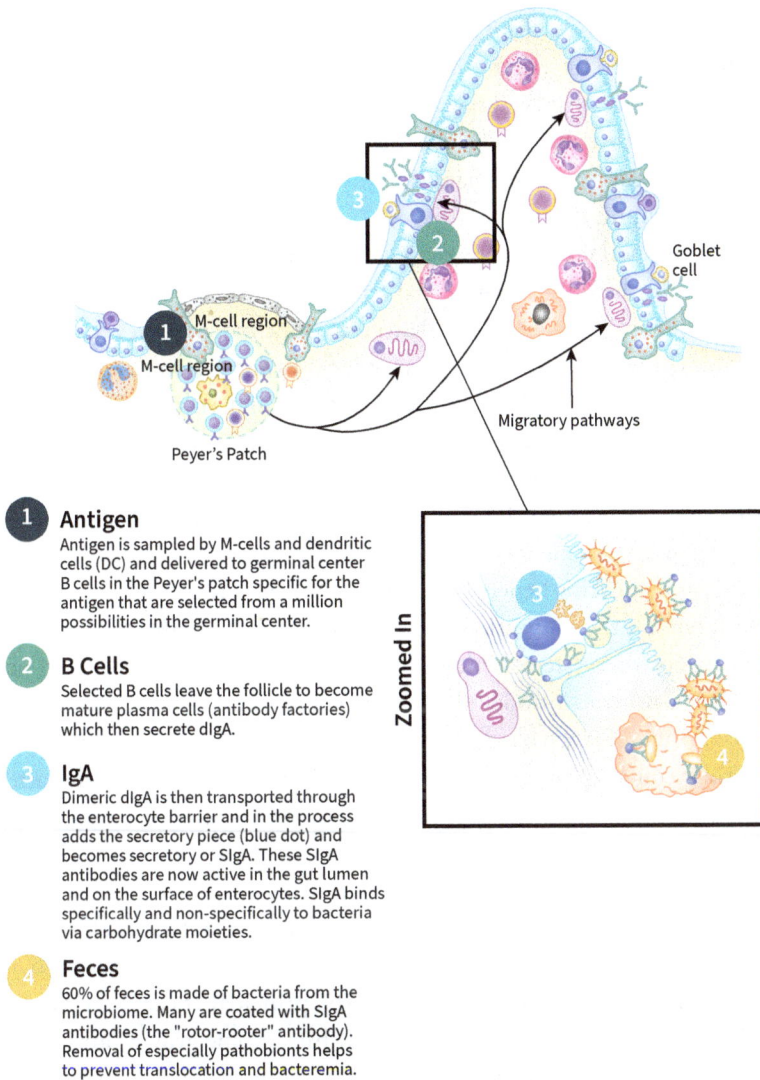

1 Antigen
Antigen is sampled by M-cells and dendritic cells (DC) and delivered to germinal center B cells in the Peyer's patch specific for the antigen that are selected from a million possibilities in the germinal center.

2 B Cells
Selected B cells leave the follicle to become mature plasma cells (antibody factories) which then secrete dIgA.

3 IgA
Dimeric dIgA is then transported through the enterocyte barrier and in the process adds the secretory piece (blue dot) and becomes secretory or SIgA. These SIgA antibodies are now active in the gut lumen and on the surface of enterocytes. SIgA binds specifically and non-specifically to bacteria via carbohydrate moieties.

4 Feces
60% of feces is made of bacteria from the microbiome. Many are coated with SIgA antibodies (the "rotor-rooter" antibody). Removal of especially pathobionts helps to prevent translocation and bacteremia.

Figure 6.6   The mucosal immune system of the GI tract and the secretion of SIgA antibodies. The villus is comprised of enterocytes and occasional Paneth and Goblet cells. The latter secrete the protective mucus that covers the gut epithelium. Enterocytes are separated by tight junctions (see insert) that when healthy prevent material from the gut lumen from passing into the lamina propria (interstitial space) that underlies the enterocyte barrier. Periodically dendritic cells (DCs) extend their pseudopods between enterocytes and sample antigens in the gut lumen. To the left of the villus is a region in which some cells differentiate into flattened M cells that overlay a lymphoid follicle called a Peyer's patch that contain germinal centers. Peyer's patches contain a collection of lymphocytes, mostly uncommitted B cells along with macrophages, some T cells, and dendritic cells that can present them with antigen. DCs and macrophages also have an intimate relationship with M cells, which serve as portals for antigens/pathogens in the gut lumen to be sampled by APCs. Antigen-specific B cells selected in the Peyer's patches then migrate to the villi to become plasma cells secreting dimeric IgA, which during its transport becomes SIgA (see insert).

Chapter 3 dIgA-producing cells in the mammary gland that trafficked from the mucosal immune system of the GI tract of the mother, and that their migration depends on CXCL13 (Table 6.3). This suggests that their specificity is directed to enteric pathogens that threaten the GI tract of the mother and are likely to threaten the GI tract of the newborn. In Chapter 3 we called this the gut-mammary gland axis. Lymphocyte trafficking plays an important role in mucosal immunity (Mikhah).

Protection at mucosal sites depends on more than neutralizing antibodies; it also involves the cytotoxic T cells that kill virus-infected cells. Except for attenuated poliovirus vaccine (see Section III), most vaccines are not delivered to the mucosal sites that are the sites of many natural infections. Those delivered at other sites depend on the migration of T and B cells to provide protection at local sites. In Chapter 3 and earlier in this chapter we indicated that the mucosal immune system of the GI tract plays an important role in immune homeostasis and the establishment of oral tolerance. Sixty percent of bacteria in the stool are coated with SIgA, in many cases through glycans found on secretory component (Figure 6.6; Bunker, SR). As previously mentioned, the system appears to discriminate and target "bad" Proteobacteria while sparing beneficial Bacteriodetes and Firmicutes.

Of recent interest is the connection between the mucosal immune system of the GI tract and the enteric nervous system, which connects to the CNS (Flayer). The microbiome-gut-brain axis (MGBA) was introduced in Chapter 5. Intestinal neurons secrete the cytokine IL-18 (Table 6.3), which when blocked renders mice susceptible to *S. typhimurium*. The GI tract mucosa also contains other cell types, such as DCs and Goblet cells; the latter produce IL-18 (Table 6.3) and secrete antibacterial peptides (Jarret, SR).

Passive Immunity

Adaptive immunity provides immune protection to the host and to the offspring. Whether through maternal antibodies stored in the eggs of reptiles/birds or through antibodies provided *in utero* or via suckling in mammals, the principal effect is the same, although mammals have provided additional features. While "home grown" antibodies protect healthy adults, they are not adequate for offspring because their **adaptive immune system** is poorly developed. If conventionally reared animals like horses, swine, cattle, and sheep are denied the chance to suckle, they die even if they are provided the essential nutrients for growth and survival, a fact that herdsmen knew thousands of years ago. While these offspring have an innate and fledgling adaptive immune system, protective passive antibodies are not supplied *in utero* (Chapter 2). Rather, they are provided only in colostrum and milk (Figure 3.3). Since human infants receive passive antibodies *in utero*, they can survive without suckling if nourishment is provided from other sources like infant formula, while conventionally reared farm animals cannot. A recent study that grew out of the COVID-19 pandemic showed that lactating mothers vaccinated with two doses of an mRNA vaccine not only have anti-spike and RBD antibodies (Appendix A-4) in their breast milk, but one-fourth also passed the mRNA vaccine to their nursing infants (Yeo). In another study of interest, an examination of masks worn by vaccinated individuals found that the masks contained COVID-19 specific IgG and IgA antibodies and these could be recovered in the nasal swabs of unvaccinated children living in the same homes as the vaccinated individuals, a new form of passive immunity (Kedl).

Postnatal immunity in mammals provides more than antibodies and potential antigens (Chapter 3). It also provides regulatory cytokines such as IL-10 and TGF-β, which suppress the development of inflammatory T cells (Figures 6.1 and 6.4) while simultaneously promoting class switch to IgA and development of the intestinal mucosa (Table 6.3; Brenmoehl). Some leukocytes are also transmitted via suckling, but they primarily act in the gut lumen and do not establish chimerism in the newborn.

Section II: Immunological Tolerance and Immunological Injury

LEARNING OBJECTIVES

1. Define central and peripheral tolerance and their relationship to autoimmune disease, allergy, and inflammatory bowel disorders.

2. Describe the role played by molecular mimicry in human disease.

3. Discuss factors that underly allergies and measures to reduce them.

4. Summarize factors that can result in autoimmunity.

The TSA and "Checkpoint Charlie": *Horror Autotoxicus* and Immunological Tolerance

B and T cells diversify their BCR and TCR specificity by somatic gene recombination during lymphogenesis in the thymus and bone marrow, respectively (Figure 6.1). Fortunately, that process does not continue for T cells after they migrate out of the thymus, while somatic gene recombination and somatic mutation continues for B cells as part of the GCRx in **secondary lymphoid tissues** (Figures 6.1 and 6.3B). This important difference between T and B cell lymphogenesis has important long-term health implications. **Central immunological tolerance** develops during T cell development in the thymus and prevents T cells from leaving the thymus if they recognize self (Figure 6.5). If somatic changes to the TCR of T cells were to continue after they left the thymus, some peripheral T cells might again recognize self, resulting in a breakdown of central immunological tolerance and leading to *Horror autotoxicus*.

With exception of the "first responder" IgM response (Panda; Figures 6.3A and 6.3C), the subsequent "better antibodies" are the product of the GCRx, which explains their delayed appearance in the **late primary response** (Figures 6.3B and 6.3D). Since somatic modifications continue in B cells, some antibodies may be generated that may again recognize self-antigens/epitopes. However, without co-recognition and help from T cells that recognize the linear peptide as foreign, B cells involved in the GCRx will never become plasma cells secreting anti-self antibodies. Therefore, the failure of T cells to recognize "self," even though mutated B cells can, provides a blocker, like "Checkpoint Charlie"[1] or a TSA airport checkpoint. These analogies demonstrate the commanding role played by T cells in "guarding the gate" for the adaptive immune system. In the healthy fetus, only self-antigens are available, so that all self-reactive T cells have been purged during thymocyte development and central tolerance have thus been established (Figure 6.5). However, fetal infections like CMV (Chapter 2) or porcine reproductive and respiratory syndrome (PRRS) virus can hijack the central tolerance mechanism. Figure 6.5A illustrates how in a fetus infected with PRRS virus, the APCs present the virus, so that it is perceived as "self." This results in thymic atrophy (Figure 6.5B). Thus, emerging peripheral T cells in the infected newborn would not recognize the virus as foreign. The infected newborn will be tolerant or "blind" to this viral pathogen and unable to mount an adaptive immune defense. Thymic atrophy (Figure 6.5B) potentially reduces the repertoire of emerging T cells and their value in immune surveillance, thus increasing the risk of other infections. Fortunately, the healthy fetal environment is sterile, so with few exceptions the development of central tolerance to a pathogen is rare. Later, we discuss autoimmunity, a condition in which immunological tolerance has failed, resulting in many well-known diseases, some appearing during the Critical Window (Chapter 3).

There are other forms of immunological tolerance not explained by events in the thymus or bone marrow that are collectively lumped together as **peripheral tolerance**. Establishing postpartum immunological tolerance appears to be strongly age dependent. Young adults who migrate from the East Coast to the Midwest, a location rich in prairie plants like ragweed, often develop type I allergy (atopy) to ragweed in 2–3 years. After several more years they can become "desensitized" (ie, they are no longer atopic), while older immigrants do not. Children born and raised in the Midwest, especially those on farms that get full exposure to ragweed and other allergens, produce IgG antibodies to these potential allergens and have a low incidence of type I allergy later in life. The BCR recognizes 3D molecular patterns, regardless of whether they are derived from a microbe, harmless plant pollen, synthetic compounds like dinitrophenyl, dyes like fluorescein, pentadecacatechol from poison ivy, or from aromatic compounds added to deodorants and perfumes. However, responsiveness to these simple molecules requires co-exposure to PAMPs or associated co-exposure to microbial products. This predicts that responses to such potential allergens require that some PAMP must be simultaneously provided as might occur during an infection. The importance of these PAMPs is now recognized by the term *adjuvant*, and they are used in the development of many vaccines (see Section III).

---

1 A former border crossing in Berlin that prevented East Germans from fleeing to the West and West Germans from infiltrating and undermining the communist government of East Germany.

Oral Tolerance and Immune Homeostasis in the GI Tract

Oral tolerance is a form of peripheral tolerance. The GI tract encounters daily a large variety of food proteins and complex carbohydrates that the developing fetus never encountered during development, so that no central tolerance exists. In addition to dietary constituents, the GI tract is exposed to more than 10^{12} bacteria from various phyla, orders, and genera, which compromise the microbiome (Chapter 5). All these foreign antigens are confronted by the GI tract's mucosal immune system (see later section). Awareness of the absence of an immune response to food constituents (ie, **oral tolerance**) dates back at least to 1909 when Besredka noted the normal absence of an immune response to cow's milk proteins. As we have mentioned above and in other chapters, the response to cow's milk proteins is common in neonates but in most cases disappears within 6–36 months, suggesting that oral tolerance has developed. Modern studies associate this with the presence of certain cytokines that expand the number of Tregs (Wang; Pabst; Figure 6.1; Table 6.2). Without such intrinsic down-regulation, the GI tract would remain in a serious state of chronic inflammation that would compromise its role in nutrition. Low-level inflammation is normal in the GI tract, but when exaggerated due to dysregulation it can become life-changing, as in the case of IBD.

A type of oral tolerance is also seen with bacteria that comprise the GI tract microbiome but it appears highly discriminatory. There is a regular response of the GI tract mucosal immune system in the form of SIgA antibodies (Appendix A-3, Table A3.1) that appears to establish immune homeostasis with Bacteriodetes and Firmicutes that characterize eubiosis while targeting Proteobacteria that are diagnostic of dysbiosis (Chapter 5). Hence the mucosal immune system discriminates between the "good" and the "bad and ugly" members of the GI tract microbiome (Chapter 5; Bunker, SR; MacPherson, SR). The mechanism underlying this discrimination awaits ongoing research.

Immunologic Injury: Molecular Mimicry, Allergy, and Autoimmunity

The host's defense against infectious disease is a delicate balance between the response to foreign substances that can cause disease and innocuous substances that do no harm, some of which may still provide a "danger" signal. We described above how the developing immune system is educated to become tolerant of itself and to react only to what is foreign (Figure 6.5A). When the system does not work as designed, *Horror autotoxicus* may occur. There are various mechanisms in play in such injury. One is "mistaken identity" that results from molecular mimicry, so the host immune system responds to eliminate the pathogen mimic that may actualy be self (see later). A second example is the inflammatory responses to a pathogen that causes bystander or "friendly fire" that can result in damage by a "cytokine storm," an expression sometimes used in the SARS-CoV-2 pandemic. Injuries range from atopic allergy, asthma, and other autoimmune diseases like rheumatoid arthritis, to multiple sclerosis, and many others (see later).

Molecular Mimicry

There are numerous examples of "antigen look-alikes" or **molecular mimics** that have been used to explain secondary diseases like rheumatic fever that affects heart muscle, because heart muscle displays epitopes that mimic part of the *streptococcal* bacteria that causes the infection. While this example has been recognized for more than 50 years and appears in many textbooks, there are many others. Another involves Guillain-Barré syndrome (GBS), which is an acute inflammatory and demyelinating disease of the central nervous system (CNS). Outbreaks of GBS have been associated with certain serotypes of *Campylobacter jejuni*. The LPS of *C. jejuni* mimics the GM1 gangliosides of the CNS and may trigger GBS (Moran). It is recognized that the A, B, and H blood group polysaccharide antigens in humans share epitopes with the LPS of certain Gram-negative bacteria, including *Neisseria gonorrhoeae*, *Neisseria meningitides*, and *Haemophilus influenza*. LPS from these bacteria also share glycolipid epitopes with the A, B, and H blood group antigens. *Helicobacter pylori*, a major cause of stomach ulcers, shares surface epitopes with the Lewis blood group antigen $Le^{x,2}$ which may explain the presence of autoantibodies to Le^x in *H. pylori* patients. Cross-reactivity often involves carbohydrate epitopes on mammalian and plant proteins, in particular galactose-α-1,3-galactose (a-gal). This observation dates to the 1930s, when immunochemist Karl Landsteine pioneered the work on blood group systems. He observed that antibodies to the group B blood group carbohydrate cross-reacted with those on mammalian proteins. This was recently shown to be the reason why some individuals develop IgE antibodies to red meat proteins, which expresses a surface glycoprotein similar but not identical to a-gal (Commins). Such cross-reactive epitopes have also been found on proteins from peanuts, shellfish, and bee venom and in ticks.

An interesting example of molecular mimicry may be the consequence of effecter immune mechanisms that evolved to eliminate worm parasites. Worm parasites were common a century ago in North America, and still abound in the less developed countries of South and Central America, Africa, and parts of Asia. Tales from grandparents describe the emergence of ascaris worms from the nostril of a child in the middle of a family dinner. The disappearance of such events in North America and Europe is an indication that the era of worm parasite infections in these parts of the world has passed. However, the propensity to respond to substances that resemble worm epitopes still exists. The anti-worm immune response and those associated with atopic allergy and asthma is believed to explain the normal physiologic role of the antibody class IgE (Table A3.1). This antibody class attaches itself to cells called mast cells and eosinophils, and when this cell-bound IgE recognizes a worm parasite or a parasite egg, it triggers these cells to release a trove of vasoactive amines, like histamine, which causes expulsion of the parasite (Figure 6.7). Figure 6.3B shows that IgE rapidly disappears from serum, which is because it quickly attaches to specific IgE receptors on basophils and eosinophils at local tissue sites (Figure 6.7). Since the major

---

2   At least 11 different blood group antigens are known in humans, including the A, B, O, and Rh systems, which are involved in many issues beyond blood transfusion.

worm parasites are largely gone from developed countries, "evolutionary inertia" appears to have shifted to environmental mimics like pollen from certain plants, notably ragweed in prairie states, cottonwoods in the Great Plains, and conifers in the Pacific Northwest. The vasoactive amines originally used to expel the parasite now cause misery through type I hypersensitivity (atopic allergy) or simply called just plain allergy and asthma. These conditions often require medical intervention, such as the use of antihistamines and various steroids. Allergy, asthma, and other immune dysregulatory illnesses in North America and Western Europe have been increasing (Chapter 5) and are correlated with lifestyle and environment changes, including the decline of helminth parasites. It seems that the **mucosal immune system** (see later section) of the respiratory tract and the GI tract are initially biased and programmed to use Th2 helper T cells (Table 6.1) that trigger production of IgE and IgA antibodies. If the "parasite mimic" is not expelled and is continuously present, the response switches to use of the Th1 T cells, resulting in inflammatory injury (Figures 6.1 and 6.4). One immunotherapeutic approach has been to desensitize the individual by promoting an IgG response. This can activate expression of inhibitory Fc receptors on mast cells, thus stopping the release of vasoactive amines that fuel allergic and asthmatic attacks.

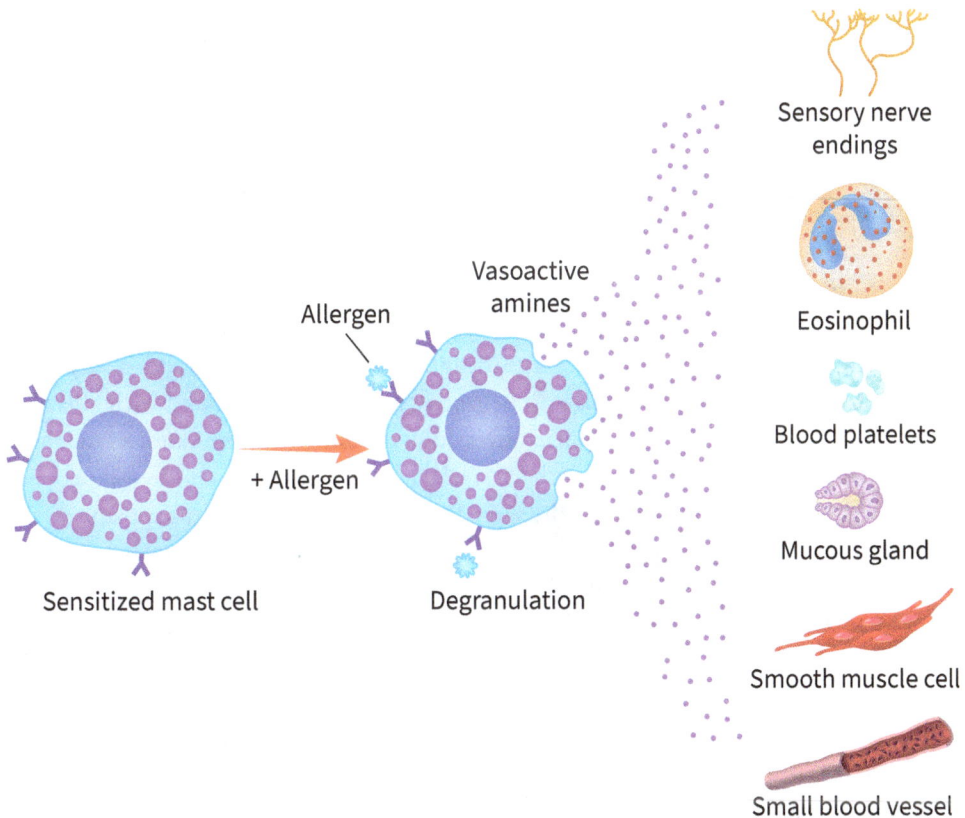

Figure 6.7   Release of vasoactive amines from a mast cell bearing an IgE antibody that can recognize the allergen. The far right depicts the various body tissues acted on by vasoactive amines that are released.

The Rise of Allergies

Theories abound to explain the rise in atopic allergy in North America and Western Europe and why children from these regions with eczema (atopic dermatitis) have a higher probability of developing seasonal allergy later in life (Mali). It may be related to a mutation in the gene encoding filaggrin or changes to the microbiome (Marrs). More than 200 million people worldwide suffer from asthma and 250,000 die each year. In the United States, asthma in children increased 3-fold from 1980 to 2001. This observation led Strachan in 1989 to propose the so-called hygiene or "dirt hypothesis" in which early exposure to noninfectious foreign antigens was correlated with reduced incidence of atopic allergy and asthma later in life, a type of peripheral tolerance, by down-regulating the switch to IgE antibodies (Strachan; Figures 6.1 and 6.3A; Table A3.1).

A study to test this hypothesis compared Hutterite and Amish farm communities (Stein). These communities are genetically related, but Hutterites use industrialized farming practices instead of the horses used by the Amish; they also have electricity to run vacuum cleaners and consequently their homes are relatively free of "dust bunnies" that contain allergens derived from fungi, bacteria, insects, and animal dander. Both groups are similar in having large families; high rates of childhood vaccination; and diets rich in fat, salt, and raw milk; children are also breastfed for a long duration. Both groups have low rates of childhood obesity and minimal exposure to tobacco and air pollution. It is important to consider family size since families with large numbers of siblings have a lower risk of developing atopy to inhalant allergens (Strachan).

Results of the study revealed that among Hutterites, the incidence of asthma was 4 times higher, allergic sensitization 4 times higher, and IgE levels in serum were 3 times higher than in the Amish. Compared to Hutterites, eosinophil levels (a measure of allergic inflammation) were much lower in Amish children, while endotoxin levels (a measure of bacterial exposure) were 4 times higher. Twenty-three cytokines, some contributing to cytokine storms (Table 6.3) were significantly lower among Amish children. This indicated a reduced level of inflammation and the discomfort associated with allergies. These observations have been supported by studies on Bavarian farm families in which younger children are allowed to live at barn level with animals. These children experience lower rates of allergy than those in the same families that lack regular exposure to the barn level environment. In such situations the reduced incidence of allergy is associated with increased levels of Treg and TGFβ (Figures 6.1 and 6.4; Schroeder). Studies in lab mice indicate that tolerance induction is favored during pre-weaning but not after weaning (Knoop). This might explain why early exposure to potential allergens reduces the risk of atopy later in life.

Another study compared the symptoms of atopic allergy, eczema, and asthma in approximately 80,000 children in two age groups in Scandinavia versus in former socialist countries of Eastern Europe. The frequency among older teenagers in Finland and Sweden was about 14%; it was about 8% in Estonia, Latvia, and Poland but only 4% in the Balkans, Russia, Georgia, and Uzbekistan. While these differences could also be ethnic, the better correlation is with a "Western lifestyle" versus one that better fits the lifestyle of the Amish and early American pioneers. As described in Chapter 5, Western lifestyle influences the constituency of the microbiome and some believe this is related to the propensity to develop allergy (Penders; McCoy).

The lower rates of allergy and asthma in Amish and farm children are attributed to repeated exposure to potential allergens, which establishes peripheral tolerance. In a laboratory model of peripheral tolerance, repeated immunization of young rabbits with bovine IgG renders them unresponsive to IgG, so when they are immunized with bovine IgA that shares many epitopes, they produce only antibodies to epitopes not shared between IgG and IgA; interestingly, this is a convenient way to make an IgA-specific antiserum. However, it is also plausible that studies comparing rural (allergen rich) versus urban (allergen poor) environments may have more to do with PAMP exposure than the specific antigen. Despite the lack of a definitive mechanism, the American Academy of Pediatrics now recommends early exposure of infants to peanut proteins as a preventive against the later development of peanut allergy, although controversy continues (Elbert, SR; Gupta).

As previously mentioned, the increase in asthma, atopic allergy, and autoimmunity is also correlated with eradication of enteric helminth worm parasites (Loke; Feehley). The "natural therapeutic effect" could be to increase the level of IgG antibodies that suppress release of vasoactive amines (Figure 6.7). However, enteric helminth infection may also lead to a higher incidence of enteric viral infection. This seems to occur when the virus and the helminth invade the same tissue (Desai). Both ascaris and *N. brasiliensis* that later migrate through the lung increase the frequency of respiratory viral infection. In the GI tract, helminth infections may damage the enteric barrier, which increases bacterial translocation (Chapter 5) and "opens the door" for the enteric virus and increases viral infection; this is a reason to treat the initial infection. It has been speculated that an enteric helminth infection could cause a shift to diversification of T cells that promote antibody production (a Th2 response) and away from a Th1 response (Table 6.1) that can cause bystander inflammation (Figure 6.4). In rodent studies, helminth infection increases the propensity for infection with West Nile virus (Desai).

Allergy to non-pathogens is not the only example of an illness that can be classified as "immunologic injury" and that has become common in highly developed countries. We mentioned in Chapter 5 that early helminth infection was correlated with a reduced risk of IBD, but the mechanism remains at the theoretical stage. We described in Chapter 5 that IBD has increased 4-fold in developed countries in the last 60 years; these are the same developed countries that have experienced an increase in allergy and asthma (Figure 5.5). Children coming from Africa that are routinely infected with worm parasites have a significantly lower chance of developing IBD when they become adults compared to those that were not infected early in life with parasitic worms. IBD is an umbrella term, but most forms involve inflammatory T cells and cytokines like INFγ and IL-17 from Th1 and Th17 cells (Table 6.3; Figure 6.4).

One of the most controversial and misunderstood forms of immunologic injury is food allergy, and for that reason it is highlighted in Chapter 8. In the eyes of the public, food allergy can be ascribed to things like food avoidance resulting from a bad experience, such as forever avoiding potato salad after a bout with *Salmonella* poisoning. Add to this psycho-physiological factors. Among these are avoiding raw oysters or sushi because such food may be foreign to the palate. Often, true immunologically based allergy can be diagnosed using skin tests, although these are less reliable for food allergy since the original contact is with the GI tract. There are several theories regarding true food allergy; the most intriguing is that human and other mammals have a food sensory system that involves cells in the GI tract, such as tuft cells and entero-endocrine cells that have communication with the CNS (Chapter 5). It is believed that these cells can sense chemicals considered noxious, which include those from certain plant families that include nut families (peanut, pistachio, walnut, and mango), many of which contain phenolic compounds. Others may sense danger in seafood that may contain toxins from microbes. Food allergies are complex and have caused some to call the issue a "can of worms." Some believe that environmental immunomodulatory factors play a role (Prescott).

Immunologic Injury Due to Autoimmunity

The health of the immune system depends on maintaining self-/non-self-discrimination, which relies on the **central** and **peripheral** tolerance mechanisms. These are important regulatory features that collectively prevent or dampen the tendency of the host immune system to recognize and attack "self." However, there is a long list of autoimmune diseases that result from a breakdown of central tolerance and/or failure to establish peripheral tolerance, as well as dysregulation of TLR signaling. Autoimmunity involves both neutrophils and eosinophils that secrete cytokines like TGF-α (Tables 6.1 and 6.3). Autoimmune diseases have a strong genetic component and can be associated with certain MHC types.

Systemic lupus, myasthenia gravis, multiple sclerosis, many forms of psoriasis, rheumatoid arthritis, Hashimoto's thyroiditis, and Graves' disease may be familiar to the public. Autoimmunity also occurs in some forms of diabetes. In myasthenia gravis, antibodies against the acetylcholine receptor block neuromuscular communication and this results in muscular weakness. In Hashimoto's thyroiditis and Graves' disease, antibodies target the thyroid gland and disturb its function. In some forms of diabetes, the target is the insulin-producing islet cells in the pancreas. In rheumatoid arthritis, connective tissue in the synovial joints is the target. Relevant to the Critical Window and the current pandemic of SARS-CoV-2 is a syndrome frequently seen in children recovering from a viral infection that is characterized by fever, shock, GI tract discomfort, and coagulation problems. This is an uncommon condition called Kawasaki disease (KD). Children infected with COVID-19 display mild symptoms compared to adults, but some later develop a multisystem inflammatory syndrome that resembles KD. Like KD, it is associated with antibodies to many self-peptides. Given the recent pandemic, parents with children recovering from COVID-19 should be alert to this syndrome.

While most autoimmune diseases are best known in adults, a number have onset *in utero* because of IgG antibodies transferred across the placenta (Chapter 2). Examples include myasthenia gravis, Graves' disease, and thrombocytopenia. In the latter, passive maternal IgG antibodies attach to fetal platelets, causing bruising and hemorrhage. In *pemphigus vulgaris*, maternal IgG antibodies attack certain antigens in the skin, producing a rash. *Erythroblastosis fetalis* was described and discussed in Chapter 2; it also belongs to this category. An example often used when discussing molecular mimicry is rheumatic fever, in which antibodies responding to a *streptococcal* infection cross-react with heart muscle (see earlier). Some forms of IBD may have a similar origin.

Broad spectrum treatment for autoimmunity involves pharmaceuticals like methotrexate that target rapidly dividing cells like those in cancer and rapidly dividing lymphocytes and inflammatory cells in autoimmunity. Currently TV and the Internet abound with ads for immunosuppressive drugs for the treatment of fundamental and cosmetic autoimmune disorders that may have some negative consequences. More targeted treatments involve the use of monoclonal antibodies (mAb) that target TNF-α or block the TNF-α receptor (Table 6.2).

Another form of immunologic injury is associated with DAMPs. DAMP occurs when tissue damage (eg, ischemia, trauma, tumors, etc.) release intracellular components into the extracellular environment. The list includes histones, certain cytokines, mitochondrial components, and others. Once freed from diseased or injured cells, some believe they may become targets for injurious autoimmune immune responses (Venereau, SR).

The Role of Viruses in Autoimmunity

We have described autoimmunity as a failure of immune tolerance to self. However, viruses may also be involved in autoimmunity (ie, *Horror autotoxicus*). Humans and other vertebrates are infected by and transmit many viruses, some of which are highly pathogenic, including HIV, smallpox, SARS-CoV-2, measles, Ebola, and Zika. Herpes viruses like *H. simplex* are characterized by cycles of latency and lytic activity (Damania), and *H. simplex* is known to produce cold sores. Another herpes virus is Epstein-Barr virus (EBV), which is characterized by the same pattern of latency and lytic behavior. EBV infects approximately 90% of humans in the world and around 50% of teenagers have antibodies to EBV where it is the causative agent of infectious mononucleosis. EBV particularly infects B cells (which are mononuclear; see Table 6.1) and can be recovered from various B cell lymphomas like Burkitt lymphoma, Hodgkin's lymphoma, nasopharyngeal carcinomas, and others. Important to this section is its association with systemic lupus and multiple sclerosis, which are both serious autoimmune diseases. EBV has developed various strategies to evade both the innate and adaptive immune system, which may interfere with mechanisms governing tolerance to self.

Section III. Vaccines and Antimicrobials

LEARNING OBJECTIVES

1. Identify differences among major categories of vaccines used for childhood vaccination.

2. Identify when adjuvants are needed and what their connection to the innate and adaptive immune systems is.

3. Identify the developments that have led to the generation of modern vaccines.

4. Describe the origin, therapeutic value, and limitations of different antimicrobials.

5. Describe the consequences of overuse of antibiotics and its relevance to MDR bacteria.

The History of Vaccination

The earliest known "vaccine" was the practice of variolation, beginning as early as the Middle Ages and known in China, India, Africa, and the Middle East as well as Europe. Variolation takes its name from *variola*, the Latin name for smallpox. Repeated outbreaks of smallpox were universal in that era, with a well-known fatality rate of about 30%. Variolation was practiced by introducing ground crusts from smallpox lesions into the nose (in Chinese practice) or onto abraded skin (in other countries). Death rates after variolation were about 1%, a risk people of the time often accepted. In Britain in the 1700s, an estimated 300,000 patients were treated over several decades by one family of physicians alone; however, famous failures included the death of a son of King George III in 1783. Cotton Mather learned of the practice from an enslaved African and advocated variolation in 1721 in response to a smallpox epidemic in Boston. George Washington mandated variolation of his troops in their winter camp at Valley Forge.

The term *vaccination* originates from an experiment by Edward Jenner, a country doctor in England, who realized that milkmaids exposed to cowpox in cattle, a virus related to smallpox in humans, never developed smallpox. The phenomenon had been reported a quarter century before Jenner by a farmer in Yetminster, England. At the time smallpox was the scourge of humanity, causing millions of deaths and leaving survivors with facial scars that would remain with them for life. While his experiment is considered medically unethical today, Jenner used the ingredients of cowpox pustules to "vaccinate" (derived from the Latin *vacca*, meaning "cow") a young boy in 1796. He subsequently challenged the boy with the live smallpox virus from a pustule, and the boy never developed smallpox. Jenner's dangerous experiment was criticized, and its conclusions were initially rejected by the Royal Academy of Science. Despite the reluctance to accept the findings of the country doctor, his observation was eventually accepted by the medical community and vaccinating individuals before the onset of a disease became widely accepted practice and was much expanded in the 20th century. It is noteworthy that Thomas Jefferson congratulated Jenner and requested the vaccine. Napoleon released English prisoners to honor Jenner. In 1840 the British government banned variolation but made vaccination free under the Vaccination Act. A revised act in 1853 made childhood vaccination mandatory and fined those who failed to comply £1.

Vaccination has virtually eliminated smallpox around the world. The last case was reported in Somalia in 1977. The success of Jenner's experiment depended on certain parts of the cowpox and smallpox viruses, called "epitopes," that are shared by both viruses. Antibodies can be cross-reactive with multiple epitopes, and this also explains molecular mimicry (see Section II).

Current events (in 2022) have circled back to the cowpox and smallpox story and the two orthomyxoviruses that constitute *Vaccinia* and *Variola*, respectively. Another orthomyxovirus that was only described in the late 20th century is monkeypox (found in several species, not just monkeys). The recent increase in human monkeypox cases prompts us to recall that *Vaccinia* has been shown to be protective against infection by monkeypox. In the United States there are now three vaccines with an indication for prevention of monkeypox, two of which produce local infection at the inoculation site. The third is a recombinant, attenuated *Vaccinia* virus that is live but unable to establish an infection. Two doses of this replication-incompetent vaccine are required for protection, and no infectious pustule is produced on the skin of the recipient.

As a result of Jenner's experiment and the advances that followed, vaccination, especially the infants, became standard practice worldwide. It has reduced to almost zero in the United States the incidence of measles, whooping cough, tetanus, diphtheria, and polio and has helped contain outbreaks of influenza. Pursuing this practice, parents are instructed to follow a certain regimen of immunization for their children (Table 6.4). Angst, concerns, and misunderstanding about childhood vaccination persist and are discussed in the final chapter (Chapter 8).

TABLE 6.4   CDC Recommended Childhood Vaccination Schedule

Birth to 18 Months: Vaccines With Multiple Doses Required			
DTaP	4 doses	At 2, 4, 6 months and 15–18 months	
Hib	4 doses	2, 4, 6 months and 12–15 months	
PCV15, PCV20	4 doses	2, 4, 6 months and 12–15 months	See CDC for special considerations for high-risk groups
IPV	3 doses	At 2 and 4 months and 6–18 months	
Rotavirus	2 or 3 doses (depending on vaccine version)	2, 4, and possibly 6 months	
Hepatitis B	3 doses	Birth, 1–2 months, 6–18 months	
Hepatitis A	2 doses	12–18 months	First dose at 6 months if in high-risk group

(Continued)

TABLE 6.4 CDC Recommended Childhood Vaccination Schedule *(Continued)*

Birth to 18 Months: Vaccines With Single Dose	
MMR	12–18 months
Varicella	12–18 months
Hepatitis A	12–18 months

18 Months to 18 Years: Single Doses, Boosters, or Multiple Doses		
DTaP booster	4–6 years old	
Tdap (booster for DTaP in older children)	11–12 years	A less reactive version used in children 7 years or older and adults
IPV	4–6 years	
MMR	4–6 years	
Varicella	4–6 years	
Meningococcal	11–12 years and 16 years	May be started in infancy in high-risk patients such as those with HIV, sickle cell disease, asplenia
HPV	11–12 years	

Tdap, DTap and dTaP are modern versions of DTAP.

Vaccine Contraindications/Cautions	
Rotavirus—contraindicated	Severe combined immunodeficiency
Rotavirus—caution	Other immunodeficiency, HIV (if CD4 cells are below a set criteria)
MMR and Varicella—contraindicated	Immunocompromised, HIV if very low CD4 cells
Live attenuated influenza—contraindicated	Immunocompromised, HIV, asplenia, asthma with wheeze ages 2–4 years
Live attenuated influenza—caution	Renal failure and dialysis, heart or lung disease, diabetes

A full vaccination schedule with detailed discussion of vaccines, ages, contraindications, and catch-up doses and recent COVID recommendation is available at: www.cdc.gov/vaccines/schedules/downloads/child/0-18yrs-child-combined-schedule.pdf.

Adapted from Centers for Disease Control and Prevention, "Recommended Child and Adolescent Immunization Schedule for Ages 18 Years or Younger," U.S. Department of Health and Human Services, 2023.

In Chapters 1 and 5, we described the role that bacteriophages play in the diversity of life forms on planet Earth. We mentioned that these can cause lysis of bacteria they infect, the mechanism of which is described in Appendix A-1. While the vaccine approach was on its way in the 20th century, there were still efforts in the 1920s to build on the "bacteriophage theory" of D'Herelle, who believed that bacteriophages could be selected to attack bacterial pathogens and thereby be used as a means to therapeutically control the spread of targeted bacterial infections (AAI Newsletter). (Refer to Appendices A-1 and A-2). While conventional vaccines have taken the limelight, bacteriophage therapy may have a place in combating mycobacterial infection (see "Hard Nuts to Crack," below). Cystic fibrosis (CF) is a pulmonary disease associated with thickened airways and alterations in the CFTR genes (see Appendices A-1 and A-2). CF patients and others experience mycobacterial infections including *M. avium* and *M. abscessus* and some success has been reported in a patient with *M. abscessus* (Nick). Bacteriophage therapy may be valuable in treating CF-associated infections. This involves engineered bacteriophage that can lyse the mycobacteria. The success of the therapy has numerous hurdles to cross, such as a host immune response to the bacteriophage and development of resistance by mycobacteria for the engineered bacteriophage.

Renewed interest in phage therapy has been fueled by the alarming increase in MDR bacteria, which are tied to antibiotic use and overuse. The World Health Organization predicts that as many as 10 million people may die annually from MDR bacteria by 2050 (WHO Joint News Release). As we will discuss in Chapter 8, some are concerned by the threat of an "antibiotic winter" when there will be no antibiotics that confront MDR bacteria (Blaser). Therefore, renewed interest in phage therapy has quickened in the last 7 years. One of the areas it is being tried in is agriculture (see Appendix A-2).

Vaccine Development, Diversity, and Administration

The original smallpox vaccine developed by Jenner was a live cowpox virus related to the smallpox virus through shared epitopes, but cowpox does not cause the smallpox in humans. The use of a related live virus was replaced with what are called **attenuated vaccines** that owe their origin to the chance experimental outcome of studies by the famous microbiologist Louis Pasteur. Pasteur allowed a culture of bacteria responsible for causing cholera to grow for a long time (this is often attributed to accident, perhaps because Pasteur went on vacation to Switzerland). While the historical facts may be fuzzy, it is true that the long-cultured bacteria were no longer able to produce cholera in rabbits (ie, they had become "attenuated"). Attenuation through long-term culture became the norm to produce many live viral vaccines such as the MMR vaccine (measles, mumps, and rubella; Table 6.4) and the oral polio, chicken pox, and hepatitis A vaccines. The genetics underlying the attenuation process is partially described in Appendix A-1.

In the case of bacterial pathogens like *C. tetani*, diphtheria, and whooping cough, attenuated organisms are not used because of the danger they may revert to a pathogenic form and because the killed bacteria are equally effective. Killed vaccines, or so-called **inactivated vaccines**, can be prepared in various ways, often using formalin. This is the historically "quick and dirty" method used for their preparation and it is used in many veterinary vaccines.

Some vaccines are not composed of the entire organism but only "parts" of the pathogen. The latter are called **subunit vaccines**. Toxins produced by a bacterial pathogen, poisonous snakes, or arachnids, can be chemically converted to a modified form that is no longer toxic but can still stimulate immunity to the native toxin. These are called *toxoids*. This is the case with the vaccine for *C. tetani* that we have used as an example in Section II of this chapter. There are also **conjugate vaccines**, containing epitopes from several strains of a pathogen that have been chemically united. These and subunit vaccines are more expensive to prepare but can be more effective because they focus the attention of the immune system on an epitope or epitopes of several strains that are most likely to lead to a protective immune response. Using subunit vaccines can eliminate certain unwanted side effects when the whole bacteria or virus is used, including unwanted inflammation and eventual scarring at the site of infection, which all those old enough to have received a smallpox vaccine will appreciate.

Composite vaccines include the DPT (or DTaP) vaccine, which includes killed diphtheria (D), killed pertussis (P), and tetanus toxoid (T). Including all three into a single vaccine reduces the number of injections, frequency of screaming children, and anxiety of the parents, while simultaneously providing an adjuvant effect (see later) that increases vaccine efficacy but may cause discomfort due to inflammation at the injection site. Adjuvants act by stimulating PAMPs (see section on innate immunity and Table 6.2). For example, the cell wall of *Bordetella pertussis*, the organism responsible for whooping cough and the "P" in DPT, is especially recognized by TLR4 (Table 6.2) and therefore activates a strong immune response to all constituents of the composite DPT vaccine. Of course, this strong response may also cause unwanted bystander inflammation, causing a lesion and pain. The modern version of this "trivalent" vaccine is called DTaP or Tdap, in which the added "a" refers to the inclusion of an acellular version of pertussis, which while lacking some of the adjuvant effect of the whole bacterium, does away with the bystander damage that sometimes occurred with the original DPT vaccine (Table 6.4). There are other examples of negative bystander effects in vaccines, such as the first experimental vaccine for respiratory syncytial virus (RSV). This vaccine was composed of formalin-inactivated RSV and unexpectedly, in the vaccine trials, it had the secondary effect of markedly causing more severe symptoms after RSV infection than in the placebo controls. Thus, the vaccine did not reach approval (see Chapter 7). Currently there are several proposed vaccines based on subunit proteins from this virus, but none have completed trials and licensure.

Valency is often used to describe certain vaccines; DPT and Tdap are referred to as "trivalent" vaccines, since they protect against three pathogens. You may also hear about 13- or 23-valent pneumococcal conjugate vaccines (eg, PCV13; Table 6.4). *Pneumococcus* is short for *Streptococcus pneumoniae*, which are bacteria that occur in many forms (called serotypes) and differ in the capsular polysaccharides that comprise the bacterial cell wall. A 13-valent pneumococcal vaccine is a conjugate of 13 different serotypes, while PPSV23 contains 23 serotypes (Table 6.4). In the case of polio, types 1, 2, and 3 comprise the trivalent oral polio vaccine (OPV).

Conjugated polysaccharide vaccines deserve a bit of note. The vaccine for *H. flu* bacteria (Hib) is a conjugated polysaccharide and was developed for children. The polysaccharide epitope is chemically coupled to a protein, resulting in a more vigorous and protective response than when infants received the isolated polysaccharide. The greater effectiveness is the result of a T cell response to the carrier protein. The development of *H. flu* vaccine entirely altered the practice of pediatrics. In the author's memory, infants and toddlers with fever were sources of great anxiety because a busy practitioner would encounter cases of *H. flu* meningitis with some regularity. Even with early recognition and vigorous antibiotic treatment, mortality was up to 15% and many survivors had neurologic damage. Younger pediatricians have never seen this disease, just like practitioners of the current era have never dealt with paralytic polio or diphtheria that were reduced to rarity through use of childhood vaccination.

The administration of killed vaccines such as DTAP, Hib, IPV, and Hepatitis B (Table 6.4) differs from the schedule for the MMR vaccine (measles, mumps, rubella). These are only given once during an early period of life, although a booster is recommended at 4–6 years of age, which is a short window to account for deferential immune system development (see Chapter 8). The same applies to the OPV. The reason for their one-time usage is that attenuated viral vaccines like the MMR and OPV vaccines continue to replicate in the host for a few weeks or longer, providing continued stimulation and long-term protection. Measles and OPV best mimic the natural disease and persistent immune response. By contrast, mumps vaccine appears overly attenuated, resulting in short-lived protection that (along with vaccine avoidance in some groups) can explain the periodic outbreaks of mumps on college campuses. A review of mumps cases in the last 15 years shows continued low-level presence of mumps cases in the United States, many associated with localized outbreaks and about one-third in children with up-to-date vaccination status (Shepersky).

Since killed, conjugated, and subunit vaccines are non-living, they do not replicate in the host and are rapidly degraded. Therefore, it is necessary they be given multiple times during childhood (Table 6.4). This is also why in adults a tetanus "booster" is advised every 10 years, and especially after "stepping on a rusty nail in the garden" (a good source of *C. tetani*).

There are additional reasons why vaccines are given at multiple times. First, infants are born with transplacentally acquired serum IgG (Chapter 2) and this passive IgG may include antibodies to the antigens of the pathogens in vaccines. This IgG can partially interfere with the vaccine by removing it from circulation or reducing the amount available to properly stimulate the immune system. Thus, childhood vaccinations (except Hep B) are delayed until about 8 weeks of age. Passive SIgA antibodies obtained through suckling should not interfere with the response to injected vaccines since they remain in the gut and do not enter the bloodstream of the infant (Chapter 3). It is possible that SIgA in breast milk could interfere with the oral polio vaccine (OPV), which is no longer used in the United States. Secondly, infants first exposed to the vaccine antigen will make a predominantly IgM antibody of unimpressive protective value. Subsequent doses initiate a GCRx, which leads to a robust IgG response and fosters strong memory B and T cell populations (Figures 6.1 and 6.3). The percentage of infants with protective levels of IgG rises with each booster, approaching 100% efficacy after the third dose of DTaP. Finally, and despite that MMR-attenuated vaccine replicates, they are given three times to reflect differences in neonatal immune competence as well as to avoid interference by passive IgG acquired *in utero*.

Vaccines for influenza A present an additional challenge. Influenza virus is an RNA virus, and this group of viruses are notorious for their ability to "change their spots" in a manner that resembles the many serotypes of pneumococcus (Figure 6.2). Most produce benign infections, but the 1918 variant may have resulted in the death of 50 million people, and it infected one-third of the human population. The more recent influenza H1N1 "swine flu" of 2009–2010 caused the death of 12,500 among 61 million infected. This new virus was a cause of great anxiety, but eventually did not cause an especially severe seasonal outbreak. In the United States, approximately 8% of Americans have symptomatic influenza each year.

Infections vary in number and severity, and as many as 60,000 Americans can die from seasonal influenza in a severe year. The influenza A virus has the remarkable ability to use various chromosomal elements to produce new variants. Because of this, the annual flu vaccine must be reconstructed each year at the CDC to match prediction models of the variants that are expected to be prevalent (Li). Currently research is underway to create a true polyvalent or "universal" influenza vaccine, which might result in some unemployment at the CDC but could make the world safer from an influenza A pandemic. A number of these target the universal stalk of the virus spike. SARS-CoV-2, responsible for the COVID-19 pandemic, is another RNA virus, which belongs to a different family (Betacoronaviridae; Appendix A-4) and is believed to "change its spots" or "spikes" at a lower rate than influenza A. Nevertheless, annual booster vaccinations may be needed for the same reason as for influenza A. Most influenza vaccines are injected, inactivated antigens. However, there is a licensed live attenuated influenza vaccine available in the United States that is administered as a spray into the nose. The relative merits of this route are still debated, and there are several contraindications, some based on risks and some based on absence of evidence in the at-risk population.

In recently years an influenza A variant carried especially by migrating waterfowl, has spread to domestic chicken and turkey flock forcing millions to be euthanized. It has now been found in dairy cattle and dairy farm workers, suggesting mutation to a zoonotic variant. It would not be unreasonable, as done in Norway, to immunize dairy workers against this bird flu variant.

The Role of Adjuvants

Those with military experience understand that the job of the adjutant officer is to serve as an aid to the commanding officer; the term *adjutant* and *adjuvant* have a common Latin origin. Gaston Ramon, a French veterinarian associated with the Pasteur Institute, noted that vaccines worked better if inflammation was produced at the site of injection and inflammation is the first feature of the host response to a pathogen (Section I). Substances like tapioca, agar, and starch oil can cause inflammation and protein-based vaccines worked best if first precipitated with aluminum salts, often called alum. In Section I, we described that PRRs, such as TLRs (Table 6.2) that recognize PAMPs, are needed to activate the immune system. Attenuated vaccines or those that comprise whole bacteria display PAMPs, such as DTAP, so an adjuvant is not required. However, subunit vaccines or toxoids are devoid of PAMPs. In addition to alum, TLR agonists like lipid A and CpG oligonucleotides are popular adjuvants. The advent of a new generation of vaccines, such as mRNA vaccines used for COVID-19, led to the use of lipid nanoparticles (LNP; Appendices A-1 and A-4), which have adjuvant and other valuable properties.

However, adjuvants can also have negative effects. Since they are designed to produce inflammation, it is not surprising that some individuals suffer painful and even allergic reactions when an adjuvant evokes a "cytokine storm" (Table 6.3). This has been experienced with the Shingrix (shingles) vaccine in individuals with a propensity for developing allergic responses; similar negative responses were encountered in a small number of patients receiving new COVID-19 vaccines.

The Story of Polio Vaccines: A Useful Model

While as many as 15 vaccines are available for childhood immunization (Table 6.4), we have used only a few of the most common as examples in explaining vaccine diversity and the rationale of the current childhood vaccination schedule. A group that deserves mention are the polio vaccines. Polio is caused by a virus normally acquired by mouth that ends up in the nervous system and was the scourge of America, especially from 1930–1960. For many the disease was asymptomatic, but in 1% of children and one in every 75 teenagers, it resulted in paralytic poliomyelitis. President Franklin Roosevelt was a well-known victim. Still today, the baby boom generation contains a number who limp, wear leg braces, or are confined to wheelchairs as a result of this childhood disease. The development of two successful vaccines, one comprised of the inactivated virus that is injected (IPV; Table 6.4) is called the Salk vaccine, while an attenuated oral version (OPV) is called the Sabin vaccine; both honor their designers. Both were major success stories in the battles against polio. The Sabin vaccine was one of the first successful attempts to precisely deliver the vaccine to the place where the virus first enters the system, namely, the GI tract. Pathogens like polio gain access to the host by breeching the host's "soft" mucosal columnar epithelium in the respiratory, GI tract, and urogenital systems (see above "Mucosal Immune System"). While pathogens entering through the cornified epithelium of the skin encounter IgG class antibodies, those entering mucosal surfaces encounter SIgA (Figure 6.6). OPV was the first **mucosal vaccine** designed to immunize the site of viral entry (the GI tract), and it played a pioneering role in our understanding of what is now called the mucosal immune system (see Section II and Figure 6.6).

Originally both vaccines (IPV and OPV) were used in America, although since 2000, only the IPV is used (Table 6.4). Worldwide, as part of the global initiative of eliminating polio from planet Earth, OPV is used. Readers may be familiar with the role of the Gates Foundation, the World Health Organization (WHO), and the United Nations Children's Fund (UNICEF) in this endeavor. Pakistan, Nigeria, and Afghanistan now remain the only endemic countries for the disease. The OPV vaccine is used worldwide because it can be painlessly administered by untrained staff, is cheaper to produce than IPV, and targets the original source of the infection, the GI tract. However, OPV has one or more disadvantages. Most concerning, and something shared with all attenuated vaccines, is that there remains a possibility that the virus can revert to a virulent form and produce the disease (Mateen; Bandyopadhyay). There have been 76 such cases from 2005–2013. The danger is increased since the reverted live virus is shed in the feces, which has been recently detected in the sewage system of New York City, which reported a polio outbreak. A second observation is that while OPV provided protection, the number of vaccinated individuals who develop serum antibodies varies from 60–90% whereas 100% of those receiving IPV develop serum antibodies. Given that the vaccine is still protective, this could be due to virus-specific T cells that migrate to the mucosa. Furthermore, OPV stimulates the development of mucosal antibodies like SIgA that would not be detected in serum but would still provide protection; the effectiveness of both depends on T cells. So, while OPV is the gold standard for the worldwide polio eradication program, only IPV is used in America (Table 6.4).

The mention of OPV invites discussion of mucosal vaccines in general, the use of which presents various challenges such as accurate control of dosage and knowing if they are equally taken up and processed. Because of these uncertainties, most approved vaccines designed to promote immunity at mucosal sites are still injected into muscles, IPV being an example. These are still effective since lymphocytes stimulated at one site migrate to other sites, including the mucosa.

Maternal Vaccination

Many vaccine-preventable diseases cause illness and even death in pregnant women and their infants. A healthy mother always has the best chance of delivering a healthy child and caring for it postpartum. In previous chapters we indicated that the newborn immune system is incompletely developed and therefore responds poorly to childhood vaccines. We also described how in healthy primates like humans, IgG antibodies are actively transported into the developing fetus and can provide passive immunity *in utero* and for up to 5 months after birth. Hence, immunizing the mother while she is pregnant offers a means to protect both mother and offspring. However, immunizing the mother postpartum with vaccines that generate serum IgG antibodies will have little value for the infant, since IgG is a trivial portion of the antibodies in breast milk where approximately 90% are SIgA and are not absorbed/transferred into the blood of the suckling infant. However, oral vaccines that target the GI tract/mucosal immune system can be beneficial since the lymphocytes stimulated in the GI tract subsequently migrate to the MG and secrete SIgA into breast milk; this is the gut-MG axis (see "Mucosal Immune System" and Chapter 3). This has proven successful for protecting piglets from viral infections of the GI tract epithelium. In humans, it is part of OPV vaccine administration.

Deciding on the time during pregnancy to vaccinate the mother depends on whether the concern is primarily for the health of the mother or whether the major concern is for the offspring. Vaccinating the mother at 28–32 weeks results in optimal transfer to the fetus. In the case of influenza, which is a threat to the mother and her offspring, vaccination should be timed to the seasonal outbreak of influenza for the country of residence. In any case, there is no approved influenza vaccine for infants younger than 6 months of age, so maternal vaccination is the only route for providing protective antibodies to the offspring. Studies show that maternal vaccination reduces the incidence of influenza by 60% and reduces the risk of hospitalization for influenza-like illness in the first 6 months of infant life.

Globally, tetanus claims over 100,000 newborns each year in underdeveloped countries. Vaccinating mothers with an adjuvant-free tetanus toxoid vaccine (not DTAP or Tdap; see above) can lead to a more than 90% reduction in neonatal death due to tetanus. In all countries, pertussis is common among the general population, and when death occurs from pertussis it is usually before 6 months of life, which is before infants have developed immunity from the Tdap vaccination regimen (Table 6.4). Immunizing pregnant women with Tdap or a tetanus toxoid vaccine in the third trimester may generate passive antibodies that interfere with the effectiveness of the Tdap childhood vaccination regimen, but the risk of disease does not justify withholding vaccination of the pregnant mother.

The story for *Streptococcus pneumoniae*, an important cause of otitis media and pneumonia, is more of a mixed bag, since various studies show that while immunization during pregnancy raises antibody levels in the mother and infant, it does not appear to reduce the disease risk for infants younger than 6 months of age The same appears to be true for *Haemophilus influenza* (the HiB vaccine; Table 6.4) in developed countries, where levels of the pathogen are low. However, HiB vaccination may be valuable for pregnant women in underdeveloped countries where children are not routinely vaccinated like they are in the United States.

COMMON VACCINE-PREVENTABLE DISEASES OF CHILDHOOD

Measles (rubeola): Measles virus briefly infects the respiratory tract after exposure, but rapidly spreads to distant sites via the bloodstream, including to the lymphoid tissues. The distinctive clinical illness includes fever, cough, rhinorrhea, conjunctivitis, and rash. About 0.1% of patients have severe CNS involvement (encephalitis), and slightly more have less destructive CNS issues such as seizures. As late as 1990, UNICEF estimated that 1 million deaths per year in developing countries were due to measles and its complications.

Mumps: Mumps virus infects multiple tissues but is most noted for inflammation and swelling of the salivary glands, especially the parotid glands (parotitis). Other glands that may be affected include testes (where inflammation is known as orchitis) especially in post-pubertal males. Other occasional target tissues are ovaries, pancreas, and breasts. Viral meningitis is probably present in most patients. Prior to vaccines, most children were infected prior to puberty.

Rubella (German measles): Infection can be asymptomatic, or produce rash, fever, malaise, and enlarged lymph nodes. The disease itself was less feared than the syndrome of congenital rubella that occurred when a pregnant woman was infected. The fetal outcome varied from death and miscarriage to severe fetal anomalies including deafness, rash at birth, cataracts, and profound developmental neurologic impacts.

Varicella (chicken pox): This illness was formerly extremely common, with over 90% of children infected by 10 years old. The clinical syndrome included fever and an itchy rash. Scratching could lead to secondary bacterial infection of open skin lesions. The disease had much worse impact in immunocompromised children, with potentially fatal multisystem infection. Thus, possible varicella cases had to be carefully excluded from hospital settings where immunocompromised children might be affected.

Poliomyelitis: The virus replicates in the GI epithelium, usually with no symptoms. In less than 1% of patients, attack on CNS motor neurons leads to temporary or permanent weakness of the muscles innervated by that motor neuron group. In a few of those with muscular weakness, the muscles of respiration are involved, which is potentially fatal. People of the authors' generation usually have had one or a few acquaintances with a weakened and atrophied arm or leg as result of the disease.

Diphtheria: This disease Is a bacterial infection (*Corynebacterium diphtheriae*) of the mucosa of the upper airway. The infection induces a thick inflammatory coating (pseudo membrane) that can fatally obstruct the airway. In addition, the organism secretes an exotoxin that can severely or fatally impair cardiac, renal, and neural function. In the 1920s, prior to vaccine development, it caused about 15,000 deaths per year in the United States.

Pertussis (whooping cough): Prior to vaccine availability, pertussis was even more deadly than diphtheria. It is caused by infection of the respiratory epithelium by *Bordetella pertussis*. The illness is characterized by cough with prolonged coughing spells, followed by a loud inspiratory "whoop." It is a very significant risk for younger infants, as they may suffer respiratory arrest or have repeated hypoxic spells due to the intense spasms of cough that prevent adequate inspiration. Nonrespiratory complications include seizures, blindness, deafness, and brain damage. Vaccine to pertussis is usually given in a combination that also includes vaccines to tetanus and diphtheria.

Herd Immunity and the Anti-Vaccination Movement

The success of childhood vaccination regimens in the United States and elsewhere is based on the concept of **herd immunity**, a term that attracted public attention during the COVID-19 pandemic. It has been proven that if the immunization of all children born into a population is continued for decades, the level of immunity is so high that the contagion cannot gain a foothold since both the number of infected individuals and the number of unprotected individuals is tiny. The WHO and other groups have steadily worked to achieve that objective and globally the rate of immunization has risen from 20% in 1980 to 86% in 2018 (Zerhouni). This has been the guiding principle for control of childhood diseases (Table 6.4). If everyone participated, almost all childhood diseases could be eliminated, just like polio and smallpox in the United States and, in the case of smallpox, in the entire world. Herd immunity is the reason certain vaccines like the oral polio vaccine (OPV) are no longer on the list of recommended vaccinations in the United States, since no cases of polio have been reported there until recently. The recent outbreak in New York City could be due to (1) residents in religious/ethnic enclaves who have stopped vaccinating their children, or (2) recent immigrants who have received the OPV, which then reverted to virulence.

The switch to IPV is also the reason why immunization of pregnant women with IPV and *Haemophilus influenza* is currently not recommended in countries like the United States. However, vaccination regimens must be enforced in other countries because it cannot be guaranteed that herd immunity has been achieved. When too many have not been vaccinated, the possibility of an epidemic increases. Examples include enclaves like Orthodox Jewish communities in New York and other communities who oppose vaccination for religious reasons. Herd immunity and consequent disease control can be easily lost by nonadherence to vaccination guidelines. We have witnessed this in America in the last 15 years and it is the reason this goal cannot be reached for SARS-CoV-2. Much false and counterproductive information has been spread through social media and by politicians.

Myths and misinformation (Chapter 8) have contributed to the COVID-19 pandemic by creating an "infodemic."

"Hard Nuts to Crack"

Vaccines are still not the panacea solution to all infectious diseases. The world's most lethal and debilitating infections include malaria, TB, and HIV. The concept that recovery from natural infection with a pathogen or after receiving a vaccine results in protective immunity does not work for all diseases. Malaria causes millions of deaths worldwide, including more than 627,000 deaths in 2020, mostly of African children under 5. Unlike viral and bacterial infections that are a threat to children in America, malaria is the result of a eukaryotic intracellular parasite that presents itself in various life cycle forms, in Asia, Africa, and Central and South America. Malaria and TB have been a "hard nut to crack," but several new vaccines are now in trial. The history of malarial vaccines is reviewed by Sinnis and Fidock (2022). HIV remains a problem because, as we have discussed, it disables the host's immune system. However, HIV can now be controlled by antiviral drugs (see next) and new vaccines show promise.

Modern Vaccine Technology

While conventional vaccines have taken up to 20 years to develop, a DNA vaccine for SARS-CoV-1 was completed in 20 months, for H5 influenza in 11 months, H1 influenza in 4 months, Zika in 3.5 months, and various new SARS-CoV-2 vaccines in less than 1 year. The details regarding new vaccines are provided in Appendix A-1, and their effectiveness in the case of COVID-19 is discussed in Appendix A-4. The explosion of molecular genetic technology in 1990 and beyond greatly facilitated the purification of viral and bacterial subunits. When Chinese scientists published the genome of SARS-CoV-2, the virus responsible for the COVID-19 pandemics, modern tools allowed molecular geneticists to produce the "spike protein" of this virus *in vitro*, and within a few weeks it was marketed to scientists for use as a subunit viral vaccine. The availability of this product has proven valuable in creating subunit vaccine model structures based on 3D electron microscopy. Other approaches involve delivering the gene encoding the spike protein of SARS-CoV-2 using a non-pathogenic virus, like adenovirus type 5, as a vector. Others incorporate mRNA encoding the spike protein of SARS-CoV-2 into lipid nanoparticles (LNP). The LNP is then taken up by various cells of the host, the mRNA released and the encoded spike protein synthesized and the spike protein is transiently expressed; these are called mRNA vaccines. They were first investigated in animal studies more than a decade ago and their first use in humans was to combat the SARS-CoV-2 virus. The details of modern vaccine development are provided in Appendix A-1.

In addition to new vaccines, there are other therapeutic treatments now in use that include use of passive antibodies and antiviral drugs. The modern therapeutic use of passive antibodies, in particular the development and use of monoclonal antibodies (mAb), is covered in Appendix A-1. Treatment with antiviral drugs fits best into the category of pharmaceuticals like antibiotics and is discussed in the next section.

Section IV. Protection Through Use of Antimicrobials

LEARNING OBJECTIVES

1. Describe the natural origin of antibiotics and their natural function.
2. Describe the overuse of antibiotics and the dangers involved.
3. Be familiar with important applications of antivirals and their mechanisms of action.

The Antibiotic Revolution: The Miracle Cure?

Bacteria like *C. tetani* can also be killed by substances made by other bacteria and fungi. The Actinomycetes bacteria that live in the same soil as *C. tetani* protect themselves against *C. tetani* using molecules called **antibiotics** ("substances that destroy other life"). These have no relationship to **antibodies** made by mammals and other vertebrates, though the close similarity of the two terms may be confusing to the public (see Chapter 8). Medical science seized on this discovery in 1929 when Professor Alexander Fleming accidentally allowed a culture of bacteria to be contaminated with ordinary bread mold called *Penicillium*, which promptly killed the bacteria. This discovery was of such significance that a nationwide search was conducted to find the most productive mold. Moldy Mary's cantaloupe won the prize when offered to the USDA laboratory in Peoria, Illinois. It produced 50,000 units/ml of mold compared to Fleming's bread mold, which produced only 4 units/ml. Subsequently, scientists grew that fungus and extracted **penicillin**, the first antibiotic. However, many antibiotics are a natural product extracted from the soil bacteria Actinomycetes, so named because these bacteria resemble fungi. Synthetic derivatives have been regularly made by pharmaceutical chemists. Within the group Actinomycetes are the Streptomyces, from which over 500 compounds have been isolated, including two of the earliest and best known, streptomycin and actinomycin; these include over 23 unique classes. Table A3.3 lists a number of common antibiotics, the chemical families to which they belong, and their effectiveness against Gram-positive and Gram-negative bacteria.

The use of antibiotics has done wonders in alleviating human suffering, disease, and death. Half of the over 700,000 people who died in the Civil War died of bacterial infection, and in WWI, more people died of infection by bacteria than from bullets. With the introduction of penicillin in 1942, the death rate among allied soldiers in WWII was reduced by 90%. Death by bacterial infection in the Korean War was less than 2%. However, a major difference between the treatment of a bacterial infection and the treatment of viral infection is that **antibiotics** have no effect on the viral infection. However, they may help to prevent secondary bacterial infection. Viral infections can only be controlled by antibodies that neutralize the circulating virus, by the cytotoxic T cells that kill the virus-producing cells, and in a few cases like HIV, by using antiviral drugs.

Despite the overwhelming value that antibiotics have had for medicine and veterinary medicine, their widespread use created several problems because antibiotics were being prescribed for all kinds of human maladies, including viral infections, for which antibiotics have no effect. In 2005 it was judged that 75% of antibiotic prescriptions in the United Kingdom were prescribed to treat viral infections (Blaser, SR) and a third of antibiotic presecription in outpatients settings in the US were not appropriate in 2010 and 2011(Mather). It has been estimated that more than 90 million cases of Salmonella gastroenteritis have cost 3 billion Euro in the European Union and $2.7 billion in the US for treatment of patients, the control of which is compromised by MDR variants (Mather). Overuse of antibiotics has led to the emergence of multidrug resistant (MDR) bacteria, which also involves methicillin-resistant *Staphylococcus aureus*, or MRSA, as it is known to the public (Furuga). Intestinal bacteria, serve as reservoir of MDR bacteria called a **resistome** that caries antibiotic resistance (**AR**) genes that can be horizontally transferred to other bacteria (see HGT; Salyers; Appendix A-1). Resistant microbes often described as "superbugs", have become increasingly difficult to control We referred to this group of bacteria in Chapter 5 as the **resistome**. The CDC indicates that 23,000 people die annually from MDR bacteria and the WHO describes it as the main cause of about 1.8 million deaths worldwide (Wikipedia; Antimicrobial resistance).

Concern about overuse of antibiotics has also focused on the feeding of antibiotics to poultry and swine to promote weight gain. This practice uses very low doses in a program known as **sub-therapeutic antibiotic therapy** (STAT), and the antibiotics used were originally called **antibiotic growth promotors (AGP)**. Some consider them to be a source of MDR bacteria (Spoor). The STAT program and its many variations remain contentious within the medical community and alternatives have been a challenge for producers that provide meat in the United States and globally. Eliminating the use of antimicrobials could have a devastating effect on the food supply if alternative solutions do not become available. These changes would also impact pharmaceutical companies, since 50% of all the antibiotics they produce are used in STAT programs.

Some have warned that overuse of antibiotics could increase the problem of MDR bacteria and could lead to "antibiotic winter" (ie, a period in which there are no natural or synthetic antibiotics left that can combat bacterial infection). This is of major concern to the antibiotic industry, which recognizes that the "golden age" of antibiotic discovery ended some years ago and that Actinomycetes had been "over-mined" as a source of natural antibiotics (Lewis). As a result, few new natural antibiotics were discovered in the last 35 years; only six have been approved in the last 20 years but none against Gram-negative bacteria. Over-mining of natural sources like soil bacteria *Streptomyces* has been replaced by large-scale screening of synthetic compounds. GlaxoSmithKline and AstraZeneca concluded in 2015 that this approach was unsuccessful. The low success rate in finding new antimicrobials has been dubbed the antimicrobial resistance crisis. Some investigators have now turned to other members of life's pyramid (Chapter 1) such as nematodes that like actinomycetes, live in the soil, and would need similar protection from soil bacteria. This has led to the discovery of certain retinoids, analogs of Vitamin A that act against the negatively charged membranes of Gram-negative bacteria but seem less likely to expand the resistome (Chapter 5). In any case, the future of antibiotic discovery will be challenging and may involve use of bacterio-phages (Chapter 5). The molecular genetics of how antibiotic resistance develops and the transfer of AR genes is described in Appendix A-1.

MDR Pathogens: Origin, STAT, and Bi-Directional Transfer

The global increase in the frequency of MDR pathogens has added 21–34 billion dol-lars to the cost of healthcare and caused a 2–3.5% decrease in global domestic product (Sprenger; Zurek). Americans are familiar with *E. coli* and *Salmonella* from outbreaks that have resulted in the recall of ground beef, eggs, and leafy vegetables and customer lawsuits. *E. coli* 0157:H1, which thrives in cattle, has been a common culprit. Zoonotic spread can result during food processing and through transfer by insects and farm and factory workers. House fly and bush fly transmission is well documented in Japan, Australia, and Kansas. Horizontal gene transfer (HGT; Appendix A-1) is especially frequent among Gram-negative enterobacteria (phylum Proteobacteria, Chapter 5) but also in *Enterococcus* and *Clostridia*. Such was the case involving the house fly/bush fly incident caused by a transposon carried by *Enterococcus* (Zurek).

MDR bacteria like MRSA, *C. difficile*, *Salmonella*, and *E. coli* have impacted human health through vertical transmission of antibiotic-resistant strains, for example cephalosporin-resistant *E. coli*. The STAT ban in Denmark resulted in a 60% reduction in MDR *E. coli*, leading the WHO to conclude that cephalosporins, fluoroquinolones, and macrolides (Table A3.4) should not be used in STAT programs (Aarestrup). Fluoroquinolones have been affectively used to treat *Salmonella* infection but were only used in early STAT programs. Some insight comes from studies of resistance to vancomycin (often used to treat *C. difficle*). This is a glycopeptide like avoparcin (Table A3.4), which is used as an AGP. Researchers followed the presence of the antibiotic-resistant (AR) gene for vancomycin after its use in turkeys and obtained the following data on the frequency of this AR gene: 50% of turkeys carried the AR gene, 39% of turkey farmers, and 20% of turkey-processing line workers, but only 14% of the local community (van den Bogaard). Similar data suggesting transfer from chickens to humans have been reported (Levy). A study by Mather challenges popular views attributing local animal reservoirs as a source of *Salmonella* and MDR bacteria in humans. Distinct populations of MRSA isolates have been demonstrated by complete sequencing of the MDR genes (Hau, Allue-Guardia, et al.; Hau, Haan, et al.). Whole microbe gene sequencing is currently fast and routine and can accurately determine the sources of MDR microbes. This important step should be taken in both the veterinary and public health sec-tors. In the absence of microbial genetic sequence information, the question of the direction of transfer and blame seems to reside with the media, not on molecular genetics.

Antiviral Drugs

The emergence of viral disease as a major threat to health is reminiscent of the threat posed by (a) pathogenic bacteria responsible for the plague of the Middle Ages, (b) enteric epidem-ics like cholera and typhus, (c) respiratory epidemics like pneumonia and TB, (d) sexually transmitted diseases like syphilis and gonorrhea, and (e) foodborne pathogens like *C. botulinum*, *Salmonella*, and pathogenic *E. coli*. In the last 50 years, emerging diseases caused by viral pathogens have dominated the scene. At present, the WHO lists eight viral diseases (including COVID-19) that are prioritized for emergency treatment (Lu, SR). In modern history, the 1918 influenza pandemic killed 50 million, HIV has killed 35 million, and by 2021, COVID-19 had killed over 7 million worldwide, including more than 1.2 million in the United States. The surge in emerging viral disease has multiple origins, such as climate change that increases the number and diversity of biting insects that serve as vectors for viral disease, globalization that allows localized outbreaks to spread, and contraction of infected wildlife habit that brings wildlife into closer contact with human populations. The appearance of the beta coronaviruses (SARS-CoV-1, SARS CoV-2, and MERS) had a zoonotic origin and jumped to new hosts lacking established immunity, allowing them to rapidly expand their numbers. Rapid nucleic acid replication (Figure 6.2; Appendix A-1) increases the opportunity for spontaneous mutants to appear. Outbreaks like the COVID-19 pandemic come at a times when medical science was ill-prepared. This is similar to historic bacterial epidemics that occurred when pan-specific antimicrobials were not available. In general, medical science is best prepared to deal with pathogens like influenza and monkey pox, which have a previous history of causing human disease. A major problem lies with those for which humans have had no previous experiences, SARS-CoV-2.

Many believed that since antibiotics have no effect on viral infections, only the host immune system could be protective against viral disease. However, in the case of HIV, the virus attacks and kills the helper T cells, so other measures were considered. Thus, efforts turned to antiviral drugs, the same principle behind the use of antibiotics. Like antibiotics, antivirals interrupt the metabolic processes of viruses, which means preventing viruses from reproducing themselves inside host cells. Such pharmaceuticals have allowed many individuals infected with HIV to live a closer to normal life, so antivirals are now being applied to other viruses. The appearance of HIV, Ebola, Zika, and the Betacoronaviridae triggered efforts to develop to antiviral drugs that could (a) block the viral receptor, (b) inhibit the proteases needed for viral entry into cells and viral protein maturation, and (c) inhibit viral polymerases (RdRp; Lu). A number of these can now be delivered to their targets using engineered mAbs (Appendix A-4). Table A3.4 is an incomplete list of approved antiviral drugs and their mechanism of action.

Understanding the approaches to developing antiviral drugs involves understanding how viruses enter cells and the features of their reproduction. Most emerging viruses are enveloped and are equipped with a fusion protein system that makes it possible for them to enter cells. This typically consists of a surface subunit (SfS) and a transmembrane subunit (TimS). SfS is responsible for binding to cell receptors and TimS for fusion with cellular membranes. In the case of HIV, it is CD4 on Th2 helper T cells, but the chemokine receptor CXC5 is a co-receptor. Helper T cells are required for the infected individual to make antibodies that can protect against HIV by blocking cell entry; this is called viral neutralization. In the case of HIV, these helper T cells are killed or lose their function (resulting in immunodeficiency), so that typical antiviral vaccines have little chance of success.

One approach is to block the cell-binding site or render deficient the role of the fusion proteins needed for entry. This is the strategy of many antiviral drugs such as Fostemsavir, Albuvirtide, Maraviroc, and Ibalizumab (Table A3.4). Antivirals currently in trial are aiming at the same target for SARS-CoV-2 and other emerging viruses. Viral entry can also require the help of host proteins, like the enzyme furin, to gain entry. Thus, protease inhibitors constitute another approach. Many viruses including SARS-CoV-2, MERS, Ebola, Zika, and HIV contain furin cleavage sites. Hence, blocking this proteolytic event would block entry. Saquinavir (Table A3.4) is one of many antivirals that are crafted to inhibit proteases.

RNA-dependent RNA polymerases (RdRp) have been known for some time. They catalyze RNA synthesis from RNA templates, resulting in virus genome replication. The catalytic domains of RdRps are highly conserved among various viruses, especially those from the same genus. Therefore, drugs that can inhibit the action of RdRps could be considered as quasi-pan-specific virus inhibitors.

Suggested Readings (SR)

Bunker JJ, Erickson SA, Flynn TM, et al. Natural polyreactive IgA antibodies coat the intestinal microbiota. *Science*. 2017;358:320–332.

Elbert NJ, Kiefte-de Jong JC, Voortman T, et al. Allergenic food introduction and risk of childhood atopic disease. *Plos One*. 2017;12: e0187999. doi:10.1371/journal.pone.0187999.

Jarret AR, Jackson R, Duizer C, et al. Enteric nervous system derived IL-18 orchestrates mucosal barrier immunity *Cell*. 2020;180:50–63.

Lu L, Su S, Yang H, Yang S. Antivirals with common targets against highly pathogenic viruses. *Cell*. 2021;184:1604–1620.

Macpherson AJ, Koeller Y, McCoy KD. The bilateral responsiveness between intestinal microbes and IgA. *Trends Immunol*. 2015;36:460–470.

Venereau E, Ceriotti C, Bianchi ME. DAMPs from cell death to new life. *Frontiers Immunol*. 2015;60:422. doi:3389/fimmu.2015.00422.

References

Aarestrup FM. The livestock reservoir for antimicrobial resistance: A personal view on changing patterns of risks, efforts of intervention and the way forward. *Phil Trans R Soc B*. 2014;370:20140085. doi:10/1098/rstb.2014.0085.

Bandyopadhyay AS, Modlin JF, Wenger J, Gast C. Immunogenicity of new primary immunization schedules with inactivated poliovirus vaccine and bivalent oral polio vaccine for the polio endgame: A review. *Clin Infect Dis*. 2018;67(Suppl. 1):S35–S41.

Benoit M, Desnuses B, Mage JL. Macrophage polarization in bacterial infections. *J Immunol*. 2008;181:3933–3739.

Blaser MJ. Missing microbes: How the overuse of antibiotics is fueling modern plagues. 2015. Picador, Henry Hunt and Company, New York

Brenmoehl J, Ohde D, Wirthgren E, Hoeflich A. Cytokines in milk and the role of TGF-β. *Best Pract Res Clin Endocrinol Metab*. 2018;33:47–56.

Brogden NK, Mehalick L, Fischwer CL, Wertz PW, Brogden KA. The emerging role of peptides and lipids as antimicrobial epidermal barriers and modulators of local inflammation. *Skin Pharmacol Physiol*. 2012;25:167–181.

Butler JE, Sinkora M, Wang G, Stepancova K, Li Y, Gai X. Perturbation of thymocyte development underlies the PRRS pandemic: A testable hypothesis. *Front Immunol*. 2019;10:1077. doi:10.3389/fimmu.2019.01077.

Cohen KW, Linderman SL, Moodie Z, et al. Longitudinal analysis shows durable and broad immune memory after SARS-CoV-2 infection with persisting antibody responses and memory B and T cells. *Cell Rep Med*. 2021;2:100354. doi:10.1016/j.xcrm.2021.100354.

Commins SP, Platts-Mills TAE. Anaphylaxis syndromes related to a new mammalian cross-reactive carbohydrate determinant. *J Allergy Clin Immunol*. 2009;124:652–657.

Crosby CM, Kronenberg M. Invariant natural killer T cells: Front-line fighters in the war against pathogenic microbes. *Immunogenetics*. 2016;68:639–648.

Dale BA, Fredricks LD. Antimicrobial peptides in the oral environment: Expression and function in health and disease. *Curr Issues Mol Bio*. 2005;7:119–133.

Damania B, Kenney SC, Raab-Traub N. Epstein-Barr viruses: Biology and clinical disease. *Cell*. 2022;185:3652–3670.

Derakhshani H, Fehr KB, Sepehri S, et al. *Invited review*: Microbiota of the bovine udder: Contributing factors and potential implications for udder health and mastitis susceptibility. *J Dairy Sci*. 2018;101:10605–10625.

Desai P, Janova H, White JP, et al. Enteric helminth coinfection enhances most susceptibility to neurotropic flaviviruses via a tuft cell IL-4 receptor signaling axis. *Cell*. 2021;184:1214–1231.

Feehley T, Stefka AT, Cao S, Nagler CR. Microbial regulation of allergic responses to food. *Semin Immunopath*. 2012;34:1–27. doi:10.1007/s00281-012-0337-5.

Flayer CH, Sokol CL. Nerves of steel: How the gut nervous system promotes a strong barrier. *Cell*. 2020;180:15–22.

Furuga EY, Lowy FD. Antimicrobial-resistant bacteria in the community setting. *Nature Rev*. 2006;4:36–45.

Gupta M, Sicherer SH. Timing of food introduction and atopy. *Preven Clin Dermat*. 2017;35:389–405.

Guthmiller JJ, Wilson PC. It's hard to tech an old B cell new tricks. *Cell*. 2020;180:18–19.

Hau SJ, Allue-Guardia A, Rusconi B, et al. Single nucleotide polymorphism analysis indicates genetic distinction and reduced diversity of swine-associated methicillin-resistant *Staphylococcus aureus* (MRSA) ST5 isolates compared to clinical MRSA ST5 Isolates. *Front Microbio*. 2018;9:2078. doi:10.3389/fmicb.2018.02078.

Hau SJ, Haan JS, Davies PR, Frana T, Nicholson TL. Antimicrobial resistance distribution differs among methicillin-resistant *Staphylococcus aureus* sequence type (ST)5 isolates from health care and agricultural sources. *Front Microbiol*. 2018;9:2102. doi:10.3389/fmicb.2018.02102.

Imokawa GA. A mechanism underlying the ceramide deficiency in atopic dermatitis expression of a deacylase enzyme that cleaves the N-acyl linkage of sphingomyelin and glucosylceramides. *J Dermatol Sci*. 2009;5:1–9.

Kedl RM, Hsieh E, Morrison TE, et al. Evidence for aerosol transfer of SARS-CoV-2-specific humoral immunity [published ahead of print April 28, 2022]. medRxiv. doi:10.1101/2022/04.28.2274443.

Knoop KA, Gustafsson JK, McDonald KG, et al. Microbial antigen encounter during a preweaning interval is critical for tolerance to gut bacteria. *Sci Immunol*. 2017;2:eaao1314. doi:10.1126/sciimmunol.aao1314.

Levy SD, Fitzgerald GB, Macone AB. Spread of antibiotic-resistant plasmids from chicken to chicken and from chicken to man. *Nature*. 1976;260:40–42.

Lewis K. The science of antibiotic discovery. *Cell*. 2020;181:29–43.

Li C, Hatta M, Burke DF, et al. Selection of antigenically advanced variants of seasonal influenza viruses. *Nat Microbiol*. 2016;1(6):16058. doi:10.1038/nnmicrobiol.2016.58.

Lluis A, Depner M, Gaugler B, et al. Increased regulatory T cell numbers are associated with farm milk exposure and lower atopic sensitization and asthma in childhood. *J Allergy Clin Immunol*. 2014;133:551–559.

Loke P, Lim YA. Helminths and the microbiota: Parts of the hygiene hypothesis. *Parasite Immunol*. 2015;37:314–323.

Mali SS, Bautista DM. Basophils as fuel to the flame of eczema itch *Cell*. 2021;184:294–295.

Marrs T, Flohr C. How do microbiota influence the development and natural history of eczema and food allergy? *Pediatrics Inf Dis*. 2016;35:1258–1261.

Mateen FJ, Shinohara RT, Sutter RW. Oral and inactivated poliovirus vaccines in the newborn: A review *Vaccine*. 2016;31:2517–2524.

Mather AE, Reid SWJ, Maskell DJ, et al. Distinguishable epidemics with different host of the multidrug resistant zoonotic pathogen *Salmonella typhimurium* DT104. *Science*. 2013;341:1514–1517.

McCoy KD, Koeller Y. New developments providing mechanistic insight into the impact of the microbiota on allergic disease. *Clin Immunol*. 2015;159:170–178.

Mikhak Z, Agace WW, Luster AD. Lymphocytes trafficking to mucosal tissues. In: Mastecky J, Strober W, Russell MW, Kelsall BL, eds. *Mucosal Immunology*. Cambridge, MA: Academic Press; 2015:805–830.

Moran AP, Prendergast MM, Appelmelk BJ. Molecular mimicry of host structures by bacterial lipopolysaccharides and its contribution to disease. *FEMS Immunol Med Microbiol*. 1996;16:105–115.

Nami-Mancinelli E, Vivier E. Advancing natural killer therapies against cancer. *Cell*. 2022;185:1451–1454.

Nick JA, Dedrick RM, Gray AL, Vladar EK, Smith BE, Freeman KG, Malcolm L C. Host and pathogen response to bacteriophage engineered against Mycobacterium absecessus lung infection. *Cell* 202; 185:1860–1874.

Pabst O, Mowat AM. Oral tolerance to food proteins. *Mucosal Immunol*. 2012;5:232–239.

Panda S, Ding JL. Natural antibodies bridge innate and adaptive immunity. *J Immunol*. 2015;194:13–20.

Penders J, Stobberingh EE, Brabdt PA, Thijs C. The role of the intestinal microbiota in the development of atopic disorders. *Allergy*. 2007;62:1223–1236.

Prescott SL. Role of dietary immunomodulatory factors in the development of immune tolerance. In: Brandtzaeg P, Isolauri E, Prescott SL, eds. *Microbial-host interactions: Tolerance versus allergy. Nestle Nutr Inst Workshop Ser Pediatr Program*. 2014;64:185–200.

Salyers AA, Gupta A, Wang W. Human intestinal bacteria as reservoirs for antibiotic resistance genes. *Trends Microbiol*; 2004;12:412–416. doi:10.1016/j.tim.2004.07.oo4.

Schroeder PC, Illi S, Casaca VI, et al. A switch in regulatory T cells through farm exposure during immune maturation in children. *Allergy*. 2017;72:604–615.

Shepersky L, Marin M, Zhang J, Pham H, Marlow MA. Mumps in vaccinated children and adolescents: 2007–2019. *Pediatrics*. 2021;148(6):e2021051873. doi: 10.1542/peds.2021-051873.

Sinkora M, Sinkorova J, Cimburek Z, Holtmeier W. Two groups of procine TCRγ/δ thymocytes behave and diverge differently. *J Immunol*. 2007;178:711–719.

Sinnis P, Fidock DA. The RTS,5 vaccine—a chance to regain the upper hand against malaria? *Cell*. 2022;185:750–754.

Sokal A, Chappert P, Barba-Spaeth G, et al. Maturation and persistence of the anti-SARS-Cov 2 memory B cell response. *Cell*. 2021;184:1201–1231.

Spoor LE, McAdam PR, Weinert LA, et al. Livestock origin for a human pandemic clone of community-associated methicillin-resistant *Staphylococcus aureus*. *mBio*. 2013;4:1–6.

Sprenger M, Fukuda K. New mechanism, new worries. *Science*. 2016;381:1263–1264.

Stein MM, Hrusch CL, Gozdz J, et al. Innate immunity and asthma risk in Amish and Hutterite farm children. *N Eng J Med*. 2016;375:411–421.

Strachan DP. Hay fever, hygiene and household size. *Brit Med J*. 1989;299:1259–1260.

van den Bogaard AE, Jensen LB, Stobberingh EE. Vancomycin-resistant Enterococci in turkeys and turkey farmers. *N Engl J Med*. 1997;337:1558–1589.

Wang S, Charbonnier, L-M, Rivas MN, et al. MyD88 adapter-dependent microbial sensing by regulatory T cells promotes mucosal tolerance and enforces commensalism. *Immunity*. 2015;43:289–303.

Wikipedia; Antimirobial resistance. http://en.wikipedia.org/wiki/Antimicrobial_resistance

World Health Organization Joint News Release. New report calls for urgent action to avert antimicrobial resistance crisis. April 29, 2019. https://www.who.int/news/item/29-04-2019-new-report-calls-for-urgent-action-to-avert-antimicrobial-resistance-crisis.

Zerhouni E. GAVI, the vaccine alliance. *Cell*. 2019;179:13–17.

Zhang O-Y, Yan ZB, Meng Y-M, et al. Antimicrobial peptides: Mechanism of action, activity and clinical potential. *Mil Med Res*. 2021;8:48. doi:10.1186/s40779-021-00343-2.

Zurek L, Ghosh A. Insects represent a link between food animal farms and the urban environment for antibiotic resistance traits. *Appl Environ Microbiol*. 2014;80:3562–3567.

Chapter Reviewers

Richard Goldsby Thomas Walton Memorial Professor of Biology Emeritus, Amherst College

John C. Cambier Emeritus Head of immunology and microbiology, University of Colorado Medical School and National Jewish Hospital

Mark Stinski Emeritus Professor, Department of Microbiology and Immunology, Carver College of Medicine, The University of Iowa

Figure Credits

Fig. 6.2: Adapted from Selma Gago et al., "Extremely High Mutation Rate of a Hammerhead Viroid," *Science*, vol. 323, no. 5919, p. 1308. Copyright © 2009 by American Association for the Advancement of Science.

Fig. 6.4: Adapted from Gillian Fitzgibbon and Kingston H. G. Mills, "The Microbiota and Immune-Mediated Diseases: Opportunities for Therapeutic Intervention," *European Journal of Immunology*, vol. 50, no. 3, p. 328. Copyright © 2020 by John Wiley & Sons, Inc.

Fig. 6.5b: John E. Butler et al., "Perturbation of Thymocyte Development Underlies the PRRS Pandemic: A Testable Hypothesis," *Frontiers in Immunology*, vol. 10, no. 1077. Copyright © by John E. Butler et al. (CC BY 4.0) at https://www.frontiersin.org/journals/immunology/articles/10.3389/fimmu.2019.01077/full.

Fig. 6.7: Adapted from Thomas J. Kindt, Barbara A. Osborne, and Richard A. Goldsby, *Kuby Immunology*, p. 373. Copyright © 2006 by Macmillan.

Fig. 6.7a: Copyright © 2021 Depositphotos/Pikovit.

Fig. 6.7b: Copyright © 2020 Depositphotos/macrovector.

Fig. 6.7c: Copyright © 2017 Depositphotos/Achiichiii.

Fig. 6.7d: Copyright © by Cvallesv (CC BY-SA 4.0) at https://commons.wikimedia.org/wiki/File:2._Allergic_response.tif.

Fig. 6.7e: Copyright © 2013 Depositphotos/edesignua.

Fig. 6.7f: Copyright © 2018 Depositphotos/fandijki.

The Bumpy Road of Progress

The Certainty of Uncertainty

LEARNING OBJECTIVES

1. Describe typical problems and weaknesses of lay publications of medical science.

2. Discuss the meaning of "falsification" of a hypothesis and actions that should follow.

3. Describe several types of clinical studies and the strength of evidence they provide.

4. Explain the difference between scientific fact and hypothesis or explain why you cannot describe the difference.

5. Discuss examples of medical decisions faced by parents and practitioners.

Evaluating Evidence: What Everyone Should Know

Individuals want to make the best possible health decisions for themselves and their families. A generation ago, that meant consulting one's physician or one of a few widely read household references on health. Today we have a deluge of easily accessible and frequently free information from electronic sources. Unfortunately, only some of this information is valid and helpful; a large fraction is misleading, perhaps reflecting limited understanding of the author, or purposely wrong because of indifference to truth or because the intent is malign. A large portion of more valuable scientific literature is available online but behind a paywall and thus likely to be economically inaccessible to those without access to an academic or industry account.

This chapter offers some general guidance on how to wade through the mud to get to sound footing. To demonstrate how the path to understanding meanders, we will note some examples of literature on the coronavirus pandemic of 2020. As this text is being written, much is still unknown about the treatment and control of this virus. It is likely that some of the studies described will later be confirmed and broadly accepted, but others will be shown to be misleading. Our discussion is not meant to tell readers what to believe but to help them to understand how "facts" in medical science come to be accepted and used to direct the care of patients.

Hype and Uncertainty

News media are not always accurate portrayers of scientific issues, as they have a tendency to hype stories and to avoid issues of uncertainty. We all see news items that begin with some equivalent of "A new study shows. ..." Some of these stories highlight new knowledge that will soon impact healthcare for the better. Unfortunately, many of these stories are attention-grabbing flashes that fade and have no obvious impact over time—that is, they are mere clickbait. Although promotion of impressive-sounding but ultimately incorrect information is especially a problem in mass media, similar problems exist in media aimed at medical professionals that purport to describe recent scientific publications. How can apparently "real science" sound so impressive but turn out to be minimally important or even wrong? The reasons lie within the nature of scientific inquiry and publications but also within the nature of the lay media. We will deal first with the simpler issue, the information available to the media.

Most scientific/medical stories in the traditional and electronic media are not written by the scientists involved. Often they originate as press releases from public relations staff (perhaps with some scientific background) at universities and private companies. The tendency of companies to hype their work is easily understandable. They stand to gain awareness of their brands, increased sales of current or future products, and higher stock value. Less obvious are the reasons for hype originating in the universities; since the university is usually not selling a product based on the science, there must be other reasons for hype. Universities want to maintain their reputations of importance; stated in the simplest of terms, having important scientists doing important work demonstrates their importance. This drive for status is a monetary reality in the academic world. Important institutions are better able to entice donations; win grants from governmental agencies, foundations, and industry; and be part of multicenter trials that provide outside funding. University media relations staff are likely tasked to increase the placement of stories about the institution; thus, more press releases are churned out on progressively smaller incremental additions to scientific knowledge. Stories about science are unlikely to appeal to lay media unless they can be portrayed as important; as a result, press releases are prone to overstate the importance and certainty of the work and, where human diseases are involved, to exaggerate its immediate therapeutic impact either subtly or flagrantly. Media are not likely to publish a story on a pilot study in an obscure field that might possibly, in a decade or two, lead to practical medical applications, or might just as well fade into obscurity as other studies refute it.

Two features of scientific progress are hard for traditional media to convey to the public: (1) It is incremental, and (2) it does *not* generally proceed by definitively proving a hypothesis.

Scientists understand that progress is incremental, that knowledge gradually accumulates to support or refute a theory. James Watson and Francis Crick did not just wake up one day and discover the structure of DNA and its central role in all living things (see Appendix A-1). They built their discovery on the work of many earlier biochemists, geneticists, and crystallographers without whom they would not have succeeded. Stories about incremental progress are not of much appeal to modern media, hence the tendency to inflate the meaning of published studies.

The thoughtful scientist also knows the purpose of research is not to directly "prove" an idea but to show that arguments against the idea, when tested, fail. In the language of science, the ideas being tested are called **hypotheses**. Scientific investigation begins with observations of nature for which someone proposes an explanatory hypothesis. What should follow is testing of the hypothesis against alternative hypotheses (note that the plural is hypotheses). An inaccurate hypothesis can generally be proven false by observation or experiment, but even an accurate hypothesis cannot be directly proven to be true. The scientist must be open to alternative hypotheses until experiments discredit them; the favored hypothesis is held increasingly likely if it cannot be shown to be false, but alternative hypotheses are clearly shown to be false. In the formal language used to describe this issue, the scientist attempts to falsify the hypothesis. Once falsified, the hypothesis must usually be discarded and alternative hypotheses considered. In laboratory science, where control of all known variables may be feasible, it is usually possible to carefully design studies that can falsify a hypothesis. These concepts were first described in this way by the Austrian philosopher Karl Popper 90 years ago (Popper, SR).

Unfortunately, the ability to perform studies that can definitively falsify hypotheses in human medicine is sometimes limited. Many studies are impractical or unethical to perform in humans or are too costly. The absolute necessity to adhere to the ethics of human research is a frequent limitation, since obviously humans cannot be controlled or put at risk in experiments in the same way as one may manipulate cell cultures or mice (HHS, SR). The limitations of research on humans mean that published studies are only as strong as the limitations allow. Many medical decisions must be made with imperfect knowledge, as we discuss later. Over time new knowledge may falsify even a generally accepted hypothesis. This evolution of our scientific understanding often is not understood by the public, causing confusion that can lead to mistrust. The potential for mistrust was demonstrated during the COVID-19 pandemic when the CDC and other authorities adjusted their statements and guidelines in response to newly emerging information.

The Hierarchy of Evidence: Weak Versus Strong

Because science is not static, but changes as our understanding increases, decisions to change our behavior or medical care must be made very carefully. Careful decision-making requires that the available data must be scrutinized for reliability, and the possible outcome of change in medical practice must be assessed not only for potential benefit but for the harm that may result from change. Frequently all risks are not known when a decision is made, lending further importance to careful evaluation. The concept of a hierarchy of strength of evidence can aid in such decisions. For decisions about the use of published literature to guide care of patients, a hierarchy of evidence quality from strongest (1) to weakest (5) typically has steps such as the following:

1. Randomized, prospective trials with comparison to adequate control
2. Non-randomized, uncontrolled observations of groups exposed (or not) to an intervention of interest
3. Case reports or a series of reports
4. Information gained from animal models (Appendix A-2)
5. Background information, opinion of experts, computer models

Table 7.1 provides a simple overview of study design and strength. This concept is often presented as a pyramid of evidence quality. Below we add details on some of these types of publications. Note that the list of evidence levels above does not include whether the work is published in a peer-reviewed journal. As you may have seen during the pandemic, mass media often seem to judge the reliability of research by whether it is published in a peer-reviewed journal. Although the most reputable journals are peer-reviewed, there are certainly journals with much poorer content that also use peer review, but the rigor of review may vary markedly. Readers who wish to critically assess the strength of a study need to review its actual details rather than simply noting where it is published. Those who form an opinion without close review of the primary literature (and possibly the actual underlying data) are only repeating the opinions of others.

TABLE 7.1 Comparisons of Common Types of Publications

Type	Strength	Weakness	Examples
Randomized, placebo controlled, blinded comparisons	Controls bias from multiple sources; most likely design to be reproducible	Not always ethical or feasible	Trials of COVID-19 vaccines. Large numbers given vaccine or placebo in blinded fashion.
Observational studies	Rapid results; may provide signal of possible effect	Large bias may be introduced by the non-random treatment decision; frequently not reproducible	Early observational studies suggesting benefit of hydroxychloroquine in COVID-19
Case reports	Source of new hypotheses	Bias as above; very often not reproducible	
Opinion of experts, Animal models, Computer simulations	May be the only information available	Poor predictive value over time; poorly predictive of risk/benefit ratio	Computer models of epidemic course Internet "experts"

Authors of literature reviews may sometimes be insufficiently rigorous in the application of evidence grades. Insufficiently rigorous reviews of published data can erroneously value the reputation of the author and the perceived quality of the journal (eg, as measured by the journal's impact factor) and incorporate the unknown biases of the reviewer. Such reviews obviously should carry much less weight in the decision-making of health professionals than more rigorous compilations (such as those sponsored by medical associations or such organizations as the Cochrane Library) that clearly state the methods used to grade and weight the available evidence (see Cumpston, SR). The tsunami of online journals developed over the last 2 decades has increased the availability of questionably credible publications.

Some authors describe another level (or two) of strength of evidence, in addition to the list above, based on summation of available evidence when there are a sufficient number of published trials. A first additional level would be formal review of available randomized controlled trials. A second level might be **meta-analysis**, a structured compilation of available data from randomized controlled trials that includes statistical evaluation of the total available data, in distinction to the statistical analysis of the individual data sets reported in the included publications (Haidich, SR; Murad, SR).

The stronger the design of a study, the greater the likelihood that the study results (1) will be reproducible by other investigators, (2) will not be falsified by thoughtful experiments, and (3) will continue to be superior to alternative hypotheses. When positive studies of a hypothesis are replicated by several investigators and none have falsified it, the hypothesis may sometimes be labelled "**scientific fact**," but one should remain aware that future knowledge may alter this assessment. The issue of reproducibility has been brought to the foreground in the last few decades as the volume of publications in scientific and medical fields has exploded. Some workers in this field suggest on theoretical grounds that as much as 80% of published biomedical research may not be reproducible (see Ioannidis, 2005, SR). Indeed, more recent attempts to judge the reproducibility of medical research have shown a distressingly low rate of reproducibility in several fields. Complex studies may contain some reproducible elements while others are not reproducible. Failure of reproducibility should lead to revised hypotheses that can be further tested. Published studies are often exploratory in nature and should be so described by authors and therefore understood by readers as hypothesis-generating rather than definitive. Frank descriptions of the preliminary nature of such work would help prevent lay (and media) overstatement of the importance of the findings.

A summary of possible approaches to improving reproducibility of published work is provided in Ioannidis (2014, SR). Full discussion of these issues is well beyond the scope of this book, but readers should be aware that standards of research behavior are evolving, and expectations of journal editors are variable and changing.

Even within the evidence grades above, there are shades of value and important points of strength and of weakness. The nuances of study design and reliability may lead to disagreement even among experts in a field, but disagreements should be resolved by further investigations as the process of science proceeds (usually) in a self-correcting manner. Expert groups may summarize the available evidence as part of construction of guidelines for care. These groups need to carefully consider the nuances of study strength in this process. Interested readers can find a detailed discussion in Guyatt (SR).

The following sections illustrate common types of studies the reader may see in the literature.

Randomized Controlled Trials (RCTs)

The RCT is the gold standard to investigate the effect of an agent on people, but the details of design and performance influence its reproducibility. An obviously important detail is the nature of the control. If the study is to evaluate a treatment, the necessary control should show the outcomes in the absence of the treatment, with other factors held constant. A comparison group receiving a placebo is the preferred control group when ethical, but the investigators and the study subjects must be rigorously blinded to the individual assignments to drug or placebo. Blinding of assignment to intervention or control is a necessary feature of the higher-quality RCTs (Schulz, "Blinding in Randomized Trials"). A high-quality study precisely specifies the details of blinding in the study protocol. The blinding mechanism must be such that inquisitive study staff and subjects cannot defeat the blind to determine the assignment of any prospective or enrolled subject (Schulz, "Allocation Concealment in Randomized Trials"). There is good evidence that inadequate techniques of blinding are associated with an increase in erroneously positive results (Schulz, "Blinding in Randomized Trials"). The blinding of assignment must be maintained until all subjects have completed the study period and all assessments of subjects are complete. Similarly, the method to randomly assign subjects to the study groups must be clearly specified in the protocol and adhered to at study sites. Failure of randomization would introduce potential bias into the study.

The details of data analysis are also important. The outcomes studied must be specified in advance in the protocol, as should the analytic plan and statistical tests to be applied; otherwise, the study reproducibility may be weakened by application of multiple after-the-fact (*post hoc*) analyses, flippantly referred to as *data dredging*. In human trials, large quantities of information other than the primary outcome are often collected, but only the single, preplanned primary outcome has high probability of reproducibility. The likelihood of a positive result due to chance increases as more secondary outcomes are analyzed. This issue can be partially handled by statistical methods to correct for multiple comparisons. Despite good design, a single high-quality randomized controlled trial might fail to be reproducible. Several trials of similar design with similar subjects that also have positive outcomes are much more convincing. As a result, the usual criterion the US Food and Drug Administration (FDA) accepts to show efficacy and safety of a new drug includes positive outcome in at least 2 trials of adequate design, performance, and analysis. The trials must have generally had the same primary outcome. The FDA rarely allows decisions for drug approval based on outcomes other than the prespecified primary outcome measurement (FDA, SR).

Observational Studies

Uncontrolled observations are more likely than RCTs to fail reproducibility for several reasons. Such trials follow (observe) patients who have been exposed to some intervention decided upon by (usually) their own clinicians for reasons not controlled by the investigator; that is, the assignment to treatment or no treatment is neither controlled nor random. Someone had reasons for the assignment, and those reasons for assignment bias the outcome of the study. The treated subjects are often compared to a group that has not been treated. Observational trials of subjects exposed to some item (drug, food, pollutant, etc.) are more likely to report a true (reproducible) "effect" if the comparison group is very similar to the exposed group, but bias introduced by the non-random decisions that led to exposure cannot be eliminated. Thus, observational studies are best thought of as suggestive rather than definitive, and may be the basis for a randomized controlled trial of the intervention (for a wider discussion, see Brown). The most appropriate description of positive outcomes in observational studies is that the exposure is associated with an outcome, rather than that it causes the outcome, thus, the quote marks the author uses above for the "effect" in this situation. Even if the association is replicated in other observational trials, the possibility of bias remains, and causation cannot be inferred. Recent history should serve to illustrate this point, as a succession of agents were suggested for use against COVID-19 based on observational data, but most failed to show efficacy in randomized controlled trials.

It is quite difficult to overcome the natural human tendency to assign causation to temporal associations. As infants we learn to see cause and effect in terms of events that always follow some other event, such as the author's granddaughter learning by 10 months of age that the TV comes on when the parent points the remote control in that direction. The cause-effect relation is far less certain in the complicated realms of human behavior and health. Even the ancient Greeks and Romans knew this and described the logical fallacy "post hoc ergo propter hoc" (after this, therefore because of this). Aristotle apparently also noted that politicians were especially prone to this logical fallacy, an observation that is still true 2,300 years later. Readers of scientific literature must be aware that confusion of association and causation may slip into descriptions of study results even in excellent journals, as indeed has likely happened in the text of this book.

Case Reports and Case Series

These types of reports are similar to observational studies but with as few as one individual described, usually as a *post hoc* review of a medical episode. Sometimes the series of cases may be contrasted to the presumably known natural history of the medical problem, or to similar patients who did not have an intervention of interest. Clearly this level of evidence is weaker, and it is usually described as medical anecdote. At most, as for larger observational studies, such publications are valued mainly for generation of hypotheses.

Lesser Evidence Levels

Information of lesser credibility for decision-making in human medicine include background scientific knowledge in an area, laboratory investigations of cellular systems or animal models, computer modeling of systems, and the opinions of experts. The first years of the SARS-CoV-2 epidemic provide many examples of such information. A number of medications were suggested for use on the basis of knowledge of the cellular mechanisms of coronavirus infection or on the basis of effects of medications on viral infections (not necessarily coronaviruses) in cell culture (Chapter 6 and Appendix A-1). Most of these suggested therapies, when studied in adequate human trials, failed to have a measurable impact on any important outcome of COVID-19 infections (Appendix A-4). This train of events should not be surprising, given that even with extensive laboratory and animal study of new pharmaceuticals, a minority of such compounds are eventually shown to be effective. The vigor with which proposed medications were touted during the pandemic also demonstrates the sometimes nearly irrational attraction of investigators to their favored hypotheses. These public and contentious arguments demonstrate that as a society we do not know how to evaluate claims and counter evidence effectively. We also learn from these events the power of the fear of a disease to fuel arguments when definitive data are lacking.

The failings of computer modeling usually reflect incomplete understanding of the cellular, organ level, or organism level system being modeled. There are certainly systems of chemical or physical phenomena that can be precisely described with simple to complex computer simulations, but biological systems are usually not understood well enough to reliably predict outcomes of a drug exposure.

The opinions of experts are usually included in the list of low-level evidence. In this setting, the opinions referred to are based on synthesis of available knowledge short of adequate controlled clinical trials. For example, among proposed medications for coronavirus, we have recently seen strongly stated expert opinions both supporting and denying the utility of many potential medications. Invariably, where there is inadequate data to answer a question, argument, sometimes fierce argument, follows. In addition, absence of dispositive data also leads to changing opinions with the passage of time and availability of more data, in accordance with an aphorism applied to almost any specialty, "Ask five experts, you'll get nine opinions."

Vaccine Trials: Examples of Strong Studies

The generation of data to support the safety and efficacy of new vaccines illustrates the care that can be applied to medical studies when investigators and governmental or corporate sponsors are held to high standards. Such studies are likely to be very costly and take several years to complete. An understanding of the work that supports vaccine approval may help guide individual decision-making in regard to the acceptance of vaccines. What follows is a summary of the FDA's approach, but regulatory agencies around the world follow very similar schemes.

Chapter 6 describes the background knowledge of immunology that supports the use of immunization for protection from infectious disease. In this chapter we focus on how the scientific method is applied by clinical scientists and regulators to produce safe and effective vaccines. Globally, regulatory agencies such as the FDA evaluate both drugs and vaccines in a stepwise fashion, beginning with preliminary work and proceeding through a graduated series of human investigations. Prior to any human studies of a vaccine, the concept of the vaccine is developed in the laboratory, and the immunizing agent is shown to induce an immune response in animals. This phase of work is termed "pre-clinical." Pre-clinical work also includes demonstration that the materials to be used are not toxic in animals, that the immunizing agent can be reliably manufactured so that each dose will include the intended amount of the desired immunogen, and that multiple lots of the immunogen can be produced that are identical in structure and effect. The FDA reviews the pre-clinical data prior to allowing trials in humans to begin.

Vaccine trials in humans then proceed in three phases, as summarized in Table 7.2. A phase 1 trial typically exposes less than 100 healthy subjects to the vaccine, with an emphasis on showing safety and tolerability (ie, that adverse reactions are not unacceptably severe). A typical study would expose small cohorts of subjects to a low dose, and if no evidence of severe reactions compared to a placebo is seen, subsequent cohorts receive progressively larger doses. Measures of vaccine immunogenicity such as antibody levels are followed to help estimate the dose that might be effective in preventing disease.

TABLE 7.2   Study Phases of Drug and Vaccine Development

	Type of Study	Number of Subjects	Principal Outcomes Measured	Control Arm if Present
Phase 1	Randomized controlled trial	~100	Tolerability of vaccine or drug Safety Evidence for vaccine immunogenicity	Placebo
Phase 2	Randomized controlled trial	Several hundred	Safety Dose-ranging for determination of dose for Phase 3	Placebo if no licensed vaccine; otherwise, active control of licensed vaccine
Phase 3	Randomized controlled trial	Thousands	Efficacy Safety	Placebo if no licensed vaccine; otherwise, active control of licensed vaccine
Phase 4 or post-marketing surveillance	Varies, usually observation of treated patients	Varies, often very large population monitored for events	Usually safety	No control; usually observation of subjects treated in clinical care

Phase 2 enlarges safety testing to several hundred subjects of diverse age, health status, and ethnicity. A range of doses thought to be effective may be compared, with the aim of identifying a dose that is immunogenic but does not have excessive adverse effects. Phase 2 trials are conducted as RCTs with a control that may be an existing vaccine, if one exists, or a placebo. Immune markers of response are measured to further understand the dose that may be needed for disease prevention. Vaccines with safety issues occurring more often than once per several hundred subjects would likely be identified at this stage.

Phase 3 includes definitive trials with thousands of subjects and can lead directly to regulatory approval of the vaccine. For diseases that have long been studied and for which convincing data shows that immune markers (such as antibody) predict the protective value of the vaccine, there is no need to show directly that vaccine recipients are less likely to contract the disease than placebo recipients. In this situation, where a current vaccine is protective, use of a placebo control design would be unethical. However, it is necessary to show that the immune response to the new vaccine is not inferior to the existing vaccine used as the control. In contrast, for emerging diseases where there is no existing vaccine, there will be a need to compare to placebo to adequately understand vaccine efficacy. Examples of the placebo-controlled design in the last few decades include vaccine trials for Ebola virus, SARS, and of course the agent of COVID-19. Enough subjects must be enrolled to allow detection of a difference in infection rates between the vaccine and placebo groups; the less common the infection, the larger the trial will have to be. If the disease attack rate is very low in the general population, the studies may need to be performed in at-risk communities, such as medical workers in rural West Africa in Ebola vaccine trials. The attack rate for COVID-19 was not high in the random population, thus studies to show efficacy of the first few vaccines typically required about 30,000 subjects each in the vaccine and placebo arms. COVID is discussed in Appendix A-4.

Safety of vaccines is a critical observation in all phases of the clinical development pathway. By the time of approval, the vaccine will have been given to multiple thousands of individuals, so that serious vaccine-induced events occurring more than perhaps once in 10,000 vaccinees would likely have been seen. Depending on the danger of the targeted infection, such a safety signal could prevent approval of the vaccine unless the risk of disease is judged to outweigh the risk of the vaccine. Most regulatory agencies mandate collection of ongoing data on vaccine safety after the formal licensure, referred to as post-marketing safety surveillance. In addition, sometimes there are residual safety questions for which an agency will mandate a formal trial of some sort after licensing a vaccine, a so-called Phase 4 study. Similar caveats sometimes are attached to licensure of other medications. In Box 7.1, we show the impact of post-marketing data on changes in vaccine recommendations for oral polio vaccine and the original rotavirus vaccine. Ongoing data collection will be needed for the ultimate understanding of some of the unknowns about the COVID-19 vaccines, such as whether there are long-term and unexpected complications of mRNA or adenoviral vector vaccines. For the immediate future it seems we will not be forced to make decisions such as those made in the 18th century to accept a 1%

death rate of variation for smallpox as opposed to the 30% death rate for naturally acquired smallpox. The path to vaccine approval in the United States is further explained in USDA (SR).

BOX 7.1 Examples: Information Drives Vaccine Changes

In the 1960s, live, attenuated poliovirus vaccine (introduced by Sabin) replaced the killed Salk vaccine in the United States. The Sabin vaccine was well accepted since no injection was needed, and because it briefly replicated in the GI tract, it produced a strong immune response. Additionally, some vaccine virus might be shed in stool and serve to immunize other children or caregivers. Cases of paralytic polio due to wildtype virus fell to a handful per year in the United States. When the wildtype paralytic cases fell low enough, it became apparent that the attenuated vaccine virus caused 2–3 cases of paralytic polio per million immunized children, as discussed in Chapter 6. With this recognition, expert advice shifted back to the injected, inactivated (killed) vaccines for use in the United States, where wildtype virus is extremely rarely detected.

An example of vaccine improvement in response to vaccine tolerability involved the DTP vaccine. Broad usage of this vaccine made diphtheria, tetanus, and pertussis (whooping cough) such rare diseases that in 40 years of pediatric experience the author (LW) has never seen diphtheria or tetanus. However, recurring outbreaks (and deaths) from pertussis in unimmunized groups have shown the need for continued vaccine use. The original DTP vaccine contained killed, whole pertussis bacteria and was impressively protective; but the vaccine frequently caused swelling at the injection site in the thigh, fever, discomfort, and crying. In addition, in rare cases infants were described as developing a syndrome of declining cognitive function in the first year of life, leading to fears this decline was due to the vaccine. The neurologic syndrome is seen across infancy, without a peak of incidence near the ages of vaccine administration, and occurs with similar frequency in unimmunized children. Subsequent research revealed that a specific genetic defect in an ion channel in neuronal membranes is responsible for many such cases. Improved vaccines were developed that used only critical antigens from the pertussis organism (acellular vaccine); this vaccine is protective but with much lower rates of discomfort and fever.

Rotavirus is the main cause of infectious diarrhea in infancy and the cause of many illnesses, hospitalizations, and deaths (especially in underserved areas). A live, attenuated rotavirus vaccine was shown to be effective in large trials and licensed in 1998. Within months of its US market entry, reports appeared of infants developing intestinal obstruction (called intussusception) soon after receiving the vaccine. About 1 million doses were administered in the first 10 months after the vaccine was approved. The data on intussusception from this large number of infants was sufficiently suggestive to discontinue use of the vaccine. Compared to unvaccinated infants, the CDC estimated that there were 1–2 excess cases of intussusception per 10,000 immunized infants. A second generation of rotavirus vaccines was developed and tested even more extensively prior to approval. The second-generation vaccines have been in use since 2006 without similar adverse events.

As stated earlier, the development of a new vaccine usually takes years. The path to regulatory acceptance can be shortened, however, as demonstrated by the rapid approval in the United States, United Kingdom, and European Union of vaccines for the SARS-CoV-2 virus (Appendix A-4). A change to the usual pace of assessment at regulators is possible, as regulatory agencies generally require stepwise consideration of pre-clinical data and Phase 1 and then Phase 2 results prior to Phase 3 trials. Manufacturers are usually anxious to know that the preceding phase has been successful before incurring considerable cost in starting up the next phase. In the US Warp Speed program, the time frame was safely compressed by several means. The pre-clinical data had already mostly accumulated over the prior 10–15 years as scientists investigated novel vaccine modes for agents such as Ebola virus, Zika virus, and the coronaviruses responsible for SARS and MERS (Middle East Respiratory Syndrome). Immune targets on the coronavirus family were known, and the technology of mRNA vaccines was already worked out at laboratory and manufacturing scale. A major time savings was made by allowing real-time data analysis of the safety and immune response in the Phase 1 and 2 trials, so that the total data for each stage could be available and rapidly assessed as soon as the last subjects exited the trials. This rolling assessment allowed movement from Phase 1 to 2 and from there to Phase 3 with minimal time lag. Because of governmental cost sharing, the industrial sponsors also compressed the timeline by doing the necessary work to secure investigational sites and required ethical approvals in advance of regulatory approval to start the trials. Industry sponsors also began to manufacture sufficient stocks for the large Phase 3 trials before it was known that the stage could indeed begin. Generally, all these steps are done sequentially, with minimal work on later phases before it is clear the earlier phase has not presented an adverse safety signal.

US drug and vaccine law allows an exception to the requirement for proof of efficacy in humans in circumstances where the trials of efficacy in humans would not be ethical or feasible. It is expected that the likeliest need for this exemption would be for response or preparation for radiological exposures, toxins, or biological agents used in terrorist acts or warfare. Agents approved in this path must have safety in humans demonstrated, but the agency is allowed by the law to approve the drug or vaccine if it judges that well-controlled animal studies in relevant animal models show reasonable likelihood that the agent will produce benefit in humans. Thankfully this exemption has not been needed for production of vaccines, but several therapeutic drugs for possible bioweapons (smallpox and anthrax) have been approved by this pathway, as have several drug indications for poisons and radiation exposure.

Making Health Decisions With Imperfect Knowledge

We mentioned in Chapter 1 that making "go/no-go" decisions regarding medical treatments or choices is important but can be complicated. The next few sections will discuss areas where parents or healthcare providers use background information on medical issues and the strength of that evidence to make decisions on behalf of young children.

Infant Formula Choices

Chapter 4 summarizes the basic composition and intended uses of common types of infant formula; however, a glance at the grocery shelf may be puzzling because of the multiple formulas within each brand. Most manufacturers feature a main brand line and usually several slightly different versions promoted for specific indications. The marketing and labeling of formulas is not as tightly controlled in the United States as it is for drugs, but the field is not a complete free-for-all. FDA regulations are based on US law and specify minimum composition of formulas, the testing necessary prior to sale, and the constraints on marketing statements that can be made. In many countries, regulatory control of formulas is more extensive than in the United States and may forbid advertising to families or more strictly limit labeling and marketing statements.

Prior to sale of infant formulas in the United States, manufacturers must present evidence to the FDA that the formula supports growth of normal infants. The evidence is usually a study of growth of infants fed the new formula compared to an existing formula in a randomized, blinded, controlled trial. Sometimes a reference group of breastfed infants is included. The only statistically valid comparison will be between the two formula groups, as these are the only randomly assigned infants. The ethics of such trials require that only mothers who have already decided not to breastfeed can be approached to join the formula arms of the trial. It is held unethical to assign infants to a choice of formula versus breast, because breast-feeding is medically preferable to formula feeding. Usually feeding in the trial lasts about 4 months, with close to 200 infants (roughly an equal number of boys and girls) completing the trial to compose a statistically valid sample size. The data must show that, with 95% certainty, the studied formula fosters growth as well as the comparator. In the setting of these small trials, statistically significant growth differences between the formula-fed group and a breastfed comparison group are not typically seen. The companies must notify the FDA of intent to sell a new formula, and the FDA can respond within 90 days to block marketing if they have objections to the adequacy of the supporting growth trial, the content of the formula, the accuracy of the label, the packaging, or the production plan. Similar requirements to show a formula is suitable for infant nutrition exist in essentially every country, and formulas often require regulatory approval before the company can move toward marketing.

Manufacturers may not promote their formulas to treat any specific disease; only licensed drugs can legally be promoted as treatment for specific diseases. If a formula were promoted to treat a disease state, it would become subject to the same requirement to show safety and efficacy as for drugs. A formula may be marketed for the nutritional management of a medical condition, but not as a treatment. Some formulas are marketed for less specific complaints (not diseases), such as fussiness, colic, and spitting. This distinction between drug treatment and nutritional management may seem obscure, but it is the basis of the relation of FDA and similar global agencies to the formula manufacturers.

Manufacturers may attempt to distinguish their brands from competitors by discovering, patenting, and adding ingredients that may have special benefits. Globally, claims of benefits for cognitive development and for immune strength are most common. The evidence for these claims is usually much less compelling than is required for drug licensing. Several forces limit the strength of evidence for such claims. The large, well-controlled trials conducted for new drugs are not economically feasible given the market pricing of formula and resulting profit for manufacturers. New drugs may see global sales of tens of billions of dollars over a decade, justifying the expense of hundreds of millions for clinical trials. Infant formula does not generate profit of that scale, and the patent protection around ingredients is much weaker than for new drugs, limiting the return value of such large-scale and expensive trials. The discussion of newer formula ingredients in Chapter 4 demonstrates the lack of uniform acceptance of many of these ingredients.

Because of the usual weakness of trials of formula, a recommendation for one formula as opposed to another would have to be made on weak evidence. Most global pediatric organizations do not make recommendations for specific formulas for healthy infants because of the lack of an adequate basis for preference and because of their clear preference for breast-feeding. Parents of normal newborns who choose to feed their infants formula may be confident that formulas legally sold in their country provide adequate nutrition, but they should be aware of evidence for gaps in many areas compared to breast-feeding. They should also know that claims of extra benefits from specific formulas may not have powerful supporting evidence.

Formulas for special medical conditions require more consideration. Several regulatory mechanisms around the world are used to manage these specialized formulas. In the United States, such formulas are regulated as "exempt infant formulas" as defined in the Food and Drug Acts. These exempt formulas (previously discussed in Chapter 4) include special products for infants with inherited metabolic diseases, for premature infants, and for digestive and allergic issues (such as food or milk allergy). The FDA has the authority to block any labeling or marketing messages that it judges to be false or misleading; therefore, these formulas usually have strong evidence (controlled trials) to verify they are useful for the stated medical conditions. Similar regulations around the world tightly control the content and labeling of formula for infants with special medical needs. In a number of countries, these products are referred to as food for special medical purposes.

In the United States, a formula recall in 2022 generated much coverage in the media due to a shortage of formula reaching retail outlets. Careful reading of the media reports on the recall is necessary, as the problems of sensationalism and careless description of data are present here as in the issues discussed earlier in this chapter. Box 7.2 provides further insight into the issues involved.

From the parents' perspective, the choice of formula is best made in consultation with the infant's medical care provider. Options that may appear attractive on the Internet or in advertisements may be seriously lacking for a particular infant. The knowledge of the medical practitioner can help parents avoid poor choices, especially for infants with an underlying health condition. The medical practitioner is obligated to either understand the particular needs of an infant illness or to seek referral or consultation with a knowledgeable source.

BOX 7.2 2022 Formula Recall

Reporting on infant formula shortages in 2022 provides an example of the imprecision seen in the media that leads to misunderstanding of events. Very careful reading of media reports is necessary to disentangle what is really known from what may be inaccurately described.

A common phrasing in reports on the formula shortage was that formulas from one manufacturer were "linked" to the rare infection *Cronobacter sakazakii*. For example, an NBC News report stated: "Four cases of *Cronobacter sakazakii* infection in infants have been linked to powdered formula from an Abbott Laboratories facility in Sturgis, Michigan."* Readers should understand from this chapter that "linked" is synonymous with "associated with" rather than indicating a proven causative relationship. Although the text following the headline above pointed out that *C. sakazakii* bacteria are widely distributed in our environment, there was no clear statement that a causative relationship to the formula factory and the illness had not been proven.

For illnesses that can have food-related sources as well as other sources, proving that a particular illness was indeed caused by the food is often difficult. In the formula example, genotyping of bacteria from infected infants and of bacteria found in their households or in the formula factory may strongly suggest causation. For example, in one of the cases, a water bottle in the home that had been used for formula water was found to have the *C. sakazakii* strain that infected the infant. However, for the two infants with *C. sakazakii* strains available for testing, neither had a strain detected by environmental testing in the factory.

It is even more difficult to prove that the formula itself was not the source of infection. Such a proof requires one to prove that no formula powder produced in the factory contained the organism. Unfortunately, such proof might require that every gram of formula powder be submitted for testing, leaving none to be shipped and sold! 100% destructive testing is not possible; instead, testing regimens are designed based on understanding the minimum number of organisms that would need to be present in a feeding to cause disease. Statistical calculation can lead to a testing regimen very likely to detect if this level is present in the powder. This logic is similar to that applied to testing of municipal water supplies for coliform bacteria to ensure safety.

The manufacturer and the regulatory agency must balance the testing of formula prior to sale, the maintenance and testing of the facility to decrease the chance of passage of microbes to the formula, and the cost and availability burden that the testing program implies for the product.

* www.nbcnews.com/health/health-news/baby-formula-recall-spotlights-rare-dangerous-cronobacter-sakazakii-rcna18139. Accessed 5/27/2022.

Vaccine Decisions

The history of vaccine development, the description of the various types of vaccines, and the program for childhood vaccination were described in Chapter 6. Newer modern vaccine approaches, including for SARS-CoV-2, are described in Appendices A-1 and A-4.

Much ink and many electrons have been spilled in the last 30 years over the issue of vaccine safety, especially the proposed role of vaccines in neurologic disorders of childhood, such as autism spectrum disorder (ASD). Most such claims have never been supported by any evidence other than anecdotes. Very rare, but medically real, adverse events are associated with some vaccines (Chapter 6). Often these events are so rare that they can only be detected after several million, or even tens of millions, of children have been vaccinated. Post-marketing surveillance of adverse events is sometimes referred to as a Phase 4 trial. When these issues prove true, and the risk of the vaccine can be reasonably argued to exceed benefit, changes have been made in medical recommendations for the vaccine or for vaccination in general. Examples of such changes in vaccine licensure and recommendations based on evolving understanding of vaccine risks are described in Box 7.1.

Healthcare professionals and parents must decide issues of vaccination for children. Careful regulatory authorities, such as the FDA in the United States and the European Medicines Agency of the European Union, require careful vaccine development pathways (as described above) that produce much data about vaccine effectiveness and safety. Decision-makers (parents and healthcare professionals) should have confidence that questions of safety and efficacy have been adequately answered prior to licensure of standard vaccines. The hesitancy by many to receive vaccines for COVID-19 is less easily overcome because of the rapid development timeline of the vaccine and the short (as of this writing, less than 2 years) history of the vaccines. Hesitancy toward COVID-19 vaccination of children is fueled by the same issues and by the understanding that the risk of the disease in healthy children is orders of magnitude less than for the elderly or the chronically ill. This issue is still evolving at the time of this writing in 2023, with no global consensus over the use of these vaccines in children. For instance, the CDC and the American Academy of Pediatrics have both recommended vaccination for all children 5 years and above (the current licensed age range), but UK agencies have recommended routine use only for children who are in a clinical risk group or are in a household where they may contact an immunosuppressed person. The UK body is currently accumulating more data to guide decisions for more general childhood usage. With the same body of evidence to consider, the CDC has recommended routine administration of COVID-19 vaccines for infants beginning at 6 months of age.

Antibiotic Usage

In Chapter 6, we described the history of antibiotics, their major chemical classes, and their general application. We discussed the issue of antibiotic resistance and multidrug-resistant (MDR) bacteria. In Appendix A-1, the mechanisms that are involved are described in greater detail. In Chapter 8, we review the history of antibiotic use, their overuse, and their use in animal feed. Studies indicate that MDR bacteria are now an important cause of death worldwide, raising the need to understand the causes of the problem and explain their proper use (CDC).

Antibiotic usage is often a shared decision between parents and healthcare providers, especially in regard to their use in non-hospitalized children, where a discussion of risks versus benefit may be in order. In children critically ill with serious infections, there is less likely a need to balance risks and benefits, as the balance is strongly driven by the risk of serious infection. As noted earlier in the book, the risks of antibiotic use include the usual possibilities of any drug, such as drug allergy, side effects, or genetically determined intolerance. In addition, consideration may be given to risks that might affect the treated child and society at large. For antibiotics, this mainly revolves around the danger of promoting bacterial antibiotic resistance, as discussed in Chapter 6. Decades ago it was observed, for instance, that in countries with very loose control of penicillin-class antibiotics, pneumococcal isolates from children were very likely resistant to penicillin, more so than in countries that maintained prescription-only usage of antibiotics. Several practices are involved in the generation of resistant strains: use of antibiotics in situations where their use is futile (eg, viral infection), use of doses too low to irradicate the infection, and treatment courses too short to be effective.

Decision-making in the outpatient setting may be as simple as deciding not to prescribe antibiotics for the healthy child who has a simple upper respiratory tract infection (a cold) but can be complicated in the case of antibiotic use for bacterial otitis media (middle ear infection). The evolving treatment standards for otitis media in children demonstrate how the medical community is adapting to reduce the generation of antibiotic-resistant organisms. In the pre-antibiotic era, otitis media was a common complication of early childhood viral upper respiratory infections, manifesting as ear pain, fever, and sometimes bacterial invasion beyond the middle ear space and into the bony portion of the skull behind the ear (mastoiditis). Mastoiditis required surgical intervention to create a drainage path for what was essentially an abscess confined to the bony mastoid. When antibiotics effective against the common bacterial causes of otitis media became available, they were rapidly adopted by pediatricians to treat the middle ear infection, to speed the resolution of the fever and pain, and to prevent complications such as mastoiditis. Over time, the use of antibiotics became nearly routine in the setting of fever with upper respiratory infection, even if the appearance of the ear drum on exam was unimpressive, or even entirely normal. Some investigators, however, began to call attention to the high rate of spontaneous resolution of otitis media without antibiotic treatment. Eventually guidelines were published that emphasized restriction of antibiotics to cases with clearly diagnostic findings on examination of the ear drum. Observation rather than immediate antibiotic treatment was encouraged in milder cases, especially when unilateral. An example of the analyses leading to this reduction of antibiotic use is in Venekamp (SR).

Nutritional Decision-Making

Compared to the issues discussed above, decisions on nutrition for the otherwise well child are frequently complicated by the paucity of high-quality research. Inferences drawn from animal models and from epidemiologic studies (with inevitable confounding) must be used in the formulation of guidelines by expert panels. Consequently, significant changes in recommendations on a near decadal frequency can lead to public hesitancy to accept the changing recommendations. On the other hand, recommendations for the nutrition of children with medical problems are usually based on much better prospective, and often well-controlled studies. Thus, compared to 40 years ago, the nutritional management of the preterm infant is much improved, and the outcomes of these infants have improved as all aspects of their care have moved forward. In general, parents and healthcare professionals rely on the judgment of expert bodies for guidance. In the case of breast versus bottle in the developed world, a mother's hesitancy to breastfeed is not a sure sentence to ill health for the infant. Healthcare professionals must not lose their place as useful collaborators to the mother by being adversely judgmental of the bottle feeder, nor should they cede their advisory role to sometimes popular but poorly reasoned online advice. As with all of medicine, acceptance of patients and parents "where they are" is the starting point to a therapeutic relationship. Preemptory demands for specific behaviors are not useful. A relationship based on accurate portrayal of risks and benefits of feeding options, without exaggeration of risks or of benefits, is the path to promote gradual movement away from behavior the health professional finds to be suboptimal.

Summary

Received wisdom is like religion or the "received pronunciation" formerly prominent with BBC news readers (for a smile, see the topic "Received Pronunciation" on Wikipedia). Received knowledge systems contain fixed information, have fixed rules that must be followed, and change little over time. Actual science is definitely not in the category of received wisdom; on the contrary, scientific knowledge evolves over time and the rules are a subject of constant, sometimes very heated, debate. Some "scientific facts" can last centuries, others last a few decades or less. The scientist, healthcare practitioner, or student must be aware that yesterday's strongly supported truth may tumble at any time, requiring an adjustment to how we understand the world and how we choose the best care for patients. Analysis of less-than-perfect information is necessary to manage patients, but the concepts of a hierarchy of study strength and of reproducibility can help us avoid prematurely jumping into decisions that will likely, sooner or later, be regretted.

Suggested Readings (SR)

Cumpston M, Flemyng E, Thomas J, Higgins JPT, Deeds JJ, Clarke MJ. Chapter I: Introduction. I.1. About Cochrane. In: Higgins JPT, Thomas J, Chandler J, Cumpston M, Li T, Page MJ, Welch VA, eds. *Cochrane handbook for systematic reviews of interventions*. Version 6.4 (updated August 2023). https://training.cochrane.org/handbook/current/chapter-i#section-i-1.

Guyatt GH, Oxman AD, Kunz R, Vist E, Falk-Ytter Y, Schunemann HJ (GRADE Working Group). What is "quality of evidence" and why is it important to clinicians? *BMJ*. 2008;336:995–998. doi:10.1136/bmj.39490.551019.BE.

Haidich AB. Meta-analysis in medical research. *Hippokratia*. 2010;14(Suppl. 1):29–37.

Ioannidis JPA. How to make more published research true. *PLoS Med.* 2014;11(10): e1001747. doi:10.1371/journal.pmed.1001747.

Ioannidis JPA. Why most published research findings are false. *PLoS Med.* 2005;2(8) e124. doi:10.1371/journal.pmed.0020124.

Murad MA, Asi N, Alsawas M, Alahdab F. New evidence pyramid. *BMJ Evid Based Med.* 2016;21:125–127. doi:10.1136/ebmed-2016-110401.

Popper K. A survey of some fundamental problems. In: *The Logic of Scientific Discovery.* New York, NY: Routledge; 1992:3–26.

US Department of Health and Human Services (HHS). The Belmont Report. April 18, 1979. www.hhs.gov/ohrp/regulations-and-policy/belmont-report/read-the-belmont-report/index.html.

US Food and Drug Administration (USDA). Vaccine development 101. https://www.fda.gov/vaccines-blood-biologics/development-approval-process-cber/vaccine-development-101.

Venekamp RP, Sanders SL, Glasziou PP, Del Mar CB, Rovers MM. Acute otitis media in children. *Cochrane Database Syst Rev.* 2015;(6):CD000219. doi:10.1002/14651858.CD000219.pub4.

References

Brown AW, Ioannidis JPA. Unscientific beliefs about scientific topics in nutrition. *Adv Nutr.* 2014;5:563–65.

Centers for Disease Control and Prevention (CDC). Epidemiology of MDROs: Management of multidrug-resistant organisms in healthcare settings. 2006. https://www.cdc.gov/infection-control/hcp/mdro-management/epidemiology.html.

Schulz KF, Grimes DA. Allocation concealment in randomized trials: defending against deciphering. *Lancet.* 2002;359:614–8.

Schulz KF, Grimes DA. Blinding in randomized trials: Hiding who got what. *Lancet.* 2002;359:696–700.

Mythology, Misconceptions, and Controversies in Healthcare

LEARNING OBJECTIVES

1. Discuss the proper/improper use of antibiotics and the appearance of multidrug-resistant bacteria.

2. Discuss the proper use of pre- and probiotics during the Critical Window and beyond.

3. Provide arguments in support of vaccine therapy and discuss the dangers posed by the anti-vaccination movement.

4. Distinguish between hypotheses, programmed gullibility, and medical facts.

5. Understand both the value and danger to childhood health posed by folklore and the experience of elders.

6. Describe what is meant by epigenetic factors and how are they related to wellness in children and adults.

7. Discuss concerns about supplementation of animal foods and food labeling.

Best and Future Medical Practices in the Critical Window

The health of next and future generations depends on events in the **Critical Window** (Figure 1.1).

Childrearing practices and care for pregnant women in the **Critical Window** rely on established medical practices and emerging science-based medical research, as well as cultural traditions and religious beliefs. Those who choose a career in healthcare can expect that acceptance of medical recommendations may meet with some resistance due to myths and misconceptions, many of which are spread through social media. Medical practices are dynamic, and recommendations continually change, especially when many phenomena are not fully understood; this may cause confusion among the public. Practices based on compelling correlations but lacking causal evidence are common in pediatric practice. While medical science prefers to rely on data from empirical studies (Chapter 7), there are situations in which such experimentation cannot be done for ethical reasons. Animal models allow for hypothesis testing in these instances (see Appendix A-2). Rapidly expanding knowledge in cell and molecular biology combined with synthetic biology will play an increasing role in healthcare decisions, for which aspiring healthcare students should be prepared. SARS-CoV-1, MERS, and now SARS-CoV-2 remind us of the need to have a national healthcare plan in place for the next emerging viral pathogen, including measures to counter the amount of confusing and false information. The best practices today will undoubtedly be altered in the future, but the principle of readiness and reliance on the best scientific information should remain in the minds of all current and future providers. In this final chapter we remind students and current providers of common misconceptions that could especially impact care for women and children during the **Critical Window** ("Scientific misinformation," SR). Many also apply to the health of all adults. We live in a dangerous and confusing time in which social media and social media influencers may distort the facts and interfere with the employment of best medical practice.

Names Can Lead to Misconceptions

A name can be a source of misconceptions. The term **germ** in biology refers to "the germ of life," the sperm and egg that are the seeds from which new life begins. However, the public may only understand *germ* to mean a microscopic life form responsible for sickness and disease. When used in this context, *germ* refers to any bacteria or virus, regardless of whether it causes disease. Thus, some may interpret "germ-free" as synonymous with good health. Quite to the contrary, and as we described in Chapter 5, the "good" bacteria that comprise the microbiome are required for nutrition, for stimulating adaptive immunity and providing protection against other microbes that cause disease. **Allergy** is another term with multiple meanings. In its strictest use in medicine, it refers to a type of immunologic injury (Chapter 6). When applied in the term *food allergy*, its usage in the lay community may refer to any form of adverse reaction or distress following consumption of some food (see last section).

Some terms are confusing because of their similarity to others. **Antibiotics** can be confused with **antibodies**; the latter are made by the adaptive immune system while the former are naturally occurring chemicals made by certain soil bacteria and fungi that are poisonous to other bacteria. While both provide **internal protection** (Chapter 6), it is antibiotics, not antibodies, that are normally prescribed to control bacterial infections. There may also be word confusion about **prebiotics**, **probiotics**, and foods labeled as **organic**.

Misconceptions About the Actions and Uses of Antibiotics

Disturbing misconceptions about the value and effect of antibiotics grew out of an era when this wonder drug saved the lives of thousands of Allied soldiers in WWII and of many children and adults after the war. First, antibiotics are not toxic to viruses, an important fact that seems to be poorly communicated to the public. Some physicians continue to prescribe antibiotics for children with a "runny nose," probably largely the result of a rhinovirus infection, resulting in prescription rates that are 3 times higher in winter than summer (Suda). This practice in the United States and United Kingdom continued so that in 2014, survey work showed that over 75% of antibiotics were inappropriately prescribed for this purpose. Since then, antibiotic prescriptions written by physicians have declined, but prescriptions written by nurse practitioners and physician assistants have surprisingly increased. Some may do so because a pneumococcal infection might be lurking in children with "colds," and in rare circumstances that might be true, so not prescribing an antibiotic might be considered medical malpractice. Students, practitioners, and the public need to be aware of various concerns regarding use of antibiotics:

1. Antibiotic-resistant bacteria, now called MDR bacteria, are responsible for a great number of deaths worldwide (1.2 million in 2019), and it has been estimated that 10 million will die from MDR bacteria by 2050.
2. Exposure to antibiotics in the first 100 days of life is common in developed countries, and they can disrupt the delicate microbiome ecosystem of the GI tract in newborns (Gibson, SR; Penders) and are associated with a higher risk of atopy in childhood (Arrieta).
3. Antibiotics can alter the effectiveness of vaccines (Hagan).
4. Antibiotics continue to be used as supplements in animal feed.

Hence, antibiotics as the "wonder drug" may be too wonderful to be true without reservation.

In Chapter 6 and elsewhere, we described how overuse of antibiotics allows the "bacterial empire" to strike back so that common bacterial pathogens that had been previously controlled with penicillin, like *Staphylococcus aureus* (which causes life-threatening wound infections), became resistant to this antibiotic and its derivatives (Table A3.3). These MDR bacteria contribute to the size of the **resistome** (Chapter 5) and present a major threat to health worldwide. Patients currently preparing for surgical procedures are familiar with the term MRSA, short for methicillin-resistant *S. aureus*, since routine testing for MRSA now precedes any surgery in hospitals. Another example is long-term antibiotic therapy in adults that disturbs the microbiome and can allow pathogens like *C. difficile* to gain a foothold. We mentioned in Chapter 5 that the constituency of the GI tract microbiome is established very early in life and becomes very stable. Therefore, hysteria about antibiotic therapy can be overblown, since only continuous and long therapy would be needed to significantly alter the established microbiome. However, that may not apply during newborn development, when use of antibiotics could have negative consequences (Gibson, SR; Hagan).

In response to the appearance of resistant variants within the "bacterial empire," the "pharmaceutical empire" struck back with a plethora of new antibiotic formulations. Regardless of these efforts, bacteria slowly became resistant to the new versions, and the industry began to realize they had "overmined" the soil bacteria *Streptomyces* (the source of the original streptomycin and other antibiotics) as a source of new or chemically modified antibiotics. This caused concern that human medicine may in the future reach a point in which antibiotic-resistant, disease-causing bacteria in humans will appear more rapidly than the development of new antibiotics to counter them. Some refer to this as the "antibiotic winter," based on the phrase "nuclear winter," which emerged after the global development of nuclear weapons (Blaser, SR). Should that scenario never develop, humans must still face the threat of emerging viral epidemics and pandemics that cannot be controlled by antibiotics, something Nobel Laureate Josh Lederberg warned of more than 40 years ago. Perhaps this is one reason pharmaceutical companies have widened their research programs to include mAbs.

Because widespread use of antibiotics paralleled the appearance of MDR bacteria, another misconception emerged—namely, that antibiotics were somehow chemically modifying bacterial genes and converting them into antibiotic-resistant (AR) genes. The public and even some biologists believed this was sound logic when knowledge of gene structure, mutation, and evolution was in its infancy. In the 1950s microbiologists were not sure of what was taking place, until it was realized that bacteria with AR genes were present among soil bacteria sampled as early as the 1920s, well before the therapeutic use of antibiotics in medicine. These MDR strains existed because of selective evolutionary pressure from naturally occurring antibiotics made by fungi and *Streptomyces* living in the same environment. We explained in Chapter 6 that the rate of spontaneous mutation is very similar among bacteria and Eukaryotes, but the rapid reproduction and the small genome of bacteria and even smaller genome of viruses (and higher mutation rates) allow for genome changes 3 to 6 logs faster than in humans (Figure 6.2). Thus, **natural selection** for spontaneously mutated microbes can lead to new microbial diseases. The misconception that antibiotics are responsible for chemically modifying bacterial genes that result in new microbial infections is not supported by biomedical science.

Antibiotics used therapeutically are not the only source of antibiotics in the human environment. In Chapter 6 and below we describe the history of supplementing animal feeds with antibiotics, a program called **sub-therapeutic antibiotic therapy (STAT)**, in which the antibiotics were originally referred to as **antibiotic growth promoters (AGP)**. We describe the mechanisms of action of AGP in Chapter 6 and Appendix A-1. Next we discuss misconceptions about the STAT program and the more recent changes to this program.

STAT: Concerns, Misconceptions, and Adjustments

The STAT program was initiated decades ago based on serendipitous observations that antibiotics added to animal and poultry food increased the growth of neonates. These **AGP** accounted for 80% of all antibiotics produced in 2000 and 50% in 2018. Major concerns were that (1) these antibiotics might be transferred in the food chain, (2) MDR bacteria arising in food animals might be transferred to humans (Spoor), and (3) their overuse would increase the number of MDR bacteria on planet Earth. The original STAT program used a broad spectrum of AGP, including those used therapeutically in veterinary and medical practice. Some AGP were banned in Denmark in 2002, but the Danish ban only involved those not used in human medicine. In any case, the result was an increase in bacterial disease in piglets. To counter this response and to follow animal welfare guidelines, usage of therapeutic antibiotics increased, so that overall antibiotic use increased rather than decreased! The details surrounding this aspect of STAT history are discussed by Key and McBride (2014) and Jensen and Hayes (2014).

An array of strategies was introduced to improve STAT programs. These included the use of new antibiotics specifically designed as AGP (see later), as well as improvements in management practices, such restricting access (of animals and humans) to production facilities, implementing rodent control programs, bird-proofing facilities, cleaning and disinfecting vehicles used to haul hogs, and preparing and implementing a written bio-security plan (MacDonald; Lopez).

The most important change was the official policy that antibiotics used therapeutically in human medicine cannot be legally used as AGPs. This led to the introduction of antibiotics such as carbadox, colistin, and avoparcin. Carbadox is added to pig starter feed for control of swine dysentery (*Brachyspira hyodysenteriae*), bacterial enteritis (eg, *Salmonella*), and nasal infections (*Bordetella bronchiseptica*). Carbadox also acts as a mutagen since it induces HGT by the activation of prophages (Appendix A-1), resulting in more frequent exchange of genetic information (Bearson). Swine are an especially rich source of bacteriophage, and in the case of *Salmonella* they transfer the kanamycin AR gene. The use of carbadox, not unexpectedly, resulted in carbadox-resistant enterobacteria that obtain resistance by expressing carbapenenase that catabolizes the antibiotic. To counter this, STAT programs introduced colistin to act against carbapenenase-producing enterobacteria, but these enterobacteria can obtain a plasmid carrying the colistin AR gene (Snesrud). This led to the spread of colistin resistance and untreatable infections (Sprenger). The effects of avoparcin, carbadox, and colistin indicate the danger of applying a different antibiotic to correct problems encountered with a previous antibiotic. Also of interest is that carbapenes (eg, carbodox) are associated with the expansion of certain Bacteroides that degrade mucin glycans, resulting in the thinning of the mucosa, which makes it less protective (Hayase).

Readers need to be reminded that AR genes can be moved by HGT, and the same plasmid cassette may contain AR genes to AGP, antibiotics used in human and veterinary therapy and those required for proper metabolism (Figure A1.4). Thus, the microbial empire strikes back again (Chapter 6). Anticipation that STAT programs may eventually end has turned veterinary and animal science research in new directions. These include genetic engineering of poultry, swine, and cattle to engineer disease-resistant strains and the rebirth of phage therapy as an alternative to antibiotic therapy (see Appendix A-2).

Prebiotics and Misconceptions About Probiotics

Prebiotics are nutrients that encourage the growth of the "good" members of the microbiome (Chapter 5), but they cannot be metabolized by the infant. The best known are human milk oligosaccharides (HMOs; Chapter 3). Formula-fed infants lack HMO exposure from breast milk, but manufacturers now include synthetic HMOs (Chapter 4) in some formulas.

Probiotics are over the counter (OTC) products, a category that in many countries also includes vitamins and multiple other supplements sold by pharmacies and health food stores. Generally, these products are less strictly regulated than drugs, but must produce no harm. Some are complex extracts and mixtures (eg, herbal extracts), making it difficult to identify and purify the active ingredients that could then be tested in appropriate trials (Chapter 7) and potentially to obtain regulatory approval as pharmaceuticals. Many are steeped in mythology and folklore, such as shark fins and pangolin scales in China, poppy blossoms and ginseng in Asia, and marijuana in the Americas. Some, like poppies, have led to FDA-approved pharmaceuticals (opioids). Our purpose is not to enumerate the many examples, but only to clarify definitions. There are programs in some medical schools that address the issues of folk and Chinese traditional medicines.

The use of live bacteria as probiotics is more controversial. The therapeutic value of **probiotics** is best realized for: (1) preterm infants denied access to vaginal birth and natural colonization of their GI tract, (2) infants that for various reasons cannot suckle, and (3) patients that have undergone prolonged treatment with oral antibiotics, which can alter or diminish their normal GI tract microbiome (Chapter 5). Probiotic use among healthy adults grew eightfold between 2000 and 2014, and by 2017 it became a $48 million industry. In 1953 Kollath coined the term probiotics, meaning "promoting life." Their use has a long history (McFarland). Abraham attributed his longevity to sour milk in 4000 BC (Genesis 18:8), Plinius in 76 BC recommended fermented milk for gastritis, and Metchnikoff (the "father" of cellular immunology) in 1907 suggested milk fermented by *Lactobacillus* could ameliorate negative GI tract problems. As early as 1921 the ingestion of *Lactobacillus acidophilus* was promoted and it is still sold as "sweet acidophilus milk" in supermarkets. Hence, probiotics are most often delivered in dairy products. Yogurt is milk fermented by *Strep. thermophilus* and supplemented with *Lactobacillus* and *Bifidobacterium* (see Chapter 5). One cup (125 ml) should contain 10^6–10^9 cfu (cfu = colony-forming units) of bacteria. Many different strains of *Lactobacillus* are used, with each commercial product touting its own variants. Probiotics are also present in cottage cheese, quark, ripened cheeses (eg, Emmental, Edam, aged brick, Beer Kaese, etc.), and fermented vegetables like sauerkraut and kimchi. There are even ice creams containing *Lactobacillus* and *Bifidobacterium*.

Public misconceptions about probiotics and other OTCs are that (1) they have FDA approval as a medicine, (2) their value rests on established scientific trials (see Chapter 7), and (3) when they are ingested by healthy adults, the probiotic bacteria can substantially alter the constituency of the established GI tract microbiome. The first two concerns were clarified above. Below, we consider the third one.

Consider for a moment that a common yogurt can deliver 10^8–10^{10} bacteria in 2–4 servings. Given the size of the existing microbiome in healthy individuals, it means the probiotic organisms would be outnumbered 10,000–100,000 to 1 by the resident bacteria. If used daily, the probiotic bacteria may alter the constituency of the GI tract microbiome, but during the same period the much larger established microbiome will also be rapidly reproducing and thus maintaining dominance. The idea of gradual alterations by regular usage of probiotics is also inconsistent with evidence that probiotics encounter marked **colonization resistance** from the existing microbiota (Chapter 5; Zmora; Slashinski). The value of probiotics for healthy adults is transient and controversial and, like many other OTCs, their endorsement rests more on folklore and testimonials than evidence-based studies. The evidence of beneficial value of probiotics for certain newborns and in patients after extensive oral antibiotic treatment is much stronger.

Vaccination Hesitancy, Herd Immunity, and Global Mobility

While most understand that **herd immunity** is not restricted to the livestock industry, the term does originate in veterinary science; mass vaccination conjures up scenes from Western movies of herds of cattle and sheep being herded through "tick baths" while simultaneously being vaccinated. Add to this the scene of humans in Third World countries waiting in long lines to receive a vaccine to control an epidemic. To briefly reiterate what was stated in Chapter 6, herd immunity applies to any population of higher vertebrates that, due to vaccination or recovery from the disease, leaves only a few susceptible (non-immune) individuals that could still acquire and effectively spread the contagion. Herd immunity refers to the statistical probability that a population is protected. Herd immunity can be achieved in two ways. Before the development of vaccines in the 20th century, it was achieved by recovering from the disease. European explorers who had experienced numerous bouts with measles had "herd immunity," but Indigenous people in the West Indies and South America had not and they died in large numbers after contact with such explorers. The same story can be told for other diseases. Of course, this means of obtaining herd immunity is effective but causes many deaths and serious illness.

The second method is vaccination. The effectiveness of vaccine-induced herd immunity was demonstrated by requiring vaccination of children against diphtheria in the 1950s, polio in the 1960s, and measles in the 1970s, which virtually eradicated these diseases in the United States (Figure 8.1). The consequences of these diseases to long-term health were described in Chapter 6. Unfortunately, after about 2000, some parents were less conscientious about childhood vaccinations, and herd immunity was being lost so the incidence of measles and measles outbreaks began to rise (Figure 8.2). After 2000, the number of measles outbreaks slowly increased so that, by 2019, the United States was at risk of losing measles elimination status (Feemster). A similar trend occurred in Europe: until 2009 there was a continuous decline in cases of measles, but its incidence increased fourfold between 2010 and 2011. From 2000 to 2010, over 5 million individuals ages 2–12 in the European Union had not received the MMR vaccine (Carrillo-Santisteve). Outbreaks of measles in

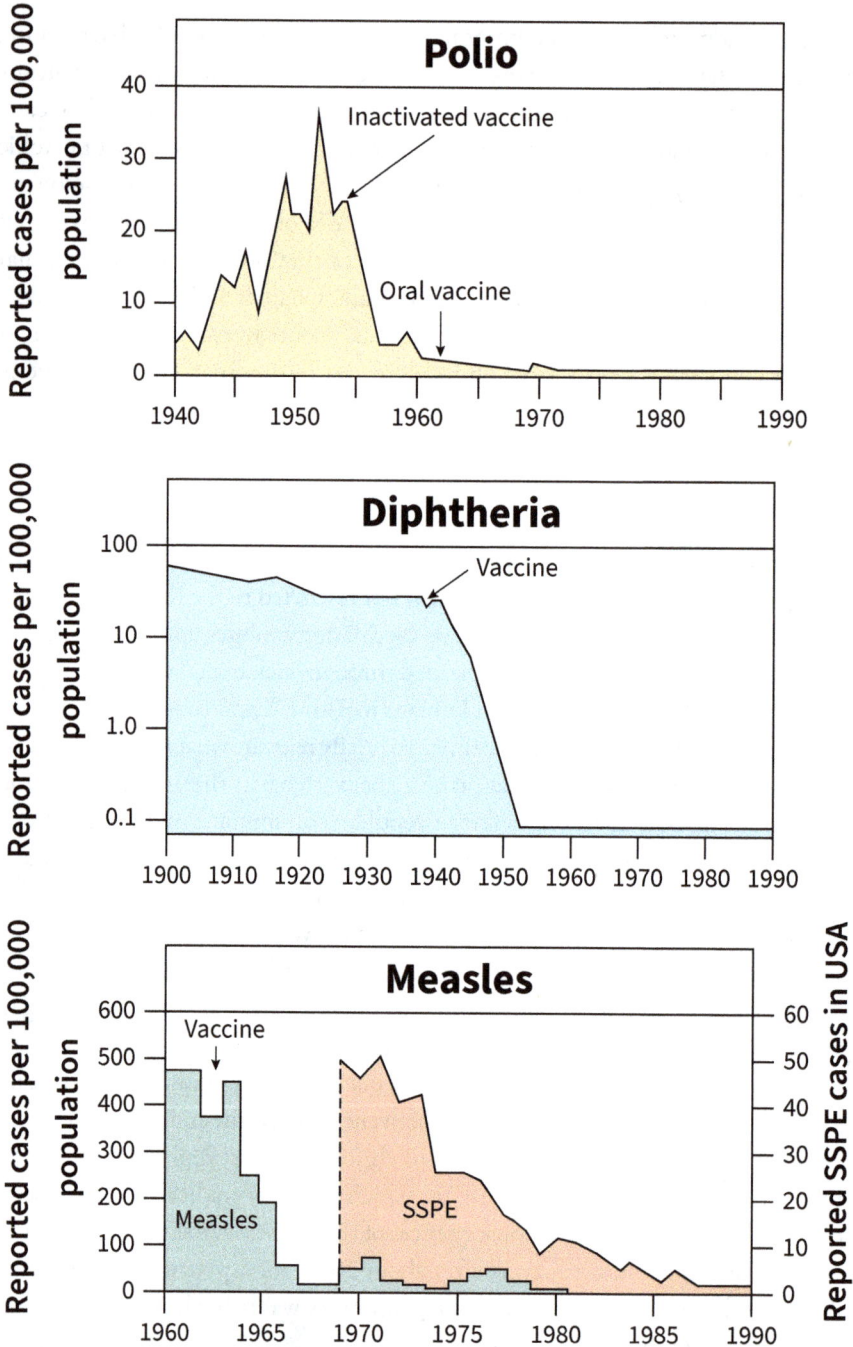

Figure 8.1   The impact of vaccines for diphtheria, polio, and measles on the incidence of reported cases of infection with these pathogens. Injected versus oral polio vaccines are discussed in Chapter 6. A sequel occurred a decade after measles infections called subacute sclerosing panencephalitis (SSPE) but does not represent a re-occurrence of measles. Once the use of the measles vaccine became standard, this secondary consequence of infection rapidly declined.

the United States from 2002 to 2014 also increased fourfold, along with the number of unvaccinated children. A study of school children showed that the risk of transmission among the unvaccinated was 70 times higher than among the vaccinated (Azimi). Studies by the WHO indicate that 95% of the population must be vaccinated to achieve herd immunity (Carrillo-Santisteve), and in the case of rubella disease can occur when vaccination rates drop below 50% (Panagiotopoulos). In the case of mumps, orchitis and parotitis can still develop in some vaccinated teenagers (Shepersky; Chapter 6). A review published in the *Journal of the American Medical Association* reported measles outbreaks. In 1,416 cases it found that 57% of individuals had not received the MMR vaccine although one-third were vaccine eligible, and 70% of those were vaccine eligible and had not used a religious or other medical exemption as an excuse (Figure 8.2; Phadke). This data supports the value of vaccination. In the United States, this is partially a result of international travel (probably also the case in Europe). Measles outbreaks in California have been linked to visitors from Asia (eg, Malaysia) and may explain the outbreak that occurred at Disney World.

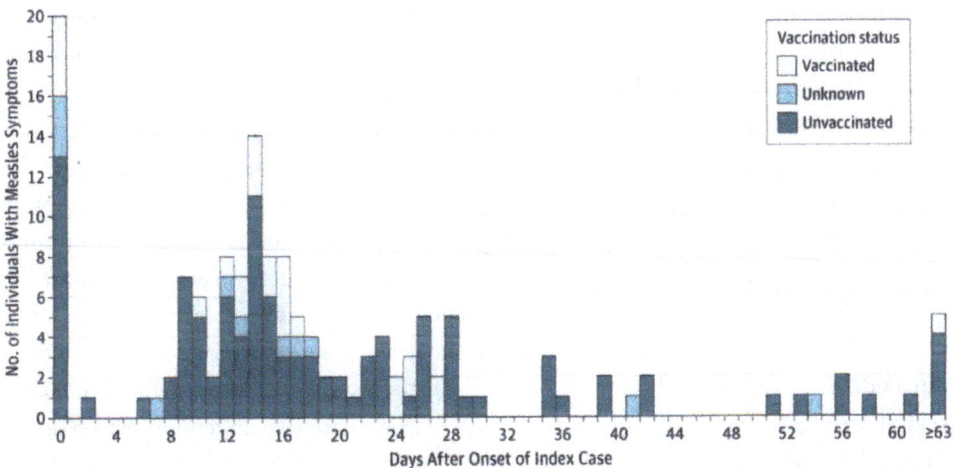

Figure 8.2   Vaccination status of individuals in measles outbreaks in the United States after declaration of the elimination of the disease. Data are from 145 cases sampled from 1,416 outbreaks from 2000–2015, for which sufficient information on symptoms onset and vaccination status was available. Re-occurrences are referenced to day 0 when the first outbreak was reported. Distribution among vaccinated, unvaccinated, and unknown is indicated in the legend. The occurrence of symptoms among the three groups in the days after day 0 are believed to be due to transmission from those initially infected. These are sometimes called "disease generations" and this repeated process extended beyond 12 weeks (Phadke).

A somewhat similar pattern has been seen with pertussis cases, but some infections have occurred in vaccinated individuals, perhaps due to waning immunity. Most recently in New York City, paralytic polio that had been virtually eliminated after 1960 (Figure 8.1) reappeared in a single case in an unimmunized man, and vaccine-related virus has been recovered from the city's sewage system (Link-Gelles). As we described in Chapter 6, the polio virus lives in the GI tract and is regularly shed in feces, which seems to be one reason for the periodic outbreaks in Asia that exclusively use the oral vaccine (OPV) that can sometimes revert to the wild type (see Appendix A-1). Its appearance in the sewage system seems to indicate that the number of infected individuals may be underestimated.

Some parents may wonder why their child should suffer the pain of needle vaccinations for diseases that they believe are no longer present. These parents and others fail to realize that the incidence of disease remained low **only because** more than 80% of eligible children had been vaccinated (ie, herd immunity; Chapter 6). The proportion of the population that needs to recover from the disease or be vaccinated depends on the disease; for SARS-CoV-2, it could be 95%. We mentioned that WHO studies recommend 95% vaccine compliance to obtain herd immunity for measles. This percentage may not be applicable to all infectious diseases. Differences depend on other factors, including (1) the route of transmission of the pathogen, (2) the stability of the pathogen's genome, and (3) the nature of microbe (eg, virus, bacteria, or eukaryotic parasite).

The most transmissible pathogens like influenza, SARS-CoV-2, and measles are spread by aerosol, so the risk that any individual will come into contact with these pathogens is very high. By contrast, intimate contact is needed for the transfer of HIV, monkeypox, and many **sexually transmitted diseases (STDs)**.

In Appendix A-4, we described how RNA viruses that have been shown to evolve to a new species (like SARS-CoV-2) often rapidly diversify their genome (Figure 6.2), since the new host has minimal immunological resistance to their "invasion." Thus, their rapidly changing genome makes them a moving target for the host immune system. Herd immunity for the alpha variant of SARS-CoV-2 may not provide immune protection against the Omicron B-5 variant, and based on the experience of earlier variants, home tests may give false negatives in infections from new variants; however, appropriately designed PCR tests (Appendix A-1) can detect the new variants. Often, symptoms are more reliable. In contrast to viral pathogens, bacterial and eukaryotic pathogens change their genomes more slowly (Figure 6.2). Because of these differences among pathogens, the percentage of vaccinated and immune individuals needed to achieve herd immunity may cover a broad range.

There are sage arguments that infection-induced herd immunity may be better than vaccination, but this is only better if the community is willing to accept morbidity and mortality and disruption of the economy. Many argue that China's stringent lockdown policies were ethical because they allowed that country to initially have a hundred-fold fewer deaths than in the United States, but they also hindered establishment of natural herd immunity. Evidence in support of this comes from the 2022 marked surge in incidence of SARS-CoV-2 in Shanghai and throughout China as lockdowns were lifted, as now seen in world news. Below we discuss the anti-vaccine movement that gained support from the Wakefield debacle, which may also have been the reason why the proportion of children receiving the MMR vaccine decreased and the incidence of measles increased (Feemster; Phadke).

Adding to the difficulty of establishing herd immunity was that beginning in the 1990s, international travel increased as did illegal immigration, and there was no guarantee that all newcomers were disease-free or had been vaccinated. The COVID-19 pandemic revealed much vaccine hesitancy in the United States. The following groups have been shown to display COVID vaccine hesitancy:

1. Approximately 33% of Americans, who consider the annual flu vaccine unnecessary or consider COVID-19 to be a hoax or the same as the flu.
2. Americans who distrust Big Pharma and don't believe a safe vaccine can be produced in a short time and that COVID vaccines were politically rushed into use in less than 1 year. Some in this group reference the disastrous Cutter incident in the 1950s involving a contaminated batch of the initial Salk vaccine.
3. African Americans, who know that in the past medical experimentation, including poorly tested vaccines, occurred without their informed consent.
4. Individuals who fear needles or who have had a negative experience after receiving a vaccine.

A combination of these factors has contributed to an **infodemic** of misinformation in American healthcare (Dube). Sadly, some suggest that the vaccine hesitancy that surfaced during the COVID-19 pandemic may have spread to failure to comply with overall childhood vaccination recommendations (Chapter 6).

The COVID-19 pandemic revealed early on that a surprising contingent of the population doubted that the vaccine adequately interrupted disease transmission. The subsequent emergence of SARS-CoV-2 virus variants supported this concern. In 2022 there were many news reports regarding cases of vaccinees that had been infected by new and emerging variants. While vaccines based on wild-type SARS-CoV-2 do not prevent reinfection, they clearly protect against severe, life-threatening disease (Appendix A-4).

Misunderstandings About Vaccination Protocols

Separate from those who are vaccine hesitant, confusion and misunderstanding exists within the public that asks why: (a) different routes/modes of administration are used (eg, oral, injected or sprayed), (b) repetitive or booster dosages are needed for some vaccines but not others, (c) vaccines cause allergy or other discomfort, and (d) it is recommended to get a flu shot be each year (Chapter 6). The 1956 Salk vaccine to combat the polio virus was injected. A few years later, the Sabin vaccine appeared; it was simply swallowed and not injected. To understand the change in administration, one must remember that the polio virus first infects the epithelial cells of the gut. While the Sabin vaccine reduced discomfort, it also delivered the vaccine to the site where viral entrance first occurs (see Chapter 6, Section I discussion of mucosal immunity). Similarly, a few attenuated influenza vaccines have been developed for use as nasal droplets or sprays and there may be more in the future; all are based on the idea of targeting the site of infection. Since the Sabin vaccine (oral polio vaccine or OPV) is an attenuated live virus like MMR, it replicates itself and therefore continues to immunize the host for some time; it is "the vaccine that keeps on giving." In Chapter 6 we outlined the advantages of the OPV but also indicated that the attenuated form may revert to virulence and produce some aspects of the disease. It can be shed in feces and could explain the recent polio case in New York City, if new emigrants had only received the OPV. Because polio had been eradicated from the United States (Figure 8.1), it was decided that the risk versus benefit analysis now favored the killed version of the virus (IPV; Salk vaccine), and in the setting of near eradication of polio, OPV administration is currently not recommended in the United States.

Since MMR replicates itself and therefore continues to immunize, why is it given more than once (Chapter 6, Table 6.4)? The level of immune development in neonates varies with age, and maternal IgG antibodies transferred *in utero* can possibly interfere with response to the vaccine. The answer to this predicament is for multiple injections to be given to increase the probability that the child will receive the vaccine when the immune system is more immunocompetent and when interference from maternal antibodies has waned (see Chapter 3).

Parents and others may ask: *If immunizing the site where the virus enters seems more natural, why inject a muscle when the site of entry and infection is elsewhere?* Intramuscular injection is simple, the dosage is easily metered, and the shoulder or thigh is an easy target during mass vaccinations. If the vaccine is injected into the muscle, dendritic cells and other APCs take up the vaccine and move it to the nearest lymph node, stimulating lymphocytes, some of which then migrate to mucosal sites like the GI tract and bronchi and secrete SIgA antibodies specific to the vaccine (see **mucosal immune system**; Figure 6.6) while others produce antibodies that enter the blood and circulate throughout the body (**the systemic immune response**; Chapter 3).

While children may fear the needle, some adults also worry about pain or other consequences associated with needle administrations. When annual flu shots are given, recipients are asked if they are allergic to the vaccine or sometimes if they are allergic to eggs. What does having a food allergy to eggs have to do with the influenza virus? The answer is that vaccine manufacturers produce the influenza vaccine by initially growing the virus in the eggs of chickens, where they grow well. When the viral protein is harvested and purified from the egg culture and placed into the final vaccine vehicle, the possibility exists that some egg protein may also be included. Beyond that, chicken eggs and influenza virus have little in common. In fact, when allergic reactions to the influenza vaccine occur, they are usually not caused by infinitesimal amounts of egg protein but by other components of the vaccine, like adjuvants.

Beyond an allergic reaction, people who have previously suffered other forms of discomfort with vaccines may delay or decline vaccination (ie, display vaccine hesitancy). You may recall from Chapter 6 that **subunit vaccines** require an **adjuvant** that can stimulate TLRs. Such stimulation produces an inflammatory response needed to initiate any immune response. Injection site pain is a well-known side effect encountered with the current shingles vaccine (Shingrix); the discomfort is caused by the inflammation produced by the adjuvant.

Chapter 7 describes the 4-phase testing regimen needed for a vaccine to gain FDA approval. Phases 1 and 2 are particularly concerned with short-term secondary complications that could result from the adjuvant. After Phases 1–3, and after a vaccine gains emergency or final approval, complications may still arise because it is nearly impossible to test representatives of all groups under all conditions or to monitor them for extended periods. That is when ongoing monitoring of adverse events (often called Phase 4, Chapter 7) kicks in. Phase 4 may continue for many years after widespread use of the vaccine. It is during this period when less common, undesirable, secondary consequences may be discovered. If these are serious, the FDA may pause or terminate the use of a vaccine until actual results are further analyzed. The public witnessed this pause with the Johnson & Johnson and AstraZeneca vaccines for SARS-CoV-2.

Many people may question why an annual flu shot is needed. This is a killed vaccine designed to stimulate neutralizing antibodies that can prevent infection but that may wane in 3–6 months. The vaccine should also generate memory B cells (Chapter 6) that in theory could extend protection for subsequent years. However, the annual influenza vaccine does not contain epitopes capable of providing protection against new or reassorted variants, such as those causing the "flu of the year" like the H1N1 variant that caused the 2009 swine flu outbreak. Therefore, the CDC or other national health agencies specify the influenza strains to be included in annual vaccines to provide protection against those strains/recombinants predicted to most likely affect the population in the upcoming influenza season. For similar reasons, modified annual COVID-19 vaccines may become routine.

The inconvenience of annual vaccines could be avoided by producing a multivalent or "universal" influenza vaccine that could provide protection against 10–20 variants or by using adjuvants that would enhance long-term immunity in the respiratory tract. While an annual influenza shot or COVID-19 shot may be recommended, previous vaccines may still provide some cross-reactivity and healthy younger members of the community often recover quickly thanks to their own natural immunity. For older individuals and those with compromised health conditions, getting the annual influenza shot is even more strongly recommended.

Hypotheses Masquerading as Facts

Chapter 7 reviewed the scientific method, the design of clinical trials, and the hierarchy of evidence principle. There is a danger that the populace may accept as "fact" what is merely a hypothesis. Here we provide two well-publicized examples that involve immunology.

The first involves breast augmentation, which in the 1950s and 1960s became popular among budding starlets who believed it could enhance their professional careers. Similar surgical procedures were employed for reconstruction in women who had undergone mastectomy because of cancer. The product used by surgeons was silicone in various forms, and Dow-Corning was a major supplier. In the 1980s, some physicians and others began to correlate breast implantation with the onset of autoimmune disease. This illustrates the danger of relying on correlation without causation. Surgical implantation causes inflammation, but autoimmunity requires the breakdown of **immunological tolerance**, which is a separate issue. Misunderstanding the difference led to a series of lawsuits, which targeted Dow-Corning Chemicals because they "have deep pockets" and lawyers pocket big rewards. Contributing to the misinformation were physicians paid by the plaintiffs who reported on correlations. A notable episode involved a charismatic plastic surgeon (Dr. "X") who dressed in 3-piece suits and wore a deliberately exposed gold watch chain. Thanks to Dr. "X," large numbers of women were convinced that they had developed autoimmunity due to Dow-Corning silicon implants. When finally forced to reveal his scientific data at an NIH meeting, Dr. "X" stated: "I was working on the data when a stiff Pacific breeze swept it out the window." Nevertheless, based on an unsubstantiated hypothesis, large rewards were paid out to the women and their attorneys. One of the co-authors of this book, who participated in the NIH meeting, was quoted in *Reader's Digest* as saying: "Dr. X appears to believe a hypothesis is the same as a fact."

A second example of hypotheses masquerading as facts, which is especially relevant to the Critical Window, involves childhood vaccination and autism spectrum disorder (ASD). The correlation was seized on by groups who were convinced that childhood vaccination regimens were responsible for the increase in ASD and that ASD was linked to the increased number of childhood vaccines being given (21 treatments as opposed to only given 2 generations ago; see Chapter 6, Table 6.4). In 2000, a socially active mother of a child with ASD mounted a campaign to reject or alter the vaccination regimen based on this hypothesis. The episode was triggered by pediatric gastroenterologist Andrew Wakefield. In 1998 he and colleagues published a paper entitled "Ileal-lymphoid-nodular hyperplasia, non-specific colitis and pervasive developmental disorder in children." This paper suggested, without evidence of causation, that the intestinal inflammation he observed in a child with ASD was the result of the childhood MMR vaccine. This ignited a firestorm that caused parents in England to decline the MMR vaccination and initiated studies that would eventually cost taxpayers millions, only to show there was no cause and effect. Later, 10 of the 13 co-authors of the article retracted their claim and Dr. Wakefield was released from his position and stripped of his medical license (Taylor, SR). Sadly, by then the damage had been done and the psychological and emotional impact remains. An enlightening and useful aspect of the debacle is a book written by Eula Bliss that deals with the psychosocial reasons humans gravitate to accepting correlation as proof of causation, regardless of the evidence (Bliss).

The Wakefield MMR debacle and the anti-vaccine movement have generated parental concerns about childhood vaccination protocols (see Chapter 6). Since it is not uncommon for children to mount a febrile response after routine vaccinations, parental concern is not uncommon. Even Benjamin Franklin had his doubts and withheld variolation (a procedure that came before vaccination; see Chapter 6) for his young son, who later died from smallpox at age 4. It is noteworthy that the risk of the mortality from variolation (3%) enormously exceeds the risk of mortality from modern vaccines. Nevertheless, vaccine opponents still believe in a causative link between "excessive vaccination" and multiple sclerosis and cancer. Even before the Wakefield story made headlines, there had been other concerns with vaccines. One of these involves thimerosal (once known by the brand name Merthiolate), a mercury-containing compound long used as a preservative (bacterial and fungal growth inhibitor) in vaccines and biological samples in general. The correlation between mercury, neurological disorder, and ASD did not go unnoticed. However, the amount of mercury received in all the vaccinations combined would be less than that obtained by eating an ocean fish. Extensive studies found no connection. A second ingredient in some vaccines is aluminum, which acts as an adjuvant and is a metal associated with neurological disorders in a few situations of high exposure and poor excretion. Extensive studies revealed that aluminum of vaccine adjuvants is rapidly removed by the kidney and offers no danger.

In addition to the impact that the Wakefield incident had on the anti-vaccine movement, there are other members of the medical community that support the movement. An Australian pathologist has promoted the view, without evidence, that mRNA vaccines (approved for SARS-CoV-2) cause autoimmunity. While there is no scientific evidence that supports this view, talk shows and YouTube still distribute such messages (see, YouTube interview: https://www.youtube.com/watch?v=yMyERFBdB4E). It is always important for medical practitioners and scientists to raise doubts about certain practices, but caution is needed when claims are at best only hypotheses, not on empirical evidence from proper clinical trials.

The better argument against a connection between childhood vaccination and ASD is that most forms of ASD develop *in utero* (Chapter 2) and thus could not be due to childhood vaccination. We speculated in Chapter 2 that gene expression in the developing fetus could be altered by environmental substances transmitted *in utero*. Since controls for *in utero* studies are unethical, suitable animal models are needed (Appendix A-2). Our message to parents is that there is no evidence that childhood vaccinations are responsible for ASD and that their children and those in the community will be healthier if the current childhood vaccination regimen (Table 6.4) is followed.

Hypotheses masquerading as facts also grew out of the COVID-19 pandemic. One was that SARS-CoV-2 is a bioterrorist weapon developed in a Chinese laboratory. The concept is old, dating back to 1320 when sheep infected with tularemia were used as a weapon to spread disease into an enemy kingdom. Nazi Germany and Japan both conducted experiments on humans using weaponized microbes, and after WWII the Soviet Union and the United States set up laboratories for this purpose. These were shut down in the 1960s when both countries recognized their danger to humanity, especially that such engineered pathogens could escape the laboratory endanger individuals in their own countries. The Chinese are fully aware of that history. The alternative origin of SARS-CoV-2, which may be more widely accepted, is that it had a zoonotic origin in Asian fruit bats, pangolins, civets, or another species as shown to be the case with related coronaviruses (see Appendix A-4). The true source of the SARS-CoV-2 virus will be difficult to prove. Nevertheless the concept of escape of SARS-CoV-2 from a Chinese laboratory, still has adherents. Paranoia about weaponized microbes also appeared after 9/11 and involved one of the co-authors (a microbiologist), who was investigated by the FBI for allegedly using his restored crop duster biplane to spread anthrax!

In summary, a list of hypotheses masquerading as facts, might also include the following:

1. Illness is caused by the use of antibiotics in animal feed.
2. There is a connection between illnesses in infants and formulas that are contaminated by bacteria during manufacturing.

3. Some viral epidemics are the result of biological warfare.
4. ASD is caused by MMR vaccines.
5. Commercial probiotics need to be used regularly by healthy individuals to maintain a healthy GI tract microbiome.
6. Genetic traits are transferred through suckling (Chapter 3).
7. Food intolerance is caused by food allergy (ie, an immune response).

It is important for students and the public not to assume that any one action or event is the cause of another event without hard scientific evidence (Chapter 7).

Programmed Gullibility

Misconceptions and conspiracies flourish through **programmed gullibility**, often called **confirmation bias**, which can pose risks to healthcare trainees and practitioners. Programmed gullibility is an intrinsic property of at least higher vertebrates and can be a positive factor in species survival (Chapter 1). Offspring of all higher vertebrates are intrinsically programmed to follow the training provided by a parent and the community that surrounds them and on which they imprint. This can form a bond of trust, which is difficult to alter as children grow up; it is accepted that fundamental beliefs and biases in children are formed before they are 10 years old. In pack animals like certain carnivores, a chain of command develops, which is essential for the survival of the pack and species. Similar dependence develops in birds so that food choices made by the fledglings depend on trust in parental judgment. The offspring of seedeaters learn to prefer seeds and insect/worm eaters learn to prefer insects and worms. Not surprisingly, in human societies, individuals have come to accept and depend on their chiefs, religious leaders, or leaders of the government (Ullrich). These bonds and allegiances are understandably difficult to break. We use the term **programmed gullibility** to describe this phenomenon.

Among human societies, the less educated are often the most gullible to folklore and to quick-fix medical remedies such as the "snake oils" and elixirs popularized in Western movies. The tradition continues today in testimonials from well-known personalities that appear on TV or on social media platforms that market products such as (1) immunosuppressive drugs that can cure cosmetic problems, (2) jellyfish proteins that improve brain function, (3) a plethora of weight loss programs, (4) supplements promoting male performance, and (5) probiotics for healthy people. Nonetheless, affluence and education are not complete preventives, as shown by acceptance in educated societies within the last century of concepts such as eugenics, frontal lobotomy for behavioral disorders, and therapies such as homeopathy and naturopathy. **Programmed gullibility** is a human trait with a long political and religious history that relies on ideologies that are often called conspiracy theories. Europeans in the 16th century rejected the potato from South America (now a worldwide staple) when their leaders promoted the belief that it was a deadly member of the poisonous nightshade family, even though there was no evidence it was killing people in South America who depend on it as a staple. It took an authoritarian German prince to change their minds.

However, too much good promotion left the Irish helpless against the potato famine. In Muslim countries, it was believed that children wet-nursed on a surrogate mother could never marry any member of the family of the wet-nurse because genetic information was transferred through suckling, and this became national policy in some countries (Chapter 3). Programmed gullibility impacts all aspects of human societies, including the education of healthcare students and practitioners.

National Priorities

The United States, the richest nation on Earth and a leader in medical science, has seen large-scale deaths and infections from SARS-CoV-2; more deaths than among American soldiers in WWII. The American population has not witnessed a pandemic for 100 years, yet pandemics are a periodic occurrence and, with international travel so rapid, epidemiologists have been warning they will become more frequent. More than 40 years ago, Nobel Laureate Josh Lederberg warned that it would be a virus. In the 1980s the American public took notice of HIV, sometimes considered a "homegrown" disease, while Ebola, Zika, SARS-CoV-1, and MERS were regarded as "foreign wars." Certainly, the most expensive healthcare system in the world would be ready if such a danger reached them! But it is too late to build a fire truck after the fire has started. The CDC clearly knew from its involvement with Ebola, Zika, SARS-CoV-1, and MERS that the next epidemic or pandemic was on the horizon.

The COVID-19 pandemic pointed to weaknesses in disease preparedness and the limits of making the public understand the risks and benefits of methods of epidemic mitigation. Developed nations that had no experience with a pandemic for a century dropped their guard. There was a lack of medical preparedness but also a lack of preparedness of governments to send a message to citizens that accurately portrayed both the knowledge and uncertainty of the situation. The problems resulting from the confusion/inconsistency of advice from governmental agencies need to be addressed and resolved. In the future, agencies and politicians need to be more aware of potential epidemics/pandemics and prepare providers and the populace for an appropriate response (Cross).

If It's Good Enough for Grandparents, It's Good Enough for Grandchildren

Societies in developed countries have the expectation that children are "automatically'" given vaccines to prevent childhood diseases. It is not unreasonable for critics to ask why their grandparents only received 0–4 vaccines and often lived into their 80s and 90s. Does this folklore have an explanation? If prior generations lived to old age by contracting the disease and then developing long-lasting immunity, why has medical research invested such time and expense to develop the MMR vaccine? During the childhood of several of the authors, it was expected that one would certainly contract measles, mumps, chicken pox, and rubella in childhood and consequently would obtain life-long immunity, shingles excluded. While immunity can indeed be established in this manner, all infections stress the child's immune system, reduce overall health, and render them more vulnerable to bacterial pathogens. Frequent infections, especially diarrheal diseases, also reduce expected weight gain in children (Figure 8.3). Studies in animal and veterinary science have long shown that infection negatively affects nutrient uptake, weight gain, and overall health, and this was one reason the STAT program was instituted (see earlier). The MMR vaccine protocol positively reduced societal disruption. Measles, mumps, and rubella infections had originally forced school absences (and sometimes school closures) in the 1940s and into the 1960s, which disrupted schooling and childcare and parental schedules, just as COVID-19 did in 2020–2021. When anti-vaccine groups wish not to vaccinate their own children, it endangers other children, disrupts society, and raises healthcare costs for the whole community.

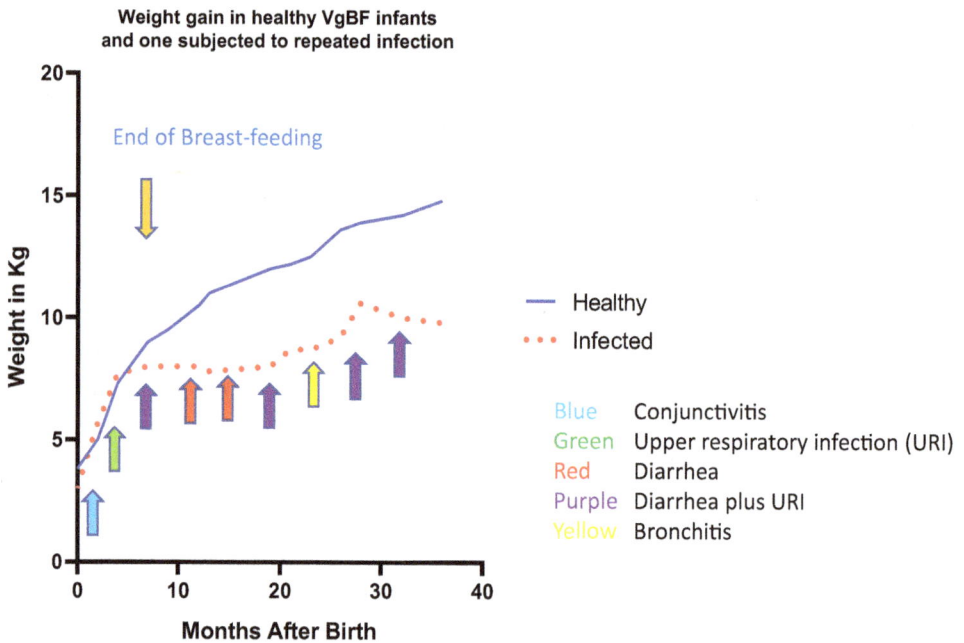

Figure 8.3   The average weight gain among healthy breast-fed infants in comparison to an infant when breast-feeding was stopped and that later suffered various bouts of illness (Mata).

Returning to a historical perspective, it should be remembered that Grandpa or Grandma may have never left the state, county, or even township in which they were born. During his time, there were few new immigrants who joined their community, who might either be bearing new diseases or have not been immunized against childhood diseases. In past times, a type of "mini-herd immunity" was established within the local community even without vaccination, since nearly everyone had contracted childhood diseases and developed immunity. We mentioned this earlier when discussing the history of European settlements in America in the 16th and 17th centuries. We now live in a world in which grandpas and grandma's descendants now travel around the world, and immigrants come from all over the world, including from countries where emerging viral diseases are common and regular vaccination protocols are absent. It is not just human carriers of pathogens that are a concern, because travelers bring invasive plants and insects. Grandpa's and Grandma's grandchildren and great-grandchildren now live in a world that, despite improvements in hygiene, are still vulnerable to pathogens and invasive life forms of all types. Finally, the folklore surrounding the generation of grandparents in America, may ignore the evidence that 100–200-year-old graveyard markers show that many children died before the age of 2 years; the sister of one of the co-authors was one of them. To avoid reoccurrences of childhood disease outbreaks, the current and evolving vaccination regimen for children needs to be followed.

Nature Versus Nurture

This age-old conundrum often arises in discussions of childhood traits and diseases. The proponents of the **nature** hypothesis strongly believe in classical Mendelian genetics and that most phenotypic traits are passed from parent to offspring. **Nurture** advocates believe that traits are shaped by pressure from the environment. We discussed in the opening chapter how genetics was the "third rail" of the triad that influences events in the Critical Window, but we also noted that environmental factors can alter gene expression and can explain some maladies. While Mendelian genetics can explain several illnesses, the reasons for others are only partially known. These include ASD, Alzheimer's in older adults, IBD, and allergy in both young and old (which has been increasing in frequency in highly developed countries; see Chapters 5 and 6). If these illnesses have a genetic basis, they may be multigenic (ie, the result of the combined effect of many genes, some not yet identified and the result of epigenetics.). **Epigenetic** or **Epigenesis** refers to changes in gene expression, that may be caused by DNA methylation, histone modification or factors provided by intracellular pathogens or cytoplasmic cell organelles; Sookoian, SR). In Appendix A-1, we used dogs as a model to explain epigenetics; 99.9% of structural genes in dogs are shared among the nearly 300 dog breeds, yet they have very different phenotypes and behavior. Unlike simple Mendelian traits that involve mutations, epigenetic traits are difficult to study, which creates problems when the principles of hypothesis testing (Chapter 7) are applied. Much evidence indicates that ASD has its origins *in utero* (Chapter 2), making it possible that some environmental modifiers transferred *in utero* may alter gene expression and cause ASD. A chronic disease that results from events *in utero* is demonstrated by individuals born small for gestational age (SGA) or large for gestational age (LGA). Causal factors for SGA and LGA can vary. Nutrient availability during gestation has been proposed as a driver of chronic disease risk by altering the physiology and metabolism of target tissues. Observed conditions linked to these proposed mechanisms include metabolic syndrome, which is a constellation of hypertension, hyperlipidemia, obesity, and insulin resistance. These not only impact the individual but also their offspring and can contribute to the health of the mother when she bears children, resulting in a generational risk. It is important that healthcare providers promote proper nutrition and lifestyle recommendations, monitor infant weight gain, support optimal maternal nutrition, and promote physical activity and breast-feeding. (Hernández; Sookoian, SR; Figure 8.3).

In Chapter 6 we described how **nurture** can be linked to allergy. We noted that children reared in an allergen-poor environment are more likely to develop allergies as they develop, and children infected with intestinal parasites early in life are less likely to develop IBD in midlife. While these only represent correlations, the American Academy of Pediatrics, based on prospective trials, recommends early exposure to peanut protein to avoid serious peanut allergies later in life.

Nurture also impacts the health of the GI tract since it influences establishment of the microbiome (Chapter 5) and may be a contributing factor. The incidence of NEC in breast-fed premature infants is less than in formula-fed infants, as the breastfed infant obtains regulatory factors through breast milk (Chapter 3) and obtains a portion of the microbiome in the same manner. Experiments involving pathogen-free piglets reared in "auto sows" on nutrient-rich milk replacers, and even with a microbiome obtained from the birth canal, gain weight poorly compared to conventionally reared piglets (Appendix A-2). This suggests that suckling provides additional factors that may influence the development of a microbiome that can generate nutrients essential for proper development (Chapter 3). Both necrotizing enterocolitis (NEC) and studies using auto sow piglets support the view that conventional birth and development play a role in neonatal development. Myths that industrialized surrogate milk can fully replace breast-feeding are unfounded, a message to be considered by professional women whose careers may interfere with their opportunity to breastfeed (Chapter 4). In discussing the auto sow system, we also showed that labile factors in colostrum, presumed to be cytokines, significantly impact *de novo* Ig synthesis (antibody production) in piglets (Figure 3.6).

The impact of **nurture** has also been studied using monozygotic twins raised in different environments. Using animal twins, an important role for oxytocin in development of the cerebrum was observed. We mentioned oxytocin in Chapter 3 as the "feel good" hormone that is recognized by oxytocin receptors and is responsible for milk release from the mammary gland. It is also associated with increased socialization. Offspring raised without suckling down-regulate oxytocin receptor expression, and compared to their identical siblings, they exhibit anti-social behavior (see Chapter 3).

Food Allergy, Intolerance, and Food Aversion— A "Can of Worms"?

Allergy or Something Else?

Understanding unwanted symptoms that can occur upon ingestion of foods requires understanding the interplay among immunology, food science, genetics, and psychology. Food aversions and avoidance may reflect a person's earlier negative experience after encounter with a particular food. The digestive discomfort that patients or parents report for their children and then ascribe to food allergy may instead have a nonimmunologic basis; eg, a response to too many beans, a wild mushroom toxin, toxins of microbial origin, or too many jalapeños. However, some symptoms have a true immunological basis (Prescott). Adverse events caused by an immune response to a food are the only food-related events that may be rightly called food allergy. Reactions to foods can result from **type I immediate hypersensitivity** mediated by IgE antibodies to food proteins, which can result in **immunological injury** (Chapter 6). Shortly after the food is eaten, the reaction can manifest with dermatitis and gastrointestinal or respiratory symptoms (hives, vomiting, wheezing, for example). Allergy to foods can also be T-cell mediated, (eg, **type IV immunologic injury**). The skin-prick test detects antigen-specific IgE, but is only reliable for **type I hypersensitivity**; it does not test for **types II–IV** immunological injury. In non-type I allergies, symptoms may not appear immediately after a meal; diarrhea is an example. The variable timing and symptoms make medical evaluation and management of suspected food allergy complicated, especially because of the absence of definitive lab tests for all forms of food allergy. In the case of food allergy suspected to be caused by Types II–IV immunologic injury, supervised oral challenge is the gold standard in diagnosing the problem causing discomfort (Merras-Salmio). If adverse responses consistently follow ingestion of a particular food, providers should encourage food avoidance until proper testing confirms the origin of the symptoms. Providers should not propose extensive food avoidances without confirmatory testing, as avoidance of multiple protein sources may have adverse nutritional consequences.

There is a known relationship between allergic dermatitis (AD, also called eczema) and food allergy and this may extend into the teenage years. In Appendix A-1, we list a varity of mAbs under various commercial names, that are effective in reducing psoriatic dermitis. AD and food allergy are both associated with lower diversity in the infant's microbiome (Chapter 5) and dysbiosis in the skin microbiome. Many children with AD do not suffer from IgE-mediated type I hypersensitivity, but they clearly have a higher frequency of atopic allergy than those without AD symptoms. Allergy is a complex medical syndrome.

Figure 3.5 indicates that compared to the gut of Group II and III mammals, the human infant gut is nearly "closed" to the indiscriminate absorption of intact dietary protein. However, some low level of uptake may continue for 3 months postpartum, and it is normal for infants fed cow's milk to develop serum IgG and IgA antibodies to cow's milk proteins that they have ingested. These classes of antibodies do not constitute or indicate type I food allergy. In fact, if these involve SIgA antibodies, they might be protective in removing ingested cow's milk proteins from the GI tract, much in the same manner that SIgA binds and removes bacteria to the feces (Chapters 5 and 6; Figure 6.6). There is evidence that immune complexes involving food proteins are cleared more rapidly than proteins alone.

Food Intolerance

One syndrome that follows ingestion of certain foods is referred to as food protein-induced enterocolitis (FPIES; Agyemany, SR). In this syndrome, ongoing exposure to an offending food results in watery diarrhea and vomiting that may reflect type II–IV hypersensitivity. FPIES often presents in infancy and self-resolves in most school children. Food triggers vary. Common triggers in the United States include oats, rice, peanuts, and milk. The offending food is often connected to the diet of the community such as fish in Spain and Italy and grains in countries in which grains comprise a major portion of the diet. As with other types II–IV hypersensitivities, skin-prick tests are typically negative. FPIES is another syndrome that has made the definition of food allergy uncertain.

Gluten intolerance is a form of food intolerance that has an immunological element, but it is not mediated by type I immunologic injury. Rather, it is linked to a deficiency in the mucosal immune system. Gluten intolerance occurs in individuals with celiac disease (also known as gluten sensitive enteropathy) and in some cases it is associated with mucosal IgA deficiency. These individuals experience abdominal discomfort and diarrhea after ingestion of grains that contain the protein gluten (typically found in wheat, barley, and rye). Ongoing exposure leads to intestinal inflammation with leaky gut syndrome and GI tract dysbiosis, which better fits into the category of IBD (Chapter 5). Individuals suffering from this syndrome must carefully control their diet and give special attention to food labeling (see last section this chapter).

Food intolerance syndromes include insufficient production of the intestinal enzyme **lactase**, which might be mistaken for immune-based food allergy (Chapter 3). Lactase converts the disaccharide lactose (milk sugar) into the monosaccharides glucose and galactose, which are readily absorbed and metabolized (except in the rare exception of infants with **galactosemia**, described in Chapter 3). Individuals with low or absent lactase may suffer digestive discomfort after milk ingestion but will have negative skin-prick tests. Only about 15% of white children in the United States are affected, but approximately 90% of Asian and Native American children have persistently low levels of intestinal lactase after infancy, which improves with age. Congenital lactase deficiency (complete absence of lactase from birth) is a rare genetic disorder and contravenes feeding of lactose-containing foods in infancy.

Preventive Strategies

A frequent misconception surrounding food allergy is that the problem can be prevented by avoidance of potential food allergens in infancy; this was once recommended by the American Academy of Pediatrics. Based on careful trials, this avoidance strategy has now been largely dropped. The expert opinion in the field now favors intentional early introduction of allergenic foods in the weaning diet, reversing the earlier recommendations (Greer; Gupta). The European Academy of Allergy and Clinical Immunology has similarly revised their guidelines on the feeding of infants and supports early introduction of potential food allergens (Halken). These changes are supported by studies comparing Amish and Mennonite children (see Chapter 6) and more recently by controlled trials of early introduction of allergenic foods. The most frequently offending allergens are from peanuts, cow's milk, and eggs. These are not uncommon allergies; for instance, the incidence of type I allergy to cow's milk in infants is 3% in America (Sicherer, SR).

The best preventive strategy to avoid food allergy and other neonatal disorders involving infectious disease is **breast-feeding** (Figure 8.3). Mothers who can breastfeed are also less reliant on infant formulas that can encounter supply chain and contamination issues. However, in situations in which breast-feeding is not an option (Chapter 3) cow's milk–based formulas are commonly used (Chapter 4). Type I allergy to cow's milk can involve production of IgE to β-lactoglobulin, a protein not found in human milk, and to caseins more prevalent in cow's milk (Table 3.1). Efforts to provide cow's milk lacking β-lactoglobulin and certain caseins have utilized CRISPR (Appendix A-1) to engineer cows that do not produce β-lactoglobulin and certain caseins (Appendix A-2). Clinical trials involving early introduction of food allergens are ongoing and may provide additional recommendations for feeding regimens within the Critical Window. There is also a familial/genetic linkage between allergic dermatitis and food allergy. When this allergic tendency is known to be a family trait, breast-feeding is recommended.

Food Allergies in Other Mammals

Food allergies and intolerance are not limited to humans. In the field of veterinary medicine, dogs are prone to allergic reactions to their food, which often includes ingredients that are foreign to the normal diet of most carnivores. Symptoms may include excessive scratching or diarrhea. Perhaps humans are causing this problem in their carnivorous pets by failing to recognize their difficulty in adapting to a food source that is unnatural to them. It might be valuable to know if this syndrome is proportionally higher in dogs and cats in developed countries, as seems to be the case for allergies in humans.

Synopsis and Conclusions

There are many reasons why individuals might reproducibly become uncomfortable after eating certain foods. We have learned much about the immune mechanisms responsible for food allergy in the last 40 years, and we hope to soon understand the mechanism of food intolerance syndromes for which we have inadequate understanding. In the meantime, practitioners will continue to hear the term **allergy** in the common, nontechnical language patients use for symptoms having nothing to do with immune-mediated food reactions. Thus, in lay usage, "food allergy" becomes an umbrella term for digestive discomfort that follows a meal. Healthcare practitioners treating "food allergy" symptoms must carefully inquire about symptoms and rely on available clinical testing before opening this "can of worms." Cow's milk and other food allergies are complex, as is their association with other atopic disorders. For a summary of reasonable size, students, neonatal providers, and counselors are recommended to a set of brief review articles contained in the free *Journal of Allergy and Clinical Immunology* issue on food allergies.[1]

---

1 "Food Allergies." *Journal of Allergy and Clinical Immunology.* 2018; 141(1): 1–81. https://www.jacionline. org/issue/S0091-6749(17)X0015-8.

Human Health and Dietary Supplementation in Food Animals

Another potential concern of adults and children is the transfer of hormones, antibiotics, and other supplements added to food animal diets. Hormones, both naturally occurring and synthetic (eg, steroids like estradiol, progesterone and testosterone) have been used in beef cattle as growth promoters (Jeong). Concerns about their transfer in the food chain are not supported by studies in humans, since estradiol given orally is quickly metabolized in humans. When given by IV, bioavailability is approximately 5% (Kuhnz) and synthetic estrogen directly injected into 19-day fetal mice causes teratology in some newborns (Henry). However 7,000 infants whose mothers took oral contraceptives while pregnant showed no teratogenic effects (Rothman). The residual amount of estradiol in the meat of treated cattle was 1,000-fold lower than the amount produced daily by humans (Jeong). Similar results apply to testosterone and progesterone, although both may accumulate in adipose tissue. Tylosin phosphate is a medical drug approved for use in beef cattle to reduce the incidence of liver abscesses caused by *Fusobacterium necrophorum* and *Arcanobacterium (Actinomyces) pyogenes*, but the consequence of its transfer to humans is unclear. As a safeguard, a veterinary feed directive (VFD) indicates that the use of medicated food containing a medically relevant drug be permitted only under the professional supervision of a licensed veterinarian and in accordance with a valid VFD. Some feed additives, such as lasalocid, monensin, bacitracin, bambermycin, and amprolium, are not considered "medically important" and do not fall under the VFD.

Of greatest concern are antibiotics added to animal feeds (see the **STAT** program discussed earlier in this chapter and in Chapter 6). The concern with STAT is not transfer to humans but the impact on MDR bacteria.

Misconceptions About Food Labeling

The labels on foods raise questions among consumers that healthcare practitioners are sometimes expected to address. It is common practice for supermarkets to use labels like "organic" for fruits and vegetables, "cage-free" for eggs, and "grass-fed" for beef. Any or all these labels may be confusing to consumers and require clarification. Guidelines for use of the term *organic* include several categories and these are treated in documents on the National Organic Program (NOP) website: https://www.ams.usda.gov/rules-regulations/organic. These and related guidelines are under the control of the Agricultural Marketing Service of the USDA (the latter sets the regulations and maintains oversight). Any marketing claims for food products must be approved by the Process Verification Program (PVP). Marketers must make an application and, if approved, compliance is verified by a third-party verification service. The website https://www.ams.usda.gov/services/auditing/process-verified-programs provides an overview of the PVP program. A more in-depth look at the various regulations and guidelines lies outside the scope of this textbook. Here we provide simple answers to questions concerning labels like "organic," to which healthcare trainees and practitioners may be asked to respond. We take no position on this issue and reserve it for those who wrote the rules.

1. In its purist form, *antibiotic free* means "no antibiotic ever." Neither AGP nor therapeutic antibiotics have been used in producing the product, whether meat, fish or eggs.
2. *Antibiotic free* might also refer to "no unsafe residues." This means that regardless of treatment of the product, no hormones or antibiotic residues are present at the time of marketing. Marketing a product without PVP approval is illegal. For example, cows that develop mastitis (recognized by "chunks" or "gargets" that appear in their milk and have a high somatic cell count) are often treated with antibiotics that can clear the infection. However, before milk from such treated animals can again be sold, it must be shown to contain no antibiotic residue.
3. *Free-range beef* means cows have all-year outside access and obtain at least 30% of their dry food from grazing. This was assumed by the public to be normal for beef cattle until "feedlots" and Kobe beef (from Japan) appeared.
4. As regards eggs, *free-range* only means the hens have access to the outside and *cage-free* means they are free to leave their cages, nothing more.
5. According to the National Organic Program (NOP), the term *organic*, when applied to eggs or other products, covers a broad range that includes many of the categories mentioned above (see consumer-friendly, https://www.ams.usda.gov/sites/default/files/media/NOP_Behind The Searl.pdf). In general, it means that animals were raised on an organic diet that did not include antibiotics or hormones. The term *antibiotic free* is the same as described in points 1 and 2 above. This also implies that dairy animals have been organically managed since the beginning of the last third of gestation. Cows requiring antibiotics to treat illness are not returned to the milking herd. *Organic* also means maintaining specific living conditions, including access to pasture for ruminants and access to the outside; direct sunlight, fresh air, and freedom of movement for all livestock; and the practice of preventive healthcare to minimize occurrence and spread of diseases and parasites.

Summary

We believe it is important for healthcare students, practitioners, and the public to be aware of misconceptions and controversies that may impact events that occur in the Critical Window of Development. The information we have presented may not agree with that channeled through the media and especially through social media. Citizens of developed Western countries are being continually exposed to promotional products by pharmaceutical firms, changes in food processing, and additives that raise health concerns. We encourage students and other readers to seek the most accurate biological and medical information. The suggested readings below, continuing education programs, and peer-reviewed publications, are good places to start. While environmental changes continue, medical practice is undergoing similar changes due to a better understanding of medical science and due to advances in molecular biology and bioengineering that offer an opportunity to address diseases in a manner never before possible.

Suggested Readings (SR)

Agyemang A, Nowak-Wegrzyn A. 2019 Food protein-induced enterocolitis syndrome: A comprehensive review. *Ann Rev Allergy Immunol.* 2019;57:261–271.

Blaser MJ. *Missing microbes: How the overuse of antibiotics is fueling our modern plagues.* New York: Picador; 2014.

Gibson MK, Crofts TS, Dantas G. Antibiotics and the developing infant gut microbiome. *Curr Opin Microbiol.* 2015;27:51–56.

Scientific misinformation: A perfect storm, missteps and moving forward. *Cell.* 2021;184:1402–1406.

Sicherer SC, Sampson HA. Food allergy: A review and update on epidemiology, pathogenesis, diagnosis, prevention, and management. *J Allergy Clin Immunol.* 2018;141:41–58.

Sookoian S, Fernández Gianotti T, Burgueño AL, Pirola CJ. Fetal metabolic programming and epigenetic modifications: A systems biology approach. *Ped Research.* 2013;73:531–542.

Taylor IE, Swerdfeger AL, Eslick GD. Vaccines are not associated with autism: Evidenced-based meta-analysis of case-control and cohort studies. *Vaccine.* 2014;32:3623–3629.

References

Arrieta M-C, Stiemsma LT, Dimitriu PA, et al. Early infancy microbial and metabolic alterations affect risk of childhood asthma. *Sci Transl Med.* 2015;7:307 ra 152. doi:10.1126/scitranslmed.aab2271.

Azimi P, Keshavarz Z, Guillermo J, Laurent C, Allen JG. Estimating the nationwide transmission risk of measles in US schools and impacts of vaccination and supplemental infection control strategies. *BMC Infect Dis.* 2020;20:497. doi:10.1186/s12879-020-05200-6.

Bearson BL, Allen HK, Brunelle BW, Soo Lee I, Casjens SR, Stanton TB. The agricultural antibiotic carbodox induces phage-mediated gene transfer in *Salmonella. Front Immunol.* 2014;5:52. doi:10.3389/fmicr.2014.00052.

Bliss E. *On Immunity: An Inoculation.* Minneapolis, MN: Graywolf Press; 2015.

Carrillo-Sentisteve P, Lopalco PL. Measles still spreads in Europe: Who is responsible for the failure to vaccinate? *Clin Microbiol Infect.* 2012;18(Suppl. 5):50–56.

Cross G, Ho JSY, Zacharas W, Jeyasekharan AD, Marazzi I. Emergency drug use in a pandemic: Harsh lessons from COVID-19. *Cell.* 2021;184:5487-5500.

Dube E, Gagnon D, MacDonald NE, et al. Strategies intended to address vaccine hesitancy: Review of published reviews. *Vaccine.* 2015;33:4191–4203.

Feemster KA, Szipsky C. Resurgence of measles in the United States: How did we get here? *Curr Opin Pediatr.* 2020;32:139–144.

Greer FR, Sicherer SH, Burks AW, and AAP Committee on Nutrition. The effects of early nutritional interventions on the development of atopic disease in infants and children: The role of maternal dietary restriction, breastfeeding, hydrolyzed formulas, and timing of introduction of allergenic complementary foods. *Pediatrics.* 2019;143:e20190281. doi:10.1542/peds.2019-0281.

Gupta M, Sicherer SH. Timing of food introduction and atopy prevention. *Clin Dermatol.* 2017;35:398–405.

Hagan T, Cortese M, Rouphael N, et al. Antibiotic-driven gut microbiome perturbation alters immunity to vaccines in humans. *Cell.* 2019;178:1312–1328.

Halken S, Muraro A, de Silva D, et al. EAACI guideline: Preventing the development of food allergy in infants and young children (2020 update). *Ped Allergy Immunol.* 2021;32:843–858. doi:10.1111/pai.13496.

Hayase E, Hayase T, Jamal MA, et al. Mucus-degrading Bacteroides link carbapenems to aggravated graft-versus-host disease. *Cell.* 2022;185:3705–3719.

Henry EC, Miller RK, Baggs RB. Direct fetal injection of diethystillbestrol and 17 beta-estradial: a method for investigation their teratogenicity. *Teratology* 1984; 2:297–304.

Hernández MI, Mericq V. Metabolic syndrome in children born small-for-gestation age. *Arq Bras Endocrinol Metab.* 2011;55:583–589.

Jensen HH, Hayes DJ. Impact of Denmark's ban on antimicrobials for growth promotion. *Curr Opin Microbiol.* 2014;19:30-36. Doi:10.1016/j.m.b.2014.05.020.

Jeong S-H, Kang D, Lim M-W, Kang CS, Jung HH J Risk assessment of growth hormones and antimicrobial residues in meat. Toxicol Res. 2010; 26:301–313

Key N, McBride WD. Sub-therapeutic antibiotics and the efficiency of U.S. hog farms. *Amer J Ag Econ.* 2014;96(3):831–850. doi:10.1093/ajac/aat091.

Kuhnz W, Gansau C, Mahler M. Pharmocokinetics of estradial, free and total estrone, in young women following single intraveneous and oral administration of 17 beta-estradial *Arzemittelforchung* 1993; 43:966–973.

Link-Gelles R, Lutterloh E, Schnabel Ruppert P, et al. Public Health Response to a Case of Paralytic Poliomyelitis in an Unvaccinated Person and Detection of Poliovirus in Wastewater—New York, June–August 2022. *MMWR Morb Mortal Wkly Rep* 2022;71:1065–1068. DOI: http://dx.doi.org/10.15585/mmwr.mm7133e2

Lopez BS. Controlling infectious diseases in animal agriculture: The best offense may be a good defense. *ImmunoHorizons.* 2022;6:730–740.

MacDonald JM, Wang S-L. Foregoing sub-therapeutic antibiotics: The impact of broiler grow-out operations. *Appl Econ Perspect Pol.* 2011;33(1):79–98.

Mata L. Diarrheal disease as a cause of malnutrition. *Am J Trop Med Hyg.* 1992;47(Suppl. 1): 16–27.

McFarland LV. From yaks to yogurt: The history, development and current use of probiotics. *Clin Inf Dis.* 2015;60 (Supp. 2):S85–90. doi10.1093/cid/civ054.

Merras-Salmio L, Kolho K-L, Pelkonen AS, et al. Markers of mucosal inflammation and cow's milk specific immunoglobulins in non-IgE cow's milk allergy. *Clin Transl Allergy.* 2014;4:8. doi:10.1186/2045-7022-4-8.

Panagiotopoulos T, Antoniadou I, Valassi-Adam E. Increase in congenital rubella after immunisation in Greece: Retrospective survey and systematic review. *BMJ.* 1999;319:1462–1467.

Penders J, Thijs C, Vink C, et al. Factors influencing the composition of the intestinal microbiota in early infancy. *Pediatrics.* 2006;118:511–521.

Phadke VK, Bednarczyk RA, Salmon DA, Omer SB. Association between vaccine refusal and vaccine-preventable diseases in the United States: A review of measles and pertussis. *JAMA.* 2016;315:1149–1158.

Prescott SL. Role of dietary immunomodulatory factors in the development of immune tolerance In: Brandtzaeg P, Isolauri E, Prescott SL, eds. *Nutrition and Immunological Homeostasis.* Switzerland: S. Karger AG; 2009:185–200.

Rothman KJ, Louik C Oral contraceptives and birth defects. *N. Engl J. Med.* 1978; 210:522–524

Shepersky L, Marin M, Zhang J, Pham H, Marlow MA. Mumps in vaccinated children and adolescents: 2007–2019. *Pediatrics.* 2021;148(6):e2021051873. doi:10.1542/peds.2021-051873.

Slashinski MJ, McCurdy SA, Achenbaun LS, Whitney SN, McGuire AL. "Snake oil," "quack medicine," and "industrially cultured organisms": Bivalves and the commercialization of human microbiome research. *BMC Med Ethics.* 2012;13:28. doi:10.1186/1472-6939-13-28.

Snesrud E, He S, Chandler M, et al. A model for transportation of the colistin resistance gene mcr-1 by ISApl1. *Antimicrob Agent and Chemo.* 2016;60:6973-6976.

Spoor LE, McAdam PR, Weinert LA, et al. Livestock origin for a human pandemic clone of community-associated Methicillin-resistant *Staphylococcus aureus.*mBio. 2013;4(4). doi:10.1128/mBio.00356-13.

Sprenger M, Fukuda K. New mechanism, new worries. *Science.* 2016;351:1263–1264.

Suda KJ, Hicks LA, Roberts RM, Hunkler RJ, Taylor TH. Trends and seasonal variation in outpatient antibiotic prescription rates in United States, 2006 to 2010. *Antimicrob Agents Chemother.* 2014;58:2763–2766.

Ullrich V. *Hitler; Downfall 1939–1945.* New York: Penguin Random House; 2020.

Zmora N, Zilberman-Schapira G, Suez J, et al. Personalized gut mucosal colonization resistance to empiric probiotics is associated with unique host and microbiome features. *Cell.* 2018;174:1385–1405.

Acknowledgments

The authors thank the following individuals for their review of this chapter and for providing critical information, especially regarding antibiotics such as AGP in animals and food labeling.

Marcus Kehrli Director, National Animal Disease Center, Ames, Iowa

Gary Onan Professor, College of Agriculture, University of Wisconsin-River Falls

David Gerleman Emeritus professor, University of Iowa College of Medicine

Figure Credits

Fig. 8.1: Charles Janeway et al., Immunobiology: The Immune System in Health and Disease, p. 34. Copyright © 2005 by Taylor & Francis Group.

Fig. 8.2: Adapted from Varun K. Phadke et al., "Association Between Vaccine Refusal and Vaccine-Preventable Diseases in the United States: A Review of Measles and Pertussis," JAMA, vol. 315, no. 11, p. 18. Copyright © 2016 by American Medical Association.

Fig. 8.3: Adapted from Leonardo Mata, "Diarrheal Disease as a Cause of Malnutrition," The American Journal of Tropical Medicine and Hygiene, vol. 47, no. 1. Copyright © 1992 by American Journal of Tropical Medicine and Hygiene.

Appendix A-1
Molecular Genetics, Biotechnology, and Bioengineering

Introduction

The major concepts in microbiology, immunology, and developmental biology featured in Chapters 1–8 arose from research in molecular and cellular biology that was heavily dependent on biotechnology. Instead of providing **learning objectives** and suggested readings (SR), in the appendices we cite the primary literature and reviews. In this appendix, we review basic and molecular genetics, the immunogenetics of adaptive immunity, and additional information on pattern recognition receptors of innate immunity. We also survey the methods employed in biotechnology and bioengineering. Finally, we review the advances made in vaccine development.

The Gene: Concept, Molecular Basis, and Mutations

Knowledge that traits were inherited and could be passed on to offspring was recognized at least 10,000 years ago by early humans, who domesticated and crossbred wild animals (Chapter 1). Throughout Eurasia, selection turned the feared wolf into the dog, while in the North, the Artic Wolf became the Alaskan malamute, a skilled seal-hunting companion and later a powerful "wheel dog" on sled teams that distributed life-saving vaccine. Further breeding and selection resulted in more than 150 dog breeds, some selected to be herders, others hunting partners, some guards and service dogs, some sniffer and rescue dogs, and others just companions. We have learned that many of the differences (**phenotypes**) among dog breeds lies with differences in gene expression, not actual changes to the genome. Farmers and animal scientists have selected animals based on phenotype to develop sheep with the best wool, cattle that produce the most milk and the best beef steaks, and swine that have larger litters and grow faster and more efficiently. The ritual of phenotype selection is played out each year at county fairs in agricultural states across America.

Domestication was a two-way agreement: food for service. Wolves no longer had to hunt for food and domesticated ruminants received a steady diet in return for milk, wool, and meat. Developing human societies obviously knew that certain traits were desirable while others were not, and they soon learned that phenotype could be controlled by breeding and selection.

It was not until the monk Gregor Mendel in Brno started experimenting by cross-pollinating peas that the idea emerged that inheritance must be controlled by certain packets of information transferred during reproduction. These packets began to be called genes; *Gen* is German for "germ of life." Some packets were more important than others (dominant) while offspring needed to inherit a larger amount of recessive genes or multiple genes for some traits to be expressed (ie, to show a certain phenotype). As biology progressed there was increasing interest in the cellular and molecular basis of these genes. During and after WWII, the Noble Laureate Linus Pauling believed that certain proteins controlled the code of life. Rosalind Franklin was the first to crystalize the biomolecule called deoxy-nucleic acid (DNA), found in the nucleus of eukaryotes, though it is also free in the cells of prokaryotes that lack a nucleus. Two biologists, James Watson and Francis Crick, with help of others, seized on her work and proposed the structure of DNA that we now understand as the molecular basis for the genetic control of all life forms. For this Watson and Crick shared the Noble Prize. Sadly, Rosalind Franklin did not share the prize, because she died before the prize was given, but some believe it was because in the early 1950s it was still a man's world. Perhaps Helen Reddy's "I Am a Woman" or the writing of Margaret Rossiter on the "Matilda Effect" brings this into focus.

The fascinating story of discovery is described in the entertaining 1955 book *The Double Helix*. Four different nucleotides, strung together like beads, formed each strand of the

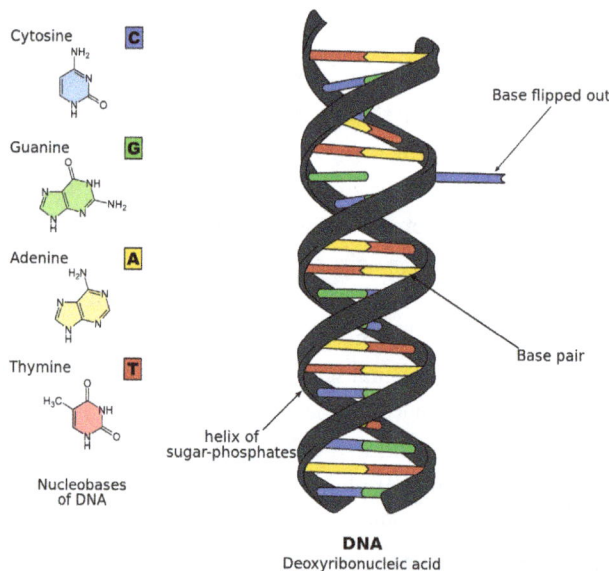

Figure A1.1A The DNA double helix and complementary nucleotide base pairing. The color-coding of nucleotide (left) then applies to the colored bars within the helix on the right. The sugar-phosphate backbone is shown as a dark ribbon. The flipped out base refers to one altered by radiation or chemically modified (see Figure A1.2).

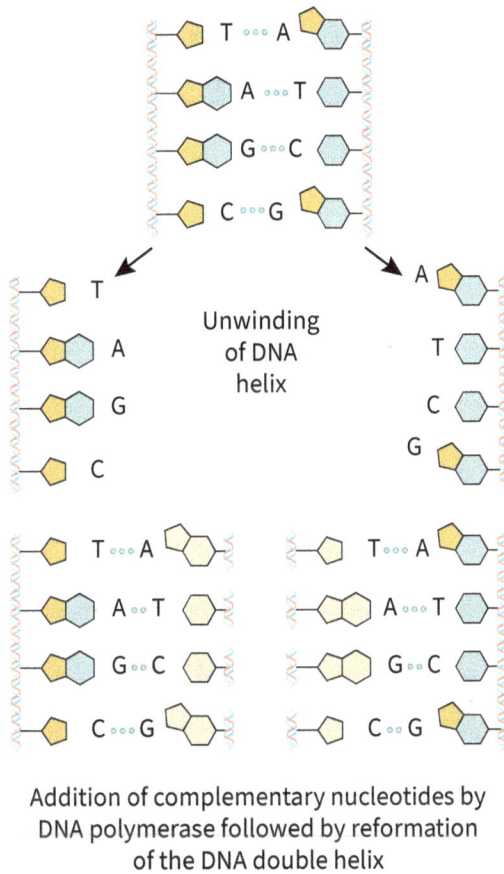

Addition of complementary nucleotides by
DNA polymerase followed by reformation
of the DNA double helix

Figure A1.1B   Nuclear events in cell division (mitosis). As life forms grow, repair, or reproduce, they duplicate their DNA. In prokaryotes this is the only means of reproduction so that by depending on mitosis, each daughter cell (or new offspring) is genetically identical to the parent cell. Figure A1.5A illustrates the pairing of complementary nucleotide bases. T = thymine, A = adenine, G = guanine, and C = cytosine. When the DNA helix (see Figure A1.1A) unwinds and complementary strands separate, DNA polymerases act and their complementary nucleotides are added, which results in replicating the original DNA. The strands then refold into the double helix form of DNA, as illustrated in Figure A1.1A.

double helix, and their exact order provided the "code of life" or genetic code. Each nucleotide is paired by hydrogen bonding: guanine with cytosine by three hydrogen bonds and adenine with thymidine by two hydrogen bonds, G-C and A-T, respectively. They are referred to as base pairs (bp; Figures A1.1A and A1.1B). Each nucleotide sequence of three (a triplet called a *codon*) is responsible for telling the metabolic machinery of the cell to select a transfer RNA (tRNA) linked to a defined amino acid. These amino acids are arranged in the same sequence as the DNA codons to yield a particular polypeptide chain. These are the building blocks for proteins that form the backbone of all life forms. Table A1.1 provides examples of how these triplet codons specify the synthesis of particular amino acids in a polypeptide chain.

TABLE A1.1 Example of the Amino Acids Specified by Each Triplet of Nucleotides in Genomic DNA

The code shown is based on inclusion of the first two nucleotides in the codon. When considering all three codons, some translations to amino acids will differ. Those with more interest in codons can consult Wikipedia. STOP codons means that translation cannot procede and the encoded gene product cannot be made.

Codon Table					
Second Position					
First Position	**T**	**C**	**A**	**G**	Third Position
T	TTT TTC Phe / TTA TTG Leu	TCT TCC TCA TCG Ser	TAT TAC Tyr / TAA STOP / TAG STOP	TGT TGC Cys / TGA STOP / TGG Trp	T C A G
C	CTT CTC CTA CTG Leu	CCT CCC CCA CCG Pro	CAT CAC His / CAA CAG Gin	CGT CGC CGA CGG Arg	T C A G
A	ATT ATC ATA Ile / ATG Met	ACT ACC ACA ACG Thr	AAT AAC Asn / AAA AAG Lys	AGT AGC Ser / AGA AGG Arg	T C A G
G	GTT GTC GTA GTG Val	TTT TTC TTA TTG Ala	GAT GAC Asp / GAA GAG Glu	GGT GGC GGA GGG Gly	T C A G

The helical chains of nucleic acids (DNA) found in the nucleus are compacted into structures called **chromosomes**, structures previously known to microscopists. The number of these chromosomes and the content of each is species dependent but does not necessarily correlate with the complexity of the organism. Humans have 23 pairs, dogs 78, fruit flies 8, cotton 52, garlic 16, mosquitoes 6, earthworms 36, hedgehogs 90, goats 60, tigers 38, carp 100, and mulberries 308. However, Eubacteria and Archaea (Chapter 1) have only one circular chromosome. Chromosomes collectively archive what is called the **genome** of an organism.

Genome size is not strictly correlated with ecological dependency or organism complexity; an onion has more DNA than a human. The minimum genome size needed to sustain a free-living existence, such as that of the Archaea (Chapter 1) appears to be around 1,500 genes. The genome of Eubacteria is small since they are parasites or symbionts (Chapter 1) and depend on nutrients provided by their complex free-living hosts. While parasitic Eubacteria can survive with 500 genes, unicellular eukaryotes like *Paramecium* or *Amoeba* require 5,000, simple multicellular eukaryotes like fruit flies need 13,000, higher plants approximately 25,000, and complex vertebrates like humans approximately 22,000.

Eubacteria and Archaea have no nuclei; their chromosomes are circular and are tethered to the cell membrane. The organization of genes in the genome of prokaryotes also differs from that of eukaryotes. In bacteria, genes are aligned end-to-end in uninterrupted fashion, so a physical map of a bacterial genome matches the peptide map they encode (ie, they are co-linear). In eukaryotes, the coding gene sequences are called **exons**; these are interrupted by non-coding sequences called **introns**. The proportion of non-coding DNA introns increases with the degree of multicellularity (Table A1.2). The origin and function of introns is not totally clear. Some may represent portions of viral/bacteriophage DNA that became integrated through the action of **intergrases** (see next section). Some may serve as sites for binding regulatory factors that control the expression of adjacent genes. We know that epithelial cells in the GI tract (enterocytes) share the same chromosomal DNA as cells in the liver, but at each site different genes are expressed. We described in Chapter 1 how the behavior of different dog breeds was the result of differential gene expression, often called **epigenetics.** If non-coding DNA is involved in gene regulation, it suggests that regulation of gene expression increases with genome size and multicellularity (Table A1.2).

The role of non-coding DNA has been best studied in bacterial and viral molecular genetics. Figure A1.3 provides an example of a cassette in the DNA of a plasmid that includes non-coding **promoter** and **repressor** DNA segments that regulate the expression of downstream structural genes within the cassette. The repressor segment also goes under the name **operator**.

Not all of the genes in eukaryotes are found in the nucleus. Another ~1% are present in organelles such as mitochondria and in the chloroplasts of plants. Those in chloroplasts account for less than 50 genes, but more like 12–16

Spontaneous deamination changes a base

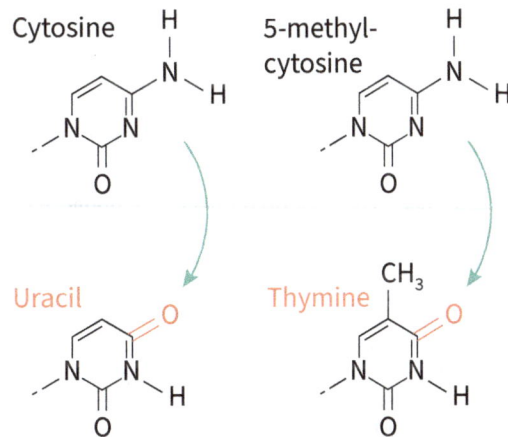

Figure A1.2   The action of activation-induced cytosine deaminase (AID) in nucleotide mutations.

in mitochondria. These are arranged in circular form like in bacteria and they also lack introns (Figure A1.4). Those in mitochondria largely encode the cytochromes and other proteins involved in the respiratory role of this organelle. Notably, some mitochondrial genes are associated with severe neuromuscular disorders (Cruz-Zaragoza). These genes of mitochondria are highly conserved and therefore they are often used to study phylogenic lineages. The origin of mitochondria is a topic in itself. It is hypothesized that mitochondria and phagolysosomes were acquired from some former free-living unicellular life forms and collectively packaged within a cell (plasma) membrane. However, there are alternative hypotheses that argue this is not true.

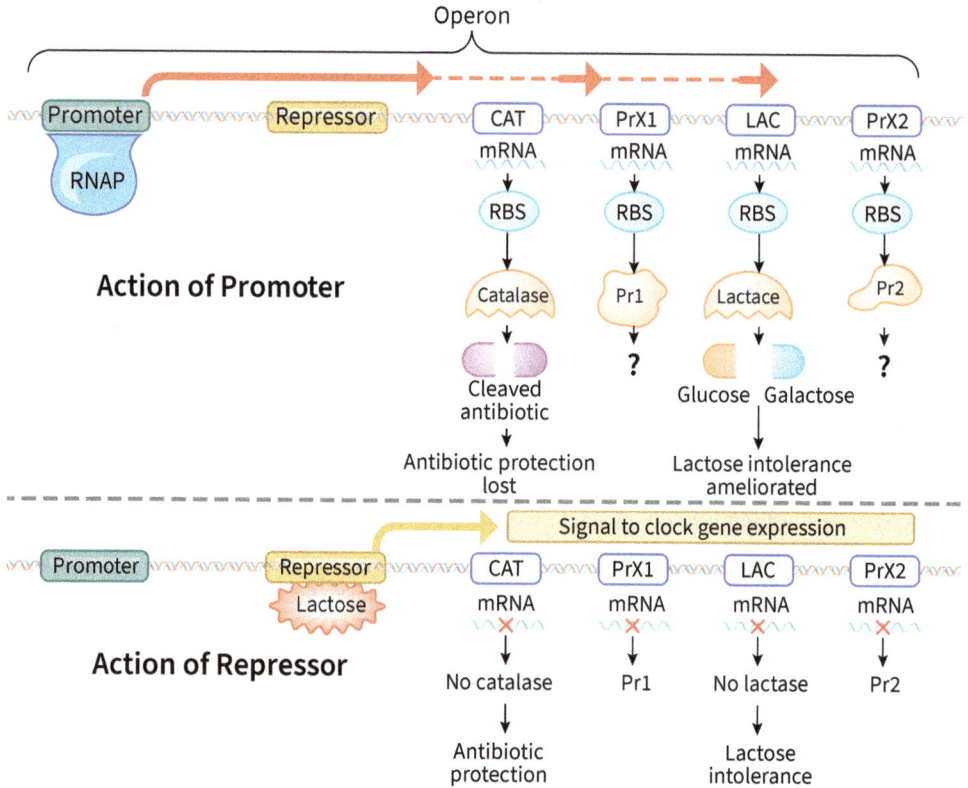

Figure A1.3 Non-coding regulatory genomic segments control gene expression. Ribonucleo-proteins (RNAP) act on non-coding promoter sequences, which promote expression of down-stream genes in the operon cassette. In this model the focus is on the CAT gene, which encodes catalase that can cleave antibiotics that are used to control pathogenic bacteria, the LAC gene, which encodes lactase that cleaves lactose and ameliorates "lactose intolerance" (Chapters 3 and 8). However, if lactose, present in ruminant milks, binds to the non-coding repressor element of the operon, catalase is not produced, the antibiotic is not cleaved, and antibiotic protection continues. The repression of LAC gene expression essentially results in lactose intolerance. In this model CAT could represent an antibiotic resistance (AR) gene; see Chapter 6. Noteworthy is that promotion and repression can have opposite effects on human health.

TABLE A1.2   The Proportion of DNA in the Genomes of Different Life Forms That Occupies Introns and Is Not Used to Encode Proteins

Life Form	Mean (%)	Range (%)
Prokaryotes	12	7–19
Protozoans	38	27–52
Fungi and Plants	68	62–72
Invertebrates	81	73–90
Chordates	86	84–88
Vertebrates	88	83–92
Humans	97	96–98

Gene Replication, Spontaneous Mutation, and Genome Change

The survival of a species depends on its ability to replicate its genes during reproduction or when tissues are repaired. Figure A1.1B illustrates how one polynucleotide strand is used as the template for the formation of the new strand. This process is mediated by the enzyme DNA polymerase. It is during this somewhat error-prone replication process that DNA's genetic code is most vulnerable to alteration. This occurs when one of the four nucleotides used to build the DNA backbone is chemically altered (Figure A1.1A). For example, cytosine can be de-aminated to become uracil, or after de-amination it can be methylated to become thymidine using the enzyme **activation-induced cytosine deaminase** (AID; Figure A1.2). We mentioned AID when discussing somatic hypermutation in B lymphocytes (Chapter 6). Fortunately, cells have a "fix-it" gene-editing system consisting of DNA repair enzymes that carry out their mission thousands of times per day and repair 99% of DNA replication errors. Were it not for these repair mechanisms, the genome and genetic code would be highly unstable. The few uncorrected errors are called **spontaneous mutations** and they occur in bacteria and in eukaryotes at a rate of ~10^{-9} per base pair (bp) per generation, although as shown in Figure 6.2 the rate can be higher in some viruses. Also, as described in Chapter 6, the number of spontaneous mutations that accumulate in a genome depends on its size, so a genome of 1,000 bp (approximately 300 genes) could accumulate 10^{-6} mutations per generation, and in humans over 70 times more. Since these only accumulate during reproduction (ie, DNA replication), the rate of DNA replication must be considered, which ranges from minutes for a virus to an hour for a bacterium and up to 13 years for humans. Consider also that a spontaneous mutation in the genome of 300 genes is much more likely to have a phenotypic effect than a genome that is 70 times greater. This can explain differences in the rate of phenotypic change among different life forms. Using this scenario, bacteria can "change their spots" 1,000 times faster than humans, and some viruses may do it a million times faster. We presented this concept in Chapter 6 to explain the evolutionary appearance of the adaptive immune system as a means of combating rapid genomic and phenotypic changes in disease-causing microbes.

In addition to the relatively similar rate of spontaneous mutation in bacteria and Eukaryotes during gene replication, there are also mutations induced by environmental agents that cause chemical changes in nucleotides (Figure A1.1A) that alter the genetic code (Table A1.1). Two of the best known are UV light and ionizing γ-radiation such as that released from a nuclear bomb and other natural and man-made activities. These changes primarily alter genes in somatic cells that regulate cell proliferation and can cause malignancies, as occurred in Japan in 1945 and at Chernobyl in 1986. Melanoma or skin cancer can be caused by UV light, especially in fair-skinned individuals in the Northern Hemisphere. Populations native to equatorial regions with darker pigmentation are protected against UV light, and this is believed to be one of the factors responsible for the lower frequency of skin cancer in certain ethnic groups. Since UV radiation is also needed to convert vitamin D, those living in northern or extreme southern regions, where sunbathing is limited to a short period, have lost their protective melanin in return for the capacity to convert vitamin D. However, these individuals place themselves in harm's way should they relocate to the beaches of

Florida or Southern California. Furthermore, the incidence of somatic and genomic muta-tion appears to increase with age while the ability to repair DNA decreases (Vijg; Kennedy)

GENETICS

Phenotype vs. genotype: The genotype represents the potential to express a certain trait encoded in the genome while the phenotype means what is expressed.

Allele: A genetic variant of a gene. There can be many for any one gene, but one genome can only accommodate two—one of maternal and the other of paternal origin.

Genetic signature and alleles: a/a = homozygous for the gene or trait; both parents have contributed the same allelic variant to the offspring's genome. a/b = heterozygous for the gene; each allele is different. -/a = one allele is a nonfunctional mutant. -/- = both alleles are nonfunctional mutants, also called a "double knockout."

Mitosis vs. meiosis: Mitosis is replication of the genomic DNA (Figure A1.1B), while meiosis is replication of the DNA after the chromosomal DNA from the ovum and sperm have interacted, which typically involves an exchange of alleles (Figure A1.5B). Meiosis is the molecular basis of sexual reproduction and diversification of the genomic repertoire.

Spontaneous vs. somatic mutation: Spontaneous mutations occur at nearly the same slow rate in bacteria and Eukaryotes as a result of errors that can occur during DNA replication during mitosis (A1.1B), including in gametic cells, and therefore are transmitted to the offspring. Somatic mutations occur during the lifetime of an individual but rarely involves gametic cells in eukaryotes. Therefore, these are not transferred to the offspring during reproduction.

Somatic hypermutation (SHM): A form of somatic mutation that is very rapid and occurs during the gene rearrangements needed to form mature B cells and T cell receptors. The result is affinity maturation, or the making of a "better" antibody (see Chapter 6). These spontaneous changes are not transmitted during reproduction (Figures A1.10 and A1.11). Each individual starts using an unaltered inherited genome.

Reproduction and Diversification of the Genome

The DNA replication illustrated in Figure A1.1B occurs each time a cell divides. This division is called **mitosis** and it constitutes the major means of reproduction for bacteria. In organisms that reproduce by mitosis only, offspring are identical to their parents. Nevertheless, the genome of these prokaryotes does not remain constant, since they rapidly accumulate spontaneous and environmentally induced mutations, and their rapid rate of reproduction allows greater opportunity for genome change (Figure 6.2). In addition to mutations, bacteria have other means of altering their genetics, which involves sharing genetic information without reproduction. Three different processes used by bacteria are depicted in Figure A1.4, all of which take the name **horizontal gene transfer** (HGT). HGT was generally believed to be restricted to prokaryotic organisms (Chapter 1), but recent evidence indicates it can occur in plants, insects, bacteria, and eukaryotes (Li et al., 2022). One mechanism of HGT, also mentioned in Chapters 1 and 5, involves the cell-to-cell transfer of small packets of circular DNA in what are called **plasmids** during a process called *conjugation*. These represent a type of episome (Figure A1.4). HGT can explain how virulence genes can transform a benign commensal *E. coli* into an intestinal pathogen. When broadly applied, epigenesis involves genes that lie outside the chromosomal genome but also includes regulatory element found in introns (Figure A1.3) that alter the chemistry of genomic nucleotides. This occurs, for example, in methylation, which can alter gene expression without altering the genetic code (Figure A1.2). In all science, there are "lumpers and splitters.", so some may make finer distinctions than those we describe in this textbook.

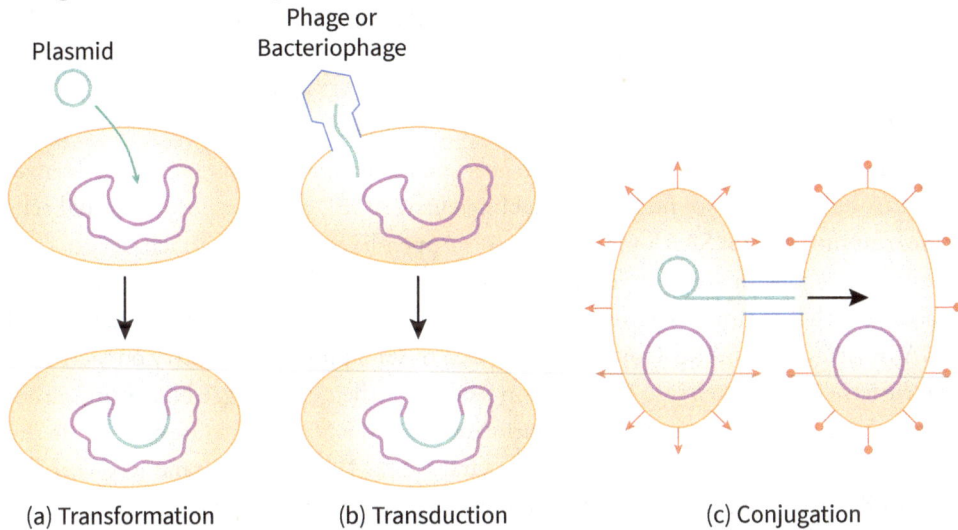

(a) Transformation   (b) Transduction   (c) Conjugation

Figure A1.4. Horizontal gene transfer (HGT) is a means whereby the genome of bacteria can change without mutation. Three processes are recognized: transformation, transduction, and conjugation. We have frequently referred to *conjugation*, in which a circular chromosome (green circle depicting a plasmid) is transferred from one bacterium to another after side-by-side enjoinment. Plasmids of unknown origin (green circle) can also enter a bacterium and their DNA (green) can become incorporated into the chromosomal DNA of the bacteria (see green insertion) a process called *transformation*. Foreign DNA can also be introduced by a bacteriophage (blue hexagon) and their DNA (green) can become part of the bacterial genome in a process called *transduction*.

Modern molecular geneticists have taken full advantage of plasmids in bioengineering in what is generically called **bacterial transformation**, which we will later discuss in the section on bioengineering. Figure A1.4 illustrates that by transduction genetic information can also be transferred by insertion of bacteriophages, a name for viruses that infect bacteria. This phenomenon (transduction) will again be mentioned in the section on bioengineering. Naked DNA can also be transferred, the origin of the original term "transformation" (Figure A1.4).

In eukaryotes, information can also be transferred using **exosomes**. Exosomes are tiny vesicles that contain lipids, chemokines, and RNA. These are distinct from structures like milk fat globules that are transferred through breast-feeding (Chapter 3). Exosomes can also exert regulatory effects, perhaps because of the RNA or the chemokines they contain. Secretion of exosomes may be stimulated by contact with certain bacteria. Exosomes secreted by enterocytes and vascular endothelial cells have been shown to regulate the activity and diversification of macrophages, sometimes called **macrophage polarization**, so macrophages diversify into subpopulations with different functions. For example, macrophages polarize into what some refer as the M1 category and secrete pro-inflammatory cytokines and have increased phagocytic activity. In the GI tract, M1 macrophages are known to limit the number of pathogenic bacteria.

Viruses and plasmids provide examples of how genes outside of the chromosomal genome can control genetic traits. However, genes contained in plasmids and some viruses can also become incorporated into the chromosomes of bacteria or eukaryotic cells, a process mediated by enzymes called **integrases**. Viruses are cell parasites and parasitism begins with a subcellular life form called a *virion*, which cannot replicate outside of a host cell. Virions are transferred from cell to cell and host to host and many carry glycoproteins in their envelope that bind cell surface molecules, enabling entry. ACE2 on respiratory epithelial cells serves this function for SARS-CoV-2 entry (see Appendix A-4). While attachment to such receptors provides an avenue to enter a cell, viruses also utilize other cell proteins for the process, which is common to enveloped viruses. Once within the cell, positive, single-strand RNA in viruses like SARS-CoV-2 are translated to viral proteins that carry out activities that turn the infected cell into a production facility for their offspring. RNA viruses either have an RNA polymerase as part of the virion or code an RNA polymerase that acts in the cytoplasm to produce multiple copies of the viral RNA. The negative strand RNA viruses have an RNA-dependent RNA polymerase (RdRp). An example is influenza virus, which must first produce a complementary version to act as mRNA (ie, have + polarity) to instruct the infected cell to make viral proteins to enable progeny virus to be constructed. In the case of **human immunodeficiency virus** (HIV) and other retroviruses, after membrane fusion and internalization of the core, reverse transcriptase converts the viral RNA to double-strand DNA. This DNA is integrated into the genome of the host cell, like what can happen during transduction in bacteria with bacteriophage DNA (Figure A1.4). Unless the gametes or germ cells are infected, these new genes are not transferred to the offspring. However, in the case of retroviruses, the integrated viral genes can negatively interfere with the normal protective genetic activity of infected host cells and by doing so facilitate spread of the virus. In HIV, this reduces the survivability of the infected T cell, thereby causing an immune deficiency disease, the reason for the name **acquired immune deficiency syndrome** (AIDS). HIV, like SARS-CoV-2, is an example of a "bad parasite" that, if allowed to go unchecked without medical intervention, can lead to the death of a substantial proportion of the host species. It is a "bad parasite" because it reduces the opportunity for the virus/parasite to reproduce, a suicide strategy.

Meiosis Allows for Genetic Diversification of Eukaryotes

In eukaryotic organisms a completely new method of passing on genetic information evolved that requires modification of the DNA duplication process during mitosis (Figure A1.5). This new means of replication required that each species occur in two different sexes, meaning that the "sexual revolution" of the 1960s was preceded by 2 billion years. We regard this as Big Bang III in the development and diversification of life on planet Earth (Chapter 1). Sexual reproduction

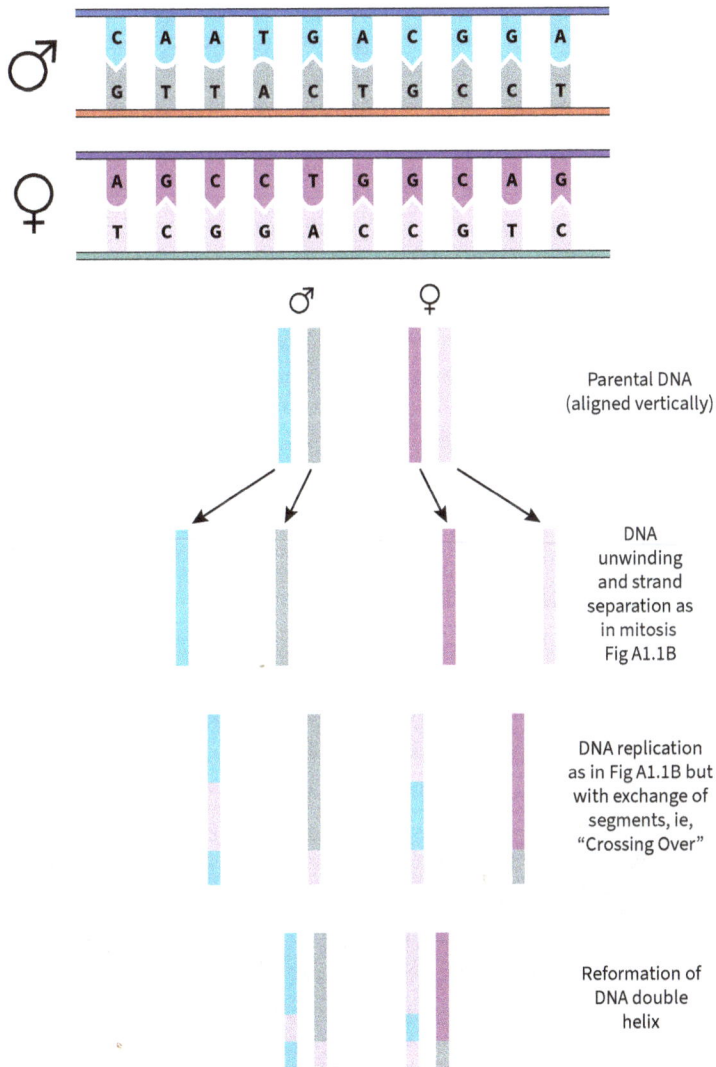

Figure A1.5   Nuclear events during sexual reproduction (meiosis). The evolutionary appearance of sexual reproduction allowed not only for duplication of DNA as in mitosis (Figure A1.1B) but for the exchange of DNA sequences among sexual partners, so that the sexual event generates offspring with genomes that differs from both parents.

requires organisms to designate certain cells exclusively for reproduction; these are called gametes, sperm cells, and egg (ovarian) cells. Figure A1.5 illustrates what occurrs during sexual reproduction. The sexual process is called meiosis. During meiosis DNA strands from maternally derived chromosomes in the egg pair with DNA strands from paternally derived chromosomes from sperm and can exchange DNA segments by the process known as "crossing over," which leads to random recombination. This assures that offspring are not identical to either parent, because each will now have a hybrid genome. Plant geneticists, especially in agriculture, used this explain what they call hybrid vigor. When this process is continued through multiple matings and generations it creates a large degree of genetic diversity within a species. When the ancestral paternal and maternal DNA pair during meiosis, the exact sequence of each gene may differ slightly. In genetic speak, these slight differences are called allelic variants or **alleles** and they are the basis for the designation of an **allotypes** (see Genetics text box). Allotypes are especially relevant when discussing the genetics of MHC (see later). Certain alleles are preferentially expressed, which explains the dominant **phenotypes** observed by early animal breeders and Gregor Mendel. For expression of a recessive trait, the same recessive allele must be provided by both parents. However, gene expression, like biology in general, is not black and white. Sometimes multiple genes encode a trait, so for example, unlike eye color, skin color in humans relies on many genes.

The evolutionary appearance of meiosis and sexual reproduction on planet Earth 1.7 billion years ago (Chapter 1) was a major evolutionary development. The diversity generated by this process prevented the extinction of entire species, but caused die-off of individuals that expressed non-survival traits.

The Genetics of Antibiotic Resistance

In Chapter 5 we mentioned **antibiotic resistance** and introduced the concept of a **resistome** and its consequences to human health. In Chapter 6 and earlier we described the enormous difference between higher vertebrates and prokaryotes in the speed by which they can alter their genome (ie, "change their spots"; Figure 6.2). The ubiquitous *Staphylococcus aureus*, the cause of wound infection and endocarditis (a major factor in heart disease) can be treated with antibiotics. However, through spontaneous mutations and HGT, it can acquire an antibiotic resistance (AR) gene (Figure A1.3). As a consequence, antibiotic therapy fails, as in the case of methicillin-resistant *S. aureus* (MRSA). This allows MRSA mutants to proliferate in a methicillin-rich environment, allowing the wound infection or endocarditis to go unchecked. We previously mentioned how *E. coli* can acquire a plasmid, allowing it to become pathogenic enterotoxigenic *E. coli* (ETEC). Benign bacteria can also acquire AR genes that result in tetracycline-resistant *E. coli* in chickens and avoparcin-resistant *Enterococcus* that can be transferred from swine to poultry and to farm workers (Chapter 8). Spontaneous mutants that carry AR genes emerge under the selective pressure of antibiotic therapy; *C. difficile* among hospitalized patients is an example.

Genes transferred by plasmids often occur in clusters called *cassettes*, and these are sometimes called **pathogenicity islands**. Figure A1.3 illustrates a cluster of genes in a cassette within a plasmid transferred by HGT. These are preceded by non-coding **promoter** and **repressor** elements.

RNA polymerase (Rnap) binds the promoter, which initiates the expression of all downstream genes in the cassette. In our model these include: (1) an AR gene encoding an antibiotic catalase, which can cleave certain antibiotics, rendering them ineffective, and (2) the gene encoding lactase, which can catabolize lactose into glucose and galactose and ameliorate lactose intolerance (see Chapters 3 and 8). In this model a high intake of lactose, such as that in cow's milk, can bind to the repressor element, which as a result blocks expression of the antibiotic resistance gene product (the catalase) and the expression of lactase, which can lead to lactose intolerance in newborns. This hypothetical model reveals the complexity of gene expression and is especially worrisome considering the many non-coding DNA segments in the genome of complex life forms (Table A1.2) that could be regulatory elements that can control gene expression and impact disease and wellness.

This model sends a worrisome message that gene clusters in bacteria can simultaneously encode favorable and unfavorable traits and that cluster activation or suppression can have both positive and negative effects, further illustrating the complexity of human disease.

Antibiotic Overuse Favors Development of a Resistome

Throughout the book we emphasize the value of antibiotics in combating bacterial pathogens while cautioning that their overuse can lead to a bacterial **resistome** (Chapter 5) and the appearance of multidrug-resistant (MDR) bacteria, which the WHO considers a worldwide threat to human health. One avenue of overuse has been the pediatric practice of prescribing antibiotics to combat the "common cold" and other viral respiratory diseases (Chapters 6–8). Other examples include the practice of requiring oral antibiotics before any dental or minor surgical procedure in patients that carry implants, which requires the administration of broad-spectrum antibiotics for undiagnosed intestinal disorders. A final example is sub-therapeutic antibiotic treatment (STAT), which adds antibiotics to the food of food animals like chickens and pigs. We describe the history of the STAT program in Chapter 8 and how in its original form it was responsible for the use of 80% of all antibiotics produced. Fortunately, the program has evolved with time, now relying on special antibiotics not used therapeutically in human or veterinary medicine.

Except for STAT, it is "damned if you do and damned if you don't," since failure to prescribe antibiotics invites medical malpractice. The ideal solution is identification of the offending pathogen combined with a new generation of antibiotics that specifically target only the offending pathogen.

Molecular and Genetic Aspects of Innate and Adaptive Immunity

Pathogen Recognition Receptors (PRRs) and Pathways in Innate Immunity

Chapter 6 described protective immunity, that starts with recognition of pathogens or other foreign biomolecules by PRRs. In the case of adaptive immunity, this begins when a broadly specific receptor, like monomeric IgM on a B cell (Chapter 6 and next section) that can recognize the foreign antigen. In the meantime, innate or "natural" IgM antibodies "put a finger in the dike" until a more effective **adaptive immune response** can mature. Producing a highly specific and efficacious antibody response takes time and **adaptive immune response** mature. This involves antigen-specific T cells to interact with antigen-specific B cells to facilitate the production of high affinity antibodies. This process also favors expansion of both antigen-specific T and B cells, which will be important for secondary responses to the offending pathogen/antigen. During this delay, protection depends on the "first responder" innate immune system.

Unlike adaptive immunity, the PRRs of the innate immune system require no maturation, their specificity is fixed and their germline is encoded. PRRs are expressed on cell surfaces, on endosomes, and within the cytosol (Chapter 6; Table 6.2). After binding a ligand, these receptors activate signal transduction pathways that converge in the nucleus. There they activate NFkB (universal transcription factor) or the TRF-3 transcription factor, leading to the production of IFNβ (a marker of inflammation; see Chapter 6) as well as inflammatory cytokines like IL-18 and antimicrobial peptides (AMP; see Chapter 6; Table 6.3). We provide limited descriptions of these pathways; for more detail see Davis; Saxena; Rietdijk; Kawasaki; Decout; and Zhang.

In Chapter 6 we introduced toll-like receptors (TLRs) as examples of PRRs that recognize pathogen-associated molecular patterns (PAMPs; Table 6.2). In addition to TLRs, there are at least four other functional clades of PRRs. These include C-type lectins receptors, retinoic acid-inducible receptors (RIG), cyclic GMP-AMP synthase (cGAS), and NOD-like receptors (NLRs). NOD is short for nucleotide-binding oligomerization domains. NLRs form a family of over 20 structurally related systems. A feature of TLRs and cytoplasmic PRRs is their binding sites, which are comprised of a motif of leucine-rich repeats (LRR; Figure A1.6A). Major TLRs (Table 6.2; Chapter 6) are found on cell surfaces but a few occur on endosomes. By contrast, RIG, cGAS and NLRs are found in the cytosol where they detect bacterial and viral products and DNA that has escaped from the endosomal compartment. We have selected three systems to review, those involving: (1) TLRs expressed on cell surfaces, (2) intracellular NLR system, and (3) intracellular cGAS-STING system.

The TLR system: The structure of a TLR is illustrated in Figure A1.6A; their specificities are described in Table 6.2. All TLRs have a similar structure that features a series of leucine-rich repeats (LLRs), the pattern of which differs among TLRs. All possess a transmembrane portion which upon PAMP binding, initiates a signal transduction cascade (Figure A1.6B). This involves many of the factors used in other cascades such as the adapter protein MyD88, various TNF receptor-associated factors (TRAFs), and various kinases (IKK; MAPk3), which ultimately leads to activation of NFkB and TRF-3 and subsequently the production of the inflammatory products described above.

The NLR system: Two major groups of NLRs are called NOD-1 and NOD-2. NOD-1 recognizes diaminopimelic acids derived from peptidoglycan (DAP) from Gram-negative bacteria, while NOD-2 recognizes dipeptides derived from peptidoglycans from both Gram-negative and Gram-positive bacteria such as muramyl dipeptide (MDP; Figure A1.6C;

Rietdijk). It was shown in a rabbit model of hypersensitivity pneumonitis (ie, alveolitis or chronic lung inflammation), that MDP given by aerosol maintained the alveolitis stimulated by aerosol exposure to a nonbacterial protein (ovalbumin). This suggested the need for a PAMP (MDP) or a Gram-positive bacteria in the maintenance of the pneumonitis (Butler 1983; Figure A1.6C).

While original studies focused on NOD-1 and NOD-2, over 22 different NLRs are now recognized (Saxena). As with TLRs, their PRRs contain various configurations of LRR. Receptor specificity differs as it does for the various TLR and the signal transduction pathways. A generic pathway for NOD-1, NOD-2, and recent variants is illustrated in Figure A1.6C. These differ in their NACHT domains, which are linked to various caspase activation and recruitment domains (CARD). These recruit the adapter protein RIP-2 and, with help of various TRAFs, proceed to activate various nuclear transcription factors, resulting in the production INFβ, cytokines, chemokines, and AMPs.

Activation of NLRs can also lead to formation and activation of **nodosomes**, also called **infammasomes** (Figure A1.6C). These are molecular complexes in the cytoplasm of activated cells, which differ in various features including phosphorylation (Davis). These complexes quite often lead to the transcription and production of IL-1B and IL-18 (Table 6.2). Activation of infammasomes may occur by contact with occupational and environmental factors like silica and asbestos or even alum used as an adjuvant in vaccines (see Chapter 6). One NLR, NLRP3, plays a role in viral immunity by helping to understand the response to double-stranded RNA from influenza and adenovirus DNA (Davis). Self-activation of infammasomes appears to have a genetic basis and more than 70 inherited mutations have been identified that can influence self-activation. These include pathologies like periodic fever syndrome, familial cold-induced auto-inflammation, and neonatal multisystem inflammation disorder.

One aspect of interest is self-activation of inflammasomes, which appears to have a genetic basis. More than 70 inherited mutations have been identified that can influence self-activation. These include pathologies like periodic fever syndrome, familial cold-induced auto-inflammation, and neonatal multisystem inflammation disorder.

The cGAS-STNG system: The cGAS-STING system (Figure A1.6D) is especially suited for the detection of cytosolic DNA, which should not be present in healthy cells but appears during viral infection, invasion by intracellular bacteria, tumorigenesis, and in the case of DNA damage (Decout). In Chapter 6 we introduced the term *DAMP* (damage-associated molecular patterns) to describe the ligand in such cases. After the PRRs of this system bind DNA, cyclic GMP-AMP synthase (cGAS) triggers a reaction that leads to the formation of GMP-AMP (cGAMP), which then binds to a molecule called stimulation of interferon gene (STING), which through subsequent steps triggers the transcription of various inflammatory substances, similar to what was described for the NLR system.

We do not discuss details of the retinoic acid-inducible gene system (RIG) but offer the results of studies with porcine circovirus-2 (PCV-2; Sinkora). This study indicated that

PCV-2 induces IFN-β, but this did not lead to activation of NFkB. Rather, PCV-2 induced IFN-β through the RIG-1/MDA pathway (Huang). Surprisingly, knocking out the RIG-1/MDA-5 system decreased rather than increased the replication of PCV-2; this study is useful because it illustrates that activation of this system by virus can also have a negative effect in the control of viral infection.

PRR Systems in Health and Disease

PRRs and the signaling pathways they generate overwhelmingly have a positive effect on human health. However, genetic/allelic variations in the NLR system are also associated with certain human maladies, and overstimulation may have negative consequences. TLR are geared to identify the type of extracellular invader (Table 6.2), while cytosolic PRRs alert the host of viral or intracellular bacterial infections like *Listeria*. As previously mentioned, they also detect DNA that does not belong outside of the nucleus unless the cell is stressed, as in tumorigenesis. PRR activation is essential for the immediate production and release of inflammatory cytokines, INFβ, and AMP (Table 6.3; Figure A1.6C). Their importance is illustrated in the case of deficiencies in certain PRRs or their allelic variants, which correlates with several disorders. These include: (1) NOD-2 polymorphism and Crohn's disease (see Chapter 5), (2) the increased risk of *H. pylori*, (3) colonic tumors in certain NOD-1 deficient mice, (4) chronic activation of STING by host DNAs, which can intensify autoimmunity, and (5) excessive INFβ production, which can cause over-reaction in autoimmunity.

While many TLRs (Table 6.2) are on cell surfaces, CLRs, RIG-1, and NOD/NLR are PRRs found in the cytoplasm. Hence, they can detect bacterial products that have evaded or escaped from the endosomal compartment. Two major groups of NLR are NOD-1 and NOD-2. NOD-1 recognizes diaminopimelic acids derived from peptidoglycan from Gram-negative bacteria, while NOD-2 recognizes dipeptides derived from peptidoglycans from both Gram-negative and Gram-positive bacteria such as muramyl dipeptide (MDP; Figure A1.6C; Rietdijk). It was shown in a rabbit model of hypersensitivity pneumonitis (ie, alveolitis or chronic lung inflammation), that MDP given by aerosol maintained the alveolitis stimulated by aerosol exposure to a nonbacterial protein (ovalbumin). This suggested the need for a PAMP (MDP) or a Gram-positive bacteria in the maintenance of the pneumonitis (Butler 1983; Figure A1.6C).

The intracellular signal transduction pathways that follow the recognition by PRRs are quite complex, and we describe here only a few features of these pathways. In the case of TLRs, so-called adapter proteins like MyD88 are required to promote signal transduction events involving various kinases, such as IRAK 1 and IRAK 4. The end product of these pathways is activation of the major DNA transcription activator, NFkB (Figure A1.6).

Activation of PRRs like NOD-1 and NOD-2 leads to formation and activation of what are called **inflammasomes**. These are molecular complexes in the cytoplasm of activated cells. There are various NLRs that differ in various features, including phosphorylation. NLRP1, NLRP3, and NLRC4 are among those studied (Davis). All result in activation of **inflammasome complexes**, quite often leading to transcription and production of IL-1B and IL-18

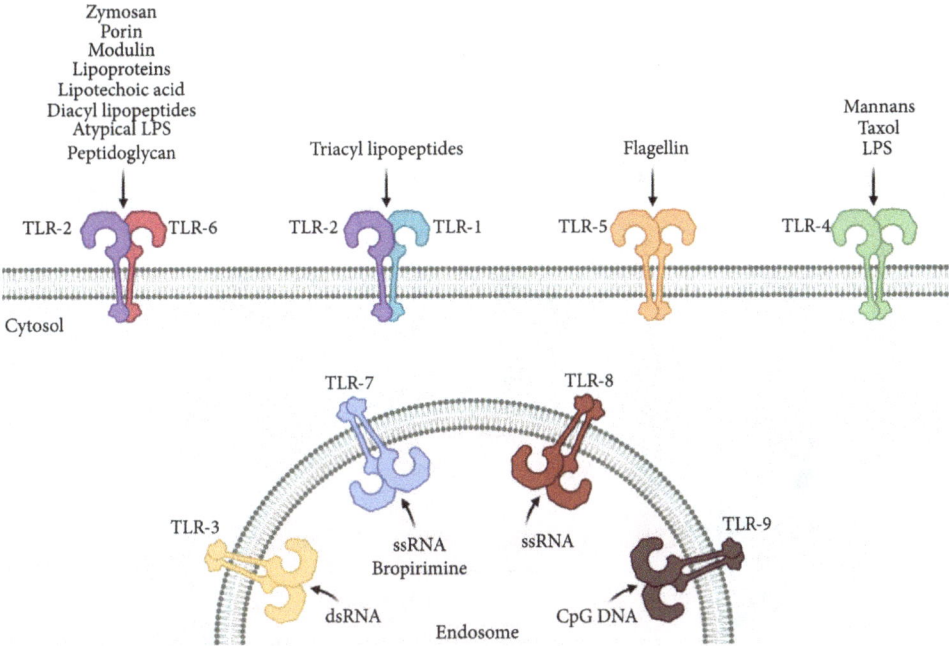

Zymosan
Porin
Modulin
Lipoproteins
Lipotechoic acid
Diacyl lipopeptides
Atypical LPS
Peptidoglycan

Triacyl lipopeptides

Flagellin

Mannans
Taxol
LPS

TLR-2   TLR-6   TLR-2   TLR-1   TLR-5   TLR-4

Cytosol

TLR-7   TLR-8

TLR-3   TLR-9

ssRNA   ssRNA
Bropirimine

dsRNA   CpG DNA
Endosome

Figure A1.6A   Toll-like receptors (TLRs) share a similar structure and are found both on the plasma membrane (eg, TLR1) and on the endosomal membrane (eg, TLR 3) and recognize different ligands (Table 6.2). TLRs are comprised of a ring of leucine-rich repeats (LRRs), an arrangement which differs among the various TLRs.

(see Table 6.3). Activation of inflammasomes may occur by contact with occupational and environmental factors like silica and asbestos or even alum used as an adjuvant in vaccines (see Chapter 6). NLRP3 plays a role in viral immunology and this pathway is becoming more important in understanding the response to double-stranded RNA from influenza and to adenovirus DNA (Davis).

One aspect of interest is self-activation of inflammasomes, which appears to have a genetic basis. More than 70 inherited mutations have been identified that can influence self-activation. These include pathologies like periodic fever syndrome, familial cold-induced auto-inflammation, and neonatal multisystem inflammation disorder.

Another innate immune pathway is one that can alert cells to foreign or damaged DNA (DAMP; see Chapter 6). This is a response to cyclic guanosine monophosphate and adenosine monophosphate synthetase, collectively called cGAS (Figure A1.6D; Zhang). Together these stimulate an interferon gene (STING), which triggers a signaling cascade that leads to secretion of type I interferons. Activation of this pathway provides an innate defense against microbial infections.

We did not discuss details of the retinoic acid-inducible gene system (RIG-1) but offer the results of studies with porcine circovirus-2 (PCV-2; Sinkora). This study indicated that PCV-2 induces IFN-β, but this did not lead to activation of NFkB. Rather, PCV-2 induced IFN-β through the RIG-1/MDA pathway (Huang). Surprisingly, knocking out the RIG-1/

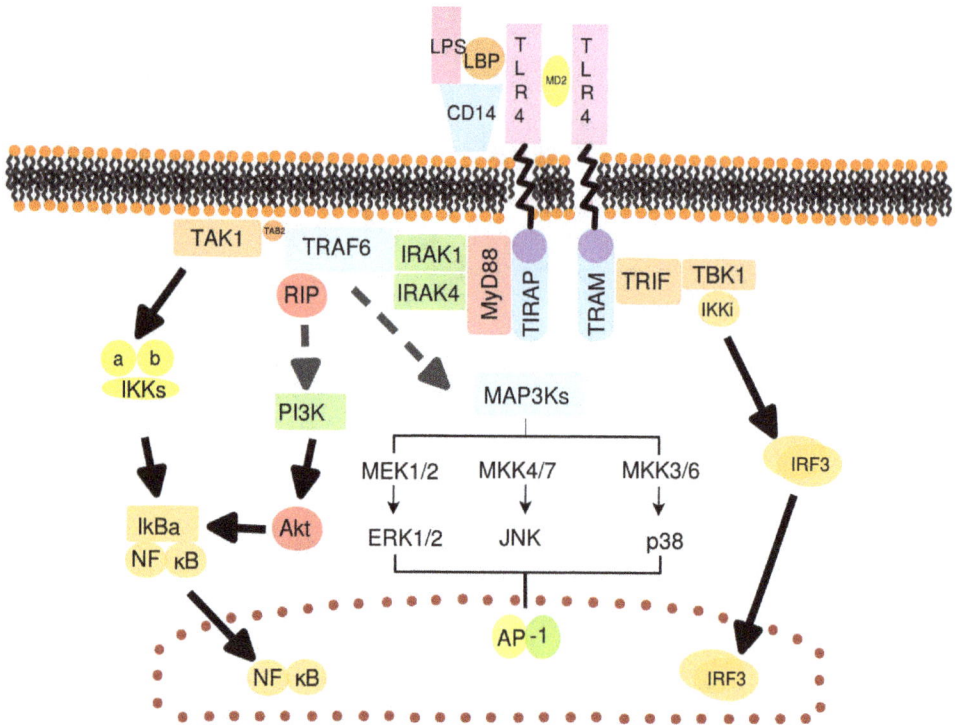

Figure A1.6B Signal transduction cascades after TLRs engage PAMPs. The binding of bacterial LPS to TLR 4 (see Table 6.2) initiates a pathway involving mediators common to most signal transduction pathways such as adapter protein MyD88, various TNF receptor-associated factors (TRAFs), RIP, various kinases (MAPK3; IKK) and others. All pathways converge on the nucleus, where NFkB and IRF-3 are activated and regulate gene expression-including those encodiing cytokines and chemokines

MDA-5 system decreased rather than increased the replication of PCV-2. This study reveals that activation by a virus can activate different innate pathways, which can have a negative effect in the control of viral infection.

We have chosen to not go into further detail regarding the intracellular pathways involved in the innate immune response because this area is dynamic and details will no doubt change as more studies are performed. In the past, studies on innate immune protection lagged behind those on adaptive immunity; currently research on the innate immune system has intensified.

Antibody and T Cell Receptor (TCR) Structure

Figure A1.7A illustrates the basic structure of various classes of immunoglobulins. Immunoglobulin is the biochemical term for any protein that has the structure and function of an antibody. The composition of the basic monomeric unit contains two heavy chains and two light chains connected through disulfide bonds. Regions called *domains* comprise the two polypeptide chains. These domains have different roles in antibody functions. In general, antibodies are "two-headed monsters": one end (the variable region) determines the specificity

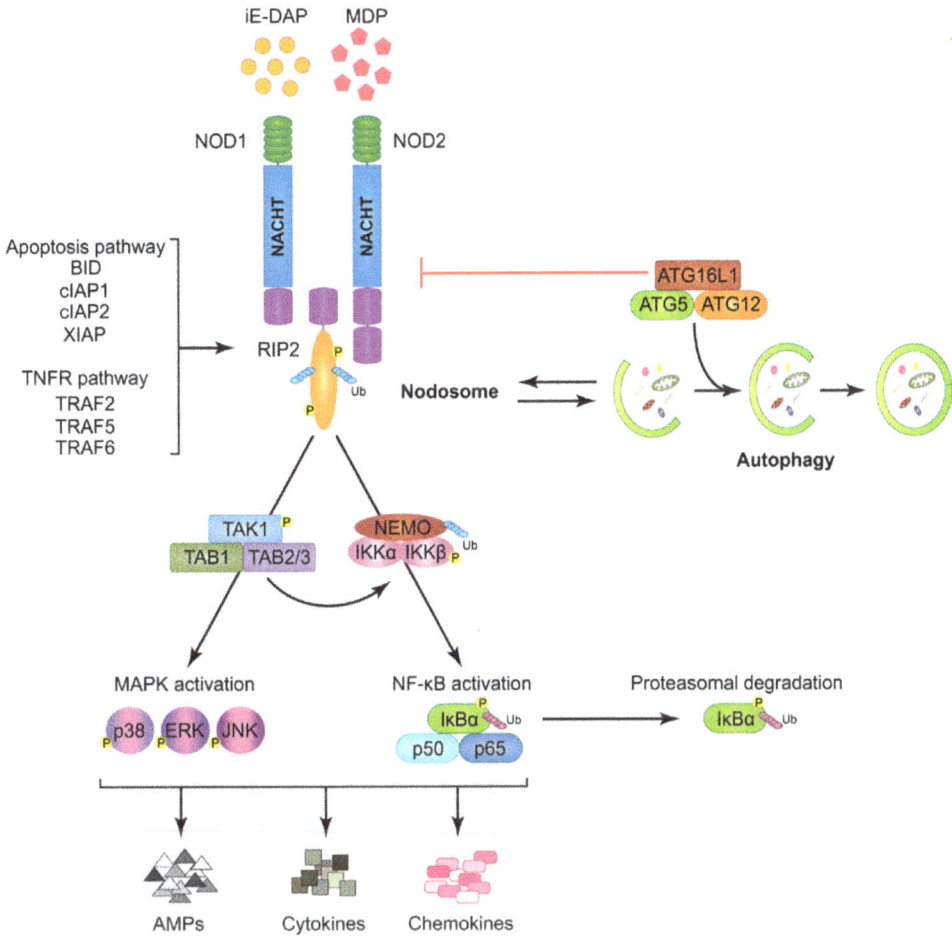

Figure A1.6C Intracellular events binding to MDP and NOD-1 binding to diaminopimelic acid peptidoglycan (DAP) from a Gram-negative bacterium. The NLRs act through NACHT domains that vary among the over 20 family members that associate with various caspase-associated recruitment domains (CARD; shown in purple), which together recruit RIP-2 and, with the help of various TRAFs and IKKs, proceed to activate NFkB and cause transcription and the production of inflammatory cytokines, chemokines, and AMP. In the case of certain NLRs, nodosome complexes, also called inflammasome complexes, are built to engage in further inflammatory events such as autophagy.

for some target antigen while the other (generally called the Fc region) mediates effector actions. These are often unique to certain antibody classes (see later section). A number of these functions were mentioned in Chapter 6 and are summarized in Table A3.1.

Most circulating antibodies are monomeric, with the exception of IgM that circulates in pentameric form (Figure A1.7B). Some versions of immunoglobulin, such as monomeric IgM and IgD, do not circulate but rather act as B cell antigen receptors (Figure A1.7A). IgA at mucosal sites is secreted as a dimer (Figure A1.7B), which becomes secretory IgA (SIgA) after transport through secretory epithelial cells like enterocytes (Figure 6.6). Differences

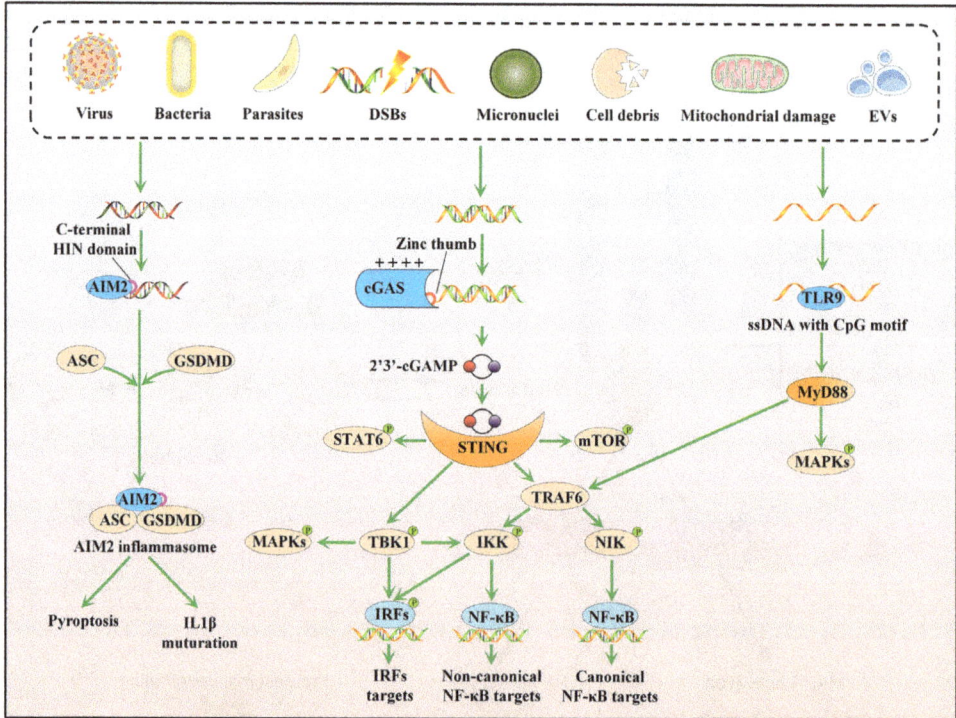

Figure A1.6D The cGAS-STING system. Cytosolic PRRs recognize cytosolic viruses, bacteria, DNA and activate cGAS, which leads to the formation of cGAMPs, which then engages STING on the endoplasmic reticulum (ER) and leads to other events that ultimately stimulate IRF, INFβ, and other regulatory cytokines.

among domains and fragments have been exploited in the engineering of antibodies for use in therapy. These will be later discussed and illustrated.

Figure A1.7C illustrates the structure and function of the T cell receptor (TCR) on α/β and γ/δ T cells in recognizing foreign peptides/antigens presented by APCs. Most of the discussion concerning T cell function and development in Chapter 6 involved α/β T cells, especially four subsets (Figure 6.4). The interaction of α/β T cells with APCs involves recognition of the peptides presented by APCs on MHC I or II (Figure A1.7C). Co-receptors like CD4 and CD8 allow for the identification of various T cell subsets involved in this process. CD4 and CD8 are among the ~300 CD markers (cluster of differentiation markers) that are expressed especially on hematopoietic cells. Using specific monoclonal antibodies for various CD markers, a particular T- or B-cell can be recognized, subsequently purified using flow cytometry (FCA) and its functions studied *in vitro* and *in vivo*. For example, Th2 helper T cells are recognized because they bear both CD4 and CD3 and NK cells because they express CD16, CD94, and CD8 (Figure A1.7C). Finer distinction among α/β T cells and NK cells and their roles in adaptive immunity can be determined by the cytokines they secreter (Figure 6. 4).

All TCRs superficially resemble the Fab portion of an immunoglobulin (Figure A1.7A), and their constant regions are disulfide bonded, like the Fab portion of heavy and light

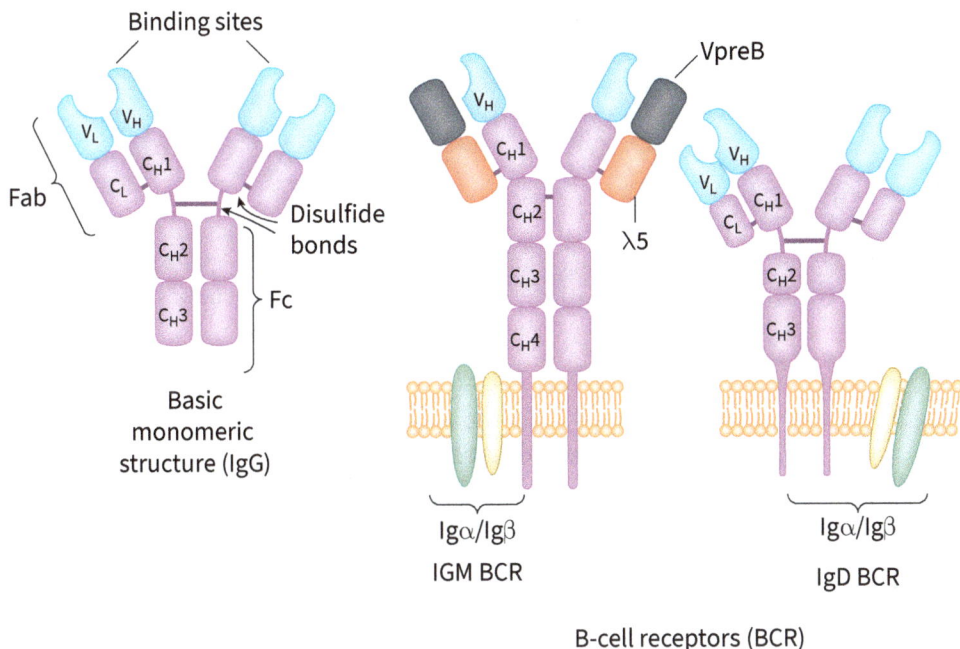

Figure A1.7A Structure of an immunoglobulin monomer secreted by plasma cells and variations of immunoglobulin structure among antibody classes. The illustration of the basic monomer which is secreted by plasma cells, shows the constituent polypeptide chains and their major fragments and domains. Monomeric IgM and IgD both serve as B cell receptors (BCRs) on the surface of B cells with segments that attach them to the cell membrane. The IgM-based BCR is found on pre-B cells but is not associated with authentic light chains; it is instead associated with VPreV and λ5, which together serve as a surrogate light chain. Exceptions to this occur in other mammals (see Appendix A-2).

chains in immunoglobulins. The γ/δ TCR is similar in structure and genetics to the α/β TCR and its γ and δ chains are also comprised of V, D, and J segments. Unlike α/β TCRs, γ/δ TCRs do not recognize peptides presented to them on MHC I and II. Rather, they are more like the BCR and recognize proteins, glycolipids, phospholipids, and other nonpeptide antigens. Structural analyses have shown that the orientation of the V and C domains of γ/δ T cells also differ from those in α/β TCRs, especially in segments that encode CDR3. CDR3 and its variations are illustrated in Figure A1.9. While γ/δ T cells constitute a very small proportion of T cells in the blood of mice and humans, they are elevated in the blood of individuals suffering from *M. tuberculosis*, *H. influenza*, and certain autoimmune diseases. Is this connected to their ability to recognize glycolipids and phospholipids expressed by these pathogens? However, γ/δ T cells in all mammals play a major role at mucosal sites, especially in the respiratory tract (Xiong). T cells, like all lymphocytes, began development as progenitors in the yolk sac and fetal liver. Prior to final development in the thymus, they are often referred to as double-positive thymocytes. Mature γ/δ appear before 55 days of gestation while α/β appear later (Appendix A-2, Figure A2.3).

Serum Antibodies

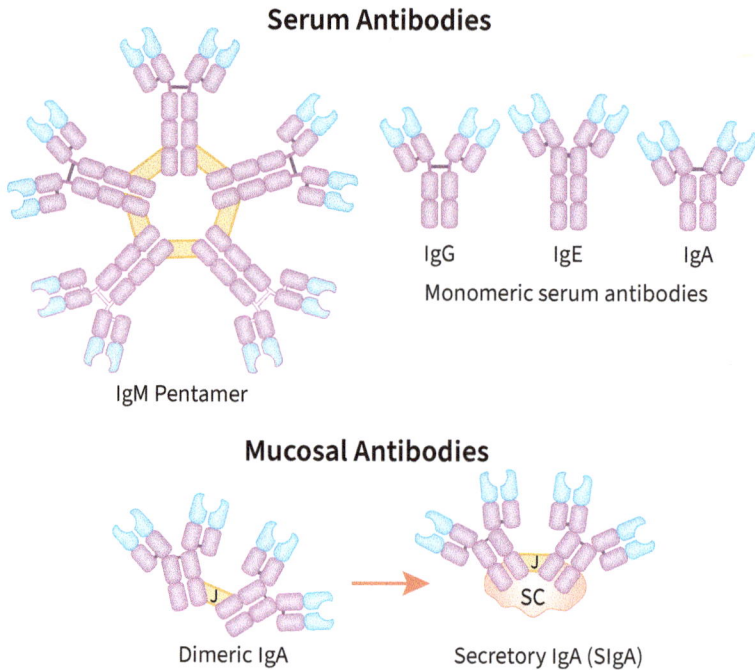

IgM Pentamer

IgG   IgE   IgA

Monomeric serum antibodies

Mucosal Antibodies

Dimeric IgA   Secretory IgA (SIgA)

Figure A1.7B Structural models of major secreted antibody classes. Monomeric IgM is rarely found in serum but rather in pentameric form. Dimeric IgA is the principal mucosal antibody and is secreted as secretory IgA (SIgA; Figure 6.6). Major classes differ in domain structure and the functions of their Fc portions (Table A3.1).

γ/δ T cells lack the CD4 co-receptor but contain a CD8 homodimer. However, this does not serve as a co-receptor (Figure A1.7C). γ/δ T cells carry the CD11b marker, which appears to facilitate their transport out of the thymus. Although γ/δ T cells normally comprise a tiny proportion of circulating T cells in mice and humans, they may comprise as much as 50% of T cells in the blood of artiodactyls, and these include three major subsets (see Appendix A-2). γ/δ T cells develop from thymocytes (as described in Chapter 6) but do not go through the receptor-editing process needed for α/β T cells. For that reason, they are the first to appear in the periphery during fetal development in species where they abound (Appendix A-2).

The variable domains of immunoglobulins are comprised of gene segments referred to as V, D, and J (Figure A1.7D). Following somatic recombination and mutation, these may encode 10^8 different antibody or BCR binding sites, each with different specificities. A similar process occurs in the formation of the TCR binding site, generating a diverse repertoire. Figure A1.7E indicates the number of quasi-duplicated V, D, and J segments that are potentially available for somatic recombination in forming the TCR binding sites for α/β T cells in mice and humans. Figure A1.7E shows that D segments in Vα do not contribute to the combinatorial diversity of the α/β TCR binding site, similar to the absence of D gene segments in the variable region repertoire of immunoglobulin light chains (Figure A1.7D). In that sense, the Vα repertoire of TCRs resemble the repertoire of immunoglobulin light chains.

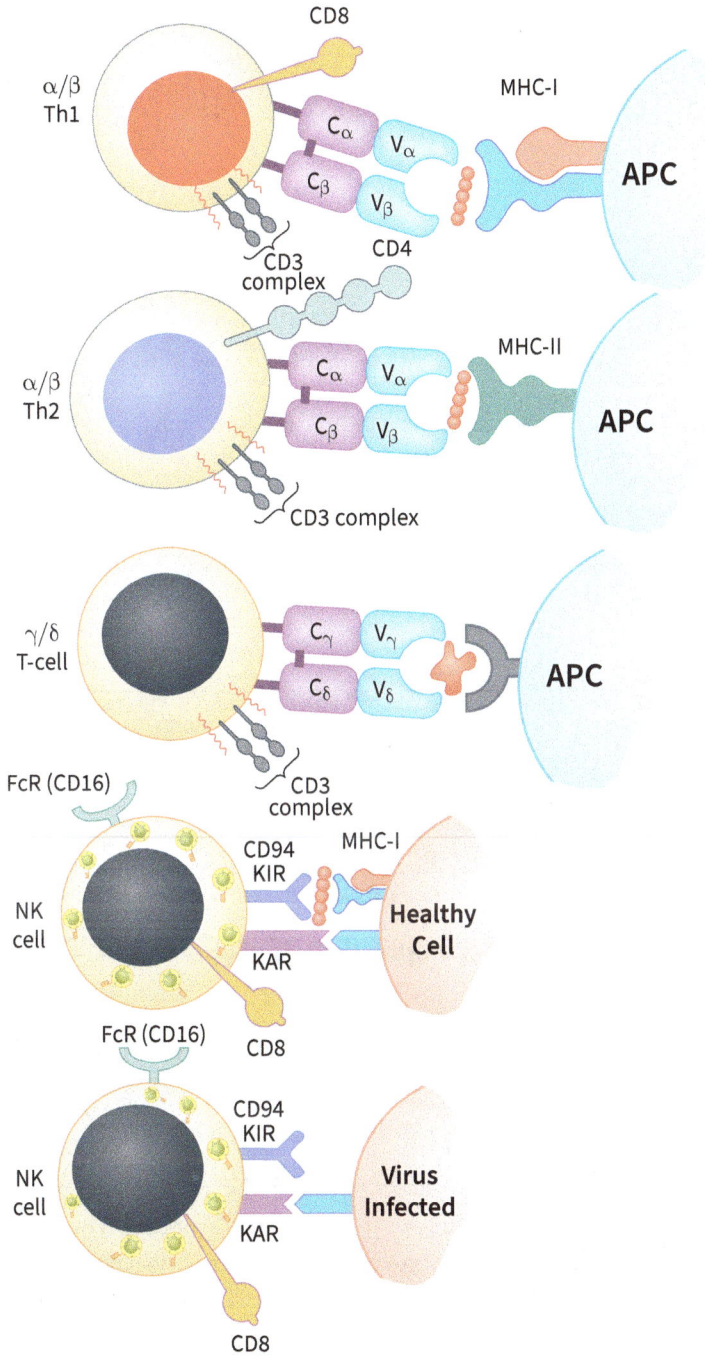

Figure A1.7C   Presentation by APCs of linear peptides to CD8 α/β TH1 and CD4 α/β TH2 T cells and to confrontational peptides to γ/δ T cells. All T cells carry the CD3 marker. The detailed features of MHC I and MHC II and the encoding loci are provided in Figure A1.9. CD94 + NK cells also recognize linerar peptides and are important in innate immunity and are able to act against virus-infected cells that have lost the ability to present viral peptides to conventional T cells (see above) and are then able to use other mechanisms to remove the virus-infected cell (see text).

α chain locus

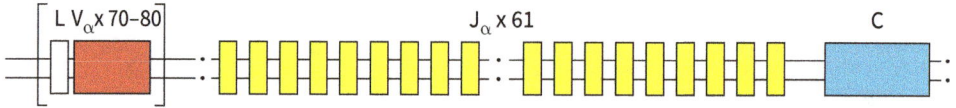

β chain locus

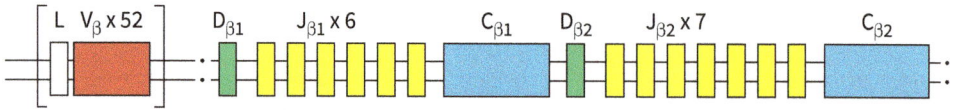

Figure A1.7D The genome encoding the α and β peptides of the human TCR. The binding site of the α/β TCR (Figure A1.7C) is encoded by a panel of >70 Va variable gene segments. These are accompanied by ~60 Ja gene segments. The binding site for the beta chain of the α/β TCR is encoded by ~50 Vβ segments and two cassettes of Vβ, Jβ, and Dβ segments assorted into duplicons, each containing a TCRβ constant region gene. During formation of the α/β TCR, these variable T cell segments are rearranged in the same manner as illustrated in Figure A1.8 for the antibody binding site.

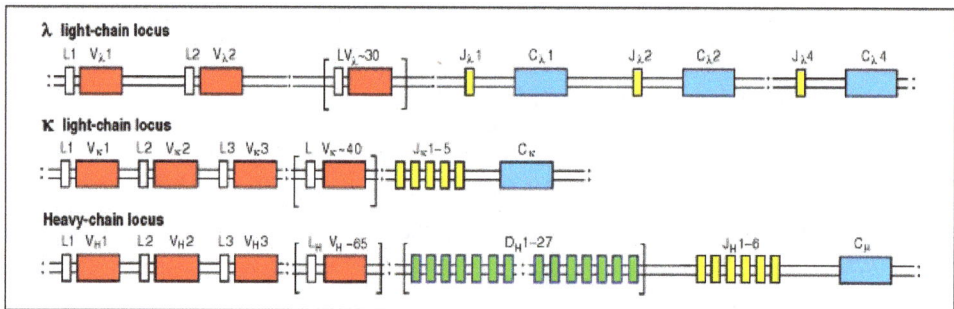

Figure A1.7E. Organization of genes available to encode the immunoglobulin λ and κ light chain loci and the heavy chain locus. Red: variable gene segments, blue: constant region gene segments, yellow: J (joining) segments, green: D (diversity) segments are shown. The number of VH, DH, and JH segments in the human genome is indicated.

In humans and mice, V and J segments encoding the α/β TCR are more diverse than those in γ/δ T cells. The full significance of this difference is unknown but it seems to follow a pattern in which the most-used isotypes are encoded from loci containing the highest number of quasi-duplicated gene segments. This pattern is also seen by the high number of Vκ light chain variants in mice that use kappa light chains in 90% of their antibodies. Similarly, there is a high number of Vγ variants in ruminants that use lambda light chains in 90% of their antibodies (Appendix A-2.).

Figure A1.7C also compares T cells to natural killer (NK) cells. NK cells were mentioned in Chapter 6 in regard to their role in innate immunity. We also mentioned them in Chapter 2 in regard to their role in the prevention of rejection of fetal hemi-allografts. Conventional

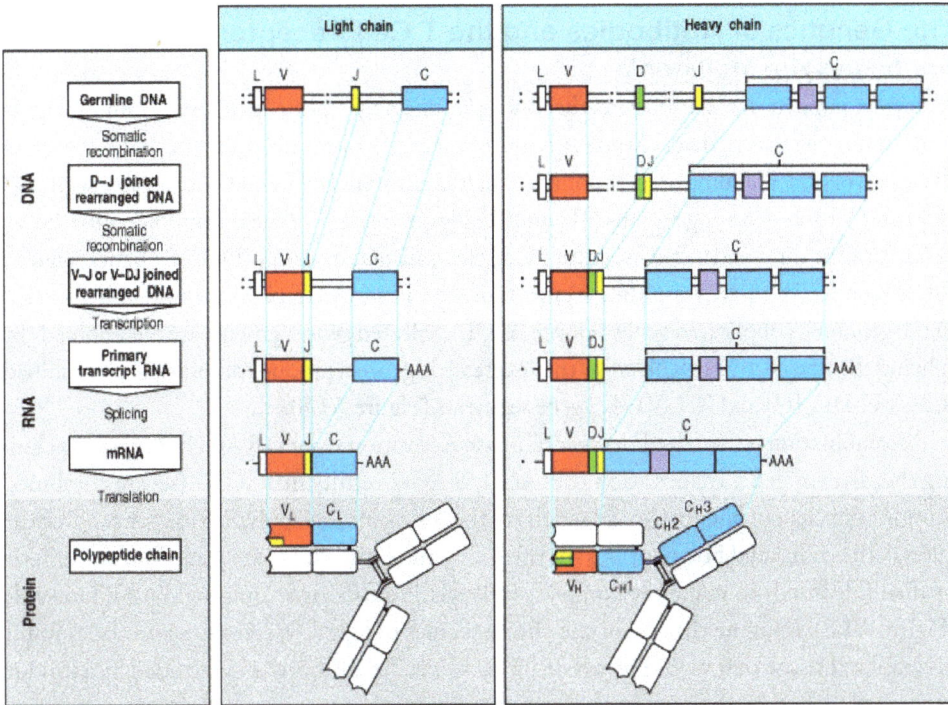

Figure A1.8. Sequential events in the synthesis of an antibody. Rearrangements of gene segments in the kappa and heavy chain loci which leads to the production of an immunoglobulin. The constant heavy chain (blue) and heavy chain hinge (purple) exons encoding IgG are also shown. The nucleotide features of each stage is shown in the left panel.

NK cells lack expression of a TCR (Figure A1.7C) but still express a homodimer of CD8 and the low-affinity Fc receptor (CD16). The latter allows them to bind immune complexes and mediate **antibody-dependent cell toxicity** (ADCC). This occurs when viral-specific antibodies become attached to the Fc receptors on NK cells like CD16, which then allows them to recognize virus-infected cells and to utilize cytokines and other effector mechanisms to destroy the cells, similarly to the action of cytotoxic T cells (CTLs). As we mentioned in Chapter 6 and shown in Figure A1.7C, NK cells express killer cell activation receptors (KARs) and killer cell inhibition receptors (KIRs). In healthy individuals, the latter interact with MHC I, which blocks their behavior as killer cells (see Figure A1.7C). However, if MHC expression is suppressed because of viral infection (see Chapter 6), it allows activation of KARs so these NK cells can now engage and destroy virus-infected cells. In these situations, NK cells can now act as CTLs.

In addition to NK cells, there are NKt cells. These are a confusing subset of NK cells that can bear either α/β or γ/δ TCRs. NKt cells frequently appear in the literature and some textbooks. Some believe these are "ghost cells" misidentified by FCA and are merely a combination of lineage T cells with NK cells. If they are contaminants, it is not surprising they share features with both NK and conventional T cells.

The Genetics of Antibodies and the T Cell Receptor (TCR)
Antibodies Are Multigenic
A concept popular in the 1960s was the "one gene, one polypeptide" principle. Immunologists were among the first to demonstrate this was not true. As illustrated in Figure A1.7A, each of these polypeptides is comprised of domains such as constant (CH and CL), variable segments (VH and VL), and joining regions (JH and JL; Figure A1.7E). In the immunoglobulin-heavy chains (and in the α and γ chains of the TCR) there are also diversity (DH) segments (Figures A1.7D and A1.7E). Genes encoding segments of the VH and VL regions are tandemly arranged in the genome as duplicated genes (Figure A1.7E). Selected gene segments are recombined (by splicing their respective mRNAs) so that expressed Igs are a product of multiple recombined [CH-VH-DH-JH] and [CL-VL-JL] gene segments (Figure A1.8).

Recombination is mediated by Recombinase Activation Genes (RAG-1/RAG-2), including the *Artemis* gene. Inactivation of RAG-1/RAG-2 results in a SCID (severe combined immune deficiency) phenotype. So much for the "one gene, one polypeptide concept" of the 1960s! The translated polypeptides for the heavy and light chains are joined intracellularly by disulfide bonds to make the complete multigenic antibody/immunoglobulin molecule (Figure A1.8). Imagine the size of the chromosomes of higher vertebrates and the amount of lymphoid tissue that would be needed if each specific antibody was encoded by a unique gene, as predicted by the "one gene, one polypeptide" theory.

Antibody Gene Segments Are Differently Recombined in B-Lymphocytes
The human genome contains approximately 100 tandemly arranged VH genes, of which about 40% are functional. It is common for loci where gene duplication is common to include numerous nonfunctional pseudogenes. In humans, there are 23 DH as well as 9JH segments. Collectively, approximately 75% of these are functional (Figure A1.7E). Quasi-random recombination of these segments results in a recombinant gene that encodes the heavy-chain contribution to the antigen binding site of a particular human antibody produced by a unique B cell clone. This [VH-DH-JH] or simply V-D-J recombination process can generate over 7,000 different heavy chains. The human VL-kappa locus has about 100 available VL genes (75% functional) and 10 VJ genes that can recombine to encode the binding site. A similar pattern involving multiple VL and JL genes is seen in the lambda light chain locus. In humans, usage of kappa and lambda light chains is nearly equally divided. The number of V, D, and J segments that encode the binding site varies widely among mammals (Appendix A-2).

Since recombined V-D-J and V-J are both needed to form the antibody's antigen binding site, random combinations of Ig variable region gene segments in both the heavy (H) and light (L) chain loci would theoretically yield a million different antibodies. An equivalent process occurs in the generation of the T cell antigen receptor (TCR) repertoire.

The various gene segments that encode antibodies, and those that encode the α and β chains of the TCR, form the **antigen binding site**, by the folding of the encoded VDJ and

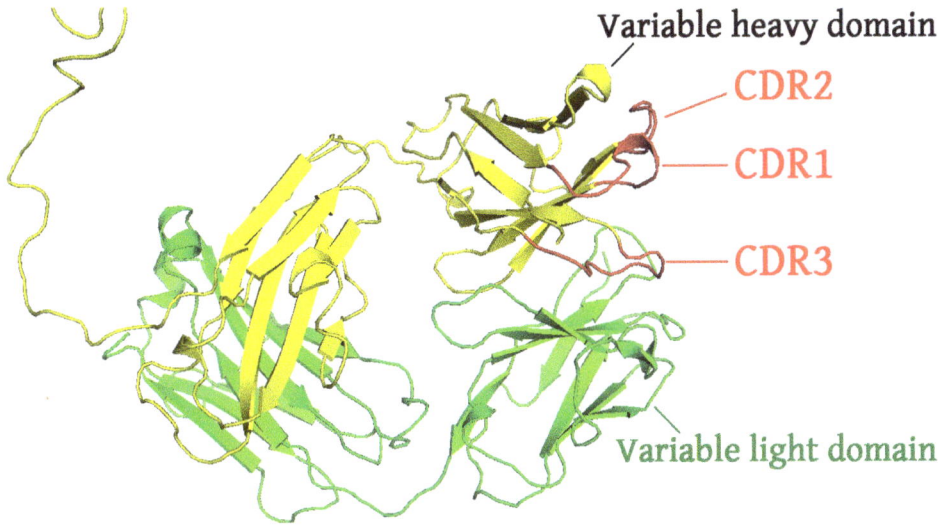

Figure A1.9   The 3D structure of polypeptides that coalesce to form the antigen binding site of antibodies that are formed by the arrangement of VH and VL gene segments (Figure A1.8). The model highlights segments encoded by CDR1(HV1), CDR2 (HV2), and CDR3 (HV3).

VJ polypeptides of the heavy and light chains in such a manner that they form a 3D pocket, ideal for recognizing conformational epitopes. These include polypeptides that encode the CDR1, CDR2, and CDR3 variable gene segments from both H and L chains and coalesce as both the BCR and TCR (Figure A1.9). In the case of antibodies, CDR1 and CDR2 are contributed by the VH or VL genes and the CDR3 region by the junction of V-D-J or V-J segments. Figure A1.10 shows the amino acid sequence encoded by rearranged and somatically mutated VH genes recovered from different B cells of the same animal. Amino acid that differ from the **consensus** are localized to the CDR1 and CDR2. Figure A1.11 shows an alignment of CDR3 regions from different B cells in the same animal, demonstrating how V-D-J rearrangements that form CDR3 also allow for insertions and deletions. Not surprisingly, CDR3 plays the major role in forming the antibody binding site (Figure A1.9), and therefore in determining antibody specificity. A similar pattern for CDR1, CDR2, and CDR3 variation is seen during formation of the TCR binding site (not shown). However, while the BCR recognizes conformational epitopes on proteins and polysaccharides, the TCR recognized linear peptides of 9–13 amino acids.

Antibody Genes Further Diversify by Somatic Hypermutation (SHM)

Somatic mutation refers to mutations that occur in cells other than gametes (egg and sperm). Some level of somatic mutation occurs in all cells and the frequency can be as much as double that of mutations that occur in gametes. In any case, these mutations are not passed on to the offspring but only impact the individual during its life time. Somatic mutation increases with age in long-lived species and can play a role in cancer and certain

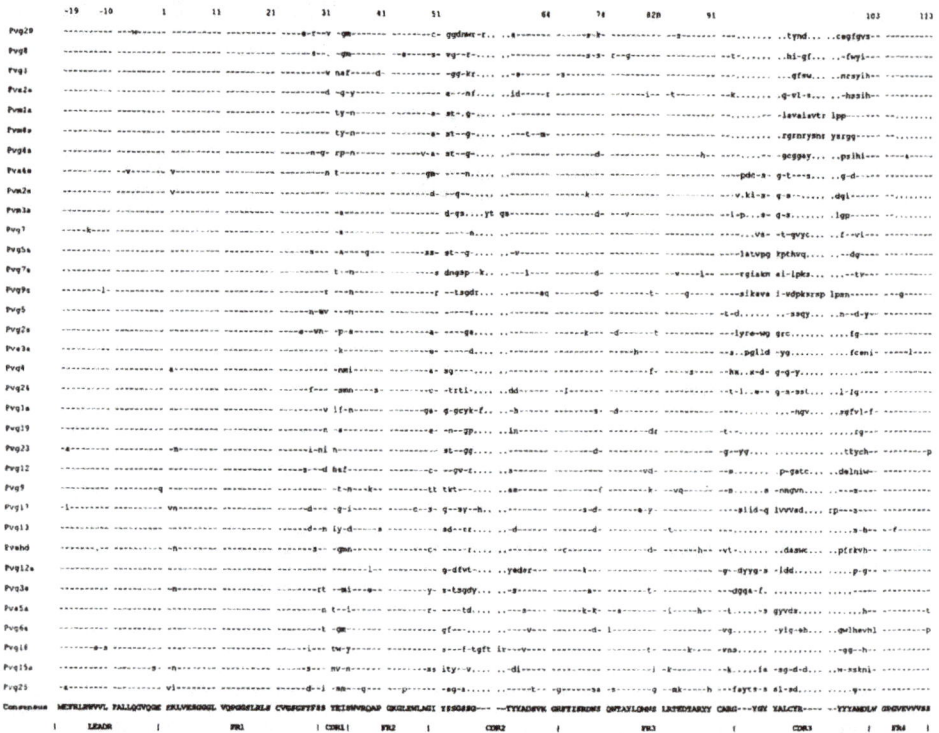

Figure A1.10   Alignment of 34 deduced amino acid sequences of VH genes recovered from individual B cells of the same animal. The demarcation of CDR1, CDR2 and CDR3 regions (see Figure A1.7D) and framework (FR) regions are shown below along with the consensus sequences for all sequences presented. Designation on the left are clone numbers. Amino acid substitutions that differ from the consensus are in bold. Note that changes are concentrated in the CDR1, CDR2 and CDR3 regions of the encoding genes.

other diseases (Vijg). However, in lymphocytes this occurs at a much higher frequency and is called **somatic hypermutation (SHM)**, resulting in changes to the **amino acid sequence** as illustrated in Figures A.10 and A1.11. We described in Chapter 6 how, after antigen contact and interaction with T cells, genes encoding the VH and VL segments in B cells are subject to SHM. One mechanism involves the action of AID (Figure A1.3). It is estimated that SHM can add 10^2 variations to the previously recombined VH and VL gene, raising the total repertoire to over 10^8 antibody variants. Ergo, somatic gene recombination and SHM in diversifying B cells can generate a repertoire that exceeds the number of genomic variants that bacteria and viruses can generate by spontaneous genomic mutation (Figure 6.2). As shown in Figure A1.10, the effect of SHM is most pronounced in the CDR1 and CDR2 regions of recombined VH genes and in the CDR3 region (Figure A1.11), which play the major role in formation of the binding site for the BCR and TCR (Figure A1.9).

CLONES	3' OF FR3	N (5')	D$_H$1 (GERMLINE) GAATTGCTATAGCTATGGTGCTAGTTGCTATAGTGAC	N (3')
npvm2:	TGT GCA AGA	GTCAAAAT	....	GAAT
npvm22	--- --- ---	GTCC	...............c..	C
npva6:	--- --- -	AG	...............aa.............	GTATCTCCAAAC
npvm20	--- --- --	GGGAGTATATT	....	AGACTGG
npvg6:	--- --- ---	GGCCT	.........gt..........	TGGGGGT
npva9:	--- --- ---	GAAGGTCT	...................a......	CCCCCCGG
npvm11	--- --G -T-	GGAAAT	....	
npvm13	--- --- ---	GGCACC	....	AC
npvg14	--- --- ---	TGT	....	AGT
npvm21	--- --G -T-	TGTGATATCAAA	....	GGAGG
npvg4:	--- --G -T	CGGG	....	ATAGGTGGTTTTTGGGGTGGTA
npvg13	--- --- ---	GGCCTTAGG	....	CACTATAAA
npva4:	--- --- ---	GTCG	....................A.....a...	GAGGG
npvm19	--- --- ---	ACA	....................A.......	TCCCCCTT
npvm12	--- --- ---	GGCATA	..........c.......A......	C
npvg8:	--- --- ---		....	TTCCGGAGGG
npvm23	--- --- ---		....	GAAGTCTCGGTGT
npvm3:	--- --- -T-	GGCCC	....	TAGGCCCC
npvm18	--- --G -	AA	....	TC
npvm9:	--- ---	GTCGAAGGTCT	....................a......	CCCGA
npvg7:	--- --- -		.........c...............	
npvm8:	--- --G -T-	GGG	....	
npvg9:	--- --- ---	GCTAGTGGC	...........A......	AATTCTCCATT
npvm15	--- --	GATTGACC		

CLONES	3' OF FR3	N (5')	D$_H$2 (GERMLINE) TGACTATAGCGGTTGCTATAGCGGTTAC	N (3')
npvm7a	--- t-G -T	GG	....	CTGCTATCCGA
npva5:	--- --- ---	GCCCTCTT	.g................	CCCACGGATTTGGG
npvm17	--- --- ---	GGCCGAGAA	....	TTGAGCCC
npvg15	--- --- g--	GGATGCG	....	GTGGG
npvg3:	--- --- ---	GGCCTT	....	GAGGGG
npvg2:	--- --- ---	GG	....	CCTTCCCCCGA
npvm10	--- --- ---	AGC	....	CCCCGTCGAGCATATCATAGG
npvm14	--- --- ---	GGCCATG	....	TGTGTGAGGATCTTG
npva3:	--- --- ---	GGCGTCGA	....	CCGATGTCGAAAGAATCCTAT
npvm1:	--- --- g--	TGGTT	....	GAGAATCCCCCC
npva2:	--- --- ---	GG	....	CCGGCCGA
npva1:	--- --- -T-		....	CCACAAGGT
npva7:	--- a-- ---	GGCTG	.......cc....	TATGAGTC
npvm5:	--- --	GAAG	....	GTAATACG
npvm4a	--- --- ---	GGCCGA	.... (inv.)	CGGGGGGGG
npvg1:	--- --- -T-	GGAATT	...tt....	ACC

Figure A1.11 Sequence differences in CDR3 account for major differences in the specificity of antibodies. Alignment of CDR3 regions of rearranged VH genes recovered from B cells from the same animal. CDR3 is composed of elements of recombined VH, DH, and JH segments. Two different DH segments, DH1 and DH2, are used in this species, and CDR3 sequences using each are indicated. Nucleotide changes in the 5' and 3' region surrounding the DH segment are extensive, so that each VDJ sequence is unique. Changes in the DH segments are due to somatic mutation. These changes influence the specificity of the antibody binding site (Figure A1.9)

Antibody Classes With the Same Specificity Have Different Effector Functions

The basic structure of an antibody is illustrated in Figure A1.7A. Figure A1.7B shows structural models for different antibody classes, also referred to as *isotypes*. The constant region of an antibody determines its class (eg, IgM, IgD, IgG, IgE, and IgA; Table A3.1). By definition, "constant" regions are not altered by somatic recombination or SHM. There are five such classes in humans (Figure A1.7B). The mRNA encoding the constant region genes is spliced to that of mRNA encoding the somatically recombined and hypermutated V-D-J gene segments (Figures A1.10 and A1.11) that encode the antibody binding site (Figure A1.9). Any rearranged and somatically mutated V-D-J can be expressed with any of the five classes. This means that while any one differentiated B cell can make only one antibody binding site, it can be expressed with different Ig classes. However, when B cells mature into plasma cells (Figures 6.1 and 6.3), the sequence encoding the binding site is hardwired into the DNA together with the constant regions encoding only one particular isotype.

Why is more than one antibody class needed? The reason is that the constant region of each class displays structural features that have different functions (Table A3.1). In Chapter 2 we noted that only IgG antibodies could be actively transported across the placenta, and in Chapter 6 we noted that IgE class antibodies that bind mast cells and eosinophils are needed to trigger type I allergic reactions. In Chapters 3 and 6, we noted that antibodies of the IgA class, which are produced by PC in the mammary gland by daughters of B cells that emigrated from the GI tract, comprise 90% of the antibodies in human colostrum and milk and, when ingested by the suckling infant, provide immune protection against pathogens of the GI tract.

Allelic Variation and Exclusion in Expression of Antibody/ Immunoglobulin Genes

Genes that encode BCR/antibody and TCR gene segments behave exactly like all other genes. There are two alleles of each gene: one of maternal origin and one of paternal origin (Figure A1.5). These can be identical (homozygous) or different (heterozygous). Unlike genes encoding eye color and many other traits, these are co-dominant. Since both are co-dominant, this creates a dilemma for individual B and T cells where antibody specificity is considered. Co-dominance would allow any one B or T cell to encode antibodies with different specificities: one protective and one causing harm. Thus, a mechanism evolved that allows only one allele to be expressed in a particular T- or B cell. This phenomenon is called **allelic exclusion**.

The T Cell Receptor (TCR) Is Multigenic

The genetic organization of the α and β chains loci encoding the TCR (Figure A1.7D) is homologous to the multigenetic pattern shown in Figure A1.7E for the variable genes that encode the B cell receptor (BCR) and the antibody binding site. Organization of the genes encoding TCR γ and δ loci is similar. Like the BCR, the recombined gene segments encoding the N-terminal segments of the TCR α, β, γ, and δ chains form the TCR in same manner as do the variable heavy and light chains of the BCR (Fig. A1.9). Figure A1.7D indicates the potential repertoire of V, D, and J gene segments available to encode the TCR α/β peptide binding site. The repertoire of variable light and heavy chain gene segments encoding the BCR is indicated in Figure A1.7E. The number of potential V, D, and J gene segments in Figures A1.7D and A1.7E are estimates for humans. These numbers vary among species (see Appendix A-2). A major difference from B cells is that, during gene segment recombination, SHM is greatly diminished after T cells immigrate out of the thymus. The significance of this difference and its importance was described in Chapter 6 and it serves as a guard against destructive autoimmune responses.

The Question of MHC Genetics

The major histocompatibility complex (MHC) provides a basis for the molecular uniqueness of all higher vertebrates. In Chapters 2 and 6 we introduced MHC and indicated that it controls tissue compatibility among individuals, including that between the fetal hemi-allograft and its mother. MHC compatibility is a critical element in tissue and organ transplantation. MHC is directly encoded, and expression is not subject to changes by somatic rearrangement or SHM; in other words, "what you see is what you get." Furthermore, there is co-dominance and no allelic exclusion. The best donor for organ transplants is an identical twin (a rare occurence) since tissue typing is not needed to find the best MHC match among donors.

The genes in the MHC locus (Figure A1.12A) encode protein complexes that are expressed on the surface of cells. There are two different types. MHC I is a heterodimer composed of a α-chain and a smaller protein called β2-microglobulin and is displayed on all cells. β2-microglobulin is invariant and encoded at a separate locus and merely provides molecular stabilization for the α-chain.β2 microglobulin is also used in the expression of other cell-surface proteins such as FcRn (Chapter 2 and Appendix A-2). MHC II is a heterodimer, composed of an α-chain (different from the α-chain of MHC I) and a β-chain. These are primarily displayed on lymphocytes and other hematopoietic cells such as macrophages, neutrophils, and dendritic cells and they serve an essential role in antigen presentation in the adaptive immune system (Chapter 6).

Allelic variations are concentrated in the α2 and α1 regions of MHC I and the β1 region of MHC II. These allelic variations cluster in the floor of the MHC binding sites (Figure A1.12B). Allelic differences in MHC are important in transplantation compatibility and are highest among identical twins and usually conserved among siblings. Genetic differences in MHC also influence adaptive immune responsiveness (see Chapter 6).

Figure A1.12A reveals there are four genes encoding the β-chain of MHC II and three encoding the a-chain of MHC II. These can be used in any combination to yield 12 different MHC II surface molecules. The MHC I locus contains three different genes for the α-chain. All can pair with the invariant β2-microglobulin. Therefore, any one individual can express 36 different cell surface phenotypes, which explains the need for tissue typing before organ transplantation. As with all genes in bacteria and eukaryotes, there are allelic variants of the α- and β-chains of MHC II and the α-chain of MHC I.

It is the extensive allelic variation among these genes in the human population that makes finding a suitable organ or tissue match for transplantation difficult. It also reinforces statements throughout the book that the immune system evolved as a self-/non-self-recognition system. As we discussed in Chapter 6, MHC I and MHC II bind and present peptides derived from pathogens and other environmental antigens to α/β T cells. Variants in the population are concentrated in the regions that are involved in peptide binding and presentation to T cells (Figures A1.7C and A1.12B). Because of allelic differences, two individuals may bind different peptides derived from a pathogen, which can explain how their immune responses can differ.

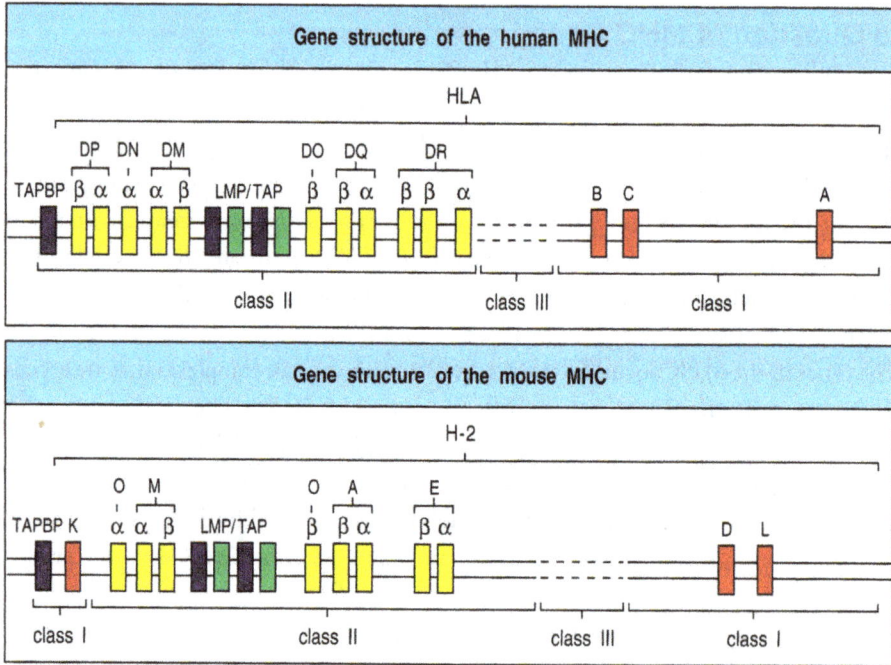

Figure A1.12A Organiziation and comparison of the MHC gene loci in human and mouse. While different nomenclature is used (HLA for human and H-2 for mouse) the encoding genes in Class I and Class II are homologs. Genes in Class III encode a variety of other proteins including complement, but these are not depicted. Allelic variation in genes encoding MHC I and MHC II are responsible for the tissue incompatibility encountered in tissue transplantation.

Biotechnology, Bioengineering, and Modern Therapy
Overview

During the last half century medical science has made enormous strides, especially in the areas of biotechnology and bioengineering. Biotechnology refers to refinements of methods and development of new tests that are orders of magnitude more rapid and sensitive than their predecessors and adaptable to automation. Our definition of **biotechnology** does not include manipulation of life, which we call **bioengineering** or creation of life components that do not exist in nature and are part of **synthetic biology** (Tan). We have selected eight biotechnical methods that have had a major impact and provide various examples of bioengineering and synthetic biology.

Biotechnical Methods
Solid-Phase Immunoassay

Prior to the mid-1970s, the methods used to measure antibodies specific for an antigen were dependent on "precipitin tests," agglutination of red blood cells and inhibition of the growth of virus *in vitro*. In the 1970s it was shown that antigens and microbes of interest could be hydrophobically adsorbed on polystyrene tubes or plates to nitrocellulose or alternatively, be

A Representative pMHC structures

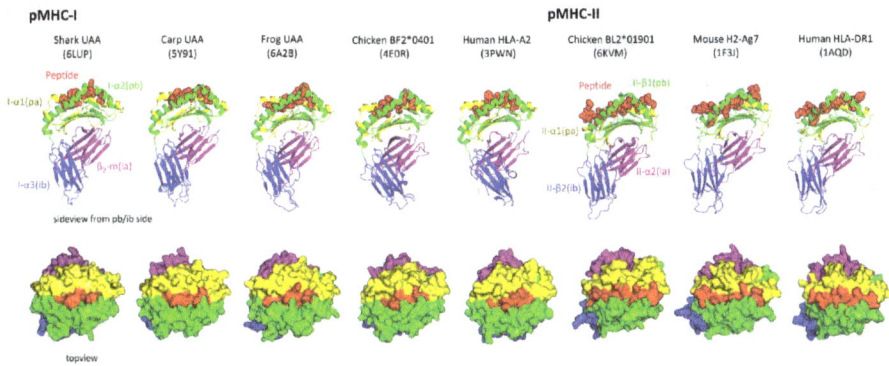

B Phylogeny of representative species

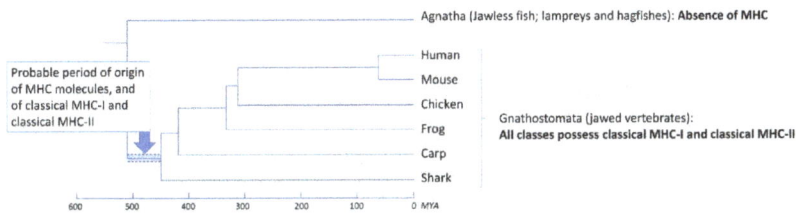

Figure A1.12B   **A)** The top row is a side-on view of models depicting the structure of MHC I in shark, carp, frog , chicken and human and MHC II in chicken, mouse, and human. In MHC I, the purple polypeptide structure is β2-microglobulin and for MHC II it is the MHC II alpha chain. The dark blue polypeptide structure is the alpha chain of MHC I and beta chain of MHC II. The green structure depicts the variable region domains of MHC I and MHC II (see text and Figure A1.7C). The linear peptides presented by an APC (see Figure A1.7C) are shown in red. The lower row shows a top-down view of MHC I and MHC II, each grasping a linear peptide (red). Note that for MHC I, the linear peptide is short (8-10 amino acids) while it is much longer for MHC II (12-16 amino acids). **B)** Phylogenetic evidence that MHC is evolutionarily conserved in vertebrates going back to teleost (boney fishes) and sharks.

chemically linked to solid phase supports. A body fluid potentially containing antibodies of interest can then be applied to the immobilized target and incubated. Thereafter, the surface is washed with a mild detergent solution, which removes unbound antibodies and other proteins. Antibodies that remain bound to the solid-phase antigen can then be detected using a **detection antibody** that is specific to the antibody class to be quantitated (see mAb section later). This **detection antibody** is conjugated to an enzyme so that the subsequent addition of the enzyme's substrate yields a colored reaction. The magnitude of the color development can be observed visually or measured in an automated spectrophotometer. The original version was called ELISA (Enzyme-Linked ImmunoSorbent Assay; Butler, 1981, 1991). The use of an enzyme-based and colorimetric detection system eliminated the hazards of using 125-I labelled antibodies as the detection antibodies and made the assay practical for general lab personel Many variations on this principle quickly followed, the most common allowing up to 96 samples to be tested in a 4-by-6-inch plastic plate. This led to rapid automation and robots so thousands of samples could be tested in 1 day. The sensitivity of these assays was 1,000 times greater than the precipitin and agglutination tests they replaced. Among the many variations is the ELISPOT method, which uses the same technology to detect and enumerate (a) individual antibody-secreting cells and (b) cells bearing certain CD markers (Appendix A-3).

DNA Sequencing

Isolation of DNA in the 1960s was laborious and efforts to sequence the product even more laborious. A breakthrough came with the Maxam-Gilbert and Sanger methods around 1977. For the Maxam-Gilbert method, isolated DNA was end-labeled with radioactive 32-P and then randomly cleaved at sites specific for each major base (A, G, C, and T). This resulted in four separate cleavage products ranging from large to small that were then electrophoretically separated in four parallel lanes on so-called polyacrylamide sequencing gels. The separated nucleotide fragments were detected in some cases by first transferring them to nylon sheets or simply wrapping the gels in saran wrap. Both were then placed in cassettes with highly sensitive photographic film and an image was obtained. The distance from the top of the gel that each labeled nucleotide had moved in the side-by-side lanes allowed the sequence to be "read." The process required 1–3 days to complete. The Sanger method used specific dideoxynucleotide fluorochromes of green, yellow, red, or blue for detection of each of the four nucleotides, A, G, T, and C. The fluorochromes were then detected with a luminometer. It was estimated that this reduced the cost of sequencing the human genome from $100,000,000 to $10,000 in a decade. Since 2010, this method has been replaced by "next gen" or high throughput sequencing using random primer for DNA synthesis with dideoxynucleotide terminators. After the sequence readout, computer analysis is used to align overlapping sequences. This has allowed for the sequencing of an entire human genome in a little over a week.

Another important application of this technology allowed for the analysis of 16S RNA found in all bacterial cells. The 16S RNA sequence is indicative of certain genera and species of bacteria and is used to determine the species constituency comprising the microbiome (Chapter 5).

Artificial DNA Synthesis

Previous *in vitro* DNA synthesis was simply DNA replication from a natural template. However, the Venter lab created a self-replicating microbe called *Mycoplasma laboratorium*. This was merely a proof-of-concept experiment to show that the short DNA sequences (ie, oligonucleotides) could be produced and used as primers for gene sequencing and especially for use in PCR (see next).

Polymerase Chain Reaction (PCR and RT-PCR)

Throughout the COVID-19 pandemic the public has become familiar with the PCR test, a highly sensitive method that can be employed to determine if an individual carries a diagnostic part of the SARS-CoV-2 genome. The technology allows a short segment of DNA to be replicated or "amplified" many times, reaching a concentration that (a) allows the product to be easily visualized or (b) readily sequenced. The technique requires a device called a **thermocycler** and the short synthetic oligonucleotides described above, which are now called "primers." Biotechnology companies have made a fortune preparing primers that can be used to sequence segments of DNA. These anneal to sequences that flank the genomic segment of DNA to be amplified. The reaction mixture contains the target DNA, the primers, a thermostable polymerase from bacteria like those that live in hot springs (*Cyanobacteria thermophiles*), and the four deoxynucleotide bases that comprise the DNA (Figure A1.1). In certain applications like SARS-CoV-2 and other RNA viruses (Appendix A-4), the sample to be tested, the viral RNA, must be first converted to DNA with reverse transcriptase and then the viral DNA strands are separated by heating and then cooled to allow the primers to anneal. This is called RT-PCR. The thermostable DNA polymerase then makes multiple copies of the DNA or the converted RNA. After the first round of duplicated DNA is generated, a high temperature is applied using the thermocycler. This causes the primers to disengage but does not damage the thermostable polymerase and the temperature is again lowered so the primers can re-anneal, and the polymerase goes back to work. For the second round, two template products are now available, for the third, four templates, and so on. Continuing this exponential amplification for 30 cycles generates a high concentration of amplified targeted DNA that can be readily sequenced as described earlier. Critical is the ability to produce the DNA primers *in vitro* (artificial DNA synthesis; see above). However, it is necessary to know the flanking DNA sequences around the target segment to which they are designed to anneal. If no product is generated in the PCR test for SARS-CoV-2, then the patient is not infected. If a product is obtained it can be sequenced to reveal whether a new variant has appeared (see section below on COVID-19).

In vitro *Eukaryotic Cell Culture*

Growing bacteria on agar plates or in large flasks is a century-old technology and easily done since each bacterium is its own complete organism. In the case of multicellular organisms, the growth of any particular cell requires "a little help from their friends" (see Chapter 1). The most successful attempts were in the growth of malignant cells, which by their very nature grow out of control and need little help. The section on bioengineering will describe how this property of malignant cells is used to produce antibodies *in vitro* and *in vivo* in animals. Nowadays, biologists have learned to culture many types of cells *in vitro* by supplying the proper cellular helpers. For example, B cell development can be studied *in vitro* by growing them on beds of fibroblast or stromal cells, a category of poorly differentiated cells that nevertheless provide the environmental help necessary to sustain nonmalignant cell culture *in vitro*.

Flow Cytometric Analysis (FCA), Also Called Fluorescence-Activated Cell Sorting (FACS)

This method allows single cells to be marked with some specific fluorescent substance, typically an antibody carrying a fluorescent marker, and passed through a laser beam (Or they can be looked at based on size and reflectance alone). This allows discrimination of cell subpopulations to (a) determine the constituency of the population being analyzed, (b) sort individual cells for additional further analyses, or (c) select them for growth and analysis *in vitro*. Using up to 20 different fluorescent labeled probes at once, each for a different molecule on the cell surface, such as some CD markers (see Table A3.2). FCA can simultaneously sort cells based on marker expression, size, and internal reflectance. Individual subsets can be recovered to study their function (eg, what cytokines they secrete) (Table 6.3) or how they interact with other cells, including their role in dealing with an infectious microbe. FCA is responsible for unraveling the complex functions of the leukocytes involved in the immune system (subsets of T cells, B cells, macrophages, and other leukocytes). For example, it can determine the proportion of T cells that carry the CD8 surface marker, which is diagnostic for cytotoxic T cells that control viral infections (Chapter 6; Table A3.2).

Single-Cell RNA Sequencing (scRNA-seq)

DNA sequencing for individual cells provides information on the genomic potential of a cell but not on how the genome is expressed (ie, the **phenotype**). Gaining information on the phenotype requires sequencing mRNA that expresses the cells **transcriptome**. Efforts began 30 years ago but have rapidly advanced. The first step is single-cell isolation, and the most primitive manual method relied on limiting dilution titration, a statistical proposition that is slow and time-consuming and may yield only 10–100 cells. Currently, laser capture microdissection (LCM) is most often applied to solid tissue (eg, a tumor). LCM typically yields less than 100 cells. For cells in circulation or those recovered by limiting dilution, cell titration can then be further separated by fluorescence-activated cell sorting (FACS; see previous section) and can yield thousands of cells (Figure A1.13). In the case of LCM and FACS, cells of interest are identified using a mAb specific to some diagnostic cell marker such as a CD marker (see sub-section on mAb technology later and Appendix A-3, Table A3.2). If they are B or T cells, they can be concurrently identified by their antigen specificity and further separated by using the specific antigen they recognize. If a specific mAb or some antigen is used for selection, they typically are biotinylated and are subsequently detected with fluorescent labeled streptavidin and sorted. These can then be labeled with commercial reagents with names like TotalSeq, which adds 3' or 5' hashtags and is loaded into a device that encapsulates each cell into an oil droplet that also contains a barcoded sequencing bead and reverse transcriptase and necessary nucleotides. cDNA synthesis occurs based on the sequence of the barcoded beads. Breaking the droplets then allows PCR amplification of the cDNA, resulting in quantities sufficient for sequencing. scRNA sequencing has many applications, especially in cancer research (Hwang; Handley). Figure A1.13 is an overview of the stepwise process. scRNA sequencing has also been modernized and has expedited mAb technology by direct cloning of paired and rearranged heavy and light chain mRNA (Banach).

Single Cell Genome Sequencing Workflow

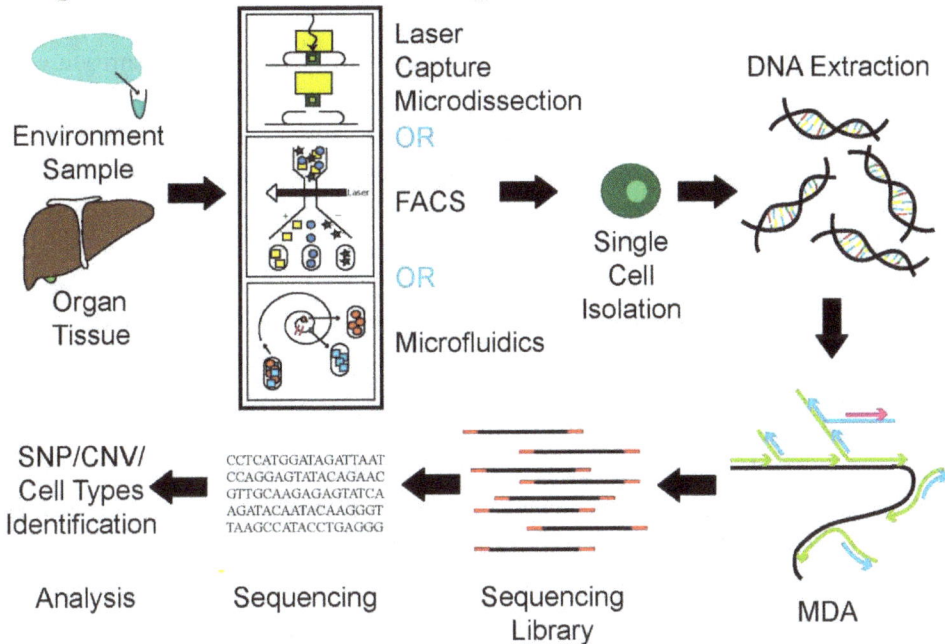

Figure A1.13 Single-cell sequencing. More than 20 slightly different methods have been described. Provided here is an overview. Tissue/cells of interest are dispersed in 96-well microtiter plates. They are cultured and cells from individual wells are collected by laser capture microdissection (LCM), or by flow cytometry (FACS) or using microfluidics, which allows for the isolation of single cells of interest and the extraction of their DNA or RNA transcripts. Multiple displacement amplification (MDA) is then applied to amplify segments of the cell's DNA or RNA, which then becomes part of a sequencing library. Sequencing and alignment of DNA segments allows relevant portions of the DNA or of RNA transcripts of the single cell to be sequenced. Fine details of the process can be found in Hwang et al. (2018).

Cryo-EM

To understand bimolecular function, knowledge of structure is important. Cryogenic electron microscopy (cyro-EM) was recently developed (Nobel Prize 2017). This is a biological molecule imaging method that uses X-ray diffraction crystallography to reveal the 3D structure of several thousand biological molecules at a resolution of three angstroms. In addition to visualization of individual bimolecular structure, the method can inform on bimolecular interactions such as viral surface receptor proteins and cell receptor structures (eg, the defining and binding of antibodies to viruses). The method in brief involves placing samples in solution or suspension on an EM grid, blotting, and flash-freezing in liquid ethane (-190°C), which traps molecules in a vitrified water layer. The samples are imaged by transmission electron microscopy (TEM) and with the aid of sophisticated computer software they are then transformed into sharp molecular structures. Since the method does not entail sample fixation or staining, structures can be visualized in their native state.

Bioengineering
Bioengineering and Synthetic Biology

Bioengineering means different things to different readers. Some may identify it with "eugenics" and experiments conducted by Nazi geneticists and physicians in the 1940s in their quest to create a mythical Aryan race of warriors. Others may consider it the use of surrogate mothers and sperm bank donors to produce more perfect offspring. Still others may understand it as efforts to replace defective genes known to be responsible for susceptibility to metabolic and infectious diseases, such as in the treatment of PKU (Chapter 2). Some may place human stem cell transfer or other forms of tissue/organ transplantation into this category. Others may understand it as genetic manipulation of embryos or somatic cells to create nucleic acids, proteins, and even bacteria that do not exist in nature. The common name for this is **synthetic biology**. This includes specific mRNAs used to develop modern vaccines and those used in CRISPR technology (see later). In Chapter 5 we mentioned the engineering of gut bacteria that do exist in nature to reduce *C. difficile* infections. Methods to develop cell-free diagnostic kits, in which the contents/reagents can be freeze-dried on paper and stored until hydrated for use, can also be regarded as synthetic. Described below are a few examples of bioengineering that are relevant to the topics mentioned in this book.

Cell Transfusion Therapy

Among the earliest examples of this procedure was the transfusion of red blood cells into newborns, since in some cases their own red cells were subject to hemolysis by maternal IgG antibodies transferred across the placenta *in utero* that recognized fetal blood group antigens encoded by paternal genes in the hemi-allograft (see Chapter 2).

In the 1960s, **organ transplantation** initially concentrated on kidneys but was rapidly expanded to other organs, success being dependent on continuing research on MHC genetics. However, in the 1980s and 1990s, transplantation was extended to the transfer of immune cells and **hematopoietic stem cells** (HSC). This now includes the transfer of cytotoxic T cells that target cancer cells in individuals with metastatic malignant melanoma and other cancers (Weber). In 25–50% of recipients, treatment results in long-lasting remission. More recently this technology has been utilized so that the TCRs of such T cells have improved specificity for certain tumors. Associated with this advance has been the use of both T and B cells with chimeric surface antigens to reduce rejection of the transferred lymphocytes. T cell therapies have also been extended to treat virus-specific diseases and are under study for treatment for Epstein-Barr virus, CMV, and certain herpes viruses. They have also been used in the treatment of HIV, and experimental studies have used transferred Tregs to control autoimmunity. A major advancement in T cell therapy involves **chimeric antigen receptor T cells** (CAR-T; see later).

HSC therapy is in routine use; the general public may recognize it as a **bone marrow transplantation**. The meaning of this term reminds readers that all the cells that become lymphocytes, neutrophils, and macrophages, as well as those that become red blood cells, have their origin in the bone marrow and arise from a common progenitor, HSC (Figure 6.1). By using targeted radiation and some mitotic inhibitors, the major portion of the recipient's HSC population is killed. This is followed by sorting to recover CD34+ cells, which are purified and then used in allotransplantation. The transferred CD34+ HSCs then repopulate the bone marrow of the patient. HSC therapy is routinely used for a wide spectrum of cancers, especially lymphocyte malignancies like leukemia, lymphoma, and various types of **multiple myeloma**. The latter is a B cell cancer that metastasize quickly and the patient becomes a factory for turning out thousands of immortal and identical plasma cells that secrete copies of the same antibody, called myeloma proteins or myeloma antibodies, which are a form of useless monoclonal antibodies (mAb). Below we will explain how medical science has used these tumor cells to generate "designer" mAbs for many different uses, including the control of the very malignant B cells that caused the original malignant tumor; "turnabout is fair play" (Carter). HSC transfer is also used in the treatment of sickle cell anemia and numerous childhood immunodeficiency diseases, like **severe combined immune deficiency** (SCID), in human infants and experimental animals. SCIDs have defects in one or more steps required for the proper development of lymphocytes and as a result cannot make antibodies and are agammaglobulinemic and T cell deficient. HSC therapy has been extended to an array of other human maladies including autoimmune disease, infantile osteoporosis, and non-Hodgkin's lymphoma.

Diagnostic Antibodies and Monoclonal Antibodies (mAb)

Diagnostic assays, such as in solid-phase immunoassay (see earlier), in the quantitation of immunoglobulins and other proteins in patient serum and the detection of CD markers on cells, depends on the use of specific antibodies to the protein or antibody isotype of interest that were raised in rabbits, guinea pigs, or sheep, that is, polyclonal antibodies. These polyclonal antibodies were produced by a spectrum of B cells, each producing an antibody of slightly different specificity for the protein or human immunoglobulin of interest and each sheep or rabbit may have responded differently. First of all their continued availability would be dependent on the life span of the producer (the sheep or rabbit). Second, these diagnostic antibody reagents needed to be subjected to time-consuming absorption on affinity matrices to remove unwanted antibodies that could interfere with accurate diagnostic measurement. Finally, each batch of polyclonal could be different. Thus, monoclonal antibody (mAb) technology was developed to overcome these problems.Bioengineering was developed so that antibodies needed in diagnostics would only recognize one specific epitope with the same affinity. Many are now universally used in FCA (see earlier).

The term mAb periodically surfaces in various chapters of this book and in the biotechnology subsection above. They are used in **biotechnology**, but their origin is a part of **bioengineering**. We described above the structure and genetics of antibodies and the myriad different specificities that can be generated. We also mentioned that in the cancer called multiple myeloma, a single plasma cell clone expands out of control and produces a myeloma protein, essentially a naturally occurring mAb. Here we describe how this disease led to a powerful technology in both medical diagnostics (biotechnology) and therapeutics.

Let's use COVID-19 as an example. Humans or susceptible vertebrates infected with a pathogen like respiratory syncytial virus (RSV), Ebola, HIV, or SARS-CoV-2 produce a broad spectrum of antibodies that recognize the virus, each with a different specificity and strength of binding (affinity). Mice immunized with the spike or S protein of SARS-CoV-2 (Appendix A-4) will make many different antibodies that bind to the S protein. mAb technology allows for selection of the B cell clones that produce antibodies that bind tightly to the S protein and can therefore be used to block binding of SARS-CoV-2 to its host cell ACE2 receptor; a process called **viral neutralization** (Appendix A-4).

Understanding the basis of mAb technology depends on knowing that normal B cells do not thrive very long when grown *in vitro* and would be more or less useless unless they also expressed genes that assured their immortality, a property of cancerous cells. In our example, to do this involves fusing B cells from mice immunized with SARS-CoV-2 with an immortalized tumor B cell line from a mouse, similar to those responsible for multiple myeloma in humans. These B cell hybrids gain the genes responsible for immortality from the tumor and the antibody specificity that recognized the SARS-CoV-2 S protein (Appendix A-4). Such hybrids can be easily grown *in vitro* and those that secrete antibodies of high affinity for the S protein can be further selected. The selected hybrid cells (now a plasmacytoma or B cell tumor) can be continuously grown in mass either *in vitro* or in the peritoneum of mice, and the mAbs they produce are regularly harvested. Since all secreted antibodies are identical and the product of a single B cell clone, they are designated as mAbs. Nowadays, most are produced using *in vitro* technology rather than having to sacrifice the mouse that was essentially given a painful cancer for the benefit of *Homo sapiens* (see animal models and Appendix A-2). Many traditional methods of mAb production have been replaced by the development of single-cell RNA sequencing (scRNA-seq; see earlier).

mAbs have become a cornerstone of many diagnostic assays such as ELISA, FCA, and ELISPOT. ELISPOT is used to detect infected cells, such as in the case of COVID-19, HIV, various cancers, and other diseases. mAbs are also being widely used therapeutically (Table A1.3). These include a mAb specific to CTLA4, a protein that captures CD80/CD86 on antigen-presenting cells (APC), a process known as *trans-endocytosis*. CTLA4 inhibits the activation of cytotoxic T cells that act against tumors and the CTLA4-specific mAb blocks this inhibition. Preventing this is one of a number of measures, for which mAbs are used in "checkpoint immunotherapies." The FDA approval of a mAb to CTLA4, which blocks the inhibition of cytotoxic T cells, is effective against metastatic melanoma (skin cancer). CTLA4 and other common CD markers are summarized in Table A3.2. The FDA has authorized use of over 40 mAbs to CDs and other markers that can block the action of cells involved in autoimmune and other disorders. Widely advertised pharmaceuticals like Humira, Skyrizi, Dupixent, and Cosentyx are examples of mAb therapies (Table A1.3).

Humanizing mAbs for Immune Therapy

mAbs that were raised in mice or mouse cells cannot directly be used in human therapy, since they represent a foreign antigen and could cause rather than alleviate disease. This danger was

TABLE A1.3   Examples of Monoclonal Antibodies Used Therapeutically*

Monoclonal	Brand	Producer	Target	Disease Targeted
adalimumab	Humira	AbbVie	TNF	Rheumatoid arthritis
bevacizumab	Avastin	Genentech	VEGD	Systemic lupus
blinatumomab	Blincyto	Amgen	CD19	Acute lymphoblastic leukemia
certolizumab	Cimzia	UCB	TNF	Crohn's disease
daclizumab	Zinbryta	Biogen	IL2R	Multiple sclerosis
infliximab	Remicade	Centocor	TNF a	Crohn's disease
ustekinumab	Stelara	Janssen	IL-12/IL-2	Plaque psoriasis
rituximab	Rituxan	Genentech	CD20	B cell lymphoma
ipilimumab	Yervoy	Bristol Meyers Squibb	CTLA-4	Metastatic melanoma
risankizumab-rzaa	Skyrizi	AbbVie	IL-23	Plaque psoriasis, psoriatic arthritis, and Crohn's disease
secukinumab	Cosentyx	Novartis	IL-17A	Plaque psoriasis and psoriatic arthritis
dupilumab	Dupixent	Regeneron	IL-4 receptor	Asthma and atopic dermatitis
benralizumab	Fascenra	AstraZeneca	IL-4R subunit	Eosinophilic asthma
guselkumab	Tremfya	Janssen	IL-23	Plaque psoriasis
efgartigimod alfa-Fcab	Vyvgart**	Fujifilm D.B.	ACR	Myasthenia gravis autoimmunity
vedolizumab	Entyvio	Takeda Pharm	α4β7	Ulcerative colitis and Crohn's disease
teplizumab	TZIED	Provention Bio, Inc	CD8	Type I diabetes

*The list provided includes only a few of over 200 mAbs that have been approved for use. An updated list is available on Wikipedia under the heading of "Therapeutic Monoclonal Antibodies."
** The Fc fragment of IgG that can block auto-antibodies to the acetylcholine receptors (ACR) in myasthenia gravis.

realized over 60 years ago when horse antibodies were used passively to neutralize the actions of toxins. Because these horse antibodies were foreign to humans, their use resulted in systemic anaphylaxis, a form of immunologic injury (Chapter 6), and it resulted in multiple deaths. Making mouse mAb safe for humans requires "humanization." This involves replacing the constant regions of the mouse antibodies with those of human antibodies; this is now a routine bioengineering procedure (Table A1.3). It is now possible to recover and culture B cells from humans infected with SARS-CoV-2 and other pathogens and produce a new generation of "humanized mAb.")

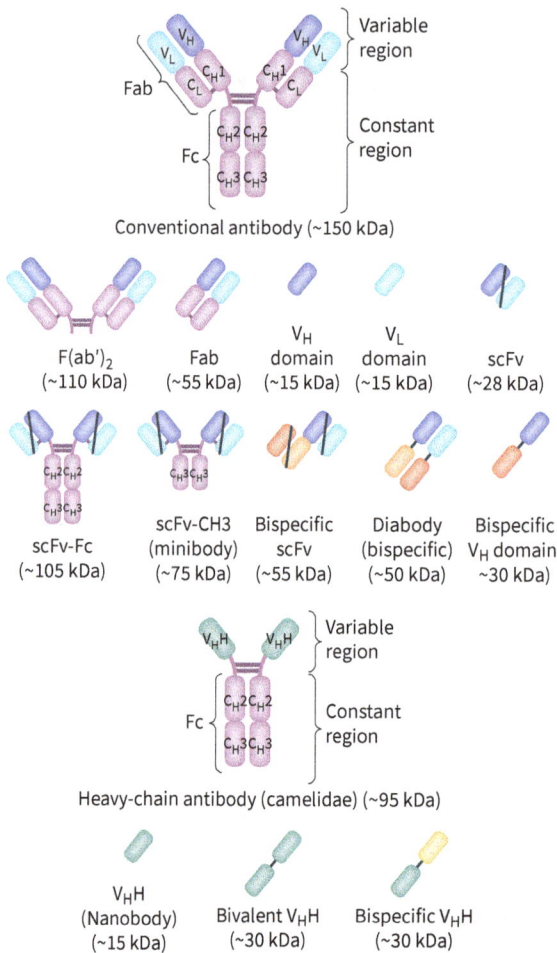

Figure A1.14 Schematic representation of antibody variants bioengineered for therapeutic use. The variants shown here are derived from conventional human and mouse antibodies and from single chain camelid antibodies. Not illustrated are "humanized" chimeric antibodies engineered from mouse mAb that bear the constant region (purple) of human antibodies.

Other Versions of Recombinant mAbs

In addition to conventional mAbs from mice, there are also mAb fragments such as those from a single or bivalent binding site fragments, or bivalent fragments with two different specificities (eg, bi-specific and camelid "nanobodies"; Figure A1.14; Marcotte). A major portion of camelid antibodies function without the need for a light chain so they are smaller (Hamer-Casterman) and have been employed to neutralize beta coronaviruses and are frequently advertised in various TV commercials. Using only the fragment containing the binding site generates a "nanobody" that is just 15 KDa, allowing their uptake and penetration into cells. These have been used in treatment of COVID-19 (Wrapp). Among the modifications are antibody fragments referred to as scFv (Figure A1.14) and the engineered chimeric antigen receptor on T cells (CAR-T cells; next section). The field of designer antibodies for therapeutic treatment has been expanded for cancer, drug delivery, oral delivery, delivery to the brain, and other selected organs (Carter).

These antibodies have numerous applications, including in therapy for multiple myeloma (van de Donk).

Chimeric Antigen Receptor T Cells (CAR-T)

T cell immunotherapy for the treatment of cancer was pioneered nearly 40 years ago and earned a Noble Prize for Allison and Honjo in 2018. This involved the recovery of lymphocytes from cancer patients, including T cells that recognized the tumor. These autologous cells were expanded *in vitro* and transfused back into the patient (Gattinoni).

This proved highly successful but had a number of weaknesses. For example, the number of tumor-specific T cells was low, as was their survival. In addition, their actions could be thwarted by an immunosuppressive microenvironment and limited by MHC restriction.

This form of immunotherapy has moved to the use of T cells with bioengineered TCRs, a technology called **chimeric antigen receptor T cells** (CAR-T cells; Zhao). There are variations, extending through as many as 5 generations of modification (Figure A1.15). In principle the new TCR is a chimera involving domains of the TCR, but with the binding site composed of the scFv (VH + VL) of an antibody (Figure A1.14) that is specific for the target of interest (eg, a tumor). The CD3 (part of the TCR complex) and the transmembrane portion of the TCR (Figure A1.7B) is retained, but co-stimulatory domains can be added including those that activate inflammatory cytokines. Thus, CAR-T cells are no longer MHC restricted and by adding co-stimulatory domains, they can be continually activated and can survive long term, with resulting positive consequences. The technology is now being applied to the treatment of multiple myeloma, cancer, and lupus (Mackensen; Finck; van de Donk). CAR-T therapy has been especially transformative in the field of oncology. It has been used to target leukemia, lymphoma, multiple myeloma, and other cancers and has received regulatory approval over the last 6 years (Finck). Recently it has been successfully used in the treatment of some autoimmune disorders, such as lupus (Mackensen), and it will likely be employed to treat other autoimmune disorders.

Engineering Bacteria

We described earlier how bacteria like *E. coli* can receive new genetic information through HGT (Figure A1.2). Plasmids are simple and usually contain less than 1,500 bp, which form a type of natural cassette into which almost any gene can be inserted. Biotech companies sell these in modified forms that are specifically designed to allow easy insertion of foreign genes. These are also engineered to include an AR gene that is expressed when a new gene has been successfully inserted, which then allows those with AR genes to survive in culture. The successful survivors can then be grown in large quantities to recover the inserted gene in large quantity. The VH and VL regions of antibodies synthesized by the many B cells of mammals can comprise 10^9 specificities (see earlier section on molecular aspects of adaptive immunity). Such technology makes it possible to selectively recover the recombinant and somatically mutated VH and VL genes from any single B cell clone for analyses (scRNA-seq sequencing). When these genes are transferred to a eukaryotic cell vector, they can be used to make "designer mAb" or designer TCR in the case of CAR-T. As an extra bargain, the technology allows many individual cloned VH and VL genes from a population of responding B cells to be sequenced to study the diversity among somatically rearranged and hypersomatically mutated VH or VL genes; this had demonstrated that these mutations primarily affect sequence changes in CDR regions (Figure A1.10). Somatic mutation also affects CDR3, but this region is also subject to nucleotide insertions and deletions in FR2, diversity segments (DH), and joining segments (JH; Figure A1.11).

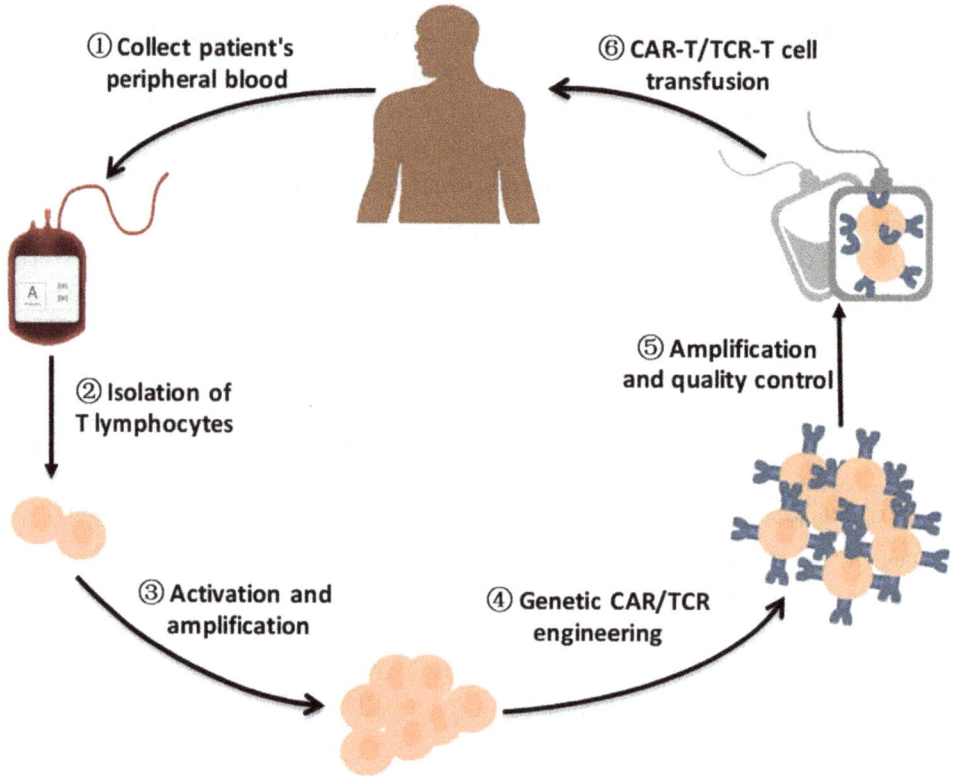

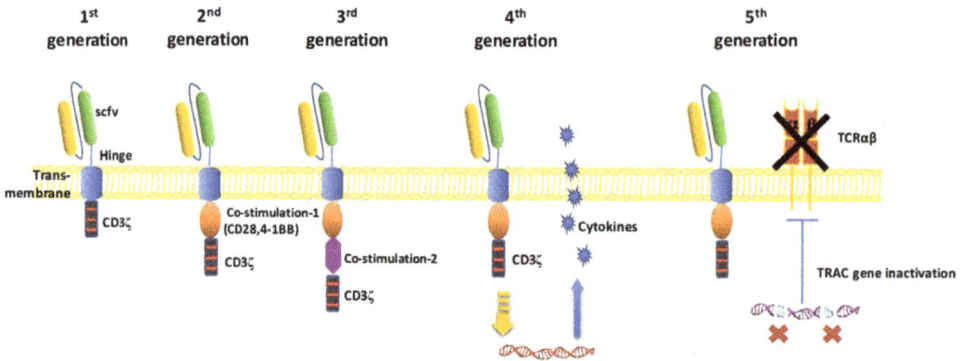

Figure A1.15   Chimeric antigen receptor T cells (CAR-T).

Expression of Eukaryotic Genes in Eukaryotic Cell Lines

E. coli–carrying plasmids can secrete the gene products encoded by the plasmid, but if they are produced by bacteria, the secreted eukaryotic gene products are likely to be improperly folded, not glycosylated, and they are often nonfunctional. Obtaining a functional product of a cloned eukaryotic gene requires synthesis by a eukaryotic cell, not by bacteria. Originally yeast cells were used but many mammalian cell lines are now used. This means the eukaryotic gene cloned and expanded using *E. coli* must be excised from the plasmid and inserted into a eukaryotic viral vector, which is then used to transform an immortal eukaryotic cell line that will be able to secrete the product of interest. An example of this technology was used to characterize the many IgG subclass variants in swine (Table A2.2). Transformed *E. coli* containing a mixture of IgG heavy-chain genes from swine were cloned and each variant recovered from separate *E. coli* clones and inserted into a benign viral vector that already contained the unusual camelid variable heavy chain gene (VHH; Figure A1.14) that is specific for a defined model antigen (ie, lysozyme). Separate viral vectors, each carrying a unique porcine constant Cγ gene, were then used to transfect a eukaryotic cell line (CHO cells) that synthesized the properly folded and now complete chimeric product, representing the swine IgG constant region and the camel VHH specific to lysozyme. The culture media from each culture was then applied to an affinity column containing lysozyme recognized by the camel VHH, and the chimeric antibodies were recovered for further study. This process recovered 11 different IgGs that could not have been purified by conventional protein chemistry (Butler, 2012). The same technology can be used to generate "designer nanobodies" (see above and Appendix A-2) humanized by using human IgG constant regions and a VHH target (eg, a tumor cell) and then used therapeutically (Marcotte).

Transgenic Animals

The house mouse (*Mus musculus*), together with field mice (*Peromyscus*) and the black rat (*Rattus rattus*), have ravaged the grain stores of human civilization for centuries while also trafficking diseases and parasites to humans. *Mus musculus* found new life in the 20th century as the species of choice for mammalian genetics and especially as an animal model for understanding the immune system (Appendix A-2). With a short gestation (21 days) and high fecundity, a plethora of inbred strains were then developed. Inbred strains are maintained by only allowing individuals of the same strain to mate and reproduce.

As early as 1974, Jaenisch and Mintz demonstrated that by inserting a foreign gene from a DNA virus into a mouse embryo, some of the offspring would express the inserted gene and, depending on dosage, some might be over-expressers. In any case, the impact of the inserted gene could be realized. However, these inserted genes were not inserted into the genome of the gametes, so they were not passed on to the next generation. Later, several other groups micro-injected the pronucleus of the developing blastocyst, but such genes became randomly inserted into the genome, and these are called **transgenic mice**. If the inserted gene was defective, these animals were called **knockouts**, but if a newly inserted gene added a function, they were called **knock-ins**. Thus, the effect of lacking a certain gene (knockout), or the function of a new functional gene (knock-in), could be studied. The use of transgenic mice greatly expanded our knowledge of the role of genes involved in obesity, heart disease, diabetes, arthritis, various cancers, aging, and Parkinson's disease. Technology has allowed the role of the various cytokines and many elements of the immune system to be understood. Animal models are discussed in Appendix A-2.

However, when injecting DNA into a mouse embryo or the gamete pronucleus, researchers could not control where the gene or genes were inserted, resulting in a very low success rate, especially when efforts were focused on a particular gene of interest. Further development involved injecting/inserting a gene into a gamete that, although being defective, could align with the wild-type gene during meiosis, a process dependent on **homologous recombination** (see Figures A1.5 and A1.16). When this was successful, the offspring would be heterozygous; they would have one nonfunctional gene at the locus paired with the functional wild-type gene. By mating littermates, one fourth of the offspring would carry the nonfunctional gene on both chromosomes, creating a knockout. Since homologous recombination that generates a knockout can be a rare event, investigators often used a marker gene to help them identify cells carrying the knockout so these cells could be used as donors for germline and somatic nuclear transfer. Homologous recombination is time consuming but was suitable in mice with a 22-day gestation and in which sexual maturity was reached in a few weeks. For large mammals with much slower reproductive rates, use of this technology was inefficient and has now been replaced by gene editing (see Appendix A-2).

Gene Editing

Experiments in altering the genome date to 1972, when Friedman and Roblin introduced a process that is now called of **gene editing**. Early approaches were awkward and too impractical to have therapeutic value, even if they were ethically allowed. The principle of the method is to create a break in both strands of the polynucleotide strands that makes up DNA—**double-strand break** (DSB) at the site where the gene exon of interest is located. At this site, the gene can be either removed or replaced. Among the early methods was the use of zinc finger nucleases. Engineered proteins that carried a DNA-binding domain targeted specific sequences in the DNA and created a DSB. This allowed either insertion of a dysfunctional knockout sequence or a knock-in gene sequence for a functional gene that encoded a new phenotype. A second method called TALEN appeared in 2010 and provided a somewhat simpler means of creating DSB, but it was still too cumbersome to be practical. Shortly thereafter a method called CRISPR-Cas9 (simply called **CRISPR**) made its appearance, and between 2013 and 2015 it was patented as the method of choice for gene editing. In 2020 its inventors received the Nobel Prize in chemistry. Neither zinc finger nor TALEN will be further discussed; instead we will focus on CRISPR and a more recent method of gene editing. CRISPR is complicated. We describe the process below but suggest that readers consult Wikipedia or detailed references and illustrations.

CRISPR technology arose from observations made in prokaryotes. CRISPR is a system naturally used by the Archaea and Eubacteria (Chapter 1) that provides a protective "cut-out device" to guard against the accumulation of potentially harmful bacteriophage genes in their genome (see Chapter 5). As mentioned in Chapter 1, a bacteriophage is a virus that infects bacteria. Over 240,000 discrete bacteriophage genomes are known and can be integrated into the bacterial genome (Chapter 5). Earlier we stated that introns are absent from prokaryotes, but this may be untrue since bacteria and some viruses contain short noncoding DNA fragments that are believed to have been left over from the action of integrases during bacteriophage and viral infections. **CRISPR** takes its name from clustered regularly interspersed short palindromic repeats. Palindromes are stem-loop nucleic acid structures that occur in over 50 forms and are found in the vast majority of bacteria. The CRISPR complex protects the bacteria by cutting out and "cleaning up" the bacterial genome that may have been "contaminated" by genes from bacteriophages and some viruses. CRISPR utilizes a small homologous RNA that can hybridize with the undesired DNA region. This is termed the *guide RNA*, and it precisely locates the region in the genomic DNA to be deleted. The large enzyme called Cas9, creates a DSB to remove the fragment. At least a dozen variants of Cas occur but the one currently used for gene editing is Cas9 (Figure A1.16). The RNA used in CRISPR gene editing is synthesized to target a particular gene in the DNA, which allows Cas9 to create a DSB at the desired location. Thereafter a repair polymerase allows for nonhomologous end-joining to repair the break, and it creates a knockout of the original gene. When a knock-in is required, a template is provided for the new gene and the DSB repaired by **homologous recombination** using direct repair polymerases (Figure A1.16). When used for gene editing in eukaryotes, the CRISPR-Cas9 complex with its specific guide RNA must be delivered by a virus. A popular choice is an adeno-associated virus (see "Viral Vector Vaccines" in this chapter and Appendix A-4). This virus is used to deliver RNA and the Cas9. A separate vector virus can be used to deliver the knock-in gene, and this can be extended to antiviral therapy (Abbott).

At the present time CRISPR gene editing in humans is only allowed for changes to somatic cells, not gametes or embryonic stem cells. However, it can be employed experimentally with stem cells if they are later destroyed. There are fewer restrictions for its use in animals or plants (see Appendix A-2). The genomes of over 50 plants have been modified by gene editing. Gene editing has also been used to improve probiotics used to create a healthy microbiome. A violation of ethical guidelines in the use of gene editing in humans brought condemnation on a Chinese investigator, who used it to knock out a receptor for HIV in embryonic stem cells and then implanted these embryos. The literature is filled with the results of many gene-editing studies carried out to provide help to individuals with neuromuscular problems and other issues. We might add that the CRISPR concept is also involved in mRNA vaccine development and immunotherapy (Appendix A-4).

In 2018 an alternative method of **gene editing** appeared, called base editing (BE; Rees). The principle is based on changing single nucleotides without needing to introduce DSB. In the CRISPR system, repair of DSB depends on homology recombination repair, which uses a donor DNA template that encodes a nucleotide containing flanked sequences homologous to regions both upstream and downstream of the DSB, reminiscent of PCR (see earlier). This homology-directed repair system is inefficient (it can only repair 0.1–5% of DSB) and can often be associated with unwanted insertions. Also, DSB can often cause translocations. BE allows for editing of 4–9 nucleotides, which is sufficient to alter single nucleotide

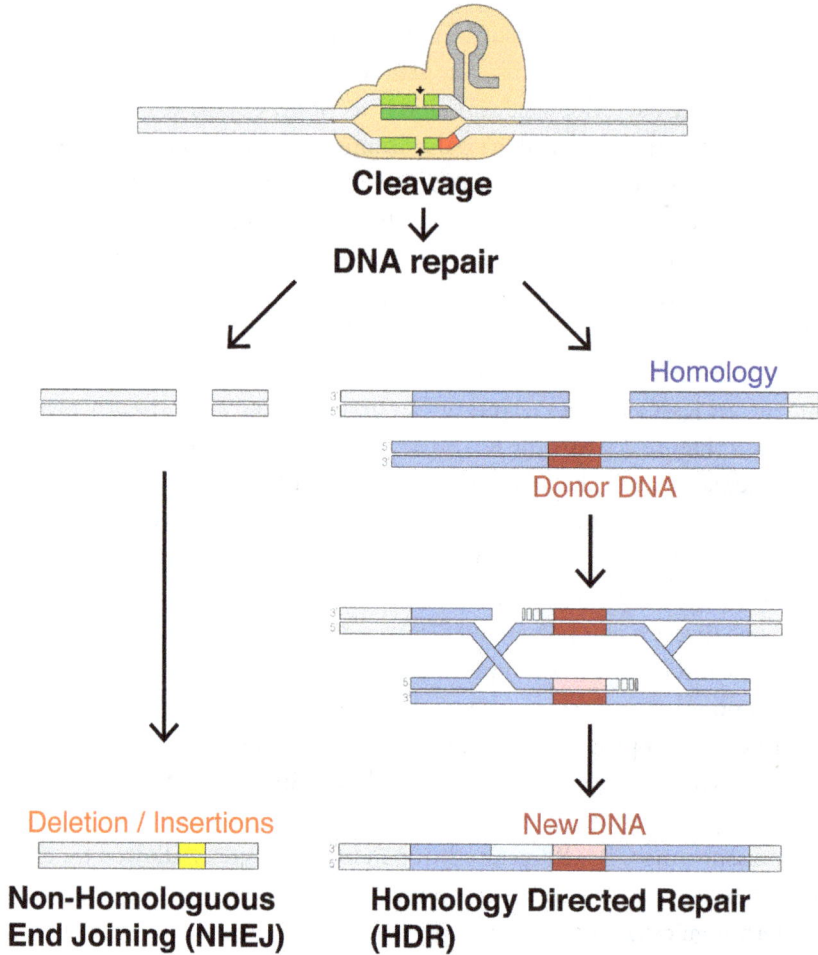

Cleavage

↓

DNA repair

Homology

Donor DNA

Deletion / Insertions

New DNA

Non-Homologuous End Joining (NHEJ)

Homology Directed Repair (HDR)

Figure A1.16   The CRISPR-Cas9 complex showing the sites where polynucle-otide changes alter the complex.

polymorphisms (SNP). Many genetic traits are controlled by SNPs. Like CRISPR, it is not allowed for genome changes in humans; however it is used in species of agricultural interest, such as pigs. For example, it is used to create leaner pigs, pigs resistant to certain diseases, and pigs with healthier heart values, which are widely used as bioprosthetic heart valves for humans (see Appendix A-2).

Evolving Immunotherapy for Allergy

Allergies or phenomena believed to have an immunological origin are "hard nuts to crack." In Chapter 6, we described the various forms of hypersensitivity, often called **immunologic injury**. In Chapter 8, we discussed controversies surrounding milk and other food allergies and forms of food intolerance that involve nonallergic phenomena. The classic Amish/Men-nonite study (Chapter 6) did not examine milk or food allergies and only provided partial laboratory findings. The study suggested that early exposure to environmental allergens leads to desensitization or tolerance. This suggests that early exposure to elements causing allergy from foods, such cow's milk protein, would reduce childhood allergy to cow's milk. However, this was not part of the Amish/Mennonite study, and our advice is to avoid this problem by breast-feeding, when this is feasible (Chapter 8). If the Strachan hypothesis (Chapter 6) applies to food allergies, then (a) the shift from breast-feeding to cow's milk formula needs to occur early on, or (b) the Strachan hypothesis does not apply to orally acquired allergy. Extending back to the 1940s, the idea of desensitization as an immunotherapeutic treatment for inhaled allergens became popular. Perhaps early exposure to an orally acquired allergen follows a different course of desensitization than that for inhaled allergens, even though the respiratory tract and the GI tract are linked through the common mucosal immune system.

Early modification of allergens for use in sensitization would currently be regarded as crude. There has been a move to recombinant DNA technology with the same purpose in mind. Major questions regarding work of this type include: (a) Will it work for only specific food allergies? (b) Can it replace the recommendation that long-term breast-feeding is the best solution? (c) Is it practical for adults with milk allergy, or only neonates? Bioengineering has created milk products for infants that cannot be breastfed, including cow's that does not make β-lactoglobulin and certain caseins. Progress in medical science will be increasingly based on understanding events at the molecular and cellular levels during development. This is a major theme throughout this textbook, and by applying new biotechnologies and bioengineering we can resolve some of these problems. Healthcare workers will need to adjust to these changes.

Modern Vaccine Development
The Shift to Modern Vaccines

Traditional vaccines, discussed in Chapter 6, depended on using killed whole bacteria, viruses, and bacterial toxins, parts of the bacteria (subunit vaccines), or attenuated viruses. (See to Appendix A-3 for acronyms used in relationship to childhood vaccines.) Attenuated viruses display the same or sufficient protective epitopes as the wild type but rarely produce disease. The oral polio vaccine (OPV) and the MMR vaccines are good examples. Whole bacteria and viruses were often used since the precise epitopes needed to stimulate a strong immune response were usually unknown unless it was a toxin. Using whole organisms is a rapid and inexpensive process compared to purifying a particular subunit by biochemical means. "Homemade" vaccines developed by using killed whole organisms were common in veterinary practice. Whole bacteria display PAMPs, so they provide a natural adjuvant needed for activation of the adaptive immune system, while subunit vaccines usually require adding a separate adjuvant. This requires additional levels of testing prior to approval, since adjuvants can result in undesirable side effects, as was experienced with some original DTP vaccines and with the current Shingrix vaccine. Attenuation of a virus is time consuming and requires clinical trials that assure that the virus does not revert to becoming virulent. We described in

Chapter 6 the merits and dangers associated with the attenuated oral polio vaccine (OPV) that is in worldwide use. In addition to examples of reversion in India and Pakistan, there are also examples of the vaccine released into feces that can then infect unvaccinated individuals in Africa or, more recently, in New York City. Thus, the development and approval of many of the conventional vaccines used in current childhood vaccination regiments required over 10 years. Testing and FDA approval was discussed in Chapter 7. This rate of development is too slow to deal with the increasing frequency of viral epidemics and pandemics (Rauch).

Advances in molecular and cellular biology have greatly reduced the development time. A SARS-CoV-1 vaccine was developed in 20 months, the Zika vaccine took 3.5 months and the vaccine for H1NI influenza took only 4 months. This pace was less than 3% of the time needed to prepare most traditional vaccines. Such rapid development has special significance for the COVID-19 pandemic. In the case of SARS-CoV-2, China released the complete genome of the virus in January 2020, less than 1 month after the Chinese recognized they were dealing with at least an epidemic, if not a pandemic, based on their previous experience with SARS-CoV-1. This information allowed molecular biologists at many pharmaceutical firms and universities to use rapid methods to produce and recover large amounts of the purified S protein (see Appendix A-4 and next) and use it to develop subunit vaccines while at the same time using parallel molecular genetic tools to develop mRNA vaccines. The fast pace of subunit recovery and use of mRNA technology was something that the pioneers of traditional vaccine development could have only dreamed about. Below we describe a number of the methods used to produce modern vaccines. It should be kept in mind that while a vaccine candidate may be developed in a relatively short time frame, today's technology scale-up and manufacturing processes still face challenges in distribution, especially in a pandemic. Manufacturing infrastructure must be available to enable large-scale production in this setting, along with skilled manufacturing technicians. The 2009 H1N1 pandemic vaccine was not widely available until after the virus's peak incidence, revealing a bottleneck in manufacturing and distribution. Given these constraints it is necessary that governments invest in preparations for emerging pandemic threats (Chapter 8) and that proper testing protocols be put in place (Chapter 7).

Modern Subunit Recovery

Traditional subunit vaccines require tedious and time-consuming biochemical purification. Rapid gene sequencing now allows the rapid cloning and identification of genes encoding epitopes of pathogens against which the immune system responds to produce a protective response. Nowadays, these sequences are cloned into suitable expression vectors and used to transfect a suitable cell line. The subunit protein is tested for its ability to induce neutralizing antibody production. While high-level expression of the target protein is achievable, downstream processing and purification can be challenging. But it is necessary in order for a subunit vaccine to reach regulatory approval. As mentioned, adjuvants are typically required for subunit vaccines. As the FDA does not license adjuvants by themselves, the vaccine immunogen-adjuvant combinations require additional approval.

Viral Vector Vaccines

This technology relies on the delivery of genes encoding one or more pathogen antigens using an unrelated "carrier virus" or vector (Rauch). The carrier virus is engineered to contain the genes that encode the epitopes deemed critical for the host to mount a protective immune response. Some may consider this a form of **nucleic acid vaccine**. The most popular carrier has been a non-replicating adenovirus vector. This allows the infected host cell to express the desired gene product, to which the host immune system can then respond. A rather large DNA segment can be incorporated into such carrier viruses, up to 8 kb, so that many segments of the pathogen genome can be included. These vaccines can be delivered intramuscularly, intranasally, intradermally, and even orally. Intranasal delivery favors a mucosal (IgA) response (Chapter 6). The ability to accept relatively large insertions is an advantage, since effective immune responses may be dependent on more than one critical epitope. Another advantage of using vector vaccines is that they carry with them the PAMPs recognized by TLRs that stimulate adaptive immunity, thus negating the need for a separate adjuvant, which is needed for most subunit vaccines (Table 6.2). Viral vector vaccines also have disadvantages. They are rather complex and comparatively cost-intensive. Furthermore, they may become integrated into the host genome, potentially resulting in immunological tolerance and potentially interference when the vector is used in repeated vaccinations. In addition to the adenovirus vector, at least five other vector viruses have been used. At the present time the FDA has approved viral vector vaccines in America for dengue fever (Dengvaxia) and SARS-CoV-2. Outside of the United States vector vaccines are being used for Ebola (licensed by Merck in Canada), and for COVID-19 (in Russia, China, India, and the United Kingdom).

DNA Vaccines

These represent another category of **nucleic acid vaccines**. DNA vaccines are bacterial plasmids in which pathogen genes have been inserted (Khan). These plasmids also contain a promoter for expression in eukaryotic cells (most often the CMV promoter) and polyadenylation signals (often from rabbit β-globin) needed for nuclear export, translation, and stability of the resultant mRNA transcript. The concept of DNA vaccines goes back to the discovery of Wolf, who used the method to express eukaryotic genes in a mouse and observed that their expression resulted in an immune response by the mouse. DNA vaccines can be delivered by needle injection or by using a helium-driven "gene gun" in which the plasmid is bound to a gold particle and is forced into the cell with the aid of a small electrical current (electroporation). Plasmids for DNA vaccines are inexpensive to prepare, and the nature of the inserted gene can easily be altered so that genes encoding the optimal epitope are expressed for recognition by the host immune system. In principle, DNA and other nucleic acid vaccines are inserted into muscle cells or given intradermally where cells transcribe, translate, and express the encoded protein. APCs like dendritic cells then carry the antigen to lymph nodes and present the foreign antigen to lymphocytes, which then initiate an adaptive immune response. In the case of intramuscular injection, myocytes probably also respond with an inflammatory reaction that recruits macrophages and other APCs, which then migrate to the draining lymph node with the expressed plasmid antigen in tow.

Despite 23 years of research, DNA vaccines have been approved for use only in veterinary medicine. First, they are poorly immunogenic, requiring that they be given with an adjuvant, unlike vector virus vaccines (Okuda). They also appear less effective when the pathogen epitope is not a protein but rather a polysaccharide, as in the case of pneumococcal and meningococcal infections. Additionally, their theoretical persistence may induce immunological tolerance to the very antigen needed for a protective immune response, especially when used in the young (Gregersen). Third, DNA vaccines provide a genetic code that depends on transcription to mRNA, which is responsible for directing the synthesis of the desired vaccine protein or peptide. Some view DNA as the curator of the genetic code and mRNA as the nucleic acid that does the hard work. So why not directly introduce the necessary mRNA (see below)? Finally, there is a delivery problem since the DNA must be delivered to the cell nucleus and it only has a minute chance of genome integration. This has been challenging and one solution mentioned above is the so-called "gene gun" technology described earlier. Despite this forceful method, the proportion of DNA that reaches the nucleus is very small.

mRNA Vaccines

The use of viral vector vaccines may result in antigen expression for a period of time too short to stimulate a robust response. A second concern is that when trafficked *in utero*, they could result in the development of **central or peripheral tolerance** to the vaccine antigen and/or the vector virus (Chapter 2; Figure 6.5A). An alternative is another **nucleic acid vaccine**. mRNA directly links the encoded gene with its expression as a protein. Therefore, mRNA vaccines eliminate one step in expressing the pathogenic epitope, to which the adaptive immune system can respond. As described earlier, the major weakness of DNA vaccines is the need to deliver the DNA to the cell nucleus. In the case of mRNA vaccines, the vaccine need only to enter the cell, not its nucleus. The principal dates to Weissman and colleagues at the University of Pennsylvania (Pardi). However, mRNA vaccines have several problems: one involves their stability and another involves delivery. Some of these problems have been resolved by using lipid nanoparticles (LNP; see later).

mRNA technology allows the bioengineer to specify exactly which protein is to be synthesized and, unlike DNA vaccines, it does not depend on the cells to transcribe DNA to the mRNA of importance. In the case of SARS-CoV-2, it is the mRNA that encodes the S protein and RBD (see below) that allows the virus to enter host cells. Technically, building such a vaccine depends on recovery of the mRNA encoding the pathogen antigen of interest and producing it *in vitro* in *E. coli*. It is then purified, a critical step since purity appears to be related to effectiveness. There are at least two current versions of mRNA vaccines: self-amplifying and non-amplifying. The former allows the host to replicate the mRNA, theoretically increasing its effectiveness by leading to production of an epitope that could stimulate an immune response. In both cases, mRNA is labile, so mRNA vaccines must be stored at extremely low temperature and not allowed to denature during delivery. To increase stability and reduce degradation, some mRNAs are delivered with associated genes that encode proteins (such as protamine) that complex and protect the mRNA.

Nanoparticle Delivery

Lipid nanoparticles (LNP) are microscopic with a diameter of 10–1,000 nanometers. They are composed of a lipid core matrix constructed from a variety of mono-, di-, and poly-glycerides stabilized with polyethylene glycol (Figure A1.17; Trollmann). The core is typically surrounded by an ionizable layer such as a phospholipid, and through pH adjustment the phospholipid can bind negatively charged biomolecules like mRNA. One approach in modern vaccine development is the use of two 50nm LNPs that form a central core (Figure A1.17). The C-terminus of the purified S protein can then be conjugated to the LNP by a glycine-serine linker and the fusion complex purified by chromatography. LNP delivery of biomolecules did not begin with their use in mRNA vaccines but with the delivery of pharmaceuticals

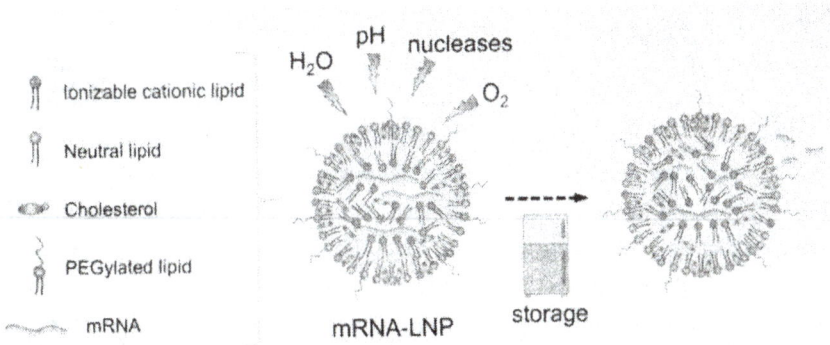

Figure A1.17   Structure of a lipid nanoparticle like those used in delivery of mRNA vaccines and some pharmaceuticals.

and with the aerosol delivery of antigens to stimulate mucosal immunity. LNP can safely pass though cell membranes and end up in the acidic environment of endosomes. This new environment allows release of their contents. We have focused on the development of mRNA vaccines and their delivery. A major challenge facing developers is the inherent instability of mRNA (Pardi; Wayment-Steele) and how degradation sites on mRNA can be protected by the coat of ionizable cationic lipids. mRNA degradation is caused by water, changes in pH, nucleases, and exposure to oxygen. If the degradation problem could be resolved, their delivery through LNP has an advantage, since the LNP is itself an adjuvant (Schoenmaker). The current solution is low-temperature storage, −15 to −25 °C for the Moderna vaccine but −60 to −90 °C for the Pfizer-BioNTech vaccine. The difference is in formulation of the LNP used, which is proprietary. The storage requirements hamper vaccine distribution, especially for the ultra-low-temp −60 to −90 °C requirement. This is manageable in highly developed countries, but it provides a hurdle for less developed countries.

Universal and Mucosal Vaccines

We mention in several chapters that (1) annual influenza A vaccines are constructed to combat the influenza variants predicted to be prevalent, and (2) the majority of antiviral vaccines are administered parenterally even though influenza, SARS-CoV-2, and other respiratory viruses target mucosal sites. Efforts to address the first concern have been to develop universal flu vaccines (Krammer). The second concern is being addressed by constructing vaccine that utilizes special adjuvants that target mucosal sites, and which stimulate cytotoxic T cells that kill virus-infected epithelial cells (Lee). More development in these directions can be expected. There are a number of novel approaches, such as using recombinant Fc-fusion proteins to increase IgA response in serum and feces by binding to Fc receptors on mucosal APC (Li, 2020).

Modern Adjuvants

Adjuvants play an important role in the performance of successful vaccines. These are biomolecules that can be recognized by TLR and other PRRs of the innate immune system, which then stimulate development of adaptive immunity (Chapter 6, Table 6.2). At this time, only seven adjuvants are approved by the FDA for use in humans, and these have been effective in stimulating antibodies that neutralize toxins, prevent virus entry, and allow for an antibody-dependent mechanism that can control the spread of bacterial infections. The next generation of vaccines will require adjuvants that (a) can stimulate CD8 cytotoxic cells, which are especially critical for control of HIV, tuberculosis, and malaria, and (b) can simultaneously stimulate CD4T cells and antibody responses at mucosal sites. This is important since many viral pathogens are first encountered on the mucosa of the respiratory and GI tracts, although many vaccines are administered parenterally so their effect at mucosal sites is secondary. Elimination of virus-infected cells at mucosal sites depends on a potent CD8 cytotoxic T cell (CLT) response. One adjuvant with promise is a carbineer-based adjuvant that can bypass aspects of cross-presentation so that dendritic cells (DCs) can directly activate specific CD8 cells (Lee).

References

Abbott TR, Dhamdhere G, Liu Y, et al. Development of CRISPR as an antiviral strategy to combat SARS-CoV-2 and influenza. *Cell*. 2020;181:865–876.

Banach M, Harley ITW, McCarthy MK, Rester C, Stassinopoulos A, Kedl RM, Morriso TE, Cambier JC. Magnetic enrichment of SARS-CoV2 antigen-binding B cells for analysis of transcriptome and antibody repertoire. Magnettochemistry 2022;8:23. doi.org/10.3390/magnetochemistry 8020023

Butler JE. The amplified ELISA: Principles of one application for the comparative quantification of subclass-specific antibodies and the distribution of antibodies and antigen in biochemical separates. In: Vunakis HV, Langone JJ, eds. *Methods in enzymology*. New York: Academic Press; 1981:482–523.

Butler JE, ed. *Immunochemistry of solid-phase immunoassay.* Boca Raton: CRC Pres Boca Raton; 1991.

Butler JE, Richerson HB, Swanson PA, Kopp WC, Suelzer MT. The influence of muramyl dipeptide on the secretory immune response. *NY Aca Sci.* 1983;409:669–687.

Butler JE, Weber P, Sinkora M, Sun J, Ford SJ, Christenson RK. Antibody repertoire development in fetal and neonatal piglets II. Characterization of heavy chain complementarity determining region-3 in the developing fetus. *J Immunol.* 2000;165:6999–7010.

Butler JE, Weber P, Wertz N. Antibody repertoire development in fetal and neonatal piglets XIII. Hybrid Vh genes and the pre-immune repertoire revisited. *J Immunol.* 2006;177:5459–5470.

Butler JE, Wertz N, Sun X-Z, Muyldermanns S. Resolution of an immunodiagnostic dilemma: Heavy chain chimeric antibodies for species in which plasmacytomas are unknown *Mol Immul.* 2012;53:140–148.

Carter PJ, Rajpal A. Designing antibodies as therapeutics. *Cell.* 2022;185:2975–2987.

Cruz-Zaragoza LD, Dennerlein S, Linden A, et al. An *in vitro* system to silence mitochondrial gene expression. *Cell.* 2021;184:5824–5837.

Davis BK, Wen H, Ting J P-Y. The inflammasome NLRs in immunity, inflammation and associated diseases. *Ann Rev Immunol.* 2011;29:707–735.

Decout A, Katz JD, Venkatraman S, Ablasser A. The cGAS-STING pathway as a therapeutic target in inflammatory diseases. *Nat Rev Immunol.* 2021;21:548–569.

Finck AV, Blanchard T, Roselle CP, Golinelli G, June CH. Engineered cellular immunotherapies in cancer and beyond. *Nat Med.* 2022;28:678–689.

Gattinoni L, Powell DJ, Rosenberg SA, Restifo NP. Adaptive immunotherapy for cancer: Building on success *Nat Rev Immunol.* 2006;6:383–393.

Gregersen JP. DNA vaccines. *Naturwissonschaften.* 2001;88:504–513.

Handley A, Schauer T, Ladurner AG, Margulies CE. Designing cell-type specific genome-wide experiments. *Mol Cell.* 2015;58:621–631.

Huang B, Li J, Zhang X, Zhao Q, Lu M, Lv Y. RIG-1 and MDA-5 signaling pathways contribute to IFN-b production and viral replication in porcine circovirus type-2 infected PK-15 cells in vitro. *Vet Immunol.* 2017;211:36–42.

Hwang B, Hyun Lee J, Bang D. Single-cell RNA sequencing technologies and bioinformatics pipelines. *Exp Mol Med.* 2018;50:96–110.

Jaenisch R, Mintz B. Simian virus 40 DNA sequences in DNA of healthy adult mice derived from preimplantatnion blastocysts injected with viral DNA. *Proc Natl Acad Sci* (USA) 1974; 1:1250–1254

Kawasaki T, Kawai T. Toll-like receptors signaling pathways. *Front Immunol.* 2014;5. doi:10.3389/fimmu.2014.00461.

Kennedy SR, Loeb LA, Herr AJ. Somatic mutation in aging, cancer and neurodegeneration. *Mech Ageing Dev.* 2011;13:118–126.

Khan K H. DNA vaccines roles against disease *GERMS* 2013; 3:26–35

Krammer F. Novel universal influenza virus vaccine approaches. *Curr Opin Virol.* 2016;17:95–103.

Lee W, Kingstad-Bakke B, Paulson P, et al. Carboneer-based adjuvants elicit CD8 T cell immunity by inducing a distinct metabolic state in cross-presenting dendritic cells. *Plos Pathogen.* 2021;17(1):e1009168. doi:10.1271/journal.ppat1009168.

Li J, Li X, Ma H, et al. Efficient mucosal vaccination of a novel classical swine fever virus E2-Fc fusion protein medicated by neonatal Fc receptor. *Vaccine*. 2020;38:4574–4583.

Li Y, Liu Z, Liu C, Shu Z, Pang L, Chen C. HGT is widespread in insects and contributes to male courtship in lepidopterans. *Cell*. 2022;185:2975–2987.

Mackensen A, Müller F, Mougiakakos D, et al. Anti-CD19 CAR T cell therapy for refractory systemic lupus erythematosus. *Nat Med*. 2022;28:2124–2132.

Marcotte H, Hammarstrom L. Passive immunization: Toward magic bullets. In: Mestecky J, Strober S, Russell MW, Kelsall BL, Cheroutre H, Lambrecht BN, eds. *Mucosal Immunoloy*. Vol. 2. Cambridge, MA: Academic Press; 2015:1403–1425. Elsevier.

Okuda K, Wada Y, Shimada M. Recent developments in preclinical DNA vaccination. *Vaccines*. 2014;2:89–106.

Pardi N, Hogan MJ, Porter FW, Weissman D. mRNA vaccines—a new era in vaccinology. *Nat Rev Drug Discov*. 2018;17:261–279.

Rauch S, Jasny E, Schmidt KE, Petsch B. New vaccine technologies to combat outbreak situations. *Front Immunol*. 2018;9:1963. doi:10.3389/frimmu.2018.01963.

Rees HA, Liu DR. Base editing: Precision chemistry on the genome and transcriptome of living cells. *Nat Rev Genet*. 2018;19:770–788.

Rietdijk ST, Burwell T, Bertin J, Coyle AJ. Sensory pathogens—NOD-like receptors. *Curr Opin Pharmacol*. 2008;8:261–266.

Saxena M, Yeretssian G. NOD-like receptors: Master regulators of inflammation and cancer. *Front Immunol*. 2014;14(5):37. doi:10.3389/fimmu.2014.00327.

Schoenmaker L, Witzigmann D, Kulkarri JA, et al. mRNA-lipid nanoparticle COVID-19 vaccines: Structure and stability. *Int J Pharm*. 2021;601:120586. doi:10.1016/j.ijpharm.2021.120586.

Sinkora M, Butler JE, Lager KM, Potochova H, Sinkorova J. The comparative profile of lymphoid cells and the T and B cell spectratype of germ-free piglets infected with viruses SIV, PRRSSV and PCV2. *Vet Res*. 2014;45:91–109.

Sun J, Butler JE. Molecular characterization of VDJ transcripts from a newborn piglet. *Immunol*. 1996;88:331–339.

Tan X, Letendre JH, Collins JJ, Wong WW. Synthetic biology in the clinic: Engineering vaccines, diagnostics, and therapeutics. *Cell*. 2021;184:881–898.

Trollmann MFW, Bockmann RA. mRNA lipid nanoparticle phase transition. *Biophys J*. 2022;121:3927–3939.

van de Donk, N. WJC, Usmani SZ, Yong K. CAR T-cell therapy for multiple myeloma: State of the art and prospects. *Lancet Haematol*. 2021;8(6):e446-e461. doi:10.1016/S2352-306(21)00057-0.

Vijg J, Dong X. Pathogenic mechanisms of somatic mutation and genomic mosaicism in aging. *Cell*. 2020;182:12–23.

Wayment-Steele HK, Kim DS, Choe, CA, Nicol JJ et al Theoretical basis for stabgilizing messenger RNA through secondary structure design. *Nucleic Acid Res* 2021; 49:10604–10617

Weber EW, Maus M, Mackall CL. The emerging landscape of immune cell therapies. *Cell*. 2020;181:46–61.

Wrapp D, De Vlieger D, Corbett KS, et al. Structural basis for potent neutralization of beta coronaviruses by single-domain camelid antibodies. *Cell*. 2020;181:1004–1015.

Wolff JA, Malone RW, Williams P et al. Direct gene transfer into mouse muscle in vivo. *Science* 1990; 247:1465–1468

Xiong N, Roulet DH. Development and selection of γ/δ T cells. *Immunol Rev*. 2007;215:15–31.

Zhang X, Bai X-Z, Chen ZJ. Structures and mechanisms in the cGAS-STING innate immunity pathway. *Immunity*. 2020;53:43–53.

Zhao L, Cao YJ. Engineered T cell therapy for cancer in the clinic. *Front Immunol*. 2019;10:2250. doi:10.3389/fimmo2019.02250.

Acknowledgments

We thank the following individuals for their careful review of this appendix and helpful suggestions.

John C. Cambier Emeritus Head, Department of Microbiology and Immunology, University of Colorado

Mark Stinski Emeritus professor, Department of Microbiology and Immunology, University of Iowa

Michael O'Hara Former Senior Scientist and Senior Program Manager, HHS/BARDA

William (Rick) Brown Director of operations, products and process support. Core Diagnostics, Abbott Laboratories, Lake Forest, IL

Figure Credits

Appendix A-2
Mammalian Diversity and Animal Models

Rationale for Appendix A-2

Much of what is known about nutrition, passive immunity, the microbiome, and the fine details governing the immune system initially had its origin in studies in other mammals. While the basic anatomy and physiology of mammals is similar, there are major differences that may help students to better understand certain aspects of human physiology and how animal models can be useful in understanding certain major concepts. We begin with a review of mammalian diversity as regards reproduction, including differences in placentation, the level of development at birth, suckling patterns, and fecundity. We then focus on the diversity of immune systems, diversity of microbiomes, and related metabolisms. We conclude by discussing animal models and animal bioengineering.

Mammalian Diversity
Classification of Mammals

Mammals are one of the four classes of vertebrates, which also include fish, amphibians, and reptiles/birds. Despite differences in appearance and lifestyle, reptiles and birds are anatomically, reproductively, and genetically quite similar. Recent paleontological evidence from China has shown that ancestral reptiles had feathers and wing structures like birds, and some ancestral forms were warm-blooded. Zoologists now consider reptiles and birds to belong to the same vertebrate class, the Sauropsida. The cataclysmic meteorite event presumed to be responsible for the demise of the large reptiles allowed their smaller and terrestrial feathered variants (birds) to survive together with small mammals. It also allowed fish to expand and diversify, and they now account for the largest number of vertebrate species. Here we only focus on class Mammalia, derived from the Latin word *mammae* for mammary gland (MG) and referring to the breast and nipple through which the mother delivers nutrients and other factors to her suckling newborn (Chapter 3).

Mammals are broadly divided into two suborders: the Protheria and the Theria (Table A2.1). The Theria are further divided into the Metatheria (renamed Marsupialia) and the Eutheria (renamed Placentalia). The former includes the

TABLE A2.1   Diversity in Reproduction and Placentation

Taxa	Fetal Development	Placentation	*In utero* IgG Transport	Maturity at Birth	Sexual Maturity	Number of Offspring	Lifespan (Years)
Protheria (Platypus)	External	NA		precocial			
Metatheria (Marsupalia)	Internal	Species-dependent	Yes, for wallabies; others may differ	altricial	Species-dependent	2–20	3–15
Eutheria (Placentalia)							
Chiroptera	Internal	UD	Yes	semi-precocial	10–14 months	1	15+
Rodentia	Internal	UD	Yes	altricial	2–12 months	4–8	2–12
Insectivora (replaced by Eutypotiphyla	Internal	UD	Yes	altricial	UD	4–8	2–4
Lagomorpha	Internal	UD	Yes	altricial	6–8 months	4–6	4–10
Ruminant Artiodactyls	Internal	cotyledonal	No	precocial	6–36 months	1–2	10–20
Suid Artiodactyls	Internal	diffuse	No	precocial	6 months	6–24	~10
Pinneipedia	Internal	zonary	Yes	precocial	5–10 years	1	~10
Carnivora	Internal	zonary	Yes	altricial	6–24 months	2-10	6–30
Cetacea	Internal	diffuse	?	precocial	Species-dependent	1	30–80
Primata	Internal	discoidal	Yes	altricial	4–15 years	1–2	20–100

UD = undefined

marsupials or "pouched mammals" that dominate Australia. The Placentalia include the many familiar mammals of the Northern Hemisphere and Africa, which zoologists classify into "meat-eaters" (order Carnivore), seals (order Pinneipedia), hooved mammals (order Artiodactyla), rodents (order Rodentia), rabbits (order Lagaomorpha), ape-like species (order Primata), bats (order Chiroptera), whales (order Cetacea), shrews and moles (Order Insectivora)and others. The separation of the Marsupialia and Placentalia is a bit confusing and somewhat controversial, since marsupials do have a simple placenta, but it is less invasive into maternal tissue than we described for human placentation (Chapter 2). The Protheria are of little concern to us in this chapter. They include the infraclass Monotremata, organisms that share many anatomical features with "true" or Therian mammals but are egg-layers, such as the duckbill platypus and spiny anteater of Australia and New Guinea.

The Marsupialia will be discussed since they are especially widespread in South America, and the American opossum is well-known to most students. Marsupials provide an interesting example of the early transition from fetal to MG nutrition. Their developing fetuses are born prematurely and transition from *in utero* placental nutrition to near-permanent attachment to the mammae; for some species this occurs inside the pouch, perhaps giving new meaning to the word "fetus." Our major focus is on the Eutheria, now called the Placentalia, and how the complexity of the placenta influences the trafficking of nutrients and other factors from mother to fetus and how this varies among mammals.

Reproductive and Developmental Diversity
Reproductive Diversity

Mammals differ from each other in the following ways: (1) placental structure, (2) placental structure and *in utero* trafficking from mother to fetus, (3) suckling patterns, (4) the number and location of mammae, (5) the composition of milks, (6) the number of offspring, and (7) the degree of maternal protection.

Differences in Placentation

Eutheria/Placentalia mammals differ in the nature of the placenta, the differences include (1) shape and contact points, and (2) the number of tissue layers that comprise the placental barrier. In rodents, and humans and other primates, the placenta has a single attachment point to the endometrium of the mother's uterus (Figure 2.1). Biologists call this condition **discoidal**. This is rather invasive and therefore complicated, as illustrated in Chapter 2. In carnivores the placenta appears as a band that surrounds the fetus, a pattern called **zonary**. In ruminants the placenta is attached to the endometrium at several points and is called **cotyledonal**, so the attachments appear like "buttons." In horses and pigs, the entire surface of the chronic epithelial layer is attached, in an arrangement called **diffuse**.

Of greater functional importance are differences in tissue complexity. The placenta is considered to be composed of six layers, three contributed by the fetus and three by the mother. Throughout the evolution of Eutherian mammals, some of these layers have been lost, while others were destroyed as fetal tissues invaded the endometrium of the mother. In Artiodactyls (ruminants, pigs, horses) all six membranes remain present, which some scientists use to explain why there is no transport of IgG from the mother to the fetus in Group III mammals (Figure 3.4). While thickness may be a factor, this is an oversimplification since trafficking depends on transport receptors like FcRn in the human placenta; FcRn has not been found in the porcine, horse, or ruminant placenta. This, rather than the number of tissue layers, likely explains the absence of *in utero* IgG transfer in some species. Interestingly, these differences (Figure 3.4) are correlated with level of maturity at birth (see later). Having a multilayered placenta, as Artiodactyls do, may reduce the level of congenital (present at birth) disease caused by infectious viruses. While some infectious microbes cross the human placenta (Chapter 2), others like PRRSV and adenovirus can also cross the thicker six-layered porcine placenta.

Of some interest is evidence that genes expressed in the placenta are the same as those expressed in the MG, perhaps suggesting an organized transfer of gene expression from placenta to MG. An obvious example is the FcRn transport receptor in the human placenta that transfers IgG *in utero* (Palmeira; Figure 2.3A). This is the same receptor used to transport IgG from blood into the milk ducts of Artiodactyls and to transport IgG across the gut epithelium in rats. FcRn is something of a "do everything" receptor for IgG and albumin transport and plays a major role in their metabolism and maintenance in all mammals (Rath). Blocking FcRn with a mAb lowers IgG and IgG immune complex levels in human serum (Blumberg). Overexpression of FcRn greatly increases serum IgG half-life, a technique for recovering large amounts of IgG antibodies from experimental animals (Kacskovics).

Maturity at Birth

Children of *The Naked Ape* (the title of an old bestseller by Desmond Morris) seem attracted to the furry offspring of other mammals, which spawned an industry that re-created animal babies as stuffed companions. These decorate their cribs and bedrooms and often comprise the major characters of children's books and television shows. In reality, many of these "fuzzy friends" where not born fuzzy. Even worse than being hairless, many are born blind.

Mammals differ as to when the transition is made from prepartum to postpartum transport of passive IgG, and this may explain differences in the maturity of their offspring at birth. Parturition is hormonally dependent and can be induced with oxytocin, suggesting that birth among different mammals is not related to the degree of *in utero* development but depends on differences in endocrine activity. Eutherian offspring like puppies, kittens, and mice are also born hairless, blind, poorly mobile, and incapable of locating the MG without help from the mother. Biologists call this condition **altricial** (Table A2.1). Many have seen a newborn foal or calf is on its feet within minutes after birth, often romping about before zeroing in on its mother's MG; such offspring are called **precocial**. This suggests that whether a species is altricial or precocial is dependent on when the endocrine system calls for birth to occur, which appears linked to placental vs. postpartum transfer of IgG. All newborn mammals that exclusively obtain IgG postpartum via colostrum and milk are precocial. These differences may have evolved because of the harsh environment faced by some newborns in which quasi-independence was needed to survive.

Interestingly, precocial vs. altricial distinction does not correlate with sexual maturity. The offspring of the "naked ape" and many primates remain for years with their mothers, and human offspring require approximately 13 years to reach sexual maturity, while rodents, rabbits, and swine can mate and produce offspring in the same year in which they were born, and carnivores require 1–3 years (Table A2.1). This suggests that other hormonal factors are at play during mammalian development and postpartum parental care. This is usually explained by the greater amount of time needed for neurological development in some mammals, which is correlated with a proportional increase in brain size, especially pronounced in humans.

Litter Size, Multiparity, and Its Consequences

Other examples of diversity relate to suckling and litter size. Marsupial offspring become immediately and continuously attached to the mammae, while Eutherian offspring suckle only when needed, sort of a self-serve system. Table A2.1 shows there are also major differences in the number of offspring resulting from a single mating (ie, litter size). We described in Chapter 1 how, in general, higher eukaryotes devote more energy to protection of their offspring, reducing the need to produce a million offspring to assure species survival by merely protecting and training a small number of offspring. Variations can range from a single offspring in most primates, to twins in sheep, to a half-dozen in rodents, up to a dozen in dogs and two dozen in certain pig breeds. Not surprisingly, litter size is also correlated with the number of mammae, which range from 2–18 and develop along two bilaterally symmetrical "milk lines." Some mammae develop only posteriorly (in ruminants, horses, and guinea pigs), only anteriorly (primates, elephants), or are continuously distributed along the milk lines (canines and swine). Humans have two mammae, since twins are not uncommon, or to alternatively assure an adequate nutrient supply for a single offspring; however, output from the two mammae can differ. If this is universally true for all mammals, one can imagine the consequences when the offspring from a litter of 20 compete for 10–16 mammae. In the opossum that may have up to 20 offspring, the premature offspring are carried in pouch in which each is continuously attached to one mammae. With only eight mammae that are permanently occupied, this means the remainder of the litter perishes; perhaps a "shot gun" strategy. This apparent wasteful process may be a positive natural selection process that favors the biggest and strongest. The situation in the kangaroo (another marsupial) is most interesting considering that the constituency of milk as regards proteins and amino acids changes during lactation, and they are therefore secreted in a programmed manner. Changes also occur in humans (Chapter 3) and appear crafted to promote different aspects of development at different times. In kangaroos, this program can operate separately on two different mammae, so the mother is able to accommodate the differing nutritional needs of two joeys of different ages.

There are other examples of mammals with multiple offspring where there is competition among the suckling neonates; the smaller and less aggressive being outcompeted, giving rise to the expression "having to suck the hind teat." Competition can mean that, for some offspring, suckling is delayed. Figure A2.1A shows that newborn piglets unable to immediately suckle obtain lower levels of passive IgG, IgA, and IgM, reducing their level of passive immune protection. Figure A2.1B shows that the amount obtained by suckling is inversely related to the degree of *de novo* synthesis by the offspring. This is most pronounced with IgG, suggesting that IgG along with labile factors in colostrum (eg, TGFβ; Figure 3.6) play a role in regulation of the developing adaptive immune system and the health of the neonate.

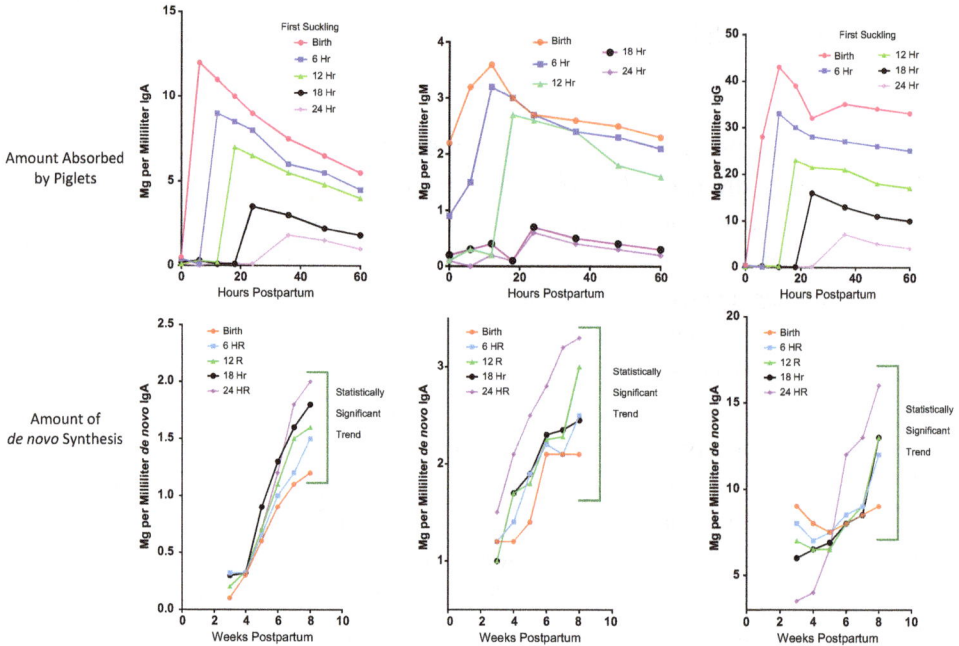

Figure A2.1 TOP: The effect of a delay in suckling on the amount of passive antibodies indiscriminately absorbed by the neonatal piglet. BOTTOM: The level of *de novo* synthesized immunoglobulins in relationship to the amount of absorbed Igs. The same colors are used for the same delay times. Legend on figure. Refer also to labile regulatory factors that influence immunoglobulin production by suckling piglets (Figure 3.3).

A curious factor that involves the MG is mate selection. Only primates and kangaroos assume an erect posture, and in human culture the MG seems to be involved in mating selection. While we try to avoid behavioral aspects, we wonder if the less conspicuous MGs of most mammals have a similar behavioral function.

A factor that may determine litter size is the mother's ability to supply the nutrients needed for her offspring. Few would question a mother bear's ability to protect her cubs, yet the normal litter size is twins. This appears related to the nutritional needs of her cubs. While brown and black bears are short-term hibernators, the body temperature and metabolism of polar bears (non-hibernators) is only moderately reduced. In any case, the mother must store enough energy to nourish the cubs that develop and are born during hibernation. Hibernation is itself an energy conservation necessity that is discussed in a subsequent section. Bats, which comprise 20% of all mammals, have a high rate of metabolism, which may explain why they can only afford nutrients for a single offspring. The mother must catch enough insects in one night to provide her own energy needs and the nutrients to produce milk for her single offspring. Some bats behave like the opossum and carry their offspring with them on their nightly forays for food, which further increases their energy requirements.

In Chapter 3 we showed that in humans, breast milk output increases during lactation and its composition changes. A question that is difficult to address is whether multiparity influences MG output and passive immunity to the sucklings. This is better addressed in controlled animal studies that show that the serum level of IgG during reproduction progressively increases with each gestation (Figure A2.2A; Klobasa). In pigs, the level of IgG in the mother's serum prepartum is directly correlated with the amount of IgG transferred to the suckling in colostrum. While first-gestation mothers accumulate 15–20 mg/ml of IgG in in their sera prepartum, this significantly increases to 18–27 mg/ml in sixth-gestation sows (Figure A2.2B). Notable is the precipitous drop in serum IgG levels 5–10 weeks prepartum, when IgG is no longer being selectively transported into the MG for eventual secretion into colostrum. Serum IgG levels rebound in the serum of the mother when "gut closure" occurs. This is when IgG in colostrum/milk is no longer indiscriminately absorbed by the suckling. This suggests a neuro-endocrine linkage between the sow MG and the enterocytes of the suckling piglets, which is most likely cytokine dependent.

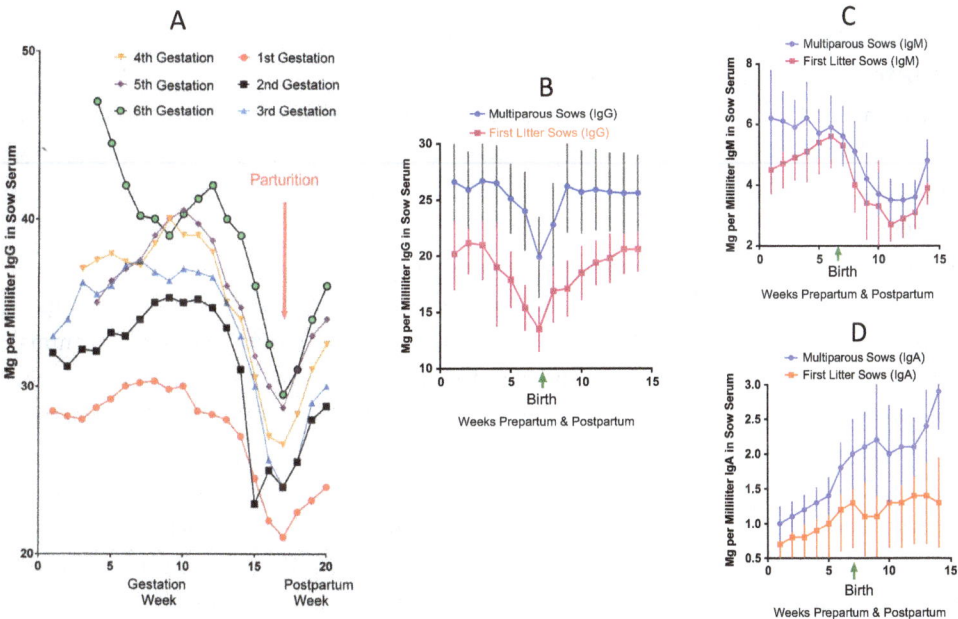

Figure A2.2   A. Serum IgG levels in first- through sixth-gestation sows prepartum and during the first 20 days postpartum when lacteal secretions are transitioning to mature milk. B. Individual variation in serum IgG levels in first- and sixth-gestation sows and restoration of serum IgG levels after gut closure. C. Individual variations in serum IgM levels in first- and sixth-gestation sows. D. Individual variation in serum IgA levels in first- and sixth-gestation sows. Legends are on the figure. In Figures B–D, error bars depict standard deviation.

Equally notable is the drop in IgM levels postpartum and their rebound postpartum, suggesting that "natural IgM antibodies" (see Figure A3.3) are also being transported into colostrum. Furthermore, serum levels of IgM are not gestation dependent (Figure A2.2C). Does this suggest a decline in "natural IgM" antibodies as the sow ages? The more vigorous production of IgA postpartum, especially in multiparous sows (Figure A2.2D) suggests that older sows provide increased mucosal immune protection to their offspring. Comparative data for multiparous women are not available.

Differences in Parenting

Mammals differ in parenting. In some cases postpartum care is extremely short, while in humans postpartum care may extend for over a decade. The degree and length of parental protection is correlated to litter size. Rodents and rabbits produce many offspring but only 10–20% survive to reproductive age. This seems like an evolutionary compromise between the random survival of early vertebrate offspring, like in fish and amphibians, and the volution to parental protection in higher vertebrates like mammals (Chapter 1). While odds are high for the very protective carnivores, they are extremely high for primates.

Diversity of Immune Systems among Mammals
Innate vs. Adaptive Immunity

The innate immune system acts as the first line of internal defense against infectious agents that display PAMPs that indicate "danger" when recognized by pattern recognition receptors (PRR) such as Toll-like receptors (TLRs; Table 6.2). Stimulation of the innate immune system causes the congregation of inflammatory cells like macrophages and neutrophils that form intracellular complexes called the **inflammasome** (Appendix A-1). These locally and momentarily stop the spread of the infection and stimulate the maturation of the adaptive immune response (Butler, 2017; see later). The diversity of the innate immune system among mammals has been less well-studied than that for adaptive immunity. However, studies indicate that TLRs are highly conserved and are present in at least all higher vertebrates. TLRs and other PRRs are present in all mammals and protection may come from innate immunity alone. Certain bats harbor viruses (rabies, Ebola, Marburg, SARS coronaviruses) and serve as viral reservoirs and vectors that can cause disease and death in other mammals such as humans, but not in the vector bats themselves. In the Egyptian *rousettus* bat, a reservoir host for Marburg virus, the innate immune system appears to be protective on its own (Larson; Randolph).

The evolutionary appearance of an internal protection system called **adaptive immunity** depends on the lymphocytes that can somatically alter the receptors that recognize infectious agents; a "game-changer" for homeothermic vertebrates (Chapter 6; Appendix A-1). Lymphocytes at various stages of development and differentiation can be identified and sorted on the basis of certain surface glycoproteins that go under the title of CD markers, short for cluster of differentiation (see flow cytometry, Appendix A-1). More than 300 CD markers are known; Table A3.2 summaries the few that are often mentioned in this textbook. Many are shared among mammals, such as CD4 that identifies helper T cells and CD8 that identifies cytotoxic T cells. Monoclonal antibodies (mAb) raised against these and other CD markers very often cross-react among various mammals and therefore may help to identify cells that have the same function as those in the lab mouse and human. Since the innate immune system is highly conserved, we shift our focus to the diversity of the adaptive immune system of mammals.

Immunoglobulin Structure and Diversity

Immunoglobulin (Ig) is the biochemical term used to describe all proteins that possess the same structure as antibodies involved in the adaptive immune response. The basic structure of immunoglobulins, the major classes of the secreted forms, and those that serve cell-bound B cell receptors (BCR) were described in Figures A1.7A and A1.7B and are summarized in Table A3.1. In Appendix A-1 we described the molecular genetics of antibody formation, including somatic gene rearrangement and mutations that influence the conformation of the antigen binding sites of the TCR and BCR. Here we describe variation among mammals in regard to these features. Table A2.2 indicates that, with the exception of IgD, all of the major classes are present in the other Eutherian mammals so far studied. As illustrated in Appendix A-1, the gene encoding IgD (Cδ) is located immediately downstream from the one encoding IgM (Cμ). Both encode monomeric Igs that function as BCRs (Figure A1.7A).

Cμ also encodes the pentameric IgM that appear approximately 3 days after antigen/pathogen exposure (Figures 6.3 and A1.7B). This is sometimes called the "natural" antibody response, which can also be considered a form of innate immunity (Chapter 6). Evidence in support of this view comes from studies using germ-free piglets in which (a) one group was infected with enterohemorrhagic *E. coli* 933D, and (b) a second group was exposed to two PAMPs (LPS & MDP; Table 6.2). Figure A2.3 shows that piglets receiving only

TABLE A2.2   Diversity of Immunoglobulin (Ig) Among Mammals

Heavy Chain Diversity									
Species	Ig Classes	Subclasses	VH	VH families	% func*	DH	% func*	JH	% func*
Human	5	4 IgG, 2 IgA	123	7	32	28	90	9	60
Mouse	5	4 IgG	~200	14	56	31	51	4	75
Rat	5	3 IgG	~300	12	37	35	71	4	100
Rabbit	4	1 IgG, 13 IgA	~100	1	< 10	11	?	6	?
Cattle	5	3 IgG	~36	1	27	23	39	4–6	~25
Swine	5	6 IgG	> 20	1	~40	4	50	5	20
Horse	5	7 IgG	50	?	< 10	40	87	8	100
Bat	5	> 4 IgG	77	?	85	> 13	> 60	9–25	~35
Opossum	4	1 IgG	26	3	80	9	?	6	33

(Continued)

TABLE A2.2 Diversity of Immunoglobulin (Ig) Among Mammals *(Continued)*

Light Chain Diversity											
Species	**Cλ**	**Cκ**	**Cλ:Cκ**	**Vλ**	**% func***	**Jλ**	**% func***	**Vκ**	**% func***	**Jκ**	**% func***
Human	?	1(2)	1:15	7	40	?	?	76	44	5	100
Mouse	3	?	1:20	3	75	40	80	169	47	5	80
Rat	4	1	~1:12	10–15	40–70	4	50	163	~50	6	85
Rabbit	5	2	~1:6	43	>2	?	?	>100	?	5	1
Cattle	3	1	20:1	63	38	8	60	25	24	3	~70
Swine	3	1	1:1	22	40	4	50	14	70	5	40
Horse	4	1	13:1	144	20	4	75	60	31	5	80
Bat**			λ>κ	>100	50–90	80	10	6	?	?	?
Opossum	8	1	2:1	64	90	8	100	122	30	4	100

** % func = Proportion believed to be functional. Assigning functionality in the IMGT system is based on sequence, but this is not based on empirical data. In many cases no reliable information is available on the proportion of variable genes that are functional.*

*** There are hundreds of bat species, and only the genome encoding antibody genes has been studied. Thus, the numbers provided are likely to vary greatly based on the species under investigation.*

Disclaimer: Because of the variability among strains within species of animals (even lab animals) and species of agricultural interest, we provide only a synopsis of what is currently understood. Those interested in finer details are encouraged to consult the most recent primary literature. Our objective in this appendix is to indicate that diversity exist among species for gene segments that encode antibody genes.

PAMPs made IgM antibodies to the entire panel of related and unrelated bacteria but also an IgA response to some members of the panel, including a strong response to *Salmonella* but no response to 933D. The latter suggests, as has Bunker, that certain IgA responses may also be innate. Noteworthy is that even though IgG accounts for about 80% of all serum immunoglobulins, there was no IgG response in piglets receiving only PAMPs, while in infected piglets, IgG responses were directed to the infecting pathogen and two cross-reactive Enterobacteria. The broad IgM response seen after exposure to the TLR ligand is the basis for using the term *natural antibodies*. This result implies that at birth piglets have plasma cells (PC) that can, without pre-exposure, recognize a spectrum of unrelated bacteria and release antibodies as early as 3 days (Figure 6.3) after encounter with a CpG, which is sustained for 2 weeks. No such IgG response is seen but an IgA response to *Salmonella* was seen. Some investigators have reported "natural" mucosal IgA responses (Bunker).

By contrast, Figure A2.3 shows that in pathogen-infected piglets, most antibodies are specific for the pathogen or other Enterobacteria and pronounced IgG and IgA responses are also seen. A complete description of the molecular and cellular aspects of B cell and antibody responses is provided in Chapter 6.

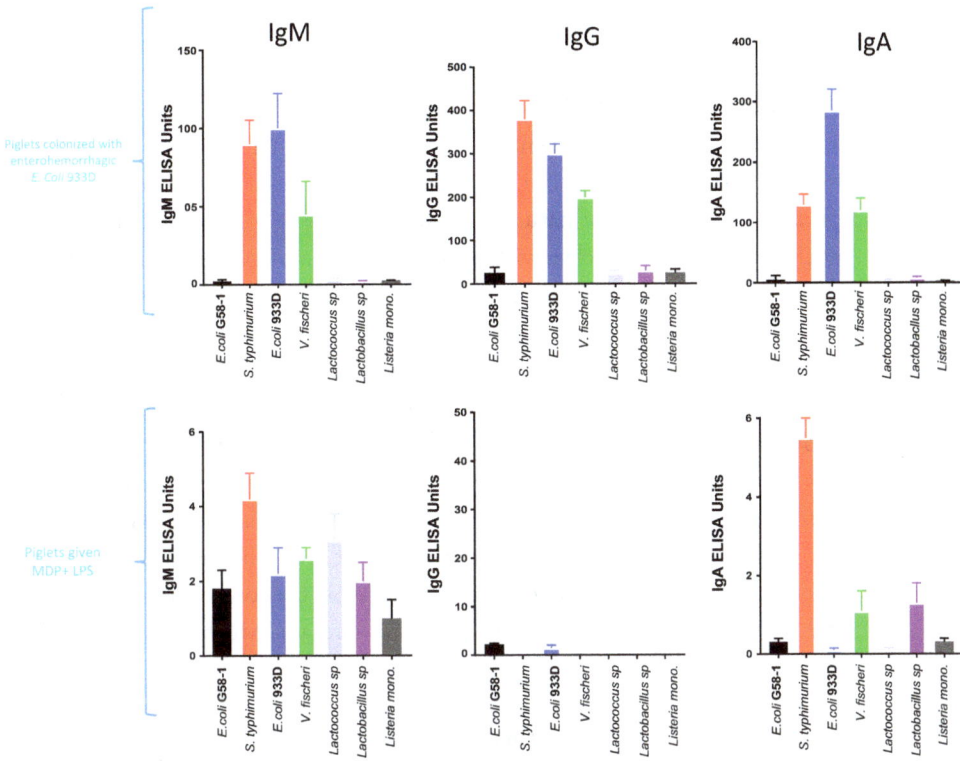

Figure A2.3   IgM, IgG, and IgA antibacterial response of germ-free isolator piglets to a panel of environmental bacteria infected with enterohemorrhagic *E. coli* 933D (top panel) or only given a mixture of two PAMPs: MDP and LPS (lower panel). Data also discussed in Chapter 6.

The phylogenetic history of IgD and IgM dates to the earliest vertebrates, where both had similar functions. It would seem that for mammals, one was enough, and IgM remained as the primary BCR on developing B cells. For that reason, the gene for IgD may be absent (Figure A2.4A) or poorly expressed in many mammals, and when present this rarely leads to a substantial number of plasma cells secreting IgD. In most, it remains membrane-bound, where it plays a secondary role to monomeric IgM, as a BCR (Figure A1.7A). Interestingly, IgD would not have been discovered so early in the pioneer days of human immunological studies were it not for an unusual single B cell lymphoma in humans.

All mammals produce and secrete IgG, IgE, and IgA antibodies, suggesting that all mammals share the same protective properties provided by these homologous antibody classes (Table A3.1). Some classes/isotypes occur in multiple forms arising from duplicated genes and are called subclasses. In addition, there are also genetic variants called allotypes, which display a number of sequence changes, but do not encode a new gene. Humans have two subclasses of IgA while rabbits have 13. However, rabbits have only one gene for IgG while other mammals have more. Pigs have six, which varies among breeds, and horses have as many as seven (Figure A.2.4, Table A2.2). The question as to whether all of these subclass variants have a unique function in each mammal is currently unresolved. Some molecular biologists believe that those encoding IgG and IgA genes reside in a "hot spot" in the genome that favors gene duplication, and that subclass similarity (Figure A2.4B) may indicate limited functional significance (Butler, 2017). This may not be true in all cases. For example, IgG3 is encoded by the most 5' proximal Cγ gene in various species, and it is the first IgG subclass to be expressed in fetal piglets (Butler and Wertz, 2006). Because of its early developmental appearance, it may also be a type of natural antibody, similar to some IgM (Figure A2.3; Bunker). Another example of a subclass with a special function is IgG1 in cattle, sheep, and goats. This IgG1 has a specialized role in passive and mucosal immunity and is overwhelmingly dominant in colostrum of ruminants (Figure A2.5). IgG1 is selectively transported from blood into the MG, secreted into milk, and absorbed across the GI tract epithelium, and may later be re-transported in the GI tract (Besser). With perhaps the exception of IgG3, IgG subclasses were not named because of their homology, but according to their order of discovery. This might be explained by the fact that initial studies focused on adult animals, and in humans and mice the recovery of different IgG subclasses came from studies on B cell plasmacytomas. Defining a universal function of IgG subtypes is therefore controversial when considering all mammals. We choose to avoid the controversy by providing Table A3.1, which focuses only on what is in known for humans. Much of the "Th1/Th2"

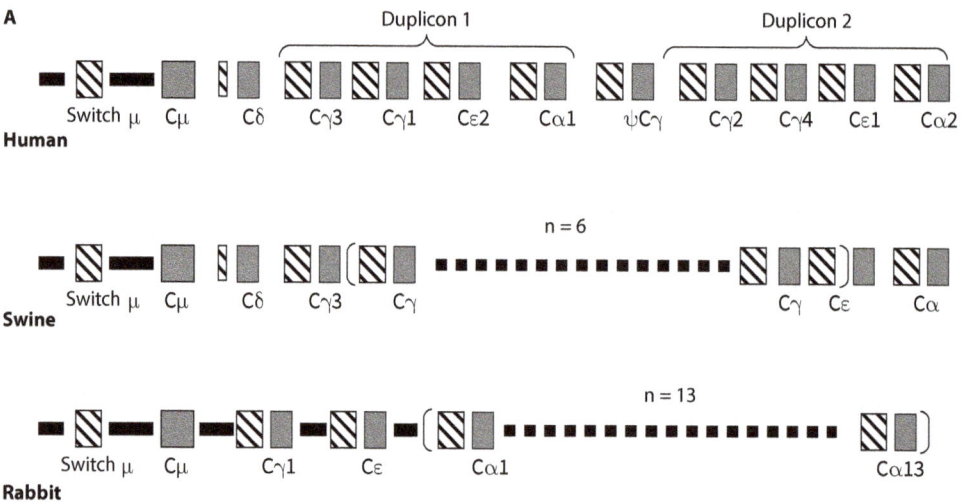

Figure A2.4A   Organization of the heavy chain constant region in three different mammals. The various constant heavy chain genes are indicated alongside their switch regions (hatched segments). These are needed in switching from the use of one isotype to another during development of a secondary immune response (Figure 6.3). Notable is the major duplication in the human constant region locus, resulting in four Cγ genes and two Cα genes. The first duplicon is initially used and Cγ3 (IgG3) is the most Cγ gene and is used first, similar to the situation in fetal piglets and the mouse (not shown). There is only one Cγ gene in rabbits but they have 13 Cα genes. Swine can have as many as six Cγ genes (Figure A2.4B). The observation from these three species supports the hypothesis that the heavy chain constant region locus is a "hot spot" for gene duplication.

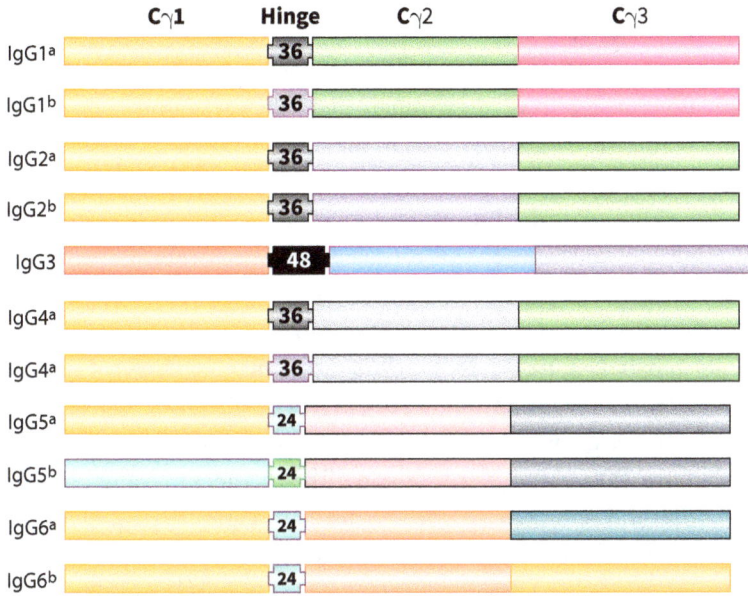

Figure A2.4B   Diagrammatic comparison of six Cγ genes and their allotypic variants from a single pig. Color-coding reflects the degree of sequence similarity among major IgG gene segments. Notable is the unshared similarity of segments in IgG3 with other subclasses and the lack of an allotypic variant.

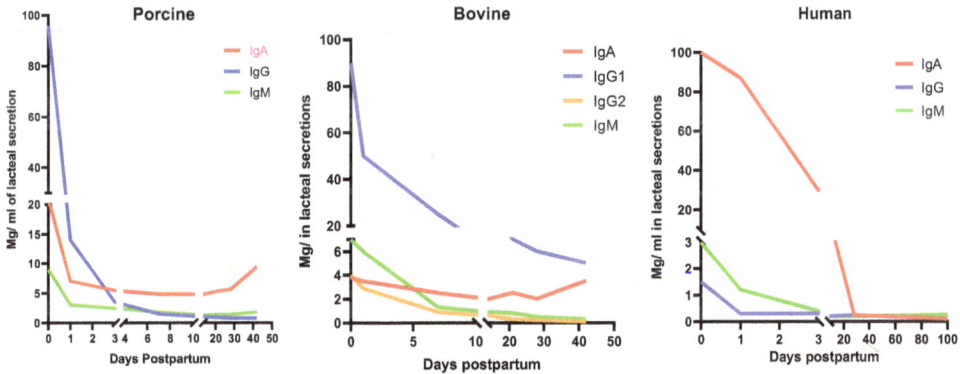

Proportion of Ig classes in colostrum (day 0) and in mature milk (day 14)

	Porcine		Bovine		Human	
	Colostrum	Milk	Colostrum	Milk	Colostrum	Milk
IgA	16	67	3.6	1.5	96	97
IgG (1)	96	14	86	74	1.3	1.8
IgM	7.1	18	6.6	6.6	2.7	1.4
IgG2	NA	NA	3.8	4.4	NA	NA

Figure A2.5   The graphs show the concentration of major Ig classes in colostrum and mature milks during lactation in three representative species. The lower table shows the proportion of each antibody class at day 0 and in mature milk at day 14. Note that IgG1 is the major Ig in the mature milk of cattle, while in swine and humans it is IgA.

dogma in the literature that relates to IgG subclass usage is based on studies in mice and cannot be easily extrapolated to other species since subclasses evolved after speciation. Only IgG3, the first downstream IgG in mammals that shares structural and developmental homology and location in the genome of many mammals, may have a universal species-wide function in the adaptive immune system.

Igs are comprised of so-called heavy and light chains (Figure A1.7A). The variable regions of both heavy and light chains form a 3D antigen binding site that recognizes conformational epitopes (Figure A1.9). Interesting is the camel family (camels, alpacas, llamas) in which approximately half of the highly functional secreted IgG does not require help from a light chain (Figure A1.14; Hamers-Casterman). In these "heavy chain only" camelid IgGs and in some IgM antibodies of cattle, a portion of the heavy chain variable region called CDR3 is greatly extended, making it possible for the heavy chain alone to form an effective 3D binding site (Pasman). The therapeutic value of "single chain" camelid antibodies and "nanobodies" was discussed in Figure A1.14.

Another feature of antibody diversity among different mammals is the number of gene segments encoding the light and heavy chain variable regions that are responsible for the antibody binding site. These differences are summarized in Table A2.2. In the heavy chain locus, the VH genome repertoire ranges from 10–360 genes, which are aligned in tandem (Figure A1.8) in mice, rats, and humans belong to many different families but in rabbits, cattle, and swine are all members of a single and phylogenetically old gene family. In all mammals, many occur as pseudogenes (defective and not functional) and do not contribute to the antibody repertoire, perhaps a reflection of a highly active site of gene duplication and selection. The number of DH segments ranges from four in swine to 28 in humans (Table A2.2). Similar variations are seen in the number of JH genes; many present as pseudogenes. Noteworthy are swine, which have only one functional JH, making them a target for producing a B cell "knockout" pig (Mendicino; see bioengineering, later).

Similar to the heavy chain locus, the light chain loci also contain multiple genes, and as many as 50% are pseudogenes (Table A2.2). The loci encoding the variable heavy and light chain genomes also appear to have been "hot spots" for gene duplication, similar to what was mentioned for the Cγ and Cα subloci of the constant region genome (Table A2.2). Another example is seen with Cλ light chain genes, where Cλ–Jλ duplicons are often repeated. Duplications of Cκ genes are exceptional, whereas duplication of Vκ and Jκ are normal, as they are for Vλ and Jλ.

Differential light chain usage represents another example of diversity among mammals. Usage of kappa is preferred 20:1 in rodents, but the near reverse is seen in cattle and horses (Table A2.2). Adult humans and swine utilize both equally; does this have functional implications?

There are also differences in how the many genes in the heavy and light chain loci are actually used to create the antibody repertoire. In swine, just four VH, two DH, and one JH rearrange to form the pre-immune repertoire, so that diversification of the antibody repertoire primarily depends on somatic hypermutation (SHM) and on deletions and additions in CDR3 (Figure A1.11). While mice and humans also use SHM, they appear to depend far more on extensive combinatorial joining of many different VH, DH, and JH genes that comprise their variable heavy chain antibody repertoire. The same appears to be true in bats (Bratsch). Rabbits, which like swine have only a single family of VH genes, also depend on SHM and CDR3 diversification, but in addition they use a process called "somatic gene conversion" in which the VH gene located in the most 3' position (Figure A1.8) is modified by translocating portions of upstream VH genes to this position, creating hybrids to generate their VH repertoire (Knight). This seems to be common practice in gallinaceous birds. Antibody repertoire diversification seems to fit the Hindu proverb, "There are many paths to the same summit."

T Cell Diversity in Mammals

In Chapter 6, we introduced the many T cell subsets: helper, inflammatory, cytotoxic (CTL) and regulatory (Treg; Figure 6.4). We also indicated there are two T cell families: α/β and γ/δ (Figure A1.7C). These two families of T cells are encoded by different genes at separate loci. The various helper, cytotoxic, and suppressor T cell subsets we described in Chapters 2, 3, and 6 are all members of the α/β family. γ/δ T cells are present in all mammals so far studied; they develop first and remain dominant during early fetal life (Figure A2.6; Sinkora et al., 2000; Stepanova). An interesting feature of γ/δ T cells is that their TCRs resemble their BCRs and recognize conformational epitopes like those found on proteins, glycolipids, and PAMPs, as opposed to the linear peptides presented by MHC to α/β T cells (Figure A1.7C). γ/δ T cells do not represent a single category (Sinkora, 2007), but two or more lineages that can be distinguished using a variety of CD and other markers (Stepanova).

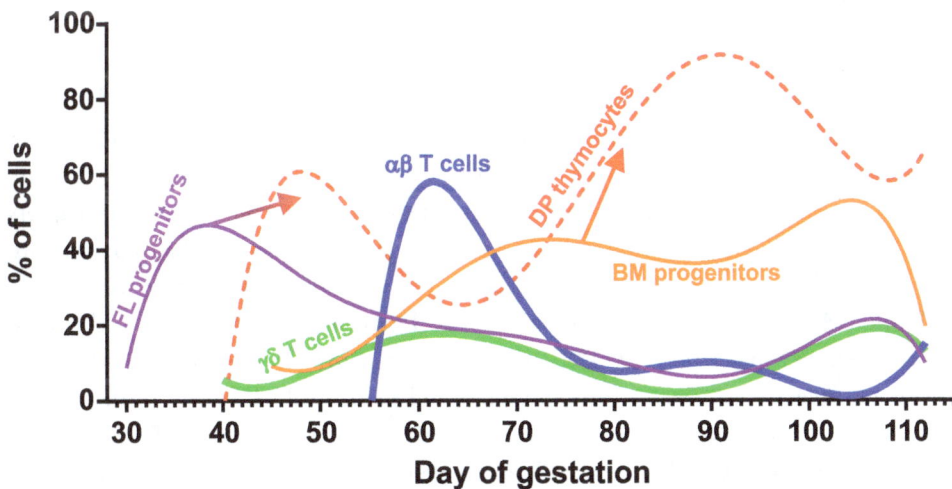

Figure A2.6   The order of T cell development in the fetal piglet. Lymphopoiesis begins in fetal liver (FL; purple) and later in bone marrow (BM; orange) from where double-positive (DB) immature thymocytes emerge (dotted red line). Notable is that γ/δ T cells (green) appear 15 days before α/β T cells (blue).

In mice and humans, γ/δ T cells comprise over 60% of all T cells in skin and mucosal sites while they are rare in blood. By contrast, in cattle and swine, they can comprise about 50% of all T cells in blood, but with age the ratio becomes more similar to that in humans and mice. Since γ/δ T cells in young swine and cattle are dominant, this might suggest they are born prematurely, but rather the opposite is true (Table A2.1). Hence, the significance of this difference and the change in distribution during development remains unresolved. Since it is speculated that γ/δ T cells play a greater role than α/β T cells in the innate immune system (Chapter 6; Appendix A-1), this might explain their early appearance during fetal development (Figure A2.6) and perhaps even their BCR-like antigen binding sites.

Diversity of Gut-Associated Lymphoepithelial Tissue (GALT)

The mucosal immune system, associated with the GI tract, is called gut-associated lympho-epithelial tissue (GALT). Most aspects of GALT are shared among all Eutherian mammals, but certain features are species or order specific. In our description of GALT in Chapter 6, we discussed lymphoid structures called Peyer's patches (PP) as regularly distributed throughout portions of the small intestine, but in many mammals similar structures are also found in the colon. In review, PP contain germinal centers (GC) like those in peripheral lymph nodes and the spleen, and they are sites for the selection of B cells, which in GALT differentiate to PC that secrete IgA. The development of PP depends on bacterial stimulation acting through TLRs and they are nearly absent from the GALT of germ-free mice though this is not universal (see later). As described in Chapter 6 and illustrated in Figure 6.6, IgA antibodies secreted by plasma cells in the GI tract are dimers and are transported intracellularly into the lumen of the GI tract by enterocytes utilizing the poly Ig receptor, a portion of which remains attached and is known as secretory component (SC, Figure A1.7B). The secreted IgA is thereafter known as SIgA. SIgA can remove enteric pathogens from the GI tract, which they specifically recognize with their antigen binding site or by the innate ability to bind non-specifically to bacteria using glycans displayed on SC (Perrier; Figure 6.6). Sixty percent of bacteria in feces are coated with SIgA either specifically bound to certain bacteria through an antibody binding site or non-specifically bound to SIgA glycans. Some have referred to these as "natural" SIgA (Bunker). In Chapters 3 and 6, we described how the precursors of the IgA-producing cells in the MG originate in the PP of the GI tract and that their specificity mainly targets gut pathogens.

While GALT, PP, and SIgA are common to all mammals and function in the same manner, certain other aspects of GALT differ among mammals. Variants of GALT have been collectively referred to as "hindgut lymphoid tissues" (Butler 2017; Butler, 2013). Examples include the sacculus rotundas and appendix in rabbits and the ileal Payer's patches (IPP) of hooved mammals. Unlike the PPs of the ileum and duodenum and the situation in germ-free mice, these develop during fetal life and tend to disappear or later transition to conventional PPs as the neonate develops (Figure A2.7). Some have described these as the mammalian equivalent of the Bursa of Fabricius, an organ found in chickens and other birds and is the site of B cell development in birds. GALT in rabbits seems to come the closest to acting like the "mammalian bursa." GALT-less young rabbits show severely curtailed B cell development, lower serum Ig levels, and less repertoire diversification. However, rabbit GALT is not the exclusive site of B cell lymphopoiesis, since it is ongoing in the bone marrow of newborn rabbits. While controversial, the IPP of sheep may serve a similar role, while in swine they appear instead to be the "mother lode" for development of the IgA-dominated immune system of the GI tract (Butler, 2017; Butler, 2016; Figure A2.7). Their removal does not affect the development of B cells or serum Ig levels since the majority of B cell development in swine occurs in bone marrow throughout life (Butler, Santiago-Mateo, et al., 2011).

Diversity in Lymphopoiesis

In humans, mice, and swine, the bone marrow is the site of B cell lymphopoiesis, which continues throughout life but gradually wanes with age, a factor contributing to reduced

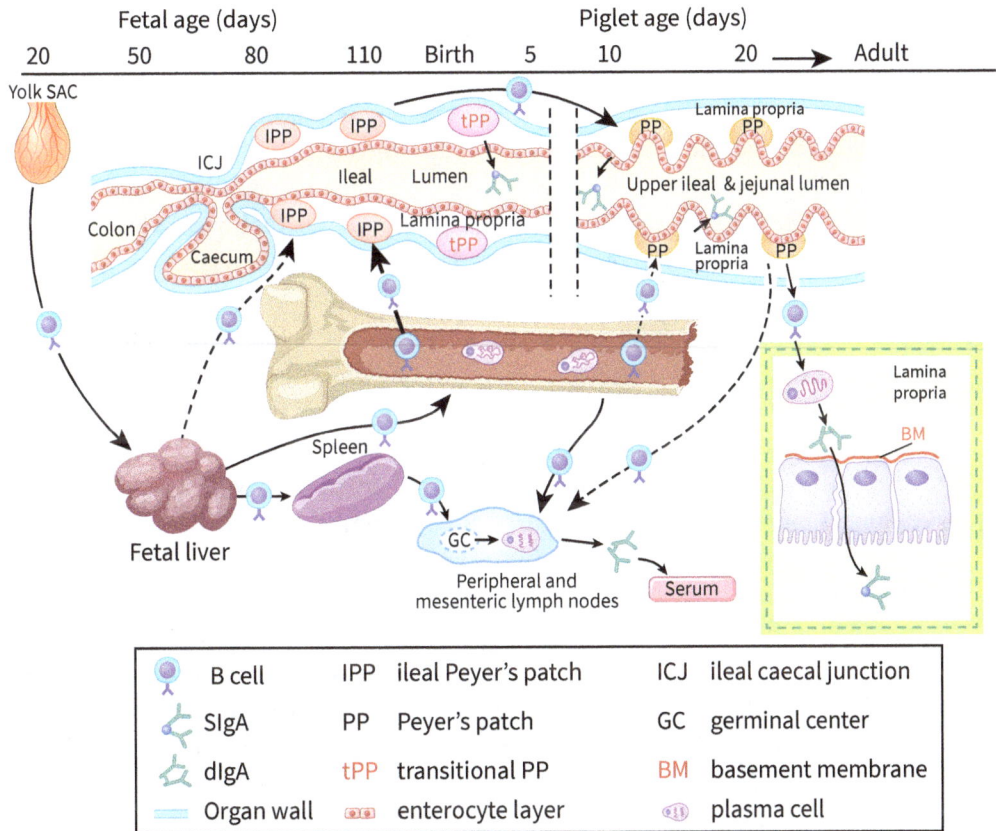

Figure A2.7 The role of the ileal Peyer's patches (IPP) in B cell and mucosal immune system development using a piglet model. B cells developing in the yolk sac migrate to the fetal liver, then to the bone marrow and eventually various lymphoid tissues. In piglets, these go first to the IPP where they give rises to the mucosal immune system. After initial development in the IPP they migrate to the Peyer's patches (PP) which become the "mother lode" for the mucosal immune system of the GI tract and other sites. These differentiate in plasma cells that produce dimeric IgA which becomes SIgA after transport through the enterocytes (See dashed green box and/or Figure 6.2 for details).

immune function in older mammals. In contrast, B cell lymphopoiesis in rabbits is perhaps more similar to that of birds, and by 8 weeks of age, early stage B cells disappear from bone marrow, which thereafter appears to be converted to a fat storage center. In cattle the spleen also appears to be a site of B cell lymphopoiesis. There is also diversity among mammals in the molecular events that occur in B cell lymphopoiesis. In mice and humans, the Cμ heavy chain of IgM is the first to be expressed on the surface of pre-B cells in association with a surrogate light chain (SLC) composed of VpreB and lambda 5 (γ5) light chains. This complex is later replaced by an authentic kappa light chain (Figure A2.6). In swine, the first Ig chain to appear on pre-B cells is a kappa light chain without any Cμ heavy chain (Sinkora, 2017; Sinkora, 2022; Figure A2.8). The first conventional BCR in swine has a kappa light chain and no SLC is used. Developing B cells in swine quickly switch to the use of lambda, leading early studies to conclude that lambda was expressed before kappa, the reverse of the situation in mice and humans. Later in fetal life, and during adulthood, kappa is again expressed and comprises 50% of the repertoire of B cells throughout adult life (Table A2.2). Among other mammals, the opossum BCR uses one of three VpreBs during pre-B cell development but then switches directly to lambda, not kappa.

Table A2.2 shows there is considerable diversity in immunoglobulins and their genes, usage, and expression. By contrast, T cell lymphopoiesis is highly conserved among mammals. As shown in Figure A2.6, γ/δ T cells are the first to develop during fetal life followed later in gestation by α/β T cells. There is a notable difference in the time needed for development, over 3 days for γ/δ cells but about 15 days for α/β cells, perhaps because of the more extensive negative and positive selection process that α/β T cells undergo (Sinkora, 2000). Like B cell lymphopoiesis in rabbits, thymic activity declines with age, being especially active during fetal development, which is consistent with the thymus's proportionally large size at that time. After birth the thymus slowly atrophies, and T cell development proportionally declines. That is one reason that the delicacy *Ris de Veau* (sweetbread) is collected from very young calves. Studying the thymus in older animals is difficult because of its small size and invasion by other tissue, which also compromises thymectomy studies. However, there are studies showing that thymic activity can be regenerated in older animals and peculiarities occur in the thymus of some mammals. Infiltration of B cells, especially those producing IgA, has been observed in a number of mammals (Butler, 1972). Lymphocyte progenitors that colonize the thymus of all mammals develop into thymocytes, which then go through various selection stages (eg, double-positive cells), before emerging as self-tolerant α/β T cells (Figure A2.6). Swine have a "confused thymus" since a sizeable proportion of progenitors start rearrangement of heavy chain immunoglobulin genes and continue to produce heavy chain VDJ transcripts while simultaneously developing into T cells (Sinkorova). These examples illustrate the diversity in lymphopoiesis among mammals, indicating that the lab mouse is not a universal model for all mammals, especially with regard to B cell development (Sinkora, 2022).

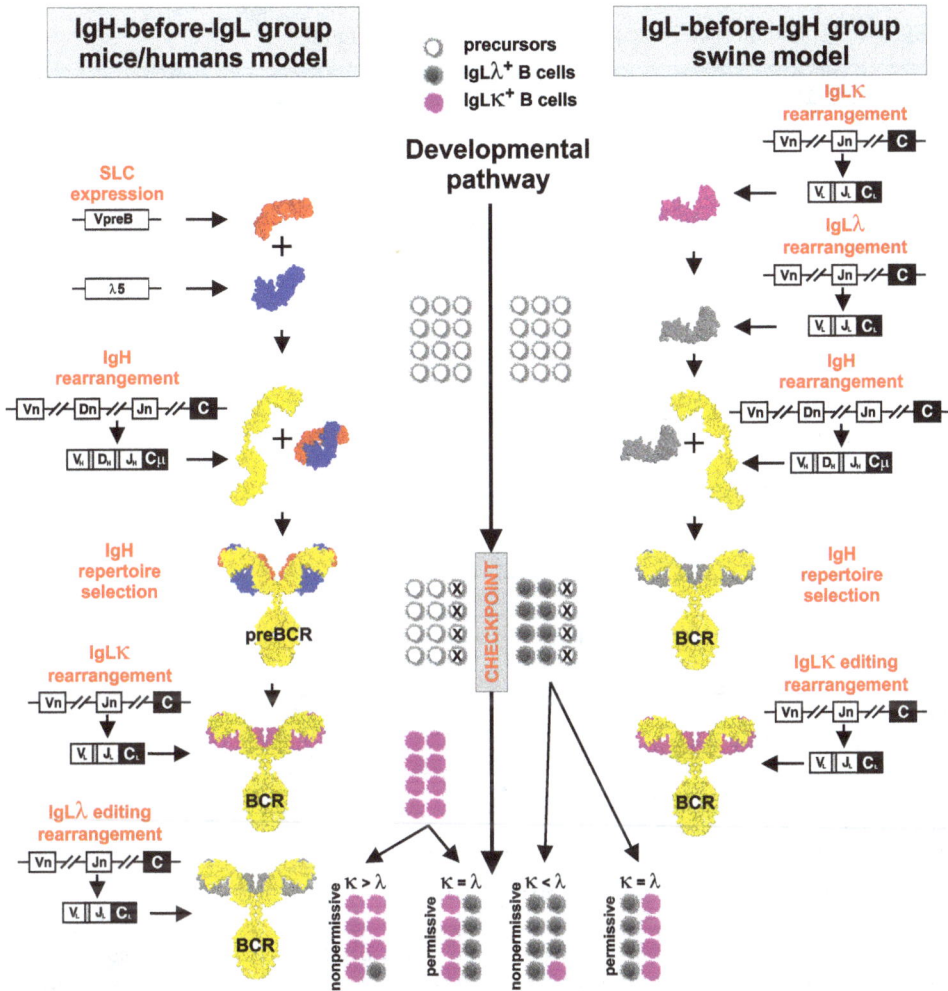

Figure A2.8   B cell development in swine in contrast with to that in mice and humans. In mice and humans (left) a surrogate light chain (SLC) composed of VpreB and lambda 5 joins with the IgM heavy chain to from the pre-B cell receptor (pre-BCR), which initially uses kappa light chains in the formation of antibodies. This gradually shifts to the use of lambda light chains. In the case of swine (right) there is no SLC, and kappa light chains alone appear first on pre-B cells. These are then joined with the IgM heavy chain to form the pre-BCR. As selection and editing continues, lambda light chains are dominant during fetal development until near the end of gestation, when kappa usage again emerges.

Diversity in Passive Immunity

The mammary gland (MG), named after the vertebrate Order Mammalia, serves multiple purposes as discussed in Chapters 3 and 4. Primarily it provides the suckling with nutrition in the form of proteins, fat, and carbohydrates. The concentration of these differs widely among mammals and is related to different lifestyles (Table A2.3). This relationship is discussed elsewhere (Butler, 2015). In lacteal secretion (colostrum and milk) there is also transfer of cells, milk fat globule

TABLE A2.3   Variation in Composition of Milk among Mammals*

Species	Fat (%) **	Protein (%)	Lactose (%)	Total Solids (%) ***
Human ****	1.6	0.6	7.0	12.4
Antelope	1.3	6.9	4.0	25.2
Donkey	1.2	1.7	6.9	10.2
Black bear	24.5	5.7	0.4	44.5
Camel	4.9	3.7	5.1	14.4
Cat	10.9	11.1	3.4	23.2
Cattle				
Brown Swiss cow	4.0	3.6	5.0	13.3
Jersey cow	5.5	3.9	4.9	12.2
Holstein cow	3.5	3.1	4.9	12.2
Deer	19.7	10.4	2.6	34.1
Dog	8.3	9.5	3.7	20.7
Dolphin	14.1	10.4	5.9	31.4
Elephant	15.1	4.9	3.4	26.9
Goat	3.5	3.1	4.6	12.0
Reindeer	22.5	10.3	2.5	36.7
Grey Seal	53.2	11.2	2.6	67.7
Whale	34.8	13.6	1.8	5.1
Norway rat	14.8	11.3	2.9	31.7
Bison	1.7	4.8	5.7	13.2
Kangaroo	2.1	6.2	trace	9.5

*Data are for mature milks. Milk composition changes during lactation in all mammals, especially during the transition from colostrum to mature milk, and may even vary among different mammae. See also Chapter 3.
** Milk of bears, deer, reindeer, seals, and whales is very high in fat, while it is low in humans, donkeys, bison, and kangaroos.
*** Total solids are a measure of density and they are high in bears, deer, reindeer, rats, and especially seals.
**** The low fat and protein content of human milk is compensated for by high levels of HMOs (Chapter 3) and lactose.
Source: Butler JE. Table 103.3, from Mucosal Immunology, Vol 2. Edited by Mestecky et al. New York: Academic Press; 2015, p. 1770.

membranes (MFGM), exosomes, and other factors (Chapter 3). Figure 3.4 illustrates differences in the transmission of passive antibodies from mother to young among some common mammals. These differences are reflected in differences in the relative concentration of major antibody classes in their colostrum and milk (Figure A2.5). In all mammals, IgG represents the refined, mature, secondary adaptive immune response that is the product of germinal center (GC) reactions in lymph nodes, the spleen, and elsewhere. IgG comprises 80–90% of antibodies in blood, and therefore represents the **systemic experience** of the mother (Butler, 1974; Butler, 2017; Butler,

2015). These are either transmitted *in utero* to the developing fetus in Group I and II mammals or only after birth through colostrum in Group III mammals (Figure 3.4). Since transfer of the maternal systemic experience has already been accomplished before birth in humans, the colostrum of humans contains less than 10% IgG, whereas in species that transfer all passive antibodies after birth, such as in Group III mammals, IgG comprises approximately 90% of all antibodies in the colostrum but the proportion rapidly declines during transition to mature milk 10 days postpartum (Figure A2.5). In Group II mammals (carnivores and rodents) that can transport some IgG *in utero*, IgG comprises only 50% of total Igs in colostrum (Figure 3.2).

IgA antibodies, like IgG, are also the result of a mature immune response, but they originate in the mucosal immune system (Figure 6.6) and their specificity is directed to pathogens or antigens encountered at mucosal sites. Hence, IgA antibodies represent the **mucosal immunological experience** of the mother and in Group I–III mammals (Figure 3.4) are exclusively transferred to the offspring in colostrum and milk produced by plasma cells (PC) in the MG. These migrate from the GI tract to the pre-lactating MG; the origin of the phrase "gut-MG axis" (see Chapter 3).

The dominant IgG in the colostrum of Group III mammals is absorbed intact by the suckling calf, foal, or piglet in the first 24 hours after birth. Absorption is indiscriminate and allows even large polymers like polyvinyl pyrrolidone to be absorbed intact. After 12 hours this indiscriminate absorption process rapidly wanes, and the GI tract epithelium undergoes what is called "gut closure" (Figure A2.1). In human infants, closure is essentially complete at birth since IgG transfer occurred *in utero*. The impact of gut closure in species like swine with multiple offspring and a limited number of MGs means that competition among piglets may delay or deny the chance to suckle, thus decreasing the newborn's ability to obtain passive immune protection (Figure A2.1). Gut closure and IgG concentration in colostrum are linked, as seen by the relative disappearance of IgG in the colostrum of cattle and swine during the transition to mature milk (Figure A2.5) and by the restoration of serum IgG levels after parturition (Figures A2.2A and A2.2B). In swine, SIgA now accounts for approximately 80% of total Igs in mature milk (Figure A2.5) and resembles the constituency of day-old human colostrum. It is notable that IgA levels in sows rapidly increase after parturition (Figure A2.2D), supporting the view that IgA plays a major role the in passive and active protection of the mucosal immune system. In swine and other mammals, dimeric IgA (dIgA) is transported from serum into mucosal sites (Figure 6.6).

In humans, gut closure is nearly complete at birth, and indiscriminate protein absorption by the GI tract of Group III mammals ends after 12–24 hrs (ie, gut closure; Figure A1.1). Meanwhile, SIgA in colostrum is ingested by all mammalian offspring, but before and after gut closure it remains protective within the newborn GI tract.

There is evidence that some IgG can be actively taken up by enterocytes after gut closure in piglets and human infants. Active and selective uptake of IgG by enterocytes in rats is mediated by a receptor called **FcRn** found on enterocytes; **Rn** = neonatal rat and **Fc** = the Fc domain of IgG that is recognized by the receptor (Rath; Chapter 2, Figure 2.3B). As mentioned above and in Chapter 2, a homolog of FcRn is also present on the syncytiotrophoblast cells in the human placenta, which can explain the *in utero* transportation of IgG to the fetus (Palmeira; Figure 2.3A).

While SIgA in swine becomes dominant after gut closure, this does not occur in ruminant artiodactyls like cattle, sheep, and goats. In these ruminants there is no switch to an overwhelming dominance by IgA in their mature milk (Figure A2.5). This led early investigators to conclude that SIgA was absent in cattle, until studies by others rejected this conclusion (Mach; Butler, 1971). IgG continues to account for more than half of the total immunoglobulin in mature cow's milk; more than 90% of which is the subclass IgG1. Unlike IgA produced by plasma cells in the MG of humans, swine, and mice, the vast majority of IgG in cow's colostrum and milk originates from the blood of the mother, which accounts for the precipitous prepartum decline in her serum IgG levels. This is followed by a restoration after gut closure (Figure A2.2). Secretion of IgG into colostrum and milk requires that it be actively transported across the capillary endothelium into the ductal fluid of the MG (facilitated by FcRn) and is then moved across the alveolar epithelial barrier to be released into milk by a yet undefined mechanism (Butler, 2015). By contrast, there is no credible evidence that IgA is transported from blood to milk in any mammal, in agreement with studies in mice (Koertge).

In ruminants, the majority of PC in the MG produce IgG1 and some may be immigrants from the GI tract. This raised the question as to whether IgG1 is some sort of ruminant mucosal antibody like IgA. Some support for this view comes from early studies demonstrating that the IgG1 that was indiscriminately absorbed prior to gut closure is later re-transported by enterocytes for secretion into the gut lumen, much like SIgA, and perhaps depends on FcRn (Butler, 2015; Besser).

Passive immunity involves more than antibodies. Fifty years ago, there was a brief uptick in interest in the transfer of lymphocytes through breast-feeding, which are taken up by the infant and presumed to help establish the infant's immune system. While this occurs, the survival of these lymphocytes in the newborn, given their MHC incompatibility, is questionable and evidence that it creates the expected chimeric offspring is lacking. What we do know, and what was described in Chapter 3, is that cytokines, antibacterial agents, and pharmaceuticals are transmitted through suckling. In isolator piglets, loss of labile factors in colostrum (presumably cytokines) results in loss of the suppression of *de novo* synthesis of all immunoglobulin classes in these piglets (Figure 3.6). This shows that in addition to suppression by purified maternal IgG (Klobasa), other factors in colostrum regulate adaptive immunity in the newborn. Presumably similar regulatory effects are mediated by factors in the colostrum of humans and other mammals. Such regulatory factors would not be available to formula-fed infants (Chapter 4) and this may have consequences for development of their immune system (Chapter 3).

The Special Case of Bats

Bats (order Chiroptera) are the only true flying mammals, and a study of their immunoglobulin genes indicates they are similar to other mammals and not birds (Table A2.2; Butler,

Wertz, et al., 2011). Similar to mice and humans, bats appear to develop their antibody repertoire using a very large number of VH, DH, and JH genes (Bratsch; Larson). Their classification as mammals is also consistent with their reproductive features (Table A2.1).

Bats are nocturnal and so they are rarely seen by diurnal humans, yet hey comprise 20% of all mammalian species. A famous mammologist at the University of Kansas claimed there were more bats per acre than birds. The worst scenario has been their established role as vectors for actual or potentially pandemic viral diseases. As mentioned earlier, these include viruses like Ebola, Marburg, and rabies, SARS-Cov-1, MERS, SARS-Cov-2, and Hendra. Many bats are resistant to the viral diseases that cause death and disease in mammals to which they transmit viruses (Larson). It has been reported that few bats die from rabies, while infected raccoons, skunks, and other carnivores do. These observations beg the question as to how this mammalian order can escape diseases that kill other mammals. Some attribute their survival to their high rate of metabolism, high body temperature, or more vigorous innate immune response. The latter view may be supported by their more vigorous secretion of type I interferons (IFN α and β), a more vigorous response by NK cells, and differences in MHC that may collectively allow for a more rapid immune response. There are reports of bats that eliminate viral infection without production of antiviral antibodies. However, caution is needed since there are over 1,000 species of bats in 21 families and their behavior and diet is diverse, so what happens in some well-studied groups may not be universal for the order. One possibility is that receptors needed by these various viruses to gain cell entrance may exist at low levels on cell surfaces or be subject to rapid turnover due to bats' higher metabolism. Receptor dependency is especially well-known in virology but may apply to bacteria as well and may have a genetic basis. As previous mentioned, some pigs lack enterocyte receptors for certain pathogenic *E. coli*, making them genetically resistant (Bosworth; Baker). It is also possible that the machinery needed to accommodate viral replication is also down-regulated in bats, thus limiting the level of cell infection that would not cause death and therefore allow them to be viral vectors. In the next section, we show that bats have a unique microbiome that is highly inflammatory, dominated by Proteobacteria, which may protect bats while a high level of Proteobacteria in humans is associated with disease and dysbiosis (Chapter 5). Discovering the mechanisms that protect these flying mammals may allow it to someday be applied therapeutically to address viral infections in humans and other mammals. Interested readers may wish to consult a forthcoming *Frontiers Immunology* article titled "The Role of Bats and Their Immune System in Structuring Host-Pathogen Interactions."

Diversity Among GI Tract Microbiomes and General Metabolism
Microbiome Overview

Phylogeny and diet influence the composition of the GI tract microbiome, and once it is established it has long-term stability (Faith). This helps explain differences in the microbiome among different human cultures/ethnicities and in different regions (Chapter 5). The impact of diet is supported by studies of around 60 mammals that indicate that microbial diversity increases progressively from carnivory to omnivory to herbivory, suggesting that the mammalian microbiome co-evolved with each mammalian order. However, data from studies on the giant panda would require modification of this simple hypothesis (see later). We include a section on hibernation and the microbiome since hibernation is **fasting**, and under this condition the diet and food supply changes, which can affect the constituency of the microbiome.

Anatomical Diversity among Mammalian GI Tracts and Its Effect on the Microbiome

The structural and physiological diversity of mammalian GI tract is correlated with the composition of its microbiome. While most recognize the stomach, small intestine, and colon as essential parts of the GI tract in omnivores like humans, herbivores have added features. In ruminants this includes a **rumen**, while other herbivores possess a fermentation segment that buds off of the extreme lower ileum, called a **caecum** (Figure A2.6). In humans and certain other omnivores, its closest evolutionary vestige is the appendix, which now seems to have a role as part of GALT in some mammals (Butler, 2013). The diversity of the GI tract among mammals has been described in many medical and veterinary textbooks. Because of these diet-correlated anatomical differences, it should not be surprising that the GI tract microbiome also differs among mammals. We highlight a few examples of the GI tract microbiome in well-studied mammals, which may be helpful in understanding the human GI tract microbiome. Examples were selected because of availability of information and because several patterns deviate from what we described as a healthy (eubiotic) or unhealthy (dysbiotic) microbiome in humans (Chapter 5).

The Ruminant Microbiome

Nutrition is part of the triad of factors that are crucial during the Critical Window of Development (Chapter 1). The ruminant GI tract microbiome is an example of a microbiome that is totally obligatory for survival. Interest in the nutritional importance of the human microbiome was preceded by many years by the studies of Hungate on microbial cellulolysis in termites that was then extended to microbial cellulolysis in ruminants and the microbial ecology of the rumen. Ruminant physiology and biochemistry were already an active session in the 1960s at the Annual Meeting of the Federation of American Societies for Experimental Biology, at a time when interest in the GI tract by human medicine was largely focused on a source of enteric pathogens. Since ruminant herbivores are a major food source, it was of great interest to understand how these animals could convert energy from plant fibers indigestible by humans to energy and growth. Much of what was originally learned about the beneficial aspects of the GI tract microbiome originated from studies of the rumen in this group of herbivores. The **rumen** is one of four pre-gastric chambers that is devoted to anaerobic fermentation that anatomically precedes the conventional elements of the GI tract of humans and other mammals (Nichei). Those lacking the pre-gastric chambers of ruminants are referred to as **monogastric** species. In almost all mammals, anaerobic fermentation is a function of the colon but some monogastric herbivores possess a **caecum**. These include rabbits, rodents, and swine, sometimes referred to as **caecotrophic** species.

The rumen contains a diverse microbial community that includes Eubacteria, Archaea, protozoans, and fungi. Archaea (see Chapter 1) may comprise up to 4% of the microbiome, but eukaryotes (protozoans and fungi) compromise only about 1% in humans. As an analogy to a climax forest, a mature or "climax" microbiome in humans is dominated by phyla Firmicutes and Bacteriodetes (Chapter 5). In ruminants, *Prevotella* (Bacteriodetes) and *Butyrivibrio* and *Ruminococcus* (Firmicutes) are dominant taxa. Hundreds of *Prevotella* species account for over 70% of the Eubacteria in the rumen across species (Mizrahi). *Prevotella* is associated with plant degradation and is also present in higher proportions in humans subsisting on a vegetarian diet. *Butyrivibrio* and *Ruminococcus* are cellulolytic bacteria. Although Archaea are also present in the GI tract of monogastric mammals, they comprise less than 1% of the microbiome. Like free-living Archaea, they utilize hydrogen released in the rumen to reduce carbon dioxide to methane. Since methane cannot be utilized for energy, it is released into the environment, making ruminants a major source of this greenhouse gas, often an issue raised by environmentalist and climate scientists. **Methanogen** species differ in the amount of methane they emit; lower emitters are often found in sheep, while *Methanobrevibacter* is a high emitter and is dominant in cattle. Differences in the composition of methanogens can also be related to diet, since corn-fed lambs release 36% less methane than wheat-fed lambs and have 30% less *Methanobrevibacter* (Popova).

The rumen microbiome supplies about 70% of the daily energy needs of ruminants, which they obtain from the degradation of cellulose, xylans, pectins, and other carbohydrates from plants that are indigestible by most monogastric mammals. In all mammals Firmicutes and Bacteriodetes convert these to SCFA. One particular SCFA is propionate and is used for gluconeogenesis and supplies ruminants with most of their daily glucose requirement, since most simple sugars in the diet are consumed by the microbes in the rumen prior to entering the small intestine. However, hyperproduction of easily fermentable carbohydrates found in processed grains can lead to acidosis. Lowering the rumen pH below 6 encourages acid-tolerant *Streptococci* and *Lactobacilli* to thrive, which lowers species diversity and creates rumen dysbiosis that can lead to severe morbidity.

Studies on the establishment of the microbiome of newborn ruminants and other nonhuman mammals provide information difficult to obtain because of manipulation associated with the birth and development of human infants. What we learn is that ruminant offspring are born functionally monogastric. In the first week of life, milk obtained by suckling bypasses fermentation in the rumen, which at this time is one-third the size of the rumen of adults (corrected for body mass). At this time, development of the GI tract microbiome follows the same pattern seen in human infants, with aerobes and facultative anaerobes of phylum Proteobacteria initially dominant. Interestingly, cellulolytic bacteria and Archaea are also present although their expansion is likely suppressed by the oxygen-rich environment, which favors Proteobacteria. Their initial presence indicates the rumen is primed very early for its eventual role. After 2 months, *Prevotella* is already dominant as the rumen microbiome develops toward a climax microbial ecosystem. An interesting observation involved *E. coli*

0157:H1, which is shed by 30% of feedlot cattle. As mentioned in Chapter 5, this *E. coli* is a threat to human health because it is a pathogen. Shifting the diet from grains to hay can result in a 100-fold reduction in the microbiome of 0157:H1 (Callaway).

The Porcine Microbiome

The offspring of non-ruminant Artiodactyls like swine can be recovered by C-section and then reared in isolators. When they are reared in this manner, studies on the development of their microbiome can be insightful. The caecum of this monogastric species (Figure A2.6) carries out fermentation, somewhat like a rumen. The microbial composition of the caecum influences host health, immunity, and nutrient recovery. As in humans, Firmicutes and Bacteriodetes predominate prior to weaning and Proteobacteria levels are higher than in healthy adults (Chapter 5). Among the Firmicutes, *Lactobacilli* are dominant in the duodenum/jejunum while *Clostridia* progressively increase in the ileum and later in the colon and caecum as *Lactobacilli* levels decline (DeRodas). In all segments of the GI tract, bacilli of various types are dominant and can account for up to 80% of the microbiome in some GI tract segments, but with 2–5% of Proteobacteria still present. One study shows a dramatic drop in *Lactobacilli* in the ileum at weaning followed by a gradual return. This has been attributed to the piglet's failure to feed at weaning, which then allows for a momentary spike in residual bacilli. The switch to solid food is characterized by a progressive increase in Firmicutes *Clostridia*, especially *Ruminococcus*. The pattern in the caecum and colon is similar but there is no "weaning" spike of bacilli and the Firmicutes *Clostridia* increases to account for about 50% of the colon and caecum microbiomes. Throughout the 2-week suckling period, bacilli are progressively replaced by the Firmicutes *Clostridia* in the ileum before slowly recovering after weaning. During this period, species diversity increases progressively in the colon and caecum but not in the duodenum or ileum.

The effects on the microbiome of breast-feeding versus formula feeding in human infants are similar to those of piglets (Chapter 5). Piglets reared on bovine colostrum had a higher abundance of *Lactobacilli* in their stomach and ileum whereas those reared on milk replacers had higher levels of Enterobacteria (phylum Proteobacteria) in the ileum compared to those reared on bovine colostrum or sow's milk (Poulsen). In these studies, the swine milk and bovine milk groups behaved similarly, suggesting that nutrients and other factors in colostrum and milk, even when of heterologous origin, influenced the development of the piglet microbiome in a similar manner. This differs sharply from the milk replacer group. This is important since cattle and swine are the major sources of meat worldwide, and these studies support the connection between feed energy conversion and its relationship to the microbiome. The enrichment of *Prevotella* in the caecum is correlated with greater energy conversion in omnivorous swine. *Prevotella* is a staple in the healthy human microbiome and has been even used as a probiotic.

Obesity is a problem in the *Homo sapiens* population, especially in developed countries, and it seems to be microbiome related (Angelakis). While diet and lifestyle play a role, differences can also be ethnic or genetic (Chapter 5). A recent public television program focused on the genetic contribution. An example of genetic-related obesity was demonstrated in the Jinhua breed of pigs in a study comparing the microbiome of Jinhua and Landrace breeds with the same diet (Xiao, 2018). The latter is a lean breed of European origin while the Jinhua is a slow-growing breed with a propensity for fat deposition and intramuscular fat deposition (back fat in producer jargon). Comparative studies showed that *Prevotella* was dominant in both the caecum and colon of the lean Landrace while Bifidobacterium was prevalent in the duodenum, ileum, and caecum of Jinhua pigs and *Lactobacilli* were dominant throughout the small intestine of Jinhua pigs. This study supports a connection between the propensity for obesity and the composition of the GI tract microbiome.

Rabbits and Other Caecotropic Mammals
When considering the microbiome of other mammals, caecotrophic mammals like rabbits, pigs, guinea pigs and other rodents should be part of the conversation. The proportionally large caecum in these species is a microbial fermentation organ. In the exclusively herbivorous rabbit family, 90% of the microbiome is comprised of Firmicutes, while Bacteriodetes comprise less than 10%; a significant difference from the human microbiome (Velasco-Galilea; Chapter 5). *Clostridia* of Phylum Firmicutes is followed by *Ruminococcus* and *Lachnospiroeae*. Genera like *Blautia* and *Coprocccous* are especially well-represented. In addition to these carbohydrate-fermenting bacteria that produce SCFA, methanogens are also present, as well as *Akkeramsia* (phylum Verrumicrobia). The latter also contribute to repair of mucosal wounds and are found in other mammals. As obligate herbivores, the rabbit family provides support for the connection between a vegetarian diet and predominance of certain taxa.

The Microbiome of Carnivores
Carnivores are the most common companion species of humans and are also monogastric, so examination of their microbiome is of special interest since they are largely meat eaters, with major exceptions (see later). Carnivores like humans lack a special fermentation organ in their GI tract outside of the colon. The mature microbiome of dogs and seals is dominated by over 80% Firmicutes and Bacteriodetes, but it may include up to 5% Actinobacteria and 3% Proteobacteria (Duysburg). Dysbiosis (Chapter 5) is known in dogs and results in diarrhea and IBD, which is often corrected by dietary fiber changes, pre- and probiotics, and even fecal microbial transfer (FMT). Harbor seals share a similar microbiome with dogs but with a higher proportion of Fusobacteria. In seals, the distribution of the various taxa seems related to their feeding location and thus the source of their food (Pacheco-Sandoval).

The giant panda is an interesting exception among carnivores because their diet has significantly diverged from the diet of other carnivores, and they feed almost entirely (99%) on bamboo. This results in very low microbiome diversity in their GI tract. The microbiome in pandas living on such a monotonous diet dramatically decreases in diversity from that during their early development with the switch from milk to only bamboo. This provides an experiment of nature to test whether diet regulates microbiome diversity or whether it is phylogenetic. During the giant panda's early stages of development, Firmicutes like *Lactobacilli* and *Clostridia* are well-represented as are Actinomyces, Proteobacteria-like *E. coli* and *Shigella*, and certain unclassified Bacteriodetes. As the diet moves to subsistence on bamboo, there is a dramatic decline in species diversity in the microbiome. In a study of nine different carnivores, an index of diversity increased as meat consumption increased, starting at an index of 1.5 in the giant pandas, moving to 3.3 in domestic cats and to approximately 4 in leopards (Guo). To test whether this occurs in non-carnivores, mice were reared on an 80% bamboo diet. Unlike in the giant panda, diversity actually increased, as it does in humans. Thus, understanding the diversity of the GI tract microbiome is complicated and depends on other factors than diet.

The Bat Microbiome

Bats (order Chiroptera) are most closely related to carnivores but possess a very different microbiome. In healthy humans, Artiodactyls, and rodents Proteobacteria comprise less than 5% of the four major phyla (see Chapter 5) and higher levels are considered a sign of dysbiosis (Table 5.1). In insectivorous bats, phylum Proteobacteria may comprise nearly half of the adult GI tract microbiome in some species (Vengust). There are seasonal changes in the bat microbiome, which is not unexpected since they are hibernators (see later section). Especially interesting are changes in the microbiome when bats are removed from the wild and placed in captivity. In the wild, insects like termites and larvae of various species rich in fat comprise their diet. The move to captivity results in a 2-fold increase in the diversity index, moving in the direction of the healthy microbiome of humans (Chapter 5; Edenborough). In captive bats this is believed to result from the change from a monotonous chitin-based diet (flying insects) to the broader diet available in captivity, and because bats living together in captivity more readily transfer their microbiome to one another.

The Microbiome in Milk and the MG

We noted in Chapters 3 and 5 that milk is not sterile, and that the bacterial microbiome is also transferred through suckling and could influence and contribute to the microbiome of the neonate. We mentioned in Chapter 3 that the dairy industry refers to the number of leukocytes in milk as the somatic cell count (SCC; Butler, 2015). This is essentially a neutrophil count and is a test for mastitis and a measure of the marketability of the milk. This phenomenon has limited relevance to the development of the neonate's healthy microbiome, but it provides insight into genetic and other causes of mastitis (Derakhshani; see Chapter 3).

Studies on the microbiota of lacteal secretions in swine have greater relevance to understanding the role of the milk microbiome in the neonate, since the only consumers are suckling piglets and pig milk is not marketed for human consumption. Using sows as a model, we learn that milk composition (Table A2.3) and its microbiome (Chen) changes during lactation. In opposition to views that milk was sterile (Chapter 3) 212 taxa have been identified, and the relative contributions of the six most abundant phyla were followed during lactation. In the first few days, Firmicutes like *Runinococcus* comprised about 50% of the microbiota, Proteobacteria accounted for 20% and Actinobacteria about 5%. During the first 5 days, Firmicutes declined but then doubled as the abundance of Proteobacteria declined. Actinobacteria levels remained constant at only about 5% of the microbiota. This study seems consistent with what has been observed in both human and bovine milk, making it a useful reference model.

The Microbiome During Hibernation

Hibernation is a phenomenon of warm-blooded animals in particular, whose inactivity in winter is coupled with metabolic depression, reduced body temperature, and lower breathing and heart rate. Hibernation is a response to limits on food supply and other environmental changes. Daily **torpor** is defined as a response to short-term seasonal effects including daily spikes in ambient temperature, sometimes called aestivation, a summertime event in very hot climates. We have included this section on hibernation since it provides a quasi-model for understanding how diet or the lack of food can influence the microbiome. Hibernation is associated with the level and constituency of the food supply. In Chapter 5, we described how diet can influence the constituency of the GI tract microbiome. These changes may resemble those seen in humans when their food supply changes during **fasting** and when hospitalized patients acquire their nutrition solely by intravenous feeding.

Hibernation is a common feature of rodents, bats, and omnivores such as bears, hedgehogs, some marsupials, one monotreme, and even one primate species in Madagascar. Hibernation may be obligate, like in ground squirrels, hedgehogs, jumping mice, marsupials, and the echidna (monotreme). In these mammals, body temperature can drop to near ambient temperature, even as low at 27°F. However, hibernation in these animals may include periodic **arousals** (see later). Both facultative and obligate hibernation are connected to food supply. The extent and depth of hibernation differs among mammals. Readers should be reminded of the biologist who tried to measure the rectal temperature of a hibernating bear, not realizing their body temperature only drops by 3–5°C, not by 30°C as in hibernating rodents (see later). In the best-studied cases, hibernation is preceded by a period of aggressive foraging, resulting in a build-up of fat stores. Fall berry pickers are familiar with sharing their favorite patch with a bear preparing for the fasting that lies ahead. Some rodents that are not "deep or long-term hibernators" vigorously collect and store seeds and nuts, should they periodically awaken hungry on a warm day. Polar bears, which are not regarded as true hibernators but **true fasters**, are an interesting example since they are also pregnant during the hibernation period, give birth near the end of hibernation, and must supply their young while fasting. Mothers typically have only two offspring to nourish, and dams can lose 15–30% of their body weight by providing nourishment to their cubs, first *in utero* and then through suckling. While bears have 1–2 offspring, their nonhibernating cousins (wolves) that live in the same environment may have half a dozen pups. However, their fecundity is also tightly correlated with the food supply; this may be a universal feature of all mammals and has been observed in Indigenous human populations. Evidence indicates the GI tract microbiome is involved in modulating metabolism during hibernation (Sommer). Bears as well as smaller seasonal hibernators consume no food for the duration of winter but benefit from urea nitrogen salvage via symbiotic gut microbes that hydrolyze urea, releasing nitrogen that can be absorbed across the gut epithelium in the form of ammonia or microbial amino acids. This contributes to maintaining a protein balance in liver, muscle, and likely other tissues (Regan).

Bats provide another example of the connection among food supply, fecundity, and litter size. Bats have a very high metabolism and typically a single offspring per pregnancy (Table A2.1), which in some cases is carried in flight by the mother during feeding. As previously mentioned, a lactating female bat must each night dine on enough insects to provide the nutrient energy to supply herself and her suckling pup during the next day when she lowers her own metabolism to conserve energy in her secluded daytime retreat. Shrews, like bats, have an extremely high metabolic rate. Shrews denied food, even during non-hibernation, may die. Readers may have encountered dead shrews during a morning walk, possibly the result of starvation. Hibernation in bats, as in other mammalian hibernators, results in a change in diet, which means a change in energy source and, as described above and in Chapter 5, a change in diet is associated with changes in the GI tract microbiome. We previously mentioned that bats have an unusual microbiome in which a high level of Proteobacteria is normal. In early spring when the emerging bats take wing to feed on insects, Proteobacteria levels are relatively high and Firmicutes low. When bats go into hibernation in late summer, the opposite is true as their dependence on a carbohydrate diet shifts to a lipid-based diet (Xiao, 2019). In addition to lowered metabolism and changes in the microbiome, hibernation may also involve immune suppression. Some suggest that the die-off of some bat species in the Northern Hemisphere due to a fungal disease called white-nosed syndrome (WNS; Blehert) may be connected with hibernation-induced immune suppression. Hibernators modulate energy metabolism and this could compromise immune function, especially considering that the immune system is second only to the nervous system in its energy requirements. In brown bears and the 13-lined ground squirrel, such depressed metabolism can last for 6 months. In Arctic ground squirrels, it can last for 9 months. During hibernation there is a reduction in anti-inflammatory cytokines (TNF-α, IFN-γ, and IL-17) and lower expression of TLR4 that responds to a danger signal presented by Gram-negative bacteria or LPS (see Chapter 6). Inflammatory cytokines (eg, IFNγ an IFNα) remain down-regulated while anti-inflammatory cytokines (IL-10; IL-4) remain up-regulated and capable of promoting protective mucosal antibody response (eg, SIgA) upon arousal. In general, it appears that all intercellular mediation is down-regulated.

While immune suppression during hibernation may occur, studies in ground squirrels provide no evidence to support suppression of the mucosal immune system of the GI tract (Kurtz). Should it eventually be proven to occur, it may not increase vulnerability to environmental microbes (bacterial and viral contagions) because these contagions survive and spread less well outside of the host during periods of low temperature. The reduced body temperature during hibernation can also slow pathogen replication since most bacterial pathogens grow slowly below 37°C (98.6°F). However, this may not apply to the fungus responsible for WNS (Blehert). Infection with WNS appears to correlate with arousal when no food (flying insects) is available. If a bat's hibernation is associated with immune suppression, such arousals could occur before the bat's immune system ramps up to a non-hibernating status.

Being omnivores, bears follow the pattern previously described for other omnivores and therefore store up on food (in this case, fruit) prior to hibernation; beware of a bear in the berry patch. Like the pattern seen with a change to a vegan diet, there is a corresponding reduction in Firmicutes and a switch to Bacteriodetes (Sommer). Studies using FMT demonstrated that the summer microbiome promoted adiposity to prepare for hibernation (see later). Thus, the hibernation microbiota had lower levels of Firmicutes and Actinobacteria but increased Bacteriodes.

Among the best-studied obligate hibernators are ground squirrels, both the 13-lined variety in the Midwest and plains states (the "golden gopher," mascot of the University of Minnesota) and the Arctic ground squirrel (Carey). Unlike bears, these rodents can lower their body temperature from 37°C (98.6°F) to approximately 5°C above freezing (40°F). Hibernation in these rodents and other small hibernators is interrupted by brief arousals in which temperatures spike to 37°C for a period of 12–24 hours. Ground squirrels feed on seeds, some bird eggs, and on insects in different developmental stages, and their metabolism during hibernation relies on stored fat deposits. Thus, pre-hibernation activity is focused on laying down fat deposits that are the primary fuel during hibernation. In humans, such an accumulation of fat deposits leads to obesity, type 2 diabetes, and insulin resistance, which does not seem to be a problem for hibernators. The absence of the normal food supply means both the hibernator and its microbiome is in fasting mode. With intake of food, the host microbiome fades and the gut mucosa on which it thrives "atrophies," resulting in reduction of villus length and crypt depth, with the total GI tract mucosal surface area resembling the undeveloped mucosa of the newborn (Figure 2.3). With the absence of food intake, the mass of the GI tract microbiome in ground squirrels is reduced and undergoes changes in certain taxonomic groups (Carey). There is a shift toward Bacteriodetes like *Prevotella* and away from Firmicutes; the latter are dependent on fiber provided by an animal's vegetarian diet. *Clostridia* and *Lactobacilli* are also reduced, and the GI tract microbiota can utilize mucins from Goblet cells, which favor specialists like *Actinobactor muciniphila*. There is also a change in the SCFA produced; butyrate is common in summer but acetate during hibernation.

The behavior of the GI tract in patients fed intravenously resembles some aspects of fasting that occurs in some mammals, but not all (Table A2.5). Intravenously fed patients down-regulate anti-inflammatory cytokines while they are up-regulated in hibernators. We present no comparative data on starving humans, but they may resemble intravenously fed patients more than hibernators. While comparison of intravenous fed patients and hibernators may be insightful, it also reveals that hibernation is not a perfect model for starvation or intravenous feeding, providing an incentive for further research and better models.

Animal Models and Bioengineering

The ideal mammalian model for humans and their diseases and maladies does not exist. The best model for any species is the species itself. However, certain mammals have been useful as models for certain physiological systems, developmental studies within the Critical Window, and studies on antibody (Ig) transport and for certain diseases (Table A2.6).

TABLE A2.5   Comparison of Host Epithelia, Immunological Behavior, and Microbiome in total Parenteral Nutrition (TPN) Patients and in Winter Fasting Hibernating Ground Squirrels

Host Feature	TPN Patients	Hibernating Ground Squirrels
Epithelial	↑ Mucosal atrophy	↑ Mucosal atrophy
	↑ Gut permeability	↑ Gut permeability
	↓ Occludin	↑ Occludin
	↓ MUC2 (ileum)	↑, ↔ MUC2 (cecum)
	↑ Enterocyte apoptosis	↔ Enterocyte apoptosis
Immune	↓ Intraepithelial lymphocytes	↑ Intraepithelial lymphocytes
	↑ Proinflammatory cytokines (IFN-γ, TNF-α)	↑ IFN-γ, TNF-α only during arousal
	↓ Anti-inflammatory cytokines (IL-10, IL-4)	↑ IL-10, ↑ IL-4
	↑TLR-4 expression	↓ TLR-4
	↓ Secretory IgA	↑ Secretory IgA
Microbiome	↓ Microbial diversity	↓ Microbial diversity
	Microbiota composition (↓ Firm, ↑ Bacter, ↑ Verruco, ↑ Proteo)	Microbiota composition (↓ Firm, ↑ Bacter, ↑ Verruco, ↑ Proteo)

Arrows indicate increased (↑), decreased (↓), or no change (↔) in TPN and hibernation, relative to control (enterally fed) levels in humans. Microbiome alterations involve Firmicutes (Firm), Bacteroidetes (Bacter), Proteobacteria (Proteo), and Verrucomicrobia (Verruco)
Modified from Carey and Assadi-Porter (2017), p. 493, Table 1.

TABLE A2.6   Animals Used in Studies on Nutrition, Protection, and Genetics

Topic	Model Species
Infant nutrition	Swine and rat
Mammary gland physiology and biology	Domesticated ruminants
Milk constituency and structure	Domesticated ruminants
Gut-mammary gland axis	Mouse, rat, and swine
Cellular transport of IgG	Mouse, rat, and domesticated ruminants
Transplantation genetics	Mouse, rat, and swine
Antibody and T cell genetics	Mouse
Microbiome	Ruminants, mouse, ground squirrel, and swine
Ontogeny of the adaptive immune system	Mouse and swine
Role of GALT*	Rabbit, mouse, sheep, and swine
Autoimmunity	Mouse
Transport and GI tract absorption of IgA	Mouse, cow, and swine
Thymus and thymocyte development	Mouse, rat, and swine
B cell development	Mouse, rabbit, and swine
Leukogenesis and lymphocyte function	Mouse
Development of suitable metal prostheses and surgical procedures	Sheep and other farm animals**

* GALT = gut associated lymphoepithelial tissue
** https://www.aofoundation.org/trauma/about-aotrauma/who-we-are
https://www.aofoundation.org/trauma
https://www.aofoundation.org/what-we-do/research-innovation/about

Choosing a Model

Understanding events in the Critical Window, which cannot be ethically addressed in humans, has led medical scientists to the use of **animal models**. However, no one mammal is an exact model for any other: "The best model for any species is always the species itself." What might be the best models for humans are other primates, but their use is highly regulated, very expensive, and heavily scrutinized by animal rights groups. Even if unlimited use of other primates was allowed, human offspring are far more altricial, and they require more than a decade to learn survival skills and even longer to obtain reproductive age (see earlier section on parenting). Furthermore, most other primates are largely herbivores, which impacts the nature of their microbiome. There are animal models for many aspects of biology, which includes psychology, exobiology, learning, aging, and other applications. Our discussions are restricted to the immunological, microbiome, and nutritional issues and only a small number of species are discussed. Some specific applications are summarized in Table A2.7.

Reliance on Rodent Models

It seems ironic that *Rattus rattus*, which spread the plague across Europe and beyond, now occupies a pivotal role as an animal model for nutritional studies and to a lesser extent in immunology. Laboratory rats (and mice) have played a key role in understanding how immunoglobulins, especially IgG, are transferred across epithelial barriers using the FcRn transport receptor (Chapters 2 and 6). The house mouse, *Mus musculus*, which eats grains, infiltrates homes, and acts as a disease vector, has become the champion model for understanding most aspects of the mammalian immune system. Their short gestation and high fecundity have allowed biologists to rapidly develop inbred strains that have proven invaluable in the study of immune systems, deficiencies, and malignancies. Their lymphocytes and other hematopoietic cells have been highly characterized, resulting in the identification of over 300 CD markers that are also found on the cells of many other mammals (Table A3.2). These have been extremely valuable in understanding lymphocyte development, cellular interactions, and the role of various cytokines and chemokines (Chapter 6). The lab mouse has also been a key player in the characterization and role of MHC in the immune response and in tissue transplantation research (Chapter 6; Appendix A-1). Malignant B cells in mice gave rise to the plasmacytomas that have played a major role in the development of monoclonal antibodies (mAbs) and mAb therapy (Appendix A-1). Rodents have also played a significant role in understanding the establishment of the microbiome (Faith) and in understanding the trafficking of lymphocytes and other hematopoietic cells. Their altricial nature (Table A2.1) makes them a quasi-model for *in utero* trafficking, but they are a less than desirable model for studies on postpartum passive immunity. The portion of the lab mouse genome containing the genes encoding antibodies is very similar to that in humans, which helps to explain how the antibody repertoire develops (Table A2.2; Sinkora, 2022). The same applies to the structure of the pre-B and B cell receptor; the former involves VpreB and a surrogate light chain

(Figure A2.8). However, not all mammals march to the same drummer, as demonstrated by B cell development in pigs.

The Importance of Non-Rodent Models

The extensive use of rodents as models has often overpowered the role played by other mammals. Below we have selected a few mammals that are used as models in medical science. We should point out that although dogs have been extensively used as experimental animals, most studies with dogs are related to physiology and not to immunology or nutrition. Therefore, they are not included.

Swine as Models

This omnivorous and monogastric species offers many advantages as a human model. Their anatomic and nutritional similarity to humans and their other shared parameters have caused some to claim that swine share 80% of their useful parameters with humans, while mice share only 10% of these parameters (Pabst). Swine offer a number of specialized rearing opportunities as well as certain surgical and bioengineering features. One feature of swine is their large litter and the ability to rear piglets in gnotobiotic and germ-free isolators as well as in specialized specific pathogen free (SPF) "auto sows" (Figure A2.9). In the latter feeding devices, piglets quickly learn to respond to Pavlovian signals (bells and whistles), which train them to know it is time to feed, and a second signal that feeding time is over and it's time for a nap. These can be programmed to limit the amount of food provided and the frequency of feeding and to include a 6-hour sleep period, similar to what would occur in naturally reared piglets. These systems have been employed in nutritional and immune regulation studies (Figure 3.6). In this manner they serve as models for preterm and vaginally born offspring. Their precocial nature (Table A2.1) allows them to be reared without their mother or surrogate mother (Butler, 2007; Splichalova). Mother-dependent species like rodents must be nursed by surrogate mothers that must be reared SPF. SPF offspring are devoid of pathogens but not of commensal bacteria. The advantage of rearing precocial offspring like swine can be summarized as follows: (1) Their responses are not influenced by *in utero* transfer of maternal antibodies. (2) The precocial offspring can be reared in SPF or in germ-free isolator facilities without a surrogate mother. (3) They can be reared entirely bacteria free not merely SPF. (4) Piglets can be infected with a pathogen on a germ-free background or colonized with a defined commensal microbiome (Figure A2.3). (5) They can be surgically manipulated at birth before being placed in isolator units. An example of the latter is represented by piglets who have had their IPP or appendix/cecum surgically removed at birth during studies to address the role of the IPP in immune system development. Comparison can then be made between those colonized with commensal bacteria or those remaining germ-free (Butler, 2007; see later).

A procedure not necessarily involving the use of isolator piglets is use of CDCD piglets (cesarian-derived, colostrum-deprived). These animals may be artificially reared on (1) cow's milk and colostrum, in so-called "artificial sows" (Figure A2.9), or (2) allowed to suckle

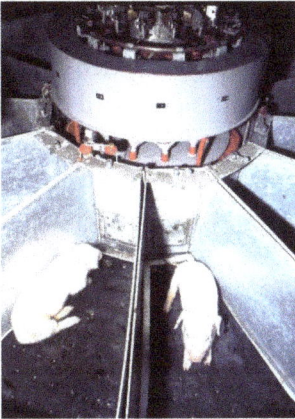

Original auto sow

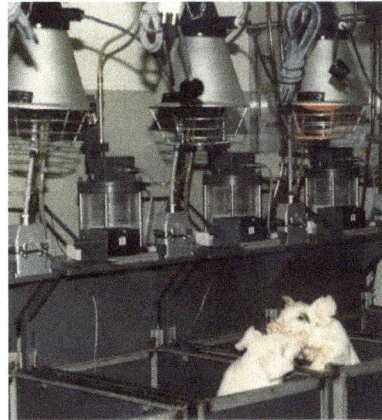

Modern auto sow

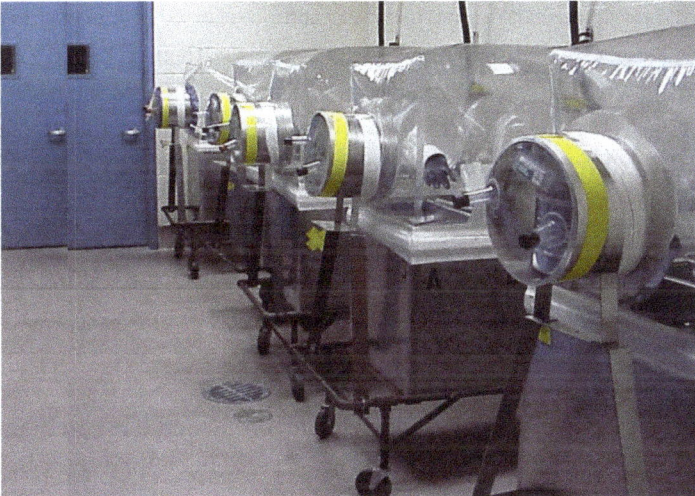

Germfree isolator facility

Figure A2.9   Examples of "auto sows" in which feeding doors open and close and piglets alerted by Pavlovian warning. Modern auto sows are computer controlled, the amount of food dispensed and eaten, automatically monitored but allowing piglets in the same study group to have periodic contact. Germ-free isolator facilities prevent any contact with environmental microbiobes or other piglets. Each facility provides different options.

a surrogate mother that in some experiments had been immunized so it provides passive antibodies during suckling. CDCD piglets are useful to determine if (1) passive antibodies in milk and colostrum provide immune protection, (2) passive antibodies interfere with the effectiveness of vaccines administered to newborn piglets, and (3) certain pathogens are transmitted through maternal contact or through suckling.

While valuable for the type of research described earlier, the swine immune system is not a good model for humans because (1) swine develop their antibody repertoire from less than 10 function VH genes, only two functional DH genes, and only one function JH gene, but which has positive ramifications for bioengineering (see later; Butler, 2017); (2) B-lymphocyte lymphopoiesis differs in that a kappa light chain is expressed before the heavy chain on the pre-B cells; (3) the BCR lacks SLC and VpreB (see earlier and Sinkora, 2022; Figure A2.8); and (4) passive antibodies are only transferred after birth in colostrum and milk (Figure 3.4).

Ruminant Models

Studies on the composition of milk and the physiology of the MG pioneered research on the physiology of the "flagship" organ of mammals. Like swine, there is no *in utero* transfer of passive antibodies (Figure 3.4), but differences between these two artiodactyls in the composition of colostrum and milk is further evidence of mammalian diversity (Figure A2.2; Table A2.3). In ruminants, a single subclass of IgG predominates, IgG1. This IgG class antibody may play a role as a secondary mucosal antibody like SIgA. In fact, after its absorption by the neonatal/calf GI tract, it can then be secreted at mucosal sites (Besser). Like swine, cattle use a small number of VH genes to form their repertoire (Table A2.2), but in addition, the CDR3 regions expressed with some bovine IgM are highly extended and can bind antigens with little help from the light chain (see earlier and Pasman). Unlike humans, domesticated ruminants use lambda light chains in approximately 95% of their antibodies and have a large Vλ repertoire (Table A2.2). Studies on the GI tract microbiome were pioneered by physiologists who studied the rumen. Given differences in the structure of the GI tract, and because of their herbivorous nature, it is not surprising that the ruminant microbiome is a poor model for humans.

Rabbits

Lagomorphs are not rodents and are entirely herbivorous, and like ruminants they are equipped with a microbial fermentation segment, the caecum. Rabbits have been used for decades to produce polyclonal antibodies for all forms of immunodiagnostics. Their effectiveness in this role may be due to their use of a single IgG subclass (Table A2.2; Figure A2.4A). Even more divergent from humans and mice is their use of a single 3' VH gene and a mechanism called **gene conversion** in the same manner as in the chicken and other gallinaceous birds. Their herbivorous lifestyle may have played a role in the diversification of the heavy chain genome, which features 13 different subclasses of IgA (Table A2.2; Figure A2.4A). Lagomorphs may serve as a model for the influence of diet on the makeup of the GI tract microbiome and its associated mucosal immune system.

Other Models

Our selection of models has been limited to a few of the most common mammals. However, guinea pigs, ferrets, armadillos, and others have also been used. One category we included was hibernators that may serve as a model for microbiome changes during fasting. Fasting hibernators may serve as a model for humans who are intravenously feeding or who are experiencing starvation (Carey). These species include ground squirrels, marmots, prairie dogs, hamster, jumping mice, some marsupials, hedgehogs, bats, and bears. We have described how studies on passive immunity, lymphocyte and antibody repertoire development, and the microbiome in non-primates can be useful. However, no species is an exact model for humans or any other mammal, as we emphasize, "The best model for any species is the species itself."

Surgical Manipulation and Bioengineering

Surgically Manipulated Research Animals

Useful animal models do not always appear in nature without human intervention. Historically, there have been minimal ethical guidelines regarding surgical manipulation of experimental animals, which dates back 200 years. In fact, colonies of beagles, miniature swine, and, of course, rodents, have specifically been bred for such use. Recently in America and elsewhere, animal rights groups and ethnologists have greatly restricted such manipulations, especially if they involve companion animals. In non-primates, thymectomy in rodents, rabbits, and lambs and removal of GALT in rabbits, sheep, and swine is allowed, along with splenectomy. In ruminants, fistulotomies can be constructed to allow investigators to directly sample activity within the rumen. Similarly, so called Thiry-Vella loops can be constructed in rats and swine that allow segments of the ileum to be brought to the body wall for the collection of contents and the administration of antigens, hormones, and other substances. Piglets have been canulated *in utero* and the canulae exposed on the body wall of the sow. This procedure has been used in various endocrinology studies and also to show that PAMPs were needed to stimulate development of the piglet's adaptive system (Butler, Klobasa, et al., 1986). In rodents, swine, and ruminants, the bile duct can be cannulated, and the cannula brought to the body wall for the convenient collection of bile and its contents. Applied to cattle, secretion of approximately 70 ml per hour has been reported. The parotid duct of large animals can also be cannulated, allowing direct monitoring of a major source of saliva (Butler, Frenyo, et al., 1986). Fortunately, parotid fluid can be directly collected from humans with a non-surgical suction cup device. Germfree isolator piglets have had their IPP removed at birth to determine if they were necessary for B cell development (Butler, Santiago-Mateo, et al., 2011). Other notable studies involved engrafting the MG to the neck of milk goats and associated attachment to the carotid blood supply to show that the organ acts independently of location; this also reduced teat contamination in experimental studies. The number of such procedures done using agricultural species is too diverse to describe, so we have highlighted only a few examples.

Bioengineering of Animals

We introduced bioengineering, the creation of transgenic "knockout" and "knockin" mouse models and gene editing, in Appendix A-1. Bioengineering of economically important animals has been done to (a) create a special purpose animal model, (b) to generate disease-resistant strains, or (c) to improve growth or quality in poultry, dairy, or other agricultural species. Gene editing in humans is not allowed if it involves changes to germline genes transmitted to the next generation, though somatic modifications such as correcting sickle cell anemia are allowed (Appendix A-1). There are few restrictions on bioengineering of other mammals so there are many genetically modified animals, especially, in species of agricultural importance. To address the demand for beef and pork, genetically modified animals that grow faster and are more disease resistant have been produced. Historically this was done by conventional breeding and selection studies, but this required many rounds of breeding. Besides being slow, it was limited to traits already in the population. Bioengineering, especially gene-editing technology, has greatly reduced the time needed to produce a "better animal," including some that did not previously exist in nature (see Appendix A-1). Domesticated ruminants and swine have received the most attention, not only for creating more productive and disease-free animals, but also for engineering them for use in medical science. This has been greatly aided by genome projects, similar to that originally undertaken for dogs and humans, but later extended to cattle, swine, and many other species. We limit our discussion to a few examples, many with relevance to human medical science (Table A2.7).

TABLE A2.7   Bioengineered Cattle, Sheep, and Swine

Species	Gene	Modification and Purpose
Swine	CFTR	Create model for study of cystic fibrosis
Swine	CD163	Remove receptor for PRRS virus to produce PRRS-resistant pigs
Swine	JH	Create porcine heavy chain antibody SCID
Swine	Ck	Create porcine kappa light chain SCID
Swine	CD13/AP-N	Remove virus receptor for TGEV
Swine	GGTA1	Impede cell surface α-galactose expression in pigs used for xenotransplantation
Swine	PAH	Create model for phenylketonuria (PKU)
Swine	Artemis	Engraft natural Artemis SCID pig for "humanization" research
Swine	TMPRSS2	Remove protease required for coronavirus cell entry
Ruminants, Swine, Fish	mUCPI	Knockout gene for myostatin to create meatier and leaner production animal
Cattle	β-lactoglobulin gene	Generate cattle lacking β-lactoglobulin in milk for use in patients with true milk allergy
Sheep	FecB	Improve lambing rates
Cattle	Celtic Pc allele	Decrease the need for de-horning (14 million/year in USA)

SCID = severe combined immunodeficiency
TGEV = transmissible gastrointestinal virus

Swine have been a chosen species for genetic modification. In the past, development of pigs that more efficiently provide meat or leaner meat was done by conventional breeding and it has resulted in over 730 breeds. Nowadays, new breeds are being bioengineered. Pronuclear injection, often called somatic cell nuclear transfer (SCNT), a method pioneered in mice (Appendix A-1), was used to create numerous lines of pigs as early as 1985. Early knockouts were generated using the zinc finger and TALEN procedures as early as 15 years ago (see Appendix A-1). Currently, modifications rely on CRISPR or base-editing technology (Appendix A-1; Wells; Song).

Genetic engineering of pigs to benefit medical research involves cystic fibrosis, a genetic disorder in children that results in many complications. The condition is the result of a mutation in the cystic fibrosis transport receptor (CFTR) gene, which encodes an ion channel transport protein that conducts chloride ions across epithelial membranes. Individuals with a mutation in the CFTR gene suffer dysregulation of fluid transport in the lungs, pancreas, and other organs. Efforts to create a mouse model by mutating the CFTR gene did not result in the human phenotype. However, knocking out the CFTR gene in swine produced the human phenotype (Rogers).

Porcine reproductive and respiratory syndrome (PRRS) virus is an RNA virus that is the cause of an annual loss to swine producers in North America and Europe of over 6 million dollars per year. Infection with the PRRS virus depends on CD163, which is required for cell entry. CRISPR was employed to create a CD163 knockout that is resistant to infection by this virus. (CD markers are reviewed in Table A3.2.) Another example was the knockout of CD13, a marker for a metalloprotease on the plasma membrane of enterocytes. This marker is the receptor for the coronavirus, and it was used to prevent transmissible gastroenteritis virus (TGEV); knocking out CD13 prevented infection by TGEV. There have been 31 different gene knockouts in pigs involving over 495 animals (Wells).

Use of pigs for xenotransplantation dates to the 1980s and involves efforts to develop an inbred strain of swine that are be more suitable donors of kidneys, hearts, and other organs for human. Heart valves and kidneys from pigs have been used on a limited scale for about 30 years. Recently the GalSafe pig was introduced, which has implication for xenotransplantation. The GalSafe pig involved a modification of cell surface protein glycosylation that is regulated by the GGTAI gene. Almost all surface proteins are glycosylated and one such moiety is α-galactose (α-gal). A common cause of the failure of porcine kidney transplants in humans is α-gal. In addition, some humans develop allergic reactions to meats bearing α-gal. Glycosylation of porcine heparin given to humans can also create problems. Hopefully, the GalSafe pig lacking the surface α-gal can provide tissue more compatible in transplantation to humans. Recently, the transplantation of an entire heart, not merely pig heart valves, made international news.

In Appendix A-1 we described the genetic manipulation of mice that prevents them from producing antibodies, experimentally creating severe combined immune deficiency (SCID). Since swine have only one functional JH (Table A2.2), mutation of this JH creates a porcine B cell "knockout" or SCID (Mendicino). Mutating the single C-kappa gene results in an animal that can only use lambda light chains. Therefore, if kappa expression is needed to generate the pre-B cell receptor in this species (Figure A2.8), the procedure creates a B cell knockout (Ramsoondar; Sinkora et al., 2022; Figure A2.6). It was envisioned that such animals could become recipients of the human immunoglobulin genome, with the goal of large-scale production of polyclonal or monoclonal human antibodies for immunotherapy.

Another tactic is to humanize a naturally occurring SCID pig resulting from mutation of the Artemis gene. These pigs have undergone zenogenetic transfer of human CD34+ hematopoietic cells (Table A3.2). Such immunologically "humanized pigs" can then be used as test beds for studies in HIV, various cancers, and even vaccine research (Boettcher).

The gene encoding myostatin controls fat deposition in swine and many vertebrates including fish. Myostatin negatively regulates skeletal growth. The controlling gene has been edited in cattle, sheep, swine, and goats to produce "meatier" animals. Knocking out this gene (mUCP1), results in market animals with less back fat (ie, leaner pigs). The same manipulation has been applied to the channel catfish (Proudfoot). Germline editing has also been used to engineer infertile Atlantic salmon, and to make improvements in tilapia, shrimp, and laying hens.

There have been a large number of gene-editing events in cattle and other ruminants for a variety of reasons, ranging from attempts to render milk less allergic to humans to improving disease resistance (van der Berg). Both SCNT and gene editing have been used. Of particular interest, and a topic mentioned in Chapters 3 and 4, concerns β-lactoglobulin found in bovine milk but absent from human milk. β-lactoglobulin is a frequent target in individuals with milk allergy (Chapters 6 and 8). Thus, milk cows lacking β-lactoglobulin have been engineered. Other targets of milk allergy are casein variants (Chapter 8). Such engineered cattle could be valuable for special cases of infants with intolerance to infant formula based on cow's milk (Chapter 4).

The Long and Short Game

In several chapters we discussed the rise in MDR bacteria and overuse of antibiotics in human medicine, and the role played by STAT, which at one time accounted for 80% of all antibiotics produced and was used as animal feed supplements. An alternative to the use of antibiotics to control pathogens in food animals is breeding and bioengineering for disease tolerance. There are many examples of tolerance/resistance to pathogens (Lopez). As we mentioned in an earlier section, certain pigs lack receptors for pathogenic *E. coli*, allowing them to remain free of diarrhea and other symptoms of the bacteria (Baker; Bosworth). Similarly, there are cattle breeds resistant to trypanosomiasis (Latre de Late; Murray), *Theileria* (Glass), and bovine respiratory disease (BRD; Bassel). There are also poultry resistant to *Salmonella* (Kogut). These observations suggest that disease tolerance is genetic. This could be approached by breeding programs in the long term and bioengineering in the short term.

Manipulation of the genome of any vertebrate species or creating new ones (synthetic biology) carries with it the danger that such disturbances could have unforeseen consequences. While knocking out CD163 or CD13 in swine has an immediate effect on virus infectivity, the normal genes may have other important roles which may be lost. What is the role of β-lactoglobulin in cattle and how does its removal affect the health of cattle? The situation and outcome become increasing complicated when knockout functions are xenogenetically replaced by those of another species. The consequences of transferring a foreign gene into a new genetic environment cannot always be predicted. It is best to consider bioengineering as short-term fix for special situations. In any case, a fix against a current virulent microbe will not prevent the appearance of spontaneous mutants of that microbe, from which the next generation of pathogens could arise (Figure 6.2). Thus, bioengineering is most successful as short-term correction of genetic traits, which buys time for the development of a more permanent fix.

The Return to Phage Therapy to Combat MDR Bacteria

We described in Chapter 6 that a century ago d'Herelle and others touted the use of bacteriophage therapy as a means to control bacterial infections. This strategy had many potential problems and was replaced by vaccines and antibiotics. However, it was recognized in the last 30 years that the use and overuse of antibiotics has allowed for the emergence of MDR bacteria, which are now considered by the WHO to be a major disease threat worldwide. One area of overuse has been in the production of food animals, in which antibiotics were supplied in their food (the STAT program). This practice accounted for approximately 80% of all antibiotics produced by pharmaceutical companies (see Chapters 6 and 8). The mechanism of antibiotic resistance was described in Appendix A-1.

Workers in agriculture were among those first to recognize that modern phage therapy might avert the predicted "antibiotic winter" (see Chapter 6), and phage therapy has now been used to reduce disease caused by *Salmonella enterica* and avian *E. coli* (Strathdee). Phage therapy has also been applied to staphylococcal infections in cattle and *E. coli* and *Salmonella enterica* in swine. Phage therapy has also been used for pets and 38 veterinary phage products are available, some now approved by the FDA (Huang), including a number used in aquaculture.

References

Angelakis E, Armougom F, Million M, Raoult D. The relationship between gut microbiota and weight gain in humans *Future Microbiol*. 2012;7:91–109.

Baker DR, Billey LO, Francis DH. Distribution of K88 *Escherichia coli*-adhesive and nonadhesive phenotypes among pigs of four breeds. Veterinary Microbiol. 1997;54:123–132.

Besser TE, Gay CC, McGuire TC, Evermann JJ. Passive immunity in bovine rotavirus infection associated with transfer of serum antibody into the intestinal lumen. *J Virol*. 1988;62:2238–2242.

Blehert DS, Lorch JM. Laboratory maintenance and culture of *Pseudogymnoascus destructans*, the fungus that causes bat white-nose syndrome. *Curr Protocol*. 2021;1:e23. doi:10.1002/epz1.23.

Blumberg LJ, Humphries JE, Jones SD, et al. Blocking FcRn in humans reduces circulating IgG levels and inhibits IgG immune complex-mediated immune responses *Sci Adv*. 2019;18:5eaax9586 doi:10.1126/sciadv.aax9586.

Boettcher AN, Li Y, Ahrens AP, et al. Engraftment of human immune cells in CRISPR/Cas9 generated Art-/-ILZRG-/l SCID pigs after *in utero* injection of human CD34+ cells [preprint only]; 2020.

Bosworth BT, Vogeli P. Compositions to identify swine genetically resistant to F18 *E. coli* associated diseases. US Patent Office, No. 7.193.072. Assignees, Biotechnology Research and Development Corporation. Peoria, IL; 2007.

Bratsch S, Wertz N, Chaloner K, Kunz TH, Butler JE. The little brown bat *M. lueifugus* displays a highly diverse Vh, Dh, and Jh repertoire but little evidence of somatic hypermutation. *Dev Comp Immunol*. 2011;35:421–430.

Bunker JJ, Erickson SA, Flyn TM, et al. Natural polyreactive IgA antibodies coat the intestinal microbiota. *Science*. 2017;358:320–332.

Butler JE. Physicochemical and immunochemical studies on bovine IgA and glycoprotein-a. *Biochem Biophys Acta*. 1971;251:435–449.

Butler JE. Immunoglobulins of the mammary secretions. In: Larsen BL, Smith V, eds. *Lactation: A Comprehensive Treatise*. Vol 3. Academic Press; 1974:217–255.

Butler JE, Frenyo VL, Whipp SC, Wilson RA, Koertge TE. The metabolism and transport of bovine serum SIgA. *Comp Immun Microbiol Inf*. 1986;9:303–315.

Butler JE, Klobasa F, Werhahn E, Cambier JC. Swine as a model for the study of maternal-neonatal immunoregulation. In: Tumbleson ME, ed. *The Swine in Biomedical Research*. New York: Plenum Press; 1986:1883–1899.

Butler JE, Maxwell CF, Pierce CS, Hylton MB, Asofsky R, Kiddy CA. Studies on the relative synthesis and distribution of IgA and IgG1 in various tissues and body fluids of the cow. *J Immunol*. 1972;109:38–46.

Butler JE, Rainard P, Lippolis J, Salmon H, Kacskovics J. The mammary gland in mucosal and regional immunity. In: Mestecky J, Strober W, Russell MW, Kelsall BL, Cheroutre H, Lambrecht BN, eds. *Mucosal Immunology*. New York: Elsevier; 2015:2269–2306.

Butler JE, Santiago-Mateo K, Sun X-Z, et al. Antibody repertoire development in fetal and neonatal piglets. XX. B cell lymphopoiesis is absent in the ileal Peyer's patches, their repertoire development is antigen dependent and they are not required for B cell maintenance. *J Immunol*. 2011;187:5141–5149.

Butler JE, Santiago-Mateo K, Wertz N, Sun X-Z, Sinkora M, Francis DL. Antibody repertoire development in fetal and neonatal piglets. XXIV. Hypothesis: The ileal Peyer's patches (IPP) are the major source of primary, undiversified IgA antibodies in newborn piglets. *Dev Comp Immunol*. 2016;65:340–361.

Butler JE, Sinkora M. The enigma of the lower gut associated lymphoid tissue (GALT). *J Leukoc Biol*. 2013;94:1–12.

Butler JE, Sinkora M. The isolator piglet: A model for studying the development of adaptive immunity *Immunol Res*. 2007;39:33–51.

Butler JE, Wertz N. Antibody repertoire development in fetal and neonatal piglets. XVII. IgG subclass transcription revisited with emphasis on new IgG3. *J Immunol*. 2006;177:5480–5489.

Butler JE, Wertz N. The porcine antibody repertoire: Variations on the textbook theme. *Front Immunol*. 2012;3:153. doi:10.3389/fimmu.2012.00153

Butler JE, Wertz N, Sinkora M. Antibody repertoire development in swine. *Ann Rev Anim Biosci*. 2017;5:255–279.

Butler JE, Wertz N, Zhao Y, et al. The two suborders of chiropterans have the canonical heavy-chain immunoglobulin (Ig) gene repertoire of eutherian mammals. *Dev Comp Immunol*. 2011;35:273–284.

Callaway TR, Carr MA, Edington TS, et al. Diet, *Escherichia coli 0157:H7* and cattle: A review after 10 years. *Curr Issues Mol Biol*. 2009;11:67–79.

Carey HV, Assadi-Porter FM. The hibernator microbiome: Host-bacterial interactions in extreme nutritional symbiosis. *Ann Rev Nutr*. 2017;37:477–500.

Chen W, Mi J, Lu N, et al. Lactation stage-dependency of the sow milk microbiota. *Frontier Microbiol*. 2018;9:945. doi:10.3389/frmicb.z018.00945.

Derakhshani H, Fehr KB, Sepehri S, et al. Invited review: Microbiota of the bovine udder: Contributing factors and potential implications for udder health and mastitis susceptibility. J Dairy Sci. 2018;101:10605–10625.

DeRodas B, Youmans BP, Danzeisen JL, Tran H, Johnson TJ. Microbiome profiling of commercial pigs from farrow to finish. *J Animal Sci*. 2018;96:1778–1794.

Duysburg C, Ossieur WP, De Paape K, et al. Development and validation of the simulator of the canine intestinal microbial ecosystem (SCIME)1. *J An Sci*. 2020;98:skz357. doi:10.1093/jas/skz357.

Edenborough KM, Mu A, Mühldorfer K, et al. Microbiome in the insectivorous bat species *Mop condylurus* rapidly converge in captivity. *Plos One*. 2020;15(3):e0223629. doi:org/10.1371/journal.pone.0223629.

Faith JJ, Guruge JL, Charbonneau M, et al. The long-term stability of the human gut microbiota. *Science*. 2013;341:1237439. doi:10.1126/science.1237439.

Glass EJ, Preston PM, Springbett A, et al. *Bos Taurus* and *Bos indicus* (Sahiwal) calves respond differently to infection with *Theilenia annulate* and produce markedly different levels of acute phase proteins. *Int J Parasitol*. 2005;35:337–347.

Guo W, Chen Y, Wang C, et al. The carnivorous digestive system and bamboo diet of giant pandas may shape their low gut bacterial diversity. *Cons Physiol*. 2020;8(1):coz104. doi:10.1093/conphys/coz-104.

Hamers-Casterman C, Aterhouch T, Muyldermanns S, et al. 1993 Naturally occurring antibodies devoid of light chains. *Nature*. 1993;363:446–448.

Huang Y, Wang W, Zhang Z, et al. Phage products for fighting antimicrobial resistance. *Microorganism*. 2022;10:1324. doi:10.3390/microorganisms10071324.

Kacskovics I, Cervenak J, Erdei A, Goldsby RA, Butler JE. Recent advances using FcRn overexpression in transgenic animals to overcome impediments of standard antibody technologies to improve the generation of specific antibodies. *Monoclonl Antibod*. 2011;3:431–439.

Klobasa F, Werhalm E, Butler JE. Regulation of humoral immunity in piglets by immunoglobulins of maternal origin. *Res Vet Sci*. 1981;31:195–206.

Knight KL, Beck RS. Molecular cases of the allelic inheritance of rabbit immunoglobulin Vh allotypes: Implications for the generations of antibody diversity. *Cell*. 1990;60:963–970.

Koertge TE, Butler JE. Dimeric M315 (IgA) is transported into mouse and rat milk in a degraded form. *Mol Immunol*. 1986;23:839–845.

Kogut MH, Arsenault RJ. Immunometabolic phenotype alteration associated with the induction of disease tolerance and persistent asymptomatic infection of *Salmonella* in chicken intestine. *Front Immunol*. 2017;8:372. doi:10.3389/fimmu.2017.00372.

Kurtz CC, Carey HV. Seasonal changes in the intestinal system of hibernating ground squirrels. *Dev Comp Immunology*. 2007;31:415–428.

Larson PA, Bartlett ML, Garcia K, et al. Genomic features of humoral immunity supports tolerance model in Egyptian rousette bats *Cell Reports*. 2021;35:109140. doi.org/10/1016/jcelrep2021.109140.

Latre de Late P, Cook EAJ, Wragg D, et al. Inherited tolerance in cattle to the *Apicomplexan Protozoan Theilera parva* is associated with the decrease proliferation of parasite-infected lymphocytes. *Front Cell Infect Microbiol*. *2021*;11. doi:10.3389/fcimb.2021.751671.

Lopez BS. Controlling infectious diseases in animal agriculture: The best offense may be a good defense. *Immuno Horizons*. 2022;6:730–740.

Mach JP, Pahud JJ, Isliker H. IgA with secretory piece in bovine colostrum and saliva. *Nature*. 1969;223:953–954.

Mendicino M, Ramsooondar J, Phelps C, et al. Generation of antibody and B cell deficient pigs by targeted disruption of the J-region gene segment of the heavy chain locus. *Transgen Res*. 2011;20:25–41.

Mizrahi I, Jami E. Review: The compositional variation of the rumen microbiome and its effect on host performance and methane emission. *Animal*. 2018;12:s220-s232.

Murray M, Morrison WI, Whitelaw DD. Host susceptibility to African trypanosomiasis: Trypanotolerance. *Advan Parasitol*. 1982;21:1–68.

Pabst R. The pig as a model for immunological research. *Cell and Tissue Research*. 2020;380:287–304.

Pacheco-Sandoval A, Schramm Y, Heckel G, et al. The Pacific harbor seal gut microbiota in Mexico: Its relationship with diet and functional interference. *Plos One*. 2019;14(8)e0221770. doi:10.1371/journal.pone.

Palmeira P, Quinello C, Silveira-Lessa AL, et al. IgG placental transfer in healthy and pathological pregnancies. *Clin Dev Immunol*. 2012;985646. doi:10.1155/2012/985646.

Pasman Y, Kaushik AK. Bovine immunoglobulin genetics. In: Kaushik AK, Pasman Y, eds. *Comparative Immunoglobulin Genetics*. Apple Academic Press; 2014:188–221.

Perrier C, Sprenger N, Corthesy B. Glycans on secretory component participate in innate protection against mucosal pathogen. *J Biol Chem*. 2006;281:14280–14287.

Popova M, Morgan DP, Martin C. Methanogenes and methanogenesis in the rumens and caecum of lambs fed two different high-grain content diets. *Appl Environ Microbiol*. 2013;6:1777–1786.

Poulsen AR, de Jonge N, Sugiharto S, Nielsen JL, Lauridsen C, Canibe N. The microbial community of the gut differs between piglets fed sow milk, milk replacer and bovine colostrum. *Br J Nutr*. 2017;117:964–978.

Proudfoot C, McFarlane G, Whitelaw B, Lillico S. Livestock breeding for the 21st century: The promise of the editing revolution. *Front Agr Sci Eng.* 2020;7:129–135.

Ramsoondar JM, Mendicino C, Phelps C, et al. Targeted disruption of the porcine immunoglobulin kappa light chain locus. *Transgen Res.* 2011;20:643–653.

Randolph HE, Barreiro LB. Holy immune tolerance, Batman! *Immunity.* 2018;48:1074–1076.

Rath T, Kuo TT, Baker K, et al. The immunologic functions of the neonatal Fc receptor for IgG. *J Clin Immunol.* 2013(Suppl 1):S9–17.

Regan MD, Chiang E, Liu Y, et al. Nitrogen recycling via gut symbionts increases in ground squirrels over the hibernation season. *Science.* 2022;375:460–463. doi:10.1126/science.abh2950.

Rogers CS, Hao Y, Rokhlina T, et al. Production of CFTR-null and CFTR-deltaF508 heterozygous pigs by adeno-associated virus-mediated gene targeting and somatic cell nuclear transfer. *J Clin In.* 2008;118:1571–1577.

Sinkora M, Sinkorová J, Cimburek Z, Holtmeier W. Two groups of porcine TCR gamma delta + thymocyte behave and diverge differently. *J Immunol.* 2007;178:711–719.

Sinkora M, Sinkorová J, Rehakova Z, Butler JE. Early ontogeny of thymocytes in pigs: Sequential colonization of the thymus by T cell progenitors. *J Immunol.* 2000;165:1832–1839.

Sinkora M, Sinkorová J, Stepanova K. Ig light chain precedes heavy chain gene rearrangement during development. *J Immunol.* 2017;118:1543–1552.

Sinkora M, Stepanova K, Butler JE, et al. Comparative aspects of immunoglobulin gene rearrangement array in different species. *Front Immunol.* 2022;13:823145. doi:10.3389.fimmu2022.823145.

Sinkorova J, Stepanova K, Butler JE, Sinkora M. T cells in swine completely rearrange immunoglobulin heavy chain genes. *Dev Comp Immunol.* 2019;99:103396. doi:10.1016/j.dci.2019.103396.

Sommer F, Stahlman M, Iikayeva O, et al. The gut microbiota modulates enteric metabolism in the hibernating brown bear *Ursus arctos. Cell Reports.* 2016;1655–1661.

Song R, Wang Y, Wang Y, Zhao J. Base editing in pigs for precision breeding. *Front Agr Sci Eng.* 2020;7:161–170.

Splichalova A, Slavikova V, Splichalova Z, Splichal I. Preterm life in sterile conditions: A study on preterm, germ-free piglets. *Front Immunol.* 2018;9. doi:10.3389/fimmu.2018.00220.

Stepanova K, Sinkora M. The expression of CD25, CD11b, SWC1, SWC7, MHC-II and family of CD45 molecules can be used to characterize different stages of γ/δ T cell lymphocytes in pigs. *Dev Comp Immunol.* 2017;36:728–740.

Strathdee SA, Hatfull GF, Mutalik VK, Schooley RT. Phage therapy: From biological mechanisms to future directions. *Cell.* 2023;186:17–31.

van der Berg JP, Kleter GA, Battaglia E, Groenen AM, Kok EJ. Developments in genetic modification of cattle and implications for regulation, safety, and traceability. *Front Arg Sci Eng.* 2020;7:136–147.

Velasco-Galilea M, Piles M, Vinas M, et al. Rabbit microbiota changes throughout the intestinal tract. *Front Microbiol.* 2018;9. doi:10.3389/fmicb.2018.02144.

Vengust M, Knapic T, Weese JS. The fecal bacterial microbiota of bats; Slovenia. *Plos One.* 2018;13(5):e0196728. doi:10.1271/journal.pone.0196728.

Wells KD, Prather RS. Genome-editing technologies to improve research, reproduction, and pro-duction in pigs. *Mol Reprod Dev*. 2017;84:1012–1017. doi:10.1002/mrd.22812.

Xiao Y, Kong F, Xiang Y, et al. Comparative biogeography of the gut microbiome between Jinhua and Landrace pig. *Sci Rep*. 2018;8:5985. doi:10.1038/s41598-018-24289-z.

Xiao G, Liu S, Xiao Y, et al. Seasonal changes in gut microbiota diversity and composition in the greater horseshoe bat. *Front Microbiol*. 2019;10:2247. doi:3389/fmicg2019.02247.

Reviewers

This appendix was reviewed and modified after comments and suggestions from the following individuals.

Mark Suter Emeritus professor, University of Zurich Veterinary School

Robert Miller Professor of biology, University of New Mexico

Hanna Carey Emeritus professor, University of Wisconsin-Madison

Tony Schountz Associate professor, Colorado State University

Figure Credits

Fig. A2.1: Generated using Prism at https://www.graphpad.com/.

Fig. A2.2: Adapted from Franc Klobasa et al., "The Influence of Age and Breed on the Concen-trations of Serum IgG, IgA and IgM in Sows Throughout the Reproductive Cycle," *Veterinary Immunology and Immunopathology*, vol. 10, no. 4, p. 359. Copyright © 1985 by Elsevier B.V.

Fig. A2.3: Generated using Prism at https://www.graphpad.com/.

Fig. A2.4a: John E. Butler and Nancy Wertz, "The Porcine Antibody Repertoire: Variations on the Textbook Theme," *Frontiers in Immunology*, vol. 3, no. 153, p. 3. Copyright © 2012 by Frontiers Media S.A.

Fig. A2.4b: John E. Butler, Nancy Wertz, and Mark Sinkora, "Antibody Repertoire Development in Swine," *Annual Reviews in Animal Bioscience*, vol. 8. no. 5, p. 265. Copyright © 2017 by Annual Reviews.

Fig. A2.5: Generated using Prism at https://www.graphpad.com/.

Fig. A2.8: Marek Sinkora et al., "Comparative Aspects of Immunoglobulin Gene Rearrangement Arrays in Different Species," *Frontiers in Immunology*, vol. 13, no. 823145, p. 3. Copyright © by Marek Sinkora et al. (CC BY 4.0) at https://www.frontiersin.org/articles/10.3389/fimmu.2022.823145/full.

Appendix A-3
Further Information and Acronyms

TABLE A3.1   Human Antibody Classes and Subclasses

Class or Subclass	Size (kD)	Serum Conc. mg/ml[a]	Serum Half-life (days)[a]	Binding Sites	Major Features
Polymeric serum IgM	~ 950	1.2	7	10	Primary natural antibody response (see Chapter 6)
Monomeric IgM	~ 180	NA	NA	2	Initial B cell receptor (BCR) on developing B cells
Monomeric IgA[b]	~ 160	3.5	6	2	Bone marrow derived; not involved in mucosal immunity
Dimeric IgA (dIgA)	~ 320	Trace	3	4	Produced by plasma cells in mucosal tissue
SIgA	~ 400	NA	NA	4	Major secreted antibody at mucosal sites; a complex of dIgA and SC
IgG1	~ 150	9	21	2	Major serum antibody transported *in utero* to the fetus
IgG2	~ 150	3	20	2	[d]
IgG3	~ 165	1	7	2	Earliest IgG produced; may act as a natural antibody
IgG4	~ 150	0.5	21	2	[d]
IgD[c]	~ 170	0.03	3[c]	2	Secondary BCR in some species
IgE	~ 190	5×10^{-5}	2	2	Responding antibody in type I allergy (atopy) and in parasitic infections

a/ Average values only. Range may vary as much as 10–50%.
b/ Monomeric IgA is a feature of humans and present in small amounts in the serum of non-primates.
c/ IgD is secreted by a few plasma cells in humans and not at all in most mammals.
d/ A unique role for this IgG subclass has not been established and it is sometimes absent in humans. The genes encoding IgG subclasses are duplicated in a number of species, perhaps suggesting this portion of the heavy chain locus is merely a "hot spot" of gene duplication, so that different subclasses may have no unique function (see Appendix A-2).

TABLE A3.2   Frequently Mentioned CD Markers

CD Marker	Source	Function
CD2	T cells, thymocytes, and NK cells	Adhesion molecule involved in T cell activation; T cell marker
CD3	Thymocytes, T cells	Marker for TCR and required for TCR expression
CD4	Helper T cells (TH1 and TH2)	Co-receptor for MHC class II
CD5	Thymocytes	Useful marker for thymocytes
CD8	Cytotoxic T-cells	Co-receptor for MHC class I
CD11a (LFA-1)	Macrophages and other leukocytes	Useful macrophage marker
CD11b (Mac-1)	Myeloid and NK cells	Integrin CR3 subunit associated with CD18
CD11c (CR4)	Myeloid cells	Integrin CR4 subunit associated with CD18
CD13	Myelomonocytic cells	Receptor for transmissible gastroenteritis virus (TGEV)
CD18	Leukocytes	Integrin subunit associated with CD11a–d
CD20	B cells	Universal B cell marker
CD21	Mature B cells	Mature B cell marker
CD25	Activated T and B cells	Receptor for IL-2
CD34	Hematopoietic precursors	Marker for stem cells and other cells
CD40	B cells or macrophages	Receptor for CD40 ligand, which promotes isotype switching
CD152 (CTLA4)	Activated T cells	Receptor for B7.1 (CD80), B7.2 (CD86); negative T cell regulator
CD163	Monocytes, macrophages	Receptor for porcine reproductive and respiratory syndrome virus PRRSV)

CD = Cluster of differentiation. Cell surface glycoproteins used to identify particular leukocytes and other cells, which can allow for their purification using flow cytometry, which makes them available for further *in vitro* studies. See Appendix A-1. Some, like CD13 and CD163, also serve as receptors for certain viruses. Many have alternative names. We stick to the CD designation here.

TABLE A3.3 Frequently Used Antibiotics and Their Biochemical Family Origins

Antibiotic	Biochemistry	Origin	Activity	Mechanism of Action
Penicillin	β-lactamase	*Penicillium*	Broad	Interferes with cell wall synthesis
Streptomycin	Aminoglycoside	*Streptomyces griseus*	Broad	Increases membrane permeability
Fluoroquinolone	Quinolone	**Synthetic**	Broad	Blocks DNA synthesis
Chloramphenicol	Amphenicol	*Streptomyces*	Broad	Interferes with protein synthesis
Erythromycin	Macrolide	*Saccharopolyspora*	Limited	Interferes with protein synthesis
Vancomycin	Glycopeptide	*Streptomyces*	Narrow	Blocks peptidoglycan synthesis
Amoxicillin	β-lactamase	**Penicillin derivative**	Broad	Interferes with cell wall synthesis
Doxycycline	Macrolide	*Micromonospora*	Broad	Inhibits protein synthesis
Gentamicin	Aminoglycoside	Mostly **synthetic**	Narrow	Alters DNA proof-reading
Tetracycline	Tetracycline family	*Streptomyces*	Broad	Interferes with protein synthesis
Cephalosporin	β-lactamase	*Cephalosporium*	Broad	Interferes with cell wall synthesis
Bacitracin	Polypeptide	*Bacillus subtilis*	Broad?	Inhibits pyrophosphate recycling
Tylosin	Macrolide	Mostly **synthetic**	Broad	Inhibits protein synthesis
Carbapenem	β-lactamase	*Streptomyces cattleya*	Very broad	Inhibits cell wall synthesis
Aureomycin	Tetracycline family	*Streptomyces*	Broad	Inhibits protein synthesis
Ciprofloxacin	Quinolone	**Synthetic**	Broad	Causes DNA fragmentation
Ampicillin	β-lactamase	Modified penicillin	Broad	Interferes with cell wall synthesis

Nearly all antibiotics are broad spectrum since there is little incentives to produce bacteria-specific forms.

TABLE A3.4 Currently Approved Antiviral Drugs[a]

Drug	Type	Target[b]	Virus[b]	Status
REGN	mAb	Viral RBD	SARS-CoV-2	EUA
LY-CoV	mAb	Viral RBD	SARS-CoV-2	EUA
Zanamivir	Small molecule	Viral membrane	IAV	Approved
Fostemsavir	Small molecule	Viral SfS	HIV	Approved
Albuvirtide	Peptide	HR1	HIV	Approved
Maraviroc	Small molecule	HIV Co-receptor	HIV	Approved
Ibalizumab	mAb	CD4 HIV receptor	HIV	Approved
Chloroquine	Small molecule	Endocytosis	HIV, Zika, and other viruses	Approved
Remdesivir	Small molecule	RdRp	Ebola, MERS, and other viruses	EUA
Favipiravir	Small molecule	RdRp	Ebola, Zika, and other viruses	Approved
Sofosbuvir	Small molecule	RdRp	Zika, SARS-CoV-2, and other viruses	Approved
Zidovudine	Small molecule	RdRp	HIV, HBV, and other viruses	Approved
Ribavirin	Small molecule	RdRp and DdDp	RSV, IAV	Approved
Saquinavir	Small molecule	Protease	HIV	Approved
Paxlovid	Small molecule	Protease	SARS-CoV-2	EAU
Molnupiravir	Small molecule	Viral RNA	SARS-CoV-2	EUA

a There are over 60 drugs in use or development. Of the approved drugs listed, some may go under other commercial names.

b/ RBD = cell binding domain; IAV = influenza A; HIV = human immunodeficiency virus; RdRp = RNA-dependent RNA polymerase; RSV = respiratory syncytial virus; HR1 = heptad repeat of fusion protein; SfS = fusion protein subunit.

EUA = emergency use authorization

TABLE A3.5   Acronyms

Administrations, Institutes, and Organizations
AAI: American Association of Immunologists

AAI: American Association of Immunologists
AAP: American Academy of Pediatrics
AMA: American Medical Association
AVMA: American Veterinary Medical Association
CDC: Centers for Disease Control, Atlanta, Georgia
CVM: Center for Veterinary Medicine, part of the USDA
EU: European Union
FDA: Food and Drug Administration (of the United States)
NADC: National Animal Disease Center, Ames, IA; part of the USDA
NIAID: National Institute of Allergy and Infectious Diseases, a division of the NIH, Bethesda, MD
NIH: National Institutes of Health, Bethesda, MD
PubMed: National Library of Medicine, which provides access to all published research to the public. A division of the NIH.
UNICEF: United Nations Children's Fund
USDA: United States Department of Agriculture. The main office is in Washington, DC, but research and administrative centers are located throughout the United States.
WHO: World Health Organization
WIV: Wuhan Institute of Virology, Wuhan, China

Acronyms for Common Childhood and Other Vaccines

DPT: diphtheria, pertussis, tetanus vaccine. See also DTaP.
DTaP: diphtheria, tetanus, acellular pertussis vaccine
HepA: Hepatitis A vaccine
HepB: Hepatitis B vaccine
Hib: *Hemophilus influenza* type b vaccine (may also be used to refer to the microorganism)
IPV: Inactivated polio vaccine
MMR: Combined measles, mumps, and rubella attenuated vaccine
OPV: Attenuated oral polio vaccine
PCV13: Pneumococcal polysaccharide 13 valent vaccine conjugated to a carrier
PPS23: Pneumococcal polysaccharide 23 valent vaccine conjugated to a carrier

General Biomedical Acronyms

ABC: ATP binding cassette
ACE2: angiotensin-converting enzyme 2
AGP: Antibiotic growth promoter
AID: activation-induced cytosine deaminase
ALA: alpha linolenic acid
APC: antigen presenting cell
AR: antibiotic resistance gene
ASD: autism spectrum disorder
BCG: Bacillus Calmette–Guérin, a live mycobacterial vaccine for tuberculosis
BCR: B cell receptor
BE: base editing
BMI: body mass index
CBF: cesarian-derived, breastfed infant
CD: Crohn's disease or cluster of differentiation (see Appendix A-1, Table A1.3)
CF: cesarean-derived, formula fed infant
CFTR: Cystic fibrosis transport gene
CMV: cytomegalovirus
CNS: central nervous system

(Continued)

TABLE A3.5 Acronyms *(Continued)*

CRISPR: clustered regularly interspersed short palindromic repeats
CSF: colony-stimulating factor
CTL: cytotoxic T cell
DAMP: damage-associated molecular patterns
DC: dendritic cell
DDT: dichlorodiphenyltrichloroethane
DHA: docosahexaenoic acid, a long chain, polyunsaturated fatty acid
DSB: double strand break
EGF: epithelial growth factor (see Chapter 6, Table 6.3, growth factors)
EHEC: enterohemorrhagic *E. coli*
ELISA: enzyme-linked immunosorbent assay
EPEC: enteropathogenic E.coli
ENS: enteric nervous system
ETEC: enterotoxigenic *E. coli*
FcRn: neonatal Fc receptor for transport of IgG
FMT: fecal microbial transplant
GBS: Guillain-Barré syndrome
GC: germinal center
GCRx: germinal center reaction
GI: gastrointestinal
GOS: Galacto-oligosaccharide, added to infant formulas to act as a prebiotic
HCQ: hydroxychloroquine
HGT: horizontal gene transfer
Hib: *Haemophilus influenzae* b
HIV: Human immunodeficiency virus
HMO: Human milk oligosaccharides
HPV: Human papilloma virus
HSC: Hematopoietic stem cells
IBD: Inflammatory bowel disease. Inclusive term that includes Crohn's disease (CD), ulcerative colitis (UC), celiac disease, and irritable bowel syndrome (IBS).
IBS: irritable bowel syndrome
Ig: Generic abbreviation for immunoglobulin, the biochemical term for antibodies
IGF: insulin-like growth factor
IVIG: intravenous immune globulin
KARS: killer cell activator receptor
KD: Kawasaki disease
KIRS: killer cell inhibitory receptor
LNP: lipid nanoparticle
LPS: lipopolysaccharide
mAb: monoclonal antibody
MCT: medium chain triglyceride
MDR: multidrug resistance
MFG: milk fat globule
MFGM: milk fat globule membrane
MG: mammary gland
MGBA: microbiome-gut-brain axis
MHC: major histocompatibility complex
MLV: Modified live virus
MMR: Acronym for the trivalent MLV vaccine for measles, mumps, and rubella
MRSA: Methicillin-resistant *Staphylococcus aureus*
MS: multiple sclerosis
NEC: necrotizing enterocolitis
NK: natural killer cell
NKt: a subset of natural killer cells
OCP: organochlorine pesticide

TABLE A3.5   Acronyms *(Continued)*

OPV: oral polio virus vaccine
PAMP: pathogen-associated molecular pattern
PC: plasma cell
PCB: polychlorinated biphenyl
PCR: polymerase chain reaction
PCV: pneumococcal vaccine
PEC: Pre-eclampsia (see Chapter 2)
PKU: phenylketonuria
PRR: pattern recognition receptor
PRRSV: porcine respiratory and reproductive syndrome virus
RBC: red blood cell, or erythrocyte
RBD: receptor binding domain
RCT: randomized controlled trial
RdPp: RNA dependent RNA polymerase
RNAp: RNA polymerase
RSV: respiratory syncytial virus
RT-PCR: polymerase chain reaction (PCR) involving conversion of RNA to DNA
SARS-CoV-2: severe acute respiratory syndrome coronavirus type 2
SCFA: short chain fatty acid
SCID: severe combined immunodeficiency disease
SCNT: Somatic cell nuclear transfer
SIgA: secretory immunoglobulin A
SNP: single nucleotide polymorphism
STAT: subtherapeutic antibiotic therapy
SYN: syncytiotrophoblast
TCR: T cell receptor
TGEV: Transmissible gastrointestinal virus, a disease of swine
TGFβ: transforming growth factor β (see Chapter 6, Table 6.3, growth factors)
TH or Th: Abbreviation for helper T cells, of which there are several varieties
THC: Delta-9-tetrahydrocannabinoid. A major active ingredient in marijuana, which is currently sold as a pharmaceutical for pain relief and epilepsy.
TLR: Toll-like receptor. Receptors found on cells of the innate immune system that recognize PAMPs and are necessary to stimulate an adaptive immune response. See Chapter 6, Table 6.2.
TNF: Acronym for tumor necrosis factor, of which there are several forms. TNF-α is part of the inflammatory immune defense provided by the innate immune system. See Chapter 6, Table 6.3, cytokines.
Treg: Regulatory T cells that can down-regulate inflammatory T cells
tRNA: transfer RNA
UC: ulcerative colitis
VC: viral bacteriophage clusters (see Chapter 5)
V-D-J: Recombined VH, DH, and JH genes responsible for the specificity of the BCR and TCR
VgBF: Vaginally born breastfed infant
VgF: Vaginally born formula-fed infant
VHH: A unique group of variable heavy chain genes in camelids (llamas, camels, alpacas, etc.) that do not need a light chain to form their BCR
VJ: Recombined VL and JL genes that contribute to the binding site of the BCR
VN: viral neutralization
VOC: Variants of concern. See Appendix A-4
VPREB: Polypeptide of developing B cells in mice and humans (see Appendix A-2)
VZV: varicella zoster virus
WT: wild type, the earliest reported microbial variant causing a disease

Appendix A-4
The COVID-19 Teaching Model

Combating Resurging Epidemics

The recorded history of human civilization and supporting paleontological data reveal that life-threatening/terminating diseases have paralleled the development of human civilization on planet Earth. The frequency of these epidemics and pandemics is likely to increase, as climate change, largely due to human activity, causes migration of populations and overcrowding. This puts diseased humans in contact with populations not previously exposed to certain pathogens, for which they have not developed some level of immunity. Overcrowding also increases human and wild animal interactions, favoring the spread of zoonotic disease, as seen with Ebola virus and various betacoronaviruses such as SARS-CoV-1 and SARS-CoV-2.

In the last 2 centuries, human societies have made major strides in the handling of human waste and assurance of safe water supplies, which has helped to control the spread of bacteria and bacterial infections. It has been stated that the greatest danger associated with nuclear attack or war, is disruption of sanitary and water systems, resulting in widespread death from disease, not nuclear fallout. Historically the greatest threat came from bacterial pathogens, which after 1940 could be controlled by antibiotics, until their overuse contributed to the spread of multidrug resistant (MDR) bacteria. The WHO claims that MDR bacteria now pose the greatest global threat to human health. Unlike bacterial infections, which to a certain extent can still be controlled by antibiotics, emerging viral diseases depend on control by the immune system and antiviral drugs. Healthcare trainees will face a new age of antiviral drug development.

Natural long-lasting protection against all infectious disease depends on the immune system. This is true for the most primitive life forms that depend almost entirely on innate and "trained innate immunity" (Chapter 6). The emergence of lymphocyte-driven adaptive immunity in higher vertebrates was a "game changer" that allowed infected vertebrate hosts to continuously and somatically generate modified receptors, expressed on lymphocytes (TCR and BCR; Chapter 6), and to secrete highly specific antibodies (the "new kid on the evolutionary block"). By somatically changing their receptors and effectors, they could keep pace with the rapid genomic changes of microbes, which are

353

thousands and even millions of times faster than genomic changes in humans (Chapter 6). Understanding this concept of adaptive immunity makes it possible to produce vaccines that can "get ahead" of pathogen spread, using preventive measures such as childhood vaccination protocols (Chapter 6). We discussed vaccines and classical vaccine development in Chapter 6 as part of "internal protection." In Appendix A-1 we discussed new developments in vaccine design, and in this appendix the use of new vaccines in combating SARS-CoV-2 infections. Understanding this strategy of disease mediation depends on understanding the virology of SARS-CoV-2, its origin, cell entry, its many variants, and the impact of spontaneous genomic change, natural selection, and the development of immune homeostasis, which allows both pathogen and host to survive. That is the reason, starting with Chapter 1, that we have focused on the broad spectrum of life's interdependence, and ecological homeostasis.

COVID-19 as Teaching Model
Epidemics and Pandemics

Chapter 1 called attention to Lederberg's prediction about emerging viral diseases, which have now taken center stage. COVID-19 started as a local **epidemic** but quickly spread to a global **pandemic**. Since it is well known to the public, it provides a teaching model for a pandemic viral disease and its medical mediation. The model teaches microbial genetics, micro-evolution, virology, the role of human behavior, the use of modern vaccines, and the importance of immunological memory in maintaining protection against viral infection. In any case, some biologists consider the zoonotic "jump" of SARS-CoV-2 to humans that resulted in the COVID-19 pandemic to be the "biggest evolutionary event in the last hundred years" (Morens). It is unlikely that this will be the last viral pandemic that earns such an honor.

The Biology of SARS-Cov-2

SARS-CoV-2 virus has infected over 500 million people, killed over 7 million worldwide including 1.2 million in the United States. The pandemic has occurred in successive waves and resulted in severe economic and societal disruption (Donthu). SARS-CoV-2 belongs to the coronavirus family, which causes upper respiratory infections and has one of the largest genomes among RNA viruses, including nine known human pathogens. The human seasonal coronaviruses are responsible for common cold–like symptoms, and like influenza, they are spread by face-to-face aerosol contact. Three new coronaviruses have emerged in the human population in the last 2 decades: SARS-CoV-1, MERS (Middle Eastern respiratory syndrome virus), and the much more contagious SARS-CoV-2, which spread worldwide (Kivrak). SARS-CoV-2 is an enveloped, single, positive-stranded RNA virus. The major virion envelope surface glycoprotein is the trimeric spike (S) protein. The S protein is depicted worldwide in cartoons, in commercials, and in the scientific literature. It contains a region called the receptor-binding domain (RBD), which allows cellular entrance by attaching to the angiotensin-converting enzyme 2 receptor (ACE2) on cells of the respiratory tract. Expression on these cells and others in the body may be influenced by sex, age, and possibly SARS-CoV-2 infection (Lima).

Mutation of the SARS-CoV-2 genome is continuous and rapid. For example, Omicron variant BA.1 was first reported in South Africa in November 2021, and a month later it had already become the major variant in the United Kingdom. The initial Omicron variant contained 58 genomic changes when compared to the genome of the Wuhan WT (Table A4.1). Thirty of these involve the S surface glycoproteins largely responsible for the attachment to the ACE2 on host cells. Subsequently the BA.2 variant of Omicron appeared and conferred higher replication efficiency in human nasal epithelial cells (Yamasoba). Thereafter, the BA-3.4 and BA.5 variants appeared, and they were among the most frequent in the United States. Almost certainly others will appear, partially due to pressure from vaccines, antivirals, and infection-induced immunity. Data show that the infectivity of the BA.2 variant is 1.4 times greater than the original BA.1 variant, and infectivity is even higher for the BA.5 variant. Subsequent variants of Omicron have somewhat higher affinity for the ACE2 receptor, which could explain their greater infectivity (Nutalai). Fortunately, antibodies cloned from antibody-producing cells from patients who received the original vaccines can still provide some level of protection (Nutalai). Understanding how genetic diversification of a virus occurs when it jumps to a new species (eg, humans) that lack any natural immunity can help students understand the continuing battle for existence of both host and virus.

TABLE A4.1   The Original SARS-CoV-2 Variants of Concern (VOCs)*

WHO label	Pango Lineage	Origin	First Report
Wuhan wild type (WT)	—	Wuhan	November 2019
Alpha	B.117	United Kingdom	September 2020
Beta	B.1351	South Africa	May 2020
Gamma	P.1	Brazil	November 2020
Delta	B.1617.2	India	October 2020
Omicron*	B.11529	Many sites	November 2021

Since 2022 nearly all SARS-CoV-2 viruses in circulation are variants of Omicron. These have Pango designations like B-1 through B-16 or use Nextstrain nomenclature and clades. We refer readers to "Variants of SARS-CoV2" available at Wikipedia, https://en.wikipedia.org/wiki/Variants_of_SARS-CoV-2#.

Altogether, the SARS-CoV-2 genome encodes 27 proteins with diverse functions involved in viral replication and packaging that includes the nucleocapsid protein (N), which binds the viral RNA, the envelope protein, and the membrane protein. Upon cellular infection and through a series of conformational changes of the S, attachment is followed by S-mediated fusion of the host and virion membranes, releasing the viral RNA into the cell to start the infection cycle (Hoffmann-1 2020). Using CRISPR (Appendix A-1) and what is called "survival scanning," it has been possible to identify factors other than ACE2 that are needed for SARS-CoV-2 infection. For the S proteins of SARS-CoV-2 to enter an epithelial cell, two proteolytic processing steps are needed. First, proteolytic cleavage of the precursor S protein is required. A second proteolytic event enhances fusigenicity of the S protein on the host cell plasma membrane or endosome, which allows the virus to enter. The latter set of events is mediated by Cathepsin L and by TMPRSS2 (Ziegler). Presumably these may differ among individuals, which may translate to differences in infectivity (Lima). SARS-CoV-2 also appears to globally disrupt splicing and translation of other proteins and their glycosylation, which affects the action of FcRn during *in utero* transfer of IgG (Chapter 2). Other factors are also involved in infectivity such as upregulation of ACE2 in smokers; smoking is a risk factor for COVID-19.

Schultze and Aschenbrenner (2021) note that SARS-CoV-2 infection is associated with release of various coagulation factors, secretion of inflammatory cytokines, and the formation of leukocyte-platelet aggregates that can lead to thrombo-embolic complications and cause death. Evidence favors a scenario that involves recognition by TLR3 and TLR7 in endosomes and includes cytosolic RIG-1 and MDA5 (Appendix A-1). A type I IFN response typically characterizes a viral infection but appears suppressed in SARS-CoV-2 infections (Acharya; Blanco-Melo; Hadjad) and in the elderly may be exacerbated by auto-antibodies to type I IFN (Bastard), which could be a factor in severe and critical infections (see later).

In Chapter 6, Table 6.1, we described the various hematopoietic cells, including those circulating in blood. One category of leukocytes, white blood cells (WBC), are designated as monocytes. These have a single kidney-shaped nucleus and they differ from the smaller lymphocytes by containing more cytoplasm with obvious organelles. These cells comprise 0.1–0.5% of all WBC and include plasmacytoid dendritic cells (pDC) that after migration into solid tissues may appear like macrophages. pDC and other forms of dendritic cells play a major role as APCs. pDCs, when stimulated through TLR2 and TLR7 pathways (Chapter 6, Table 6.2), result in production of IL-6 and type I IFN. The latter is of major importance in innate immune protection against viral infections. Neuropilin-1 (NRP-1) and Ax1 are secondary receptors for SARS-CoV-2 and activation of pDC through this pathway down-regulates type I IFN (van der Sluis). Since hospitalized COVID patients also have reduced numbers of pDCs, this could explain the increased severity of their disease.

Diversification/Microevolution of SARS-CoV-2

There is a high rate of spontaneous mutation in RNA viruses (Figure 6.2; Chapter 6), especially in coronaviruses (Hoffmann-2, 2020), despite the fact they have a proofreading enzyme (nsp14). Some virologists have been surprised by how rapidly SARS-CoV-2 accumulated mutations. However, it is known that when zoonotic pathogens "jump" to a new host that lacks internal immune protection, they rapidly diversify and reproduce. As reviewed in the portion of Appendix A-1 on genetics, most spontaneous mutation occurs during reproduction, when the DNA/RNA is duplicating; the more frequent the replication, the greater the possibility of generating new mutants. It seems possible that the pre-pandemic SARS-CoV-2 ancestors were "pre-adapted" for "jumping" to various mammals, perhaps only needing the T372A mutation (see later) to allow them to bind ACE2 in a variety of new hosts. It is to the advantage of any parasite to be contagious since it enhances survival of the species. However, becoming more virulent has its disadvantages, since "good parasites don't kill their hosts." Thus variants like Omicron often evolve to become more contagious but less virulent. This pattern seems to be the path to establishing homeostasis with their new host, allowing both to survive. This may be the case for coronaviruses that are responsible for some "common colds." Such interdependence between host and pathogen (Chapter 1) allows the host population to develop natural immunity and for mothers to supply virus-neutralizing (VN) antibodies *in utero* and later in breast milk. This hypothesis has problems when applied to highly virulent viruses like rabies and SARS-CoV-2, since they are not dependent on one species but can readily infect other mammals. Rabies is broadly distributed among the canine family and their close relatives like bats (Chiroptera). Coronaviruses are widespread, and aside from humans, bats, and pangolins, they are also common in pigs, cattle, mice, cats, dogs, chickens, deer, and hedgehogs, where they are responsible for more than respiratory diseases (Corman). SARS-CoV-2 has now been detected in one-third of deer in the Midwest.

Recognized Variants of SARS-CoV-2

More than 16 million genomes of SARS-CoV-2 (over 6 million for Omicron) have been sequenced, and the number continues to grow exponentially. An early report indicated that at least one-third of these involve glycosylation sites that can drastically affect the degree of infectivity, since they alter the structure of the trimeric S protein (Li). Over 300 million infections have been documented and sequence analyses reveal over 100 variants belonging to a minimum of six distinct lineages. For clarity, the WHO, in collaboration with the CDC, has established a Greek letter designation for the lineages designated as "variants of concern" (VOC). In the earliest research studies, they were given a "Pango" designation (Table A4.1). Current circulating SARS-CoV-2 viruses are variants of Omicron, which differs by 58 or more mutations from the Wuhan WT. These are given B- or BA-designation while some investigators designate them as Nextstrain clades (see Variants of SARS-CoV-2 in Wikipedia). In this textbook we will primarily use the early VOCs as examples in discussing mutations affecting the RBD.

In this overview we focus on mutations affecting the RBD and the S protein in which it is embedded. Mutation sites are identified according to the location of the codon in the genomic sequence. For example, in animal reservoirs of closely related coronaviruses, position 372 in the S protein encodes alanine, but in SARS-CoV-2, alanine replaces threonine; this codon change is designated A372T. It was shown that this change is associated with greater infectivity due to its higher affinity for ACE2. Early variants of the spike of the "wild type" (WT) Wuhan strain also have a change from aspartic acid at position 614 to glycine, designated D614G. *In vitro* studies show that this is associated with increased replication in human cell lines and with higher viral titers in the nasopharynx of infected patients (Kang). The alpha variant that appeared in the United Kingdom (B.117, VOC alpha; see

Table A4.1) has 17 amino changes relative to the Wuhan WT, including eight in the region encoding the S protein. Of particular interest has been the N501Y mutation (asp-tyr), which, based on computer modeling studies, is located where neutralizing antibodies, whether due to infection, vaccine, or mAbs prepared for immunotherapy, bind to the virion and block attachment to ACE2. The alpha (B.117) variant also has higher affinity for ACE2 and is associated with 40–50% greater transmission compared to D614G variants or the WT variant and can lead to more than 30% higher mortality (Supasa). The N501Y mutation and two others in the RBD (K417T; E484K) are also common to gamma variants. P.1 (gamma; Table A4.1) shares these mutations with the beta variants (B.1351; Table A4.1). All three variants that share these mutations have increased affinity for binding to the ACE2 receptor (Dejnirattisai). Not surprisingly, mutations like theses impact the effectiveness of neutralizing antibodies, which may explain their greater virulence.

Infectivity also depends on mutations in the RBD that lie outside the region that encodes the S protein, since viral entry involves more than just binding to the ACE2 receptor (Ziegler). Results from another study show that P.1 escape mutants (gamma; Table A4.1) that share these three mutations (E484K; K417 N/T; N501Y) appear less resistant to naturally acquired or vaccine-induced anti–SARS-CoV-2 responses, indicating that changes outside the RBD also influence VN (Dejnirattisai). Many variants involve glycosylation, which can also influence infectivity. Based only on *in vitro* studies, removing a critical glycosylation site (N345) impaired RBD folding, decreasing expression and infectivity (Starr).

This appendix covering SARS-CoV-2 and COVID-19 is not intended to be comprehensive, especially regarding the many Omicron variants and the specific mutation associated with each variant. Rather we hope to provide enough information and examples to illustrate the biological complexity of an emerging disease and in doing so to give students insight into the types of studies involved in the effort to understand a viral pandemic. The examples provided have focus on the S protein, RBD, and VN, since these often take priority in studies and VN is most often the major initial defense against viral infection, to which vaccine development is directed (see next section). However, we mentioned the apparent failure or misdirection of the innate immune response, especially in the transition of the infection from upper to lower respiratory tract and the development of "long COVID." It may be found that affected individuals have genetic defects in innate immunity, just like those more often documented for the adaptive immune system (Chapter 6). Such research may also explain why age-dependent waning of innate immunity makes older populations more susceptible to severe COVID-19.

The Origin of SARS-CoV-2

Coronaviruses that have led to previous epidemics in the last 2 decades (SARS-CoV-1 and MERS) had their origins in animals common to certain cultures, such as MERS in Middle Eastern camels. The COVID-19 pandemic caused by SARS-CoV-2 moved rapidly from a local epidemic in Wuhan, China, to a global pandemic; neither its origin nor the reasons for its rapid spread are entirely clear. Sadly, politics and other human behavior became involved. Wuhan is a major city in central China and has a large seafood wholesale market trading in fish and live animals, including poultry, Asian fruit bats, pangolins, marmots, and snakes. Pangolins are smuggled into Southeast Asia and sold in wet markets. In these cultures, their scales are used in traditional medicine and their meat is considered a delicacy. It is a "wet" or "on the hoof" market. It is also home to the Wuhan Institute of Virology (WIV), which has a well-known reputation for studies on coronaviruses. This raised the question as to whether SARS-CoV-2 was a laboratory escapee, originated in bats or some other wet market mammals, or had a separate origin. Initial claims by some virologists and politicians that it was an engineered virus do not seem plausible since there is no evidence that virologists at WIV were involved in studies of any closely related coronavirus (Karlsson). All previous coronavirus outbreaks have had a zoonotic origin and two of these were linked to wild animals in the wet market (Holmes).

Asian bats and pangolins, both sold in wet markets, have been a focus of efforts to identify a SARS-CoV-2–like coronavirus in these mammals. In samples collected in Yunnan province from the Horseshoe bat, *Rhinolophus*, the overall genome was approximately 90% homologous to SARS-CoV-2, but homology was relatively low in the S protein sequence. However, the bat CoV RaT613 virus showed 97% homology with SARS-CoV-2 in the S protein (Liu). Some pangolin-derived coronaviruses have RBD that are nearly identical to SARS-CoV-2 (Holmes). Currently a zoonotic origin, combined with the A372T mutation, seems most likely. If the original SARS-CoV-2 viruses can mutate and diversify as rapidly as has been observed (Table A4.1), why have they not previously been transferred to humans? The first reported infection of a human was a vendor in the Wuhan wet market on November 18, 2019. On the other hand, prior to the pandemic, the exact same virus was not found in any other species. Unfortunately, the Chinese government has been less than open and helpful in the assessment of the source of this virus.

The Host Immune Response to SARS-CoV-2

Protective immunity depends on both the innate and adaptive immune systems; the former is part of the first line of defense and its stimulation is very important in viral infection and leads to the development of the latter (see Chapter 6). Its stimulation by viral infection typically results in the release of type I IFN, which activates other innate immune functions. Protective adaptive immunity depends on VN antibodies and cytotoxic T cells that kill virus-infected cells. We shall examine each in relation to COVID-19.

The Innate Immune Response to SARS-CoV-2

SARS-CoV-2, like influenza, rapidly replicates in the nasopharynx or nares by gaining access to epithelial and other cells, by the mechanism described in the previous section. Ciliated cells in the nasopharynx are the primary target, but the issue is somewhat unresolved. This leads to an upper respiratory infection over several days, but a subset of patients develop lower respiratory tract infections, which can cause severe damage to airways, alveoli, and vasculature and leads to dependence on respirators and all too often to death. This may suggest a type of failed innate antiviral immunity in the nasal epithelium (Ziegler). Studies reviewed by Schultze and Aschenbrenner (2021) indicate that variability in expression of innate immune system components is a major contributor to differences in the disease course in COVID-19. Some individuals may continue to suffer what is called "long COVID." Exactly how SARS-CoV-2 can damage the host is a subject of much study, but misdirection of innate immunity is likely a factor.

The innate immune response to infectious agents begins with recognition by pathogen response receptors (PRRs; Chapter 6). In Chapter 6 we discussed TLRs (Chapter 6, Table 6.2) as representative PRRs, and in Appendix A-1, we extended this to additional PRRs and several intracellular pathways. The consequence of SARS-CoV-2 infection ranges from mild to critical disease. As mentioned previously, in cases of severe COVID there appears to be poor or suppressed innate immune and type I IFN responses (Hadjad). Instead, the response is often skewed toward the release of inflammatory cytokines like TNF, IL-1, IL-6, CXCLl8, and type II IFN (Chapter 6, Table 6.3), resulting in what has been vernacularly called a "cytokine storm." These "storms," also referred to as the cytokine release syndrome (CRS), may explain severe COVID and long COVID. It has been suggested that a failure of an appropriate innate antiviral response in the nasopharynx allows the infection to spread to the lower respiratory tract, which can prove fatal (Schultze). This is supported by a mouse model (Ho). Evidence is weak that replication of the virus in host tissue can alone explain disease, especially severe and critical disease. Rather, the immune response of the host and the conditions of the environment, including genetic factors, play a role in disease severity (van der Made).

Growing evidence, including the personal experiences of infected healthcare professionals, confirms that this secondary illness is not merely manufactured by social media. Symptoms may persist 7 weeks post-infection (Kao). "Brain fog" is one feature of long COVID, and in patients and mice it is associated with elevated levels of CCL11, both in plasma and cerebro-spinal fluid. Brain fog was also reported during the 1918 Spanish Flu Pandemic and in some H1N1 (influenza) infections. Systemic CCL11 administration in a mouse model caused hippocampal microglial reactivity and impaired neurogenesis (Fernández-Castañeda). As we previously indicated, long COVID symptoms seem to result from changes in the innate immune system and elevated CCL11 may be one example of this.

The role of TLRs (Chapter 6) and other PRRs (Appendix A-1) in activation of the innate immune system and release of type I interferons (IFNs) was described. As mentioned earlier, the TLR3 and TLR7 pathways are especially important in the response to viral infection of respiratory epithelial cells. In COVID-19, deficiencies in TLR3 and TLR7 are a risk factor for severe COVID. As previously mentioned, severe COVID is associated with suppressed innate immunity and poor release of type I IFNs (Hadjad). Also mentioned previously, a major source of type I IFNs is pDCs (Becker), the release of which is triggered through the TLR7 and TLR2 pathways. In hospitalized COVID-19 patients. The reduction in pDCs correlates with disease severity (van der Sluis).

The risk of fatal COVID doubles every 5 years from childhood onward, and in individuals 60–90 years of age this correlates with the increase in auto-antibodies to certain type I IFNs (Bastard). This implies that in individuals less than age 50, the production of type I IFNs and lack of hindrances to its actions protects against severe COVID.

The Adaptive Immune Response to SARS-CoV-2

Longitudinal studies indicate that durable and broad T and B cell immunologic memory develops in normal fashion after infection (Cohen; Sokal). Most encouraging is that many antibodies resulting from infection or that are vaccine-generated still bind the RBD of VOCs despite micro-evolution/diversification of SARS-CoV-2 and they can still offer protection against severe disease caused by all major variants (Table A4.1). In general, patient antibody responses target the S, N, and RBD proteins; those to S provide the greatest protection, although those to N seem most cross-reactive and are of highest affinity (Banach). Not surprisingly, mutational changes diminish the effectiveness of antibodies initially generated against the Wuhan WT strain (Table A4.1), especially in the case of the Omicron variant. Almost all of the approximately 30 vaccines in use or development target the RBD, with the goal of stimulating the production of antibodies that are cross-reactive and can competitively block attachment and penetration of the virus (ie, result in viral neutralization [VN]). As we described in Chapter 6 and reviewed earlier, VN is not the only immune mechanism involved in control and protection against viral infection, so laboratory VN tests cannot exclusively predict the efficacy of a vaccine and there is good evidence that T and B cell cross-protection is needed (Cevik). Memory B cells that supply VN antibodies may provide limited protection against Omicron variants of SARS-CoV-2, while T cell memory is more persistent (Tarke). There is also evidence that the short amino acid T cell epitopes are more cross-reactive among SARS-CoV-2 variants than are the B cell epitopes expressed by different SARS-CoV-2 variants. The B cell memory that develops (Sokal) appears to drop off, especially for the Omicron variant (Tarke), and few clones are derived from higher-affinity precursors (Mesin). T cell memory across VOC variants (Table A4.1) remains at approximately 85%, but B cell memory drops to approximately 40%. Part of the dilemma is that the frequency of B cells in blood specific for any antigen is less than 0.1% (Banach). However, their recovery from blood using magnetic enrichment indicates they possess an enriched COVID-19 repertoire and are indeed derived from memory B cells.

Immune System Avoidance by SARS-CoV-2

In Chapter 6 we noted that viruses possess mechanisms that prevent the host from ending the viral life cycle. One mechanism we described was down-regulation of MHC I, so that infected cells would be "invisible" to targeting cytotoxic T cells. Others, like some herpes viruses and the virus responsible for chicken pox (Varicella) go dormant or "into hiding" until they are awakened by some environmental stimulant. In addition to apparent SARS-CoV-2–induced type I IFN suppression, several non-structural proteins encoded in the

SARS-CoV-2 genome bind ribosomal RNA in the infected cells, which inhibits mRNA translation (Banerjee).

SARS-CoV-2 and other viruses that jump to a host that lacks natural immunity to them replicate rapidly and many genomic "escape mutant" variants quickly accumulate (Table A4.1). This is the most obvious means of immune system avoidance. As in all evolutionary events, escape mutants that can survive pressure from natural or vaccine-dependent immune responses rapidly reproduce setting the stage for the next generation of escape mutants. By this means, SARS-CoV-2 has resisted efforts by the host immune system to eliminate it as a species. As more is learned about SARS-CoV-2, we will likely learn there are additional maneuvers used by this virus to avoid elimination by the host immune system.

Controlling the COVID-19 Pandemic
Overview

There are three ways to control a microbial pandemic: (1) Allow the pandemic to run its course until there are few remaining susceptible individuals that can serve as hosts. (2) Introduce physical barriers to reduce the spread of the contagion. (3) Introduce manmade therapeutic intervention. While intervention through the use of antibiotics was highly affective for bacterial epidemics/pandemics, the only options for emerging viral diseases are effective vaccines, antiviral drugs, and changes in human behavior. Human societies are loath to employ the first option in the case of SARS-CoV-2. Like rabies, SARS-CoV-2 can survive by simply moving to a new host. Therefore, human societies typically choose the second and third options. The third option is only effective if an effective vaccine or drug can be rapidly developed and if susceptible individuals are willing to accept science, take the vaccine or the drug and help the movement toward achieving herd immunity (Chapter 6). Especially in the United States, the second option had limited success for political and religious reasons and the anti-vaccination movement has interfered with development of herd immunity.

Next we summarize the vaccines developed to combat SARS-CoV-2 as well as other measures used to control the pandemic. The biotechnology involved in the development of these vaccines was discusses in Appendix A-1.

SARS-CoV-2 Vaccines

Attenuated Vaccines

Attenuated vaccines are "the gift that keeps on giving" by continuing to grow and reproduce in the host, thus potentially providing lifelong immunity, as the childhood MMR vaccine does. Attenuated viruses have the danger of reverting to a pathogenic form, as we described for the oral polio vaccine (OPV) in Asia (Chapter 6). Hence, attenuation was considered a very risky approach for SARS-CoV-2, although it is being tested in animal models.

Subunit Vaccines

Development of these follows the same principles as traditional subunit vaccines but, as described in Appendix A-1, modern subunit recovery is more rapid and yields cleaner products; the Novavax vaccine is an example. A potential weakness of subunit vaccines is their poor immunogenicity and the need for an adjuvant, which can cause uncomfortable side effects (Chapter 6). Incorporating them into special lipid nanoparticles (LNP) modified to express TLR ligands may help (Brouwer; see Appendix A-1). Another tactic to improve subunit vaccines for SARS-CoV-2 that reduces the need for an adjuvant is the use of the naturally occurring dimers of the S protein (Dai). This improves immunogenicity, perhaps because the size of the S protein dimer allows for a greater capacity to cross-link BCRs.

Viral Vector Vaccines

This technology typically involves the use of a carrier adenovirus, the "Trojan Horse" of vaccine biotechnologists. The Russian Sputnik V, AstraZeneca (Oxford), and Janssen/Johnson & Johnson vaccines are based on this technology. Some of these have been approved totally or for emergency use worldwide and have proven effective.

mRNA Vaccines

These have been developed by several pharmaceutical/biotech firms. Those from Pfizer-BioNTech and Moderna obtained full FDA approval for adults and are gradually being extended to the pediatric population. There are efforts to produce similar vaccines such as at the State Key Laboratory in Beijing (Zhang, 2020). These seem to be the most effective vaccines and they provide better immunity than that resulting from natural infection and may explain the ineffectiveness of convalescent immune globulin (see later).

Mucosal Vaccines

Although COVID is an infection of the respiratory mucosa, all current vaccines are given parenterally, which means the stimulation of mucosal immunity to SARS-CoV-2 is a secondary consequence like that to Saulk-based IPV (see Chapter 6). We described how the Sabin OPV is designed to stimulate the GI tract mucosa, the site infected by the polio virus. All original and most current influenza vaccines are also given parenterally, so mucosal immune stimulation is a secondary consequence. We mentioned that SARS-CoV-2 vaccines and infections reliably generate better T cell than B cell memory and that T cell epitopes (short linear peptides) are more cross-reactive among variants than B cell epitopes (Kingstad-Bakke, 2022). While antibodies neutralize the virus by blocking cell entry, it is the CD8+ CTLs that eliminate the infected epithelial cells. Hence, the need exists for the development of more effective mucosal vaccines for SARS-CoV-2 and other respiratory viruses, such as those that can enrich for T cell memory and CD8+ CTLs in the respiratory mucosa.

We briefly mentioned this in Appendix A-1 under the topic "modern adjuvants," since a major challenge is the development of mucosal adjuvants. Promising results have been obtained with Adjuplex (ADJ), a carbineer-based adjuvant that is used in conjunction to

CpG; CpG is a synthetic nucleic acid PRR that is recognized by TLR 9 (Chapter 6). This has successfully been used in a mouse model for delivering influenza A nucleoprotein in a nano-emulsion to the nasal passages (Kingstad-Bakke, 2021). More recently, Kingstad-Bakke et al. (2022) have formulated an intranasal (IN) SARS-CoV-2 vaccine based on ADJ-CpG and ADG-GLA and tested it in a mouse model. Mouse immunologists recognize three categories of T memory cells. Trm memory cells are recognized by bearing CD69 and CD102. Using this means of identification, Trm memory T cells that accumulate in the airways are significantly increased when using the IN SARS-CoV-2 vaccine in mice. This IN vaccine can provide effective immunity even in the absence of VN antibodies. This proof of concept of mucosal vaccines for SARS-CoV-2 is yet to be used in human clinical trials (Chapter 7). In any case, efforts to develop mucosal vaccines that target the mucosal immune system are likely to be a wave of the future.

Effectiveness of Vaccine Therapy

There are up to 10 COVID-19 vaccines being used worldwide and perhaps another 20 in development. Some have achieved approval by the FDA, their equivalents in the United Kingdom and Western Europe, and from the WHO. Even without such approvals, vaccines like Sputnik V and Sinovac are in wide usage. In general, all are effective and have been evaluated by at least two criteria: (1) protection against symptomatic infection, and (2) protection against severe disease. The original mRNA vaccines (Pfizer-BioNTech and Moderna) provide 85–90% protection against SARS-CoV-2 WT and the Alpha variant (Table A4.1). Such protection continued for the Delta and Beta/Gamma variants when using the Pfizer-BioNTech vaccine, but it dropped off to approximately 70% with the Moderna, AstraZeneca, and J&J vaccines. However, some report Moderna produces higher antibody titers. While vaccines from Novavax, J&J, and Sinovax perform well against the Alpha variant, protection also falls off with Delta, Gamma/Delta, and Omicron. Recent studies report a similar drop off in protection against Omicron using the Pfizer-BioNTech and Moderna vaccines (Goel). Their effectiveness in VN against variants (Table A4.1) depends on amino acid changes in the S protein or the RBD. The work of Cevik (earlier) illustrates these differences. The original vaccines were based on the sequence of the Wuhan WT virus, so it is not surprising that their effectiveness wanes as new variants emerge with mutations in RBD and S protein (Tuekprakhon). It was shown that antibodies generated against Wuhan WT SARS-CoV-2 have poor VN ability against the Omicron variant, allowing it to escape and giving it the opportunity to reproduce and spread the contagion (Hoffmann, 2020; Dejnirattisai). In general, vaccine-generated antibodies using formulations based on Wuhan WT are 10–40% less effective in neutralizing Omicron. This forecasts that designing the most effective COVID-19 vaccines, will require changes in formulation as SARS-CoV-2 micro-evolves into new variants as it spreads within its new hosts. This is the type of upgrading of viral vaccines that has been common practice with the annual flu vaccine, another RNA virus. Fortunately, modern biotechnology allows for changes in formulation of mRNA and vector vaccines to be rapidly made.

A 6-month comparison of mRNA vaccines (Moderna and Pfizer-BioNtech) with subunit vaccines (Novavax) and a vector vaccine (Janssen/J&J) indicated that all individuals made memory CD4+ T cells and mRNA and the vector vaccine induced comparable CD8+ T cells. The vector vaccine induced a higher level of memory B cells. mRNA vaccines were associated with a substantial decline in serum antibody titers but comparable memory T and B cells (Zhang, 2022). We previously mentioned that linear peptide T cell epitopes are more cross-reactive or conserved among SARS-CoV-2 variants. At present, a full comparison among vaccines in use is not yet available.

The second criterion for judging vaccines is effectiveness in **preventing severe disease** (ie, infections requiring hospitalization and the need for ventilators). Using that criterion, all vaccines in current use perform in the 95% category (Cevik). Unless there are data showing a major negative response to vaccination, any major vaccine is better that no vaccine.

Contentious and Unresolved Issues

While shown to be over 90% effective, questions concerning mRNA vaccines remain and especially about events in the Critical Window. These include how long will infected cells continue to secrete the S protein that could continue to stimulate the immune system and when young children are exposed, could this lead to **peripheral tolerance** (Chapters 2 and 6), since mothers who received an mRNA vaccine transmit it in in utero or in breast milk and how long does vaccine-induced protection endure? In any case, COVID-19 Vaccines are recommended for pregnant and breastfeeding mothers (Novillo). Addressing these questions awaits long-term studies (see the discussion of Phase 4 trials in Chapter 7).

A concern that involves the effectiveness of all vaccines is their ability to stimulate immunologic memory, which in the case of respiratory diseases involves memory T and B cells at mucosal sites. Original reports stated that coronaviruses that caused the common cold insufficiently stimulated memory responses; this information was used by some to explain the frequent reoccurrence of the common cold in the same individuals, though this has been debunked. However, seasonal coronavirus antibody levels are boosted after SARS-CoV-2 infection; these cross-react with other variants but are non-neutralizing (Anderson). Of greater concern is how long memory T and B cells remain after vaccination or infection. There is clear evidence for B cell memory in the response to SARS-CoV-2 infection and mRNA vaccines (Banach); one concern is whether this extends to the various Omicron variants. Omicron carries a large number of mutations, approximately 15 in the RBD alone, which is correlated with the 10–40% reduction in neutralizing capacity by the sera of patients infected with the Wuhan WT or exposed to vaccine based on pre-Omicron variants. Originally the concern was that memory B cells were poorly developed or low in number, but recent data indicate that the memory B cells that are generated remain durable for 9 months and that 40–50% of these memory B cells are specific for the RBD and recognize the Alpha, Beta, Delta, and Omicron variants (Table A4.1). A third dose of the vaccine significantly increases their levels (Goel).

Other Medical Interventions
Antiviral Drug Therapy

The concept and use of antiviral drugs was discussed in Chapter 6 and examples were listed in Table A3.4. We will discuss these in relation to controlling COVID-19. Efforts to control SARS-CoV-2 initially involved hydroxychloroquine, Ivermectin, remdesivir, and dexamethasone. The first two have been used widely and effectively in the control of malaria and other Eukaryotic parasites (Rakedzon). Some, like favipiravir, remdesivir, and the corticosteroid dexamethasone, have been studied both *in vitro* and *in vivo* with a number of viruses including SARS-CoV-2 (Kivrak). Favipiravir (Table A3.4) was the first antiviral used in China and lowers infectivity and the risk of more serious diseases, but only when given early. Remdesivir is approved by the FDA and when properly used can reduce mortality by up to 10%, although it is known to produce several adverse side effects. Dexamethasone has only been used in ICU patients to reduce "cytokine storm" associated lung damage, thus reducing the number of patients needing to go on respirators. Chloroquine and hydroxychloroquine (HCQ) are antiparasite drugs. While originally reported to reduce viral entry and suppress inflammation, they are generally considered useless but produce only mild adverse side effects. Both have been used in *in vitro* and animal studies for several viral diseases such as HIV, hepatitis C, influenza A, and flaviviruses like dengue and Zika and some coronaviruses. Sadly, neither reduced the deaths from SARS-CoV-2 in human clinical trials. Artemisinin, derived from *Artemisia*, has also been a major weapon against malaria and *in vitro* it inhibits viral replication of hepatitis B, Epstein-Barr, virus and CMV. Used in the Ebola epidemic, artemisinin reduced deaths by 37%. Similarly, Ivermectin, which like HCQ received considerable attention during the early phase of the COVID-19 pandemic in 2020, was effective *in vitro*, but proper clinical studies showed no effect (Rakedzon). This might be anticipated since Ivermectin increases the permeability of the eukaryote cell membrane, which of course is likely irrelevant in viral infection.

Recently two antivirals designed to inhibit SARS-CoV-2 replication have been approved for emergency use (Table A3.4). Both are designed to stop the spread of SARS-CoV-2 in individuals at high risk for severe COVID-19 disease. Paxlovid™ blocks the action of the SARS-CoV-2 3C-like protease, inhibiting replication of the virus at the proteolysis stage. Molnupiravir is a ribonucleotide analog that becomes phosphorylated by host kinases and subsequently inhibits RNA viral replication. At this point, a "magic bullet" drug against SARS-CoV-2 is not yet widely available, although there is considerable activity in this area. However, some drugs have been shown to reduce the inflammatory response associated with SARS-CoV-2 infection and reduce spread of the infection if they are given early. They also reduce the spread of SARS-CoV-2 to the lungs, thus reducing lung damage and mortality and preventing long COVID. For enterprising medical science trainees, viral immunology, vaccine development, and antiviral pharmacology are good areas to pursue.

Hybrid Immunity

It should not be surprising that natural infection and vaccination produce different response/protective outlines. We previously indicated that vaccination is more effective in generating protective immunity than infection. Studies on convalescent patients that later received an mRNA vaccine provide a basis for what is called *hybrid immunity*. Studies show that following vaccination, previously infected patients generated more SARS-CoV-2 RBD memory B cells than those who were never infected and only vaccinated. Furthermore, such patients had more CD4 T cells that recognized S protein peptides than those who were only vaccinated and never infected (Rodda). This would seem to support media reports that those who have recovered from COVID-19 should thereafter be vaccinated to obtain hybrid immunity.

Passive Immune Therapy

Therapeutic treatment of COVID-19 also includes use of convalescent sera and mAb (ie, passive immunity). While introduced early in 2020 as a stopgap, convalescent serum has been of marginal value and is no longer recommended. While previous and regular exposure to human coronaviruses responsible for common colds generate antibodies that cross-react with SARS-CoV-2, they are at such low levels that they do not protect against SARS-CoV-2 (Anderson). Use of mAb was approved in only 10 months (November 2020) although they were used experimentally in mid-2020 including to treat then-President Trump. At this writing four different mAb cocktails have received approval. The use of mAb therapy for viral disease skyrocketed after 2016 and at least 115 have been approved for treatment of RSV, anthrax, rabies, Ebola, HIV; approximately 14 SARS-CoV-2 cocktails have been tested (Corti) as well as potent mAb engineered from single-sorted B cells (Figure A1.13) from convalescent patients (Andreano). Results obtained using mAb have been valuable and variable in understanding VN, since they target different epitopes in the RBD. Of interest has been that trimeric RBD occurs in two different conformations, referred to as "open" and "closed." Certain mAb bind only to the open configuration. The affinity and effectiveness of therapeutic antibodies for different VOC variants depends on the number of mutations in the RBD. Except for Evusheld, most have proven to be ineffective against Omicron (Hoffmann-2, 2022) and are not currently recommended.

Bioengineering in Combatting COVID

We described bioengineering in Appendix A-1, including CRISPR. Use of the latter *in vitro* has been shown to degrade RNA from SARS-CoV-2 and influenza A in human lung epithelial cells (Abbott).

The Take-Home Message

The international attention that COVID-19 received makes it an attractive teaching model. It provides the opportunity to review the primary research literature in virology, the origin of a pandemic disease, and the micro-genetic diversification of a pathogen that apparently "jumped" from some other mammal to humans who lacked cross-reactive immunity and therefore failed to establish homeostasis with this pathogen. Global environmental changes and the enhanced connection among human populations naturally increases exposure to emerging viral diseases (Chapter 1). This can lead to a local outbreak, but in the case of SARS-CoV-2 it led to a global pandemic. Current healthcare students need to keep in mind that COVID-19 will not be the last pandemic they encounter, they will likely someday be required to respond medically to a new pandemic. While the frequency of epidemics and pandemics may increase, modern medical science and its associated biotechnology and bio-engineering will also increase (Appendix A-1). SARS-CoV-2 revealed the need to prepare and get out ahead of the pathogen. Viral immunology in the future is likely to focus more on the formulation of vaccines that can act at the site of infections (in the case of SARS-CoV-2, the respiratory epithelium). These are tasks for researchers, but it is important to keep informed of the status and efforts to provide better protection as part of continuing medical education.

References

Abbott TR, Dhamdhere G, Liu Y, et al. Development of CRISPR as an antiviral strategy to combat SARS-CoV-2 and influenza. *Cell*. 2020;181:865–876.

Acharya D, Lui G, Gack MU. Dysregulation of type I interferon responses in COVID-19. *Nat Rev Immunol*. 2020;20:397–398.

Anderson EM, Goodwin EC, Verma A, et al. Seasonal human coronavirus antibodies are boosted upon SARS-CoV-2 infection but not associated with protection. *Cell*. 2021;184:1858–1864.

Andreano E, Nicastri E, Pacello I, Pileri P, et al. SARS-CoV-2 escape from a highly neutralizing COVID-19 convalescent plasma. *Cell*. 2021;184(11):2926–2938.e11. doi:10.1016/j.cell.2021.02.035

Banach M, Harley ITW, McCarthy MK, et al. Magnetic enrichment of SARS-CoV-2 antigen-binding B-cells for analysis of transcriptions and antibody repertoire. *Magnetochem*. 2022;8:23. doi:10-3390/magnetochemistry8020023.

Banerjee AK, Bianco MR, Bruce EA, et al. SARS-CoV-2 disrupts splicing, translation, and protein trafficking to suppress host defense. *Cell*. 2020;183:1325–1339.

Bastard P, Gervais A, Voyer TL, et al. Auto-antibodies neutralizing type I IFNs are present in 4% of uninfected individuals over 70 years old and account for ~20% of COVID-19 deaths. *Sci Immunol*. 2021;6:eabl4340. doi:10.1126/sciimmunol.abl4340.

Becker J, Kalinke U. Toll-like receptors matter: Plasmacytoid dendritic cells in COVID-19. *EMBO J*. 2022;41:e111208. doi:10.15252/embj.2022111208.

Blanco-Melo D, Nilsson BE, Lui W-C, et al. Imbalanced host responses to SARS-CoV-2 drives development of COVID-19. *Cell*. 2020;181:1036–1045.

Brouwer PJM, Brinkkemper M, Maisonnasse P, et al. Two-component spike nanoparticle vaccine protects macaques from SARS-CoV-2 infection. *Cell*. 2021;184:1188–1200.

Cevik M, Grubaugh ND, Iwasaki A, Openshaw P. COVID-19 vaccines: Keeping pace with SARS-CoV-2 variants. *Cell*. 2021;184:5077–5081.

Cohen KW, Linderman SL, Moodie Z, et al. Longitudinal analysis shows durable and broad immune memory after SARS-CoV-2 infection with persisting antibody responses and memory B and T cells. *medRxiv*. 2021; version 2:100354. doi:10.1101/2021.04.19.21255739.

Corman VM, Muth D, Niemeyer D, Drosten C. Hosts and sources of endemic human coronaviruses. *Adv Virus Res*. 2016;100:163–188.

Corti D, Purcell LA, Snell G, Veesler, D. Tackling Covid-19 with neutralizing monoclonal antibodies *Cell* 2021; 184:3086–3108

Dai L, Zheng T, Xu K, et al. A universal design of beta coronavirus vaccines against COVID-19, MERS and SARS. *Cell*. 2020;782:722–733.

Dejnirattisai W, Huo J, Zhou D, et al. SARS-CoV-2 Omicron B.1.1.529 leads to widespread escape from neutralizing antibody responses. *Cell*. 2022;185:467–484.

Donthu N, Gustafsson A. Effects of COVID-19 on business and research. *J Bus Res*. 2020;117:284–289.

Fernández-Castañeda A, Lu P, Geraghty AC, et al. Mild respiratory COVID can cause multi-lineage neural cell and myelin dysregulation. *Cell*. 2022;185:2452–2468.

Goel RR, Painter MM, Lundgreen KA, et al. Efficient recall of Omicron-reactive B cell memory after a third dose of SARS-CoV-2 mRNA vaccine. *Cell*. 2022;185:1875–1887.

Hadjad J, Yatim N, Barnabei L, et al. Impaired type I interferon activity and inflammatory responses in severe COVID-19 patients. *Science*. 2020;369:718–724.

Ho JSY, Wing-Yee Mok B, Campisi L, et al. TOP1 inhibition therapy protect against SARS-CoV-2–induced lethal inflammation. *Cell*. 2021;184:2618–2632.

Hoffman -1, M, Kleine-Weber J, Schroder S, et al. SARS-CoV-2 cell entry depends on ACE2 and TMPRSS2 and is blocked by a clinically proven protease inhibitor. *Cell*. 2020;181:271–280.

Hoffmann -2, M, Krüger N, Schulz S, et al. The Omicron variant is highly resistant against antibody-mediated neutralization: Implications for control of the COVID-19 pandemic. *Cell*. 2022;185:447–456.

Holmes EC, Goldstein SA, Rasmussen AL, et al. The origin of SARS-CoV-2: A critical review. *Cell*. 2021;184:4848–4856.

Kang L, He G, Sharp AK, et al. A selective sweep in the *Spike* gene has driven SARS-CoV-2 human adaptation. *Cell*. 2021;184:4392–4400.

Kao J, Frankland PW. COVID fog demystified. *Cell*. 2022;185:2391–2393.

Karlsson EA, Duong V. The continuing search for the origins of SARS-CoV-2. *Cell*. 2021;184:4373–4390.

Kingstad-Bakke B, Lee W, Chandrasekar SS, Suresh M. Vaccine-induced systemic and mucosal T cell immunity in SARS-CoV-2 viral variants. *Proc Natl Acad Sci USA*. 2022;119(20): e2118312119. doi:10.1073/pnas.2118312119.

Kingstad-Bakke B, Toy R, Lee W, et al. Polymeric pathogen-like particles-based combination adjuvants elicit potent mucosal T cell immunity to influenza A virus. *Front Immunol*. 2021;11. doi:10.3389/fimmu.2020.559382.

Kivrak A, Ulas B, Kivrak H. A comparative analysis for antiviral drugs: Their efficiency against SARS-CoV-2. *Int Immunopharmacol*. 2021;90:1567–5769.

Ledford H. CRISPR, the disruptor. *Nature*. 2015;522:20–24.

Li Q, Wu J, Nie J, et al. The impact of mutations in SARS-CoV-2 spike on viral infectivity and antigenicity. *Cell*. 2020;182:1284–1294.

Lima RS, Rocha LPC, Moreira PR. 2021. Genetic and epigenetic control of ACE2 expression and its possible role in COVID-19. *Cell Biochem Funct*. 2021;39:713–726.

Liu K, Pan X, Li L, et al. Binding and molecular basis of the bat coronavirus RaTG13 virus to ACE2 in humans and other species. *Cell*. 2021;184(13):3438–3451.

Mesin L, Schiepers A, Ersching J, et al. Restricted clonality and limited germinal center entry characterize memory B cell reactivation by boosting. *Cell*. 2020;190:92–106.

Morens DM, Fauci AS. Emerging pandemic diseases: How we got to COVID-19. *Cell*. 2020;182:1077–1092.

Novillo B, Marinez-Varea A. Covid-19 vaccines during pregnancy and breastfeeding: A systematic review. *J.Pers Med* 2022; 13:40. Doi. 10.3390/jpm13010040

Nutalai R, Zhou D, Tuekprakhon A, et al. Potential cross-reactive antibodies following Omicron breakthrough in vaccinees. *Cell*. 2022;185:2116–2131.

Rakedzon S, Neuberger S, Domb AJ, Petersiel N, Schwartz E. From hydroxychloroquine to ivermectin: What are the antiviral properties of antiparasitic drugs to combat SARS-CoV-2? *J Travel Med*. 2021;28:taab005. doi:10.1093/jtm/taab005.

Rodda LB, Morawski PA, Pruner KB, et al. Imprinted SARS-CoV-2–specific memory lymphocytes define hybrid immunity. *Cell*. 2022;185:1588–1601.

Schultze JL, Aschenbrenner AC. COVID-19 and the human innate immune system. *Cell*. 2021;184:1671–1688.

Sokal A, Chappert P, Barba-Spaeth G, et al. Maturation and persistence of the anti-SARS-CoV-2 memory B cell response. *Cell*. 2021;184:1201–1213.

Starr TN, Greaney AJ, Hilton SK, et al. Deep mutational scanning of SARS-CoV-2 receptor binding domain reveals constraints of folding and ACEZ binding. *Cell*. 2020;182:1295–1310.

Supasa P, Zhou D, Dejnirattisai W, et al. Reduced neutralization of SARS-CoV-2 B1.1.7 variant by convalescent and vaccine sera. *Cell*. 2021;184:2201–2211.

Tarke A, Coelho CH, Zhang Z, et al. SARS-CoV-2 vaccination induces immunological T-cell memory able to cross-recognize variants from Alpha to Omicron. *Cell*. 2022;185:847–859.

Tuekprakhon A, Nutalai R, Dijokaite-Guraliuc A, et al. Antibody escape of SARS-CoV-2 Omicron BA.4 and BA.5 from vaccine and BA.1 serum. *Cell*. 2022;185:2422–2433.

van der Made CI, Simons A, Schuurs-Hoeijmakers J, et al. Presence of genetic variants among young men with severe COVID-19. *JAMA*. 2020;324:663–673.

van der Sluis RM, Cham LB, Gris-Oliver A, et al. TLR2 and TLR7 mediate distinct immunopathological and antiviral plasmacytoid dendritic cell responses to SARS-CoV-2 infection. *EMBO J*. 2022;41:e109622. doi:10.15252/embj.2021109622.

Wikipedia. Variants of SARS-CoV-2. https://en.wikipedia.org/wiki/Variants_of_SARS-CoV-2

Yamasoba D, Kimura I, Nasser H, et al. Virological characteristics of the SARS-CoV-2 Omicron BA.2 spike. *Cell*. 2022;185(12):2103–2115.

Zhang, N-N, Li X-F, Deng Y-Q, et al. A thermostable mRNA vaccine against COVID-19. *Cell*. 2020;182:1271–1283.

Zhang Z, Mateus J, Coelho CH, et al. Humoral and cellular memory to four COVID-19 vaccines. *Cell*. 2022;185:2434–2451.

Ziegler CGK, Miao VN, Owings AH, et al. Impaired local intrinsic immunity to SARS-CoV-2 infection in severe COVID-19. *Cell*. 2021;184:4713–4733.

Reviewers

Mark Stinski Emeritus professor, University of Iowa College of Medicine

Stanley Perlman Professor of microbiology/immunology, University of Iowa College of Medicine

Michael O'Hara Senior scientist and senior program manager, HHS/BARDA

M. Suresh J. E. Butler Professor of comparative and mucosal immunology, Department of Pathobiological Science, University of Wisconsin-Madison

Wendy Maury Professor of microbiology and immunology, University of Iowa College of Medicine

Abbreviations and Glossary

Adjuvant	Substance added to a vaccine or any foreign antigen to enhance the immune response. Adjuvants are biomolecules typically of bacterial origin that are recognized by TLRs and other PRRs.
AGP	Antibiotic growth promoters. Antibiotics not used for human medicine that can be given to chicks and piglets to promote health and growth.
AID	Activation-induced cytosine deaminase. Enzyme that converts the nucleotide cytosine to uracil which can be methylated to become thymidine. Key factor in somatic mutation (SH) and antibody class switch.
Allele	The genetic variant of a gene such as those encoding blue vs. brown eye color in humans.
APC	Antigen presenting cell. Cells like macrophages and dendritic cells that present degraded portions of foreign antigens to B and T cells.
Archaea	Oldest life form on Earth. Anaerobic bacteria that do not depend on products made by other life forms.
ASD	Autism syndrome disorder. A heterogeneous group of disorders in children that impact the CNS and cognitive learning and includes Asperger syndrome.
BCR	B-cell receptor. A surface antibody of the IgM class that serves as the receptor on B cells for foreign antigens.
BMI	Body mass index. Index that measures healthy body size and growth by the ratio of weight and height.
CBF	Caesarian-delivered breastfed infant.
CD	Abbreviation for Cluster of Differentiation markers of which ~300 have been described and that allow biologists to identify the phenotype of any particular cell (see Appendix A-3 for examples).
CF	Caesarian-delivered formula-fed infant.
Chromosome	A microscopic organelle that contain the DNA double helix surrounded by regulatory and protective proteins like histones.

CMV   Cytomegalovirus. One of the few viruses that is transmitted to fetus in utero in humans and can cause serious problems.

CNS & ENS Central and enteric nervous systems, respectively.

Codon   The sequence of three nucleotides in DNA that signals and encodes the synthesis of a particular amino acid in the structure of all proteins.

CRISPR   Acronym for Clustered Regularly Interspersed Short Palindromic Repeats. A method used to edit genes in animals and plants resulting in loss or addition of gene function.

CSF   A type of cytokine essential for stimulating the growth of cells.

CTL   Cytotoxic T cell that destroys virus-infected and tumor cells.

DC   Dendritic cell. Spider-like cells with extensive pseudopods that together with macrophages, act as APCs.

Dysbiosis A condition in which bacteria that comprise the GIT microbiome are associated with disease.

Episomal   A genetic trait not encoded by chromosomal DNA and not inherited. Results from a chemical change that alters gene expression. Plasmids are an example of episomal genetics (called epigenesis).

Epitope   Any molecular structure on a protein, peptide, or cell that is recognized by and binds to TCRs and BCRs.

Eubacteria Also called "true bacteria" that thrive on products made by other life forms. Largest group of life forms on planet Earth.

Eubiosis   A condition in which the GIT microbiome is associated with a healthy host.

Exosome   Membraned micro-organelle produced by enterocytes of the GIT and endothelial cells that contains RNA and may affect macrophage activity.

FMT   Fecal microbial transplant. Gut flora transplanted from one individual to another.

GALT   Gut associated lymphoid tissue. Essentially equivalent to the GIT mucosal immune system.

GC   Germinal center. Found in lymph nodes, spleen, and Peyer's patches where T and B cells interact and B cell selection occurs.

Genome   The grand total of all genetic information in all chromosome of any one individual organism.

GIT   Gastrointestinal tract.

GOP   Galacto-oligosaccharides added to infant formulas to act as HMOs.

HIV   Human immunodeficiency virus that prevents the patient from making a protective immune response.

HMO   Human milk oligosaccharides. Secreted in human breast milk for exclusive use by the neonatal gut microbiome.

HSC	Hemopoeitic stem cells. Cells in bone marrow that give rise to various types of leucocytes including lymphocytes.
IBD	Inflammatory bowel disease. This includes Crohn's disease (CD), ulcerative colitis (UC), celiac disease and irritable bowel syndrome (BS).
Ig	Abbreviation for "immunoglobulin," which is the biochemical name for molecules functionally known as antibodies.
IgE	A class of antibody that is attached to eosinophils and mast cells which upon binding of antigen results in type I allergy.
IgG	Class of antibodies/immunoglobulins that comprise ~80% of the total immunoglobulin content of serum in mammals.
Il-1,-3 etc.	Interleukins. A family of cytokine that acts as intercellular messengers among especially leucocytes (See Appendix A-3 for examples).
INF	Interferon. A family of cytokines that act as intercellular messengers in the initial and inflammatory response to pathogens.
IPP	Ileal Peyer's patches. Lymphoid tissue associated with the lower ileum in hooved mammals.
LPS	Lipopolysaccharide. A product of Gram-negative bacteria that is recognized by TLR4.
mAbs	Monoclonal antibody. An antibody produced by a single B cell clone either as a result of bone cancer (multiple myeloma) or bioengineered in the lab. Used for diagnostics and immune therapy.
MFG	Milk fat globule. Secreted by the epithelial cells of the MG and surrounded by a membrane (MFGM).
MG	Mammary gland.
MGBA	Microbiome gut brain axis.
MHC	Major histocompatibility complex. The gene products are displayed on the surface of cells resulting in an individual-specific phenotype. MHC-I is found on all cells and MHC-II is restricted to leucocytes.
MLV	Modified live virus. Attenuated virus such as those that comprise the MMR and oral polio (tOPV) vaccines.
MMR	Acronym for the trivalent MLV vaccine for measles, mumps, and rubella that is recommended for all children in the United States.
MRSA	Methicillin resistant *Staphylococcus aureus*. A variant of this bacteria that is resistant to various antibiotics.
MS-1	Muscular dystrophy. Chronic autoimmune condition in which muscle mass and function is gradually lost.
MS-2	Multiple sclerosis. An autoimmune disease that attacks the central nervous system and is a common cause of neurologic disability in Western countries.

NEC   Necrotizing enterocolitis. Disease of the newborns that occurs in those not breastfed.

NK cell   Natural killer cell. A lymphocyte-like cell that belongs to the innate immune system and is important in the initial protection against pathogens.

PAMP   Pathogen Associated Molecular Patterns. A type of biomolecule found in bacteria and viruses but not in eukaryotic life forms.

PEC   Pre-eclampsia. A serious complication of pregnancy associated with high blood pressure and proteinuria.

Plasmid   A circular packet of DNA that can be transferred horizontally among bacteria that supplies new genetic information.

PP   Peyer's patches. Secondary lymphoid tissue distributed especially along the small intestine of the GIT. Serves as germinal centers (GC) for the mucosal immune system.

Preterm   An infant born before the normal end of gestation in humans or recovered early by Caesarian section (C-section).

Resistome   Members of the GIT microbiome that are resistant to killing by antibiotics.

SC   Part of the epithelial transport receptor of IgA and IgM that remains attached and gives rise to the terms SIgA and SIgM.

SCFA   Short chain fatty acids; acetic, propionic, butyric made by bacteria of especially Phyla Firmicutes and Bacteriodetes that are needed for the health of tight junction between epithelial cells of the GIT.

SCID   Severe combined immunodeficiency disease. A condition in mammals in which offspring lack a functional adaptive immune system. There can be multiple mechanisms involved.

SH or SHM   Somatic mutation. Mutations that occur during the lifetime in non-germline cells and are therefore not passed to the next generation.

SIgA   The antibody class produced in the largest amounts in all mammals by plasma cells associated with mucosal surfaces to which SC is added during epithelial transport.

SLE   Systemic lupus erythematosus. Autoimmune disease causing a "butterfly" rash and characterized by autoantibodies to many self proteins.

TCR   T-cell receptor found on T cells that recognizes peptides derived from foreign proteins and pathogens including those of host origin.

TGFβ   A cytokine secreted by various cells including Tregs that is necessary for switching to the production of IgA antibodies but independently down-regulates inflammatory responses.

TH   Abbreviation for helper T cell (TH) of which there are several varieties. Helper T cells activate B and T cells stimulating them to make antibodies or CTLs.

THC   Dekta-9-tetrahydrocannabinoid. A major active ingredient in marijuana currently sold as a pharmaceutical for pain relief and epilepsy.

TLR	Toll-like receptor. Receptors found on cells of the innate immune system that recognize PAMPs and are necessary to stimulate an adaptive immune response.
TNF	Acronym for tumor necrosis factor of which there are several forms. TNF-α is part of the inflammatory immune defense provided by the innate immune system.
Treg	Regulatory T cell that can down-regulate inflammatory T cells.
V-D-J	Recombined VH, DH, and JH genes that provide the specificity for the BCR and TCR.
VgBF	Vaginally born breastfed infant.
VgF	Vaginally born formula-fed infant.
VHI	Wuhan Virology Institute.
VHH	A unique group of variable heavy chain genes in camelids (llama, camels, alpacas etc.) that do not need a light chain to form their BCR.
VJ	Recombined VL and JL genes that contribute to the binding site of the BCR.

Index

A

acquired immune deficiency syndrome (AIDS), 250
Actinomyces, 104, 106, 236, 326
activation-induced cytosine deaminase, 247
adaptive immune system, 12, 14–15, 28, 47, 150–154, 253–272, 358–359
adhesion molecules, 110
Adjuplex (ADJ), 363–364
adjuvants, 147, 178, 225, 289–290, 294, 363–364
Aedes aegypti, 11
allele, 248, 252, 270–271
allelic exclusion, 270–271
allergic dermatitis (AD), 233, 235
allergies, 21, 52, 88–89, 120–123, 168–170, 214, 232–235
Allison, 282
allograft, 42–44, 149, 264, 271, 278
allotypes, 252, 309
alpha-linolenic acid (ALA), 95
alpha variant, 222, 357–358, 364–365
altricial, 16, 302, 331
American Academy of Pediatrics (AAP), 53–55, 75, 83, 91, 208, 232, 234
amniocentesis, 19
amnion, 24–25, 47, 118
aneuploidy, 23
animal models, 20–21, 329–335
  bioengineering of, 335–338
  choosing, 331
  non-rodents, 332–334
  overview, 299
  rabbits as, 334
  rodents, 331–332
  ruminant, 334
  surgical manipulation of, 335–339
  Swine as, 332–334
antibiotic free, 237
antibiotic growth promoters (AGP), 185–186, 216–217, 237
antibiotic resistance (AR), 3, 107, 185–186, 208–209, 252–253, 339
antibiotics, 14–15, 131–132, 184–186, 208–209, 215–216, 353
antibody, 14–16, 28–31, 66, 184, 214, 258–270
  ADCC, 265
  de novo synthesis of, 74, 303, 320–321
  detection, 273–274
  gene segments, 266–271
  lymphocytes/MHC and, 154–156
  mAbs, 15, 31, 171, 183, 279–281, 307, 331
  passive, 28–31, 71–72
  polyclonal, 279, 334
  structure, 258–263
  therapeutic, 15
antibody-dependent cell toxicity (ADCC), 265
antigen binding site, 152, 266, 307, 312, 314
antigen-presenting cells (APC), 37, 110–111, 164, 224, 280, 291, 356
antigens, 43–44, 115, 154, 163–166, 278, 293, 334–335
Antimicrobial Peptides (AMPs), 150
anti-vaccination movement, 182–183, 362
antiviral drugs, 35, 186–188, 353, 362, 366

Arcanobacterium (Actinomyces) pyogenes, 236
Archaea, 3–6, 9–10, 103–104, 245–246, 286, 323–324
arousals, 327–329
Artemisinin, 366
artificial DNA synthesis, 274–275
Artiodactyls, 301–302
Aschenbrenner, A.C., 356, 360
AstraZeneca, 185, 225, 363–364
attenuated vaccines, 175, 178–179, 363
autism spectrum disorder (ASD), 3, 19, 38, 46, 103, 127, 208, 226
autoimmunity, 31, 118, 170–171, 225–227, 256, 278

B

Bacilli, 103–104, 324
bacterial transformation, 249–250
Bacteriodes, 106–108, 111, 118, 131, 329
bacteriology, 103–105
bacteriophages, 9, 106, 174–175, 249–250, 287, 339
  defined, 9–10
  in GI tract microbiome, 106
  internal protection from, 14–15
Bacteroides fragilis, 113, 118, 125, 130–131
base editing, 287–288. *See also* gene editing
B cell receptor (BCR), 152–157, 163–164, 267, 307–309, 334
B cell(s), 33, 151–158, 253–254, 278–280, 314–316
BCG vaccine, 148
BCR. *See* B cell receptor (BCR)

Beta variant, 364–365
Bifidobacterium infantis, 67–69, 107–108, 119–120, 128–132, 218
bioengineering, 19–20, 272, 278–289
  animal models and, 329–335
  cell transfusion therapy, 278–279
  diagnostic assays and mAbs, 279–283
  gene editing, 286–289
  genetic defect correction, 19–20
  immunotherapy, 288
  in COVID-19, 367–368
  of bacteria, 283–285
  of eukaryotic genes, 284
  surgical manipulation and, 335–339
  transgenic animals, 285–286
Biological Big Bang (BBB), 4–5
biological development, 1–21
  emerging diseases, 10–13
  genetics and health in, 18–20
  life evolution, 3–10
  medicine, 20–21
  nutrition, 16–18
  parental care/species survival/wellness, 1–3
  protection, 13–16
biomass pyramid, 10
biotechnical methods, 272–288
  artificial DNA synthesis, 274–275
  Cryo-EM, 277–278
  DNA sequencing, 274
  eukaryotic cell culture, 275–276
  FCA, 276
  overview, 272
  PCR and RT-PCR, 274
  scRNA-seq, 276–277
  solid-phase immunoassay, 272–273
biotechnology, 272–288
blastocyst, 23–25
Bliss, Eula, 226
body mass index (BMI), 119
bone marrow, 47, 151, 163–164, 278, 315–316
Bordetella pertussis, 176, 182
Borrelia burgdorferi, 7
breast-feeding, 51–78, 235. *See also* mammary gland (MG)
  alternatives of. *See* infant formulas and later health, 53–54
  bacteria in, 68–69
  colostrum and, 68

drugs/environmental contaminants in, 75–76
  for infant growth, 62–63
  maternal diet and, 63
  options, 54–55
  pathogens in, 75
  role of, 51
  societal/economic issues and, 52–53
  supplementation, 77
Butyrivibrio, 323

C

caecotrophic, 323, 325
caecum, 322–325, 334
caesarian delivered breastfed (CBF), 118, 129
caesarian formula fed (CF), 117, 129
Campylobacter, 67, 166
carbadox, 217
Carlson, Rachel, 40
caseins, 55–56, 64, 85, 88, 235, 289, 338
Cas9 enzyme, 287
CD4, 11, 18, 146, 158, 260, 367
CD8, 146, 260, 294, 307, 365
cell lines, 280, 284, 291, 357
cell transfusion therapy, 278–279
cellular trafficking, 33
Centers for Disease Control (CDC), 20, 178, 185, 195, 208, 229, 357
central immunological tolerance, 47, 159, 163–165, 170, 292
central nervous system (CNS), 33–34, 38, 128, 166, 170, 181
certolizumab, 38
Cevik, M., 364
cGAS-STNG system, 255
chemokines, 24, 147, 149–150, 250, 331
childhood vaccinations, 71–72
chimeric antigen receptor T cells (CAR-T), 278, 282–284
Chloroquine and hydroxychloroquine (HCQ), 366
chromosomes, 3, 23, 245–246, 250, 252, 266, 286
Clostridium botulinum, 107, 187
Clostridium difficile, 107, 118, 125, 128–130, 215, 278
Clostridium perfringens, 107
Clostridium tetani, 30, 106–107, 154, 156, 158
Clustered Regularly Interspersed Short Palindromic Repeats (CRISPR), 235, 278, 286–289, 337, 355–356

Cluster of Differentiation markers (CD), 141–146, 274, 280, 306, 331
Codex Alimentarius (CODEX), 91, 95
codon, 243, 357
colonization resistance, 14, 17–18, 109–110, 113, 125, 129, 219
Colony-stimulating factor (CSF), 90
colostrum, 46–47, 60, 90, 160–161, 270, 317–320, 333–334
commensals, 69–70, 100, 104, 107, 110, 118
complement system, 147–148
composite vaccines, 176
confirmation bias, 228
conjugated polysaccharide vaccines, 176–177
conjugate vaccines, 175–176
conjugation, 249
cotyledonal, 301
COVID-19, 10–13, 75, 178, 225, 353–368. *See also* SARS-CoV-2 virus
  as teaching model, 354–362
  controlling, 362–368
  epidemics/pandemics, 353–354
  overview, 353–354, 362
CoV RaT613 virus, 359
Crick, Francis, 195, 242
CRISPR. *See* Clustered Regularly Interspersed Short Palindromic Repeats (CRISPR)
critical window, 1–21, 213–214. *See also* biological development
Cronobacter sakazakii, 207
cryogenic electron microscopy (cyro-EM), 277–278
cystic fibrosis (CF), 34, 175–176, 337
cytokines, 24–25, 72–74, 147–152, 149–150, 254–256, 328–329, 360
cytomegalovirus (CMV), 11, 17, 33–34, 75, 149, 158, 164, 278
cytotoxic T cell (CTL), 149, 151–152, 162, 265, 280–281, 307, 361

D

damage-associated molecular patterns (DAMPs), 147, 150, 171
data dredging, defined, 198
defensins, 65–66, 150
Delta-9-Tetrahydrocannabinol (THC), 27–28, 39
Delta variant, 364–365

dendritic cells (DCs), 42–43, 70, 115, 124, 224, 294, 356
de novo synthesis, 74, 303, 320–321
deoxynucleic acid (DNA), 3–4, 64, 114, 242–245, 274–277, 356–357
detection antibody, 273–274
Dexamethasone drug, 366
D'Herelle, 174, 339
dichlorodiphenyl trichloroethane (DDT), 40
Dietary Guidelines for Americans, 20
diffuse, defined, 301
Diphtheria, 181–182
discoidal, 301
DNA Sequencing, 274
DNA vaccines, 291–292
docosahexaenoic acid (DHA), 95
The Double Helix (Watson), 242
double-strand break (DSB), 286–289
Dow-Corning, 225–226
DPT vaccine, 176, 203
drugs, 37–41
    antiviral, 186–188
    contamination in milk, 75–76
    immunosuppressive, 38
    smoking/alcohol/dietary supplements, 38–39
    teratogens, 39–41
    thalidomide, 37, 46
    THC, 39
dysbiosis/dysbiotic, 69, 103, 106–107, 124–125

E

early phase primary antibody response, 152, 156
ELISPOT, 274, 280. See also Enzyme-Linked ImmunoSorbent Assay (ELISA)
emerging diseases, 7, 10–13, 187, 202
    and human behavior, 12–13
    history of, 10–12
enteric nervous system (ENS), 127–128
Enterococcus, 111, 115, 130, 186, 252
Enzyme-Linked ImmunoSorbent Assay (ELISA), 273, 280
epidemics, 10–11, 186–187, 229, 353–354, 362. See also SARS-CoV-2 virus
epigenetics, 18–19, 231, 245
epitope, 89, 152, 175 176, 267 268, 289–292, 361, 367
Epstein-Barr virus (EBV), 75, 171

erythroblastosis fetalis, 43, 171
Escherichia coli (E. coli), 64–67, 104–106, 122–124, 186–187, 252, 284, 307, 338–339
Eubacteria, 3–6, 10, 103, 245–246, 286, 323
eubiosis/eubiotic, 103, 106–107, 127, 165
eukaryotes, 3–6, 140, 251–253, 303, 323
European Academy of Allergy and Clinical Immunology, 234
European Medicines Agency, 208
European Union Commission (EU Commission), 91–92, 95
Eutheria. See Placentalia
exosome, 9, 250, 318–319
external nutrition, 51
extravillous trophoblast (EVT), 25, 36–37, 43

F

fasting, 322, 327, 329, 334–335
Favipiravir, 366
FcRn, 28–31, 38, 271, 301–302, 319, 331
fecal microbiota transplantation (FMT), 103, 126, 325, 329
fecundity, 13–14
Federation of American Societies for Experimental Biology, 322
Fidock, D.A., 183
Fleming, Alexander, 184
Flow Cytometric Analysis (FCA), 265, 275, 279
Fluorescence-Activated Cell Sorting (FACS). See Flow Cytometric Analysis (FCA)
food allergies, 18, 53, 88–89, 235, 289
Food and Drug Acts, 206
Food and Drug Administration (FDA), 76, 128, 200–201, 205–206, 224–225, 363–364
food intolerance, 233–234
food protein-induced enterocolitis (FPIES), 233–234
Franklin, Benjamin, 226
Franklin, Rosalind, 242
free-range beef, defined, 237
Friedman, 286

G

galacto-oligosaccharides (GOPs), 128
galactosemia, 44–45, 55, 87, 234
GalSafe pig, 337

Gamma variant, 358, 364
gastrointestinal illnesses, 87–88
gastrointestinal tract microbiome, 3–4, 6, 17–18, 46, 99–101, 109–111, 322–330
    bacteriology role in, 103–105
    bacteriophage role in, 105
    childhood allergy and, 120–123
    colonization in, 112–114
    developing neonatal, 131–132
    disease and, 122–126
    during hibernation, 327–329
    dysbiosis of, 119–121
    epithelial barrier of, 109–111
    ethnic/cultural influences on, 107–108
    eubiotic/dysbiotic, 103, 106
    in milk/MG, 326–327
    mucosal fungi role in, 106
    of bats, 326
    of carnivores, 325–326
    of mammals, 322–330
    of maternal-fetal connection, 101–102
    of rabbits, 325
    of reproductive tract, 111–112
    oral tolerance in, 165
    origin of, 113–118
    overview, 99–103, 321
    porcine, 324–325
    postnatal feeding and, 130–131
    pregnancy influences on, 119–121
    pre/pro/synbiotics, 128–130
    ruminants, 322–324
gene editing, 286–289
    and base editing, 287–288
    CRISPR, 286–289
    TALEN, 286–287
gene expression, 18–19, 148, 231, 246, 302
"gene gun" technology, 292
gene replication, 247–248
genes, 18–20, 121, 185–186, 241–273, 309–312
genetic defects, 19–20, 203, 358
genetics, 1, 18–20, 241–294
    changes in pathogens, 19
    concept/molecular basis of, 241–246
    congenital diseases, 44–46
    defect correction, 19–20
    diversification of eukaryotes, 251–253
    epigenetics, 18–19
    expression, 18–19
    genotype, 10
    of antibiotic resistance, 252–253

of innate/adaptive immunity, 253–272
overview, 241
phenotype, 10
replication, 247–248
reproduction, 248–250
genetic signature, 248
genome, defined, 245
genotype, 10, 33, 248
germ, defined, 214
germinal center (GCs), 115, 156, 314, 318
germinal center reaction (GCRx), 115, 156–158, 163–164, 177
GlaxoSmithKline, 185
Gluten intolerance, 234
Glycogen storage disease, 45
Goblet cells, 73–74, 115, 162, 329
Gram, Christian, 104
Gram-negative bacteria, 64–65, 104, 150, 184–187, 256, 328
Gram-positive bacteria, 65, 150, 254, 256–257
grandparents/grandchildren, 229–231
Graves' disease, 170–171
growth faltering, 63
guide RNA, 287
Guillain-Barre syndrome (GBS), 166
Gut-Associated Lymphoepithelial Tissue (GALT), 314–315

H

Haemophilus influenza, 120, 166, 181–182
Hashimoto's thyroiditis, 170
HCQ. *See* Chloroquine and hydroxychloroquine (HCQ)
Helicobacter pylori, 64, 105–106, 122, 166, 256
helper T cell (TH), 154–155, 158, 167, 187–188, 307
hematopoietic stem cells (HSC), 278–279
hemolytic disease of the newborn, 33, 43–44
herd immunity, 182–183, 219–223
hibernation, 327–329
Hib vaccine, 176–177
homologous recombination, 286–287
Honjo, 282
horizontal gene transfer (HGT), 5, 104–105, 118, 126, 217, 249, 283
horror autotoxicus, 163–165
human behavior, 12–13

human colonization, 8–9
human health, 236
human immunodeficiency virus (HIV), 10–12, 18–19, 55, 75, 187–188, 250, 366
human milk oligosaccharides (HMOs), 17, 59, 67–68, 96
human offspring, 16–17
hygiene hypothesis, 8, 91, 120–121
hypothesis/hypotheses, 193–210. *See also* scientific literature
as facts, 197, 225–228
defined, 195
evidences, 193–200
falsified, 195
hygiene, 8, 91, 120–121
media role in, 194–195
nature *versus* nurture, 231–232

I

Ileal-lymphoid-nodular hyperplasia, non-specific colitis and pervasive developmental disorder in children (Wakefield), 226
ileal peyer's patches (IPP), 315, 332, 335
immune-privileged sites, 42
immune system, 15–16, 46–47, 139–188
adaptive, 150–154
AMPs, 150
at birth, 47
autoimmunity, 171
B cells, 151–158
cytokines and chemokines, 149–150
innate, 146–150
lymphocytes, 154–156
memory, 157
mucosal, 160–161
of mammals, 307–319
overview, 140–146
passive, 162–163
response to microbes, 157–160
response to SARS-CoV-2, 359–362
self-/non-self-discrimination, 140
T cells, 150–152
tolerance, 163–165
immunoglobulin, 307–312
allelic exclusion of, 270–271
immunoglobulin A (IgA), 16, 59, 69–70, 124, 152–156, 233–234, 319–320
immunoglobulin E (IgE), 28, 90, 120, 156–157, 166–168, 233, 309

immunoglobulin G (IgG), 15, 69–70, 152, 177, 233, 285, 301–303, 319–321
immunoglobulin M (IgM), 44, 150, 152–154, 259, 306, 308–310
immunological tolerance, 47, 159, 163–164, 225, 291–292
central, 47, 159, 163–165, 170, 292
peripheral, 164–165, 168–170, 292, 365
immunologic injury, 165–171, 233, 288
allergies, 168–170
autoimmunity, 170–171
molecular mimics, 166–167
immunologic memory, 148, 157, 361, 365
immunology, 140–146
immunosuppressive drugs, 38
immunotherapy, 15, 283, 287–288, 338, 358
Inactivated polio vaccine (IPV), 179, 180, 363
inactivated vaccines, 175
infammasomes, 147, 255, 256–258
infant formulas, 83–97
choices, 205–207
composition/regulation of, 91–95
consequences of, 89–91
for allergies, 88–89
for gastrointestinal illnesses, 87–88
for metabolic diseases, 87
for premature infants, 86–87
history of, 83–86
in special medical situations, 86–89
recent additions to, 95–97
short-term versus long-term issues, 89
soy-based, 86–88
infectious disease, 36–37
inflammasome, 306
inflammasome complexes, 256
inflammation, 147
inflammatory bowel disorders (IBD), 2, 19, 38, 150
inflammatory T cells, 43, 90, 124, 150, 169, 313
infodemic, 21, 223
innate immune system, 14–15, 47, 146–150, 258–259, 307, 360
innate *versus* adaptive immunity, 306
Insulin-like growth factor (IGF), 73, 90

integrases, 10, 245, 250, 287
Interferon (INF), 113–114, 150, 255,
    257, 321, 360
interleukins (Il-1,-3), 24
internal protection, 14–16, 51, 63,
    103, 127, 139–188, 214, 306.
    See also immune system
intranasal vaccine (IN), 364
intrauterine growth restriction
    (IGR), 44
introns, 245
Ioannidis, J.P.A., 197
Ivermectin, 366

J

Jaenisch, R., 285–286
Jefferson, Thomas, 172–173
Jenner, Edward, 172–173, 175
Jinhua pigs, 325
Johnson & Johnson, 225, 363
*Journal of the American Medical
    Association*, 221

K

Kawasaki disease (KD), 170–171
Key, N., 217
killed vaccines. *See* inactivated
    vaccines
Kingstad-Bakke, B., 364
knock-ins, 285
knockouts, 285, 337

L

Lachnospiroeae, 325
α-Lactalbumin, 65
lactase, 45, 54–55, 73, 88, 90, 234,
    253–254
lactation, 57–62, 72–73, 115, 303,
    318
Lactobacillus/Lactobacilli, 69, 111–
    113, 128–131, 218, 323–326,
    329
lactoferrin, 64–65, 96–97
β-Lactoglobulin, 65
Lagomorphs, 334
laser capture microdissection
    (LCM), 276
late phase primary responses, 156,
    163
Lederberg, Josh, 216, 229, 354
life, 3–10
    ancestors/descendants, 10
    establishment of, 3–5
    forms on Earth, 3–5
    human colonization, 8–9
    pyramid and interdependence
        of, 5–10
    subcellular forms of, 9–10

lipid nanoparticles (LNP), 293–294,
    363
lipopolysaccharide (LPS), 64–65,
    150, 152, 166, 328
Listeria monocytogenes, 35, 43, 110,
    114, 256
lymphocytes, 150, 154–156, 180,
    224, 278–279, 320, 356
lymphopoiesis, 315–317
lysozyme, 65–66, 109, 285

M

M. abscessus, 175
M. avium, 175
M. tuberculosis, 261
macrophage polarization, 250
major histocompatibility locus
    (MHC), 42–43, 67, 140,
    154–156, 270–272
malaria, 7, 35, 183, 366
mammalian diversity, 299–338
    at birth, 302–303
    classification of, 299–301
    immunoglobulin and,
        307–312
    in lymphopoiesis, 315–317
    in parenting, 306
    in placentation, 301–302
    in T Cell, 313–314
    litter size/multiparity and,
        303–306
    of GALT, 314–315
    of GI tract, 322–330
    overview, 299
    reproduction, 301–306
mammary gland (MG), 16, 55–63
    anatomy and physiology of,
        55–59
    functional changes in, 60–61
    microbiome of, 326–327
    passive immunity and, 69–76
    structure of, 55–56
Marsupialia, 299–301
mastitis, 54, 68–69, 237, 326
mastoiditis, 209
Maternal and Child Health Bureau,
    20
maternal-fetal connection, 23–47.
    See also placenta
    allograft incompatibility, 42–44
    establishment of, 23–25
    GI Tract changes, 46–47
    immune system changes, 46–47
    microbiome of, 101–102
    non infectious diseases, 44–46
    nutrient supply/fetal growth/
        postnatal, 25–27
    transfer mechanisms, 27–41

Mather, Cotton, 172
mature milk, 60
Maxam-Gilbert method, 274
McBride, W.D., 217
measles, mumps and Rubella vaccine
    (MMR), 33–34, 177, 221–224,
    229–230, 289, 362
Measles (rubeola), 181
medicine, 20–21
meiosis, 20, 248, 251–253, 286
memory T cells (Trm), 114, 157,
    364–365
Mendel, Gregor, 18, 43, 231, 242,
    252
meta-analysis, 197
metabolic diseases, 87, 206
Metatheria. *See* Marsupialia
Metchnikoff, 218
Methanobrevibacter, 323
Methanogen, 323
methicillin resistant *Staphylococcus
    aureus* (MRSA), 107, 185–186,
    215, 252
microbes, defined, 10
microbiome, 6, 17–18, 99–131,
    322–330
microbiome-gut-brain axis (MGBA),
    130
Middle East Respiratory Syndrome
    (MERS), 204, 229, 354,
    358–359
milk, 63–69
    bacteria in, 68–69
    caseins, 64
    condensed/concentrated, 84–85
    contaminants in, 75–76
    for infant growth, 62–63
    HMOs, 67–68
    Lactoferrin, 64–65
    MFG, 66–67
    microbiome of, 326–327
    α and β-Lactoglobulin, 65
milk allergy, 88–89
milk banks, 53–54
milk fat globule membranes
    (MFGM), 66–67, 77, 96, 317
milk fat globules (MFG), 57, 66–67,
    96
Mintz, B., 285–286
misconceptions/controversies,
    213–238
    antibiotics, 215–216
    critical window, 21, 213–214
    food allergy/intolerance/aversion,
        232–235
    food labeling, 236–237
    human health, 236

names leading to, 214
national priorities, 229
of prebiotics/probiotics, 218–219
programmed gullibility, 228–229
STAT program, 216–217
vaccines, 219–225
mitosis, 46–47, 248, 251–253
mitosis versus meiosis, 248
MMR vaccines, 289
molecular mimics, 166–167
Molnupiravir, 366
monoclonal antibodies (mAbs), 15,
31, 171, 183, 279–283, 307,
331
monogastric species, 322–324, 332
mRNA vaccines, 183, 292–293, 363
mucosal fungi, 106
mucosal immune system, 127–128,
160–161, 167, 179, 289, 319,
364
mucosal immunologic experience,
69–70, 319
mucosal vaccine, 179
multicellularity, 4, 272
multidrug-resistant (MDR) bacteria,
14–15, 131–132, 186
multiple myeloma, 279
multiple sclerosis (MS), 124, 128
Mumps, 181
Mus musculus, 285, 331
mutations, 46, 157, 231, 283,
356–358
in SARS-CoV-2, 356–358
SHM, 248, 267–270, 313
spontaneous, 247–248, 252
mutualism, 6, 100
Mycoplasma laboratorium, 274–275
myoepithelial cells, 56–57

N

N. brasiliensis, 169
The Naked Ape (Morris), 302
National Institutes of Health (NIH),
226
National Library of Medicine
(PubMed), 157–158
National Organic Program (NOP),
236–237
national priorities, 229
natural killer (NK) cells, 25, 31,
36–37, 42–43, 149–150,
260–262, 321
natural selection, 216, 303, 354
nature, 231–232
nature versus nurture, 231–232
necrotizing enterocolitis (NEC), 54,
65, 77, 86–87, 90

Neisseria gonorrhoeae, 166
NOD-like receptors (NLRs), 147,
254–258
nodosomes, 255
non-infectious diseases, 44–46
non-rodent models, 332–334
Novavax, 363–364
nucleic acid vaccine, 291–292
nucleotides, 242–243
nucleus, 3–4, 242, 244–245, 292–
293, 356
nurture, 231–232
nutrition, 1, 16–18, 20, 63
decision-making, 209–210
external, 51
of human offspring, 16–17
overview, 13
supply/fetal growth/postnatal,
25–27
transfer and microbiome role,
17–18

O

Omicron variant, 355, 357–358,
364–365
operator segments, 245
opsonization, defined, 148
oral polio vaccine (OPV), 69, 72,
179–181, 182, 222–224, 290,
362–363
oral therapeutic immune globulin, 15
oral tolerance, 73, 112, 162, 165
organ allograft, 42
organic, defined, 237
organic foods, 214
organochlorine pesticides (OCP), 40
organ transplantation, 271, 278
oxytocin, 56–57

P

pandemic, 10–11, 353–354. *See
also* SARS-CoV-2 virus
paracellular transport, 58
parasitism, 7–8
parental care/species survival/well-
ness, 1–3
parturition, 56, 111, 114, 302, 319
passive antibodies, 28–31
passive immunity, 12, 14–16, 69–76,
162–163
pasteurization, 54, 75, 90, 132
Pasteur, Louis, 175
pathogen-associated molecular patterns (PAMPs), 31, 127, 147,
152, 176, 289, 306, 307
pathogenicity islands, 253

pathogens, 19, 33–35, 75, 103–110,
215, 332–333
pattern recognition receptors (PRR),
147, 253–260
Pauling, Linus, 242
PaxlovidTM, 366
pemphigus vulgaris, 171
penicillin, 184, 209, 215
peripheral tolerance, 164–165,
168–170, 292, 365
Pertussis (whooping cough), 182
Peterson, 16
Peyer's patches (PP), 115, 124,
314–315
Pfizer-BioNTech, 364
pharmaceuticals, 37
phenotype, 10, 242, 248, 252, 276,
337
phenotype *versus* genotype, 248
phenylketonuria (PKU),
44–45, 87
phocomelia, 37
placenta, 27–41, 301–302
cellular trafficking, 33
drugs transfer in, 37–41
establishment of, 23–25
FcRn in, 28–31, 38, 271, 301–
302, 319
infectious disease changes in,
36–37
nutrient supply/fetal growth/
postnatal, 25–27
passive antibodies, 28–31
pathogens/congenital infections
in, 33–35
regulatory factors, 31–32
Placentalia, 299–301
plasma cells (PCs), 59, 152, 156,
279–280, 309, 319–320
plasmids, 9–10, 104, 249–250,
291–292
Plasmodium, 35
Plinius, 218
Poliomyelitis, 181
polyacrylamide sequencing gels, 274
polychlorinated biphenyls (PCBs),
40
polyclonal antibodies, 279, 334
Polymerase Chain Reaction (PCR),
274
Popper, Karl, 195
porcine reproductive and respiratory
syndrome virus (PRRSV), 11,
160, 302
prebiotics, 67, 69, 77, 218–219
precocial, 16, 302, 332

preeclampsia (PEC), 27, 32, 43, 119–120
premature infants, 77–78, 86–87
preterms, 77–78, 86–87, 117, 131, 210, 218, 332
preventing severe disease, 365
Prevotella, 105–107, 111–112, 119–120, 125, 323–325, 329
primary CMV, 34. *See also* cytomegalovirus (CMV)
primary lymphoid tissues, 47, 151
primers, 275
probiotics, 218–219
Process Verification Program (PVP), 236
programmed gullibility, 228–229
prokaryotes, 3, 5, 35, 245–246, 287
    Archaea, 3–6, 9–10, 103–104, 245–246
    Eubacteria, 3–6, 10, 103, 245–246
promoter segments, 245, 252, 291–292
protection, 1, 13–16, 20
    and fecundity, 13–14
    by immune system, 15–16
    from antibiotics and bacteriophages, 14–15
    internal, 14
    overview, 13
    pathogens, 19
proviruses, 10

R

Ramon, Gaston, 178
Randomized Controlled Trials (RCTs), 198
Rattus rattus, 331
receptor-binding domain (RBD), 357–359
recombinant DNA technology, 289
Recombinase Activation Genes (RAG), 266
recombination, 163, 266–267, 286–288
recurrent CMV, 34. *See also* cytomegalovirus (CMV)
red blood cells (RBCs), 33, 43–44
regulatory factors, 31–32, 72–74
regulatory T cell (Treg), 25, 42–43, 73, 115–116, 124, 151, 278, 313
Remdesivir drug, 366
repressor segments, 245, 252–253
resistome, 131–132, 185, 215, 252–253
respiratory syncytial virus (RSV), 12, 176, 280, 367

Rhinolophus (Horseshoe bat), 359
ribonucleic acid (RNA), 10, 12, 33, 158, 188, 250, 274–277, 287, 366–367
RNA-dependent RNA polymerases (RdRp), 188, 250
Roblin, 286
rodent models, 331–332
Roosevelt, Franklin, 179
Rossiter, Margaret, 242
Royal Academy of Science, 172
RT-PCR, 275
Rubella (German measles), 181
rumen, 322–323
ruminants, 322–324, 334
Ruminococcus, 106, 113, 119, 121, 125, 126, 323–325

S

Sabin vaccine. *See* oral polio vaccine (OPV)
Saccharomyces boullardii, 129–130
Salk vaccine. *See* Inactivated polio vaccine (IPV)
Salmonella, 35, 65–66, 104–105, 110, 186–187, 217, 308, 338–339
Salmonella enterica, 339
Salmonella typhosa, 35
Sanger method, 274
SARS-CoV-2 virus, 10–13, 75, 157, 182–183, 222–225, 280, 321, 353–368
    antiviral drug therapy for, 366
    bioengineering in, 367–368
    biology of, 354–356
    diversification/microevolution of, 356–357
    hybrid immunity, 367
    immune response to, 359–361, 361–362
    mAbs for, 280
    mutation of, 356–358
    origin of, 358–359
    passive immune therapy for, 367
    PCR test for, 275
    vaccines for, 200–204, 362–365
    variants of, 355, 357–358, 364–365
    viral vector vaccines for, 363
Schultze, J.L., 356, 360
scientific fact, 197
scientific literature, 193–210
    case reports/series, 199
    evidences, 193–200
    for health decisions, 204–210
    for vaccine trials, 200–204

hype/uncertainties in, 194–195
hypotheses, 195
media role in, 194–195
observational studies, 199
peer-reviewed journals for, 196–197
RCTs in, 198
secondary lymphoid tissues, 156, 160, 163
secretory immunoglobulin A (SIgA), 16, 70, 90–91
self-recognition system, 4
severe combined immunodeficiency disorder (SCID), 33, 68, 279, 337–338
sexually transmitted diseases (STDs), 222
sexual reproduction, 251–253. *See also* meiosis
Shigella, 104, 110–111, 326
Shingrix vaccine, 178, 289
short chain fatty acids (SCFA), 17, 67–68, 90, 109, 115–118, 127–128, 323, 329
short-term versus long-term issues, 89
Silent Spring (Carlson), 40
Single-Cell RNA Sequencing (scRNA-seq), 276–277
single nucleotide polymorphisms (SNP), 287–288
Sinnis, P., 183
Sinovax, 364
solid-phase immunoassay, 272–273
somatic cells, 68, 247, 278, 287
Somatic hypermutation (SHM), 151, 248, 267–270, 312
somatic mutation, 20, 157, 163, 248, 267–268, 283
Spanish Flu, 11, 360
specific pathogen free (SPF), 332
spontaneous mutations, 247–248, 252
spontaneous *versus* somatic mutation, 248
Sputnik V, 363–364
Staphylococcus aureus, 69, 107, 118, 185, 215, 252
Staphylococcus epidermidis, 118
State Key Laboratory, 363
Strachan, D.P., 120–122, 168, 289
Streptococcus mutans, 107, 185, 216, 252
Streptococcus pneumoniae, 176, 181
Streptococcus thermophilus, 128, 218

sub-therapeutic antibiotic therapy (STAT), 185–186, 216–217, 230, 236, 253, 338
subunit vaccines, 175, 224, 291
surgical manipulation, 335–339
surrogate light chain (SLC), 316
surrogate milks, 83–86
survival, 1–2, 42–44, 86, 162, 228, 320–322
Swine, 332–334
symbiosis/symbionts, 6, 9, 17, 69, 99–100
synbiotics, defined, 129
synthetic biology. *See* bioengineering
systemic experience, 318
systemic immune response, 224
systemic immunologic experience, 69–70
systemic lupus erythematosus (SLE), 125

T

TALEN, 286–287
T cell(s), 31, 150–152, 151, 364–365
   helper, 154–155, 158, 167, 187–188, 307
   inflammatory, 43, 90, 125, 147, 169, 313
   memory, 114, 157, 364
   regulatory, 25, 42–43, 73, 115–116, 124, 151, 278, 313
T cell receptor (TCR), 149, 152, 163, 258–268, 307, 314
Tdap vaccine, 176
teratogens, 39–41
thalidomide, 37, 46
THC. *See* Delta-9-Tetrahydrocannabinol (THC)
therapeutic antibodies, 15
thermocycler, 275
thermostable DNA polymerase, 275
thymus, 47, 151, 163–164, 262, 316
toll-like receptors (TLRs), 65, 147, 178, 254–257, 306, 360
torpor, defined, 327
TotalSeq, 276–277
toxoids, defined, 175
Toxoplasma gondii, 35
trained immunity, 148, 157
transcriptome, 276
trans-endocytosis, defined, 280
transfer RNA (tRNA), 243
transforming growth factor β (TGFβ), 42–43, 73–74, 77, 90, 121, 150

transgenic animals, 285–286
transgenic mice, 148, 285
transition milk, 60
transmission electron microscopy (TEM), 277
trophoblast, 25, 29, 35–36, 39, 43
true bacteria. *See* Eubacteria
true fasters, 327
tumor necrosis factor (TNF), 24
Tylosin phosphate drug, 236
type I immediate hypersensitivity, 90, 120, 164, 167, 233–235, 270
type IV immunologic injury, 233
types II–IV immunological injury, 233–234

U

ulcerative colitis (UC), 126
United Nations Children's Fund (UNICEF), 52, 166, 179
University of Kansas, 321
University of Minnesota, 16
USDA. *See* U.S. Department of Agriculture (USDA)
U.S. Department of Agriculture (USDA), 53, 184, 203, 236
US Warp Speed program, 204
uterine NK cells (nNKs), 42

V

vaccines/vaccination, 15, 172–184, 219–225, 289–294
   adjuvants role in, 178, 294
   decisions, 207–208
   development/diversity/administration, 175–178, 289–290
   DNA, 291–292
   effectiveness of, 364–365
   for grandparents/grandchildren, 229–231
   herd immunity, 182–183
   hesitancy, 34, 219–223
   history of, 172–175
   LNP role, 293–294
   maternal, 180–182
   misunderstandings about, 223–225
   modern, 183, 289–290
   mRNA, 183, 292–293, 363
   OPV, 179–181
   preventable diseases, 181–182
   subunit, 175, 224, 290
   trials, 200–204
   universal and mucosal, 294

viral vector, 291, 363
Vaginal formula feeding (VgF), 114, 118, 129
Vaginally born and breastfed (VgBF), 101–102, 107, 118–119, 130–131
variable heavy chain (VHH), 285
variants. *See* specific variants
Varicella (chicken pox), 181
varicella-zoster virus (VZV), 11–12
V-D-J recombination, 266–267, 269
veterinary feed directive (VFD), 236
Vibrio cholera, 110, 122
viral neutralization (VN), 187, 280, 361
viral vector vaccines, 291, 363
virions, defined, 158, 250
virus-neutralizing (VN) antibodies, 357

W

Wakefield, Andrew, 226–227
Washington, George, 172
Watson, James, 195, 242
weak *versus* strong evidence, 195–198
Weissman, D., 292–293
wellness, 2
whey, 55–56
white blood cells (WBC), 356
Wilson, Woodrow, 13
World Health Organization (WHO), 14, 20, 52, 63, 175, 179, 185–187, 339
Wuhan Virology Institute (WHI), 359
Wuhan WT variant, 355, 357–358, 364–365

X

X-ray diffraction crystallography, 277

Y

Yersinia pestis, 12–13

Z

Zika virus, 11, 33
zonary, 301
zoonotic diseases, 11
zymogens, 148

www.ingramcontent.com/pod-product-compliance
Lightning Source LLC
Chambersburg PA
CBHW080657220326
41598CB00033B/5238